3rd edition

microbiology and infectious diseases

National Medical Series

In the basic sciences

anatomy, 3rd edition
the behavioral sciences in psychiatry, 3rd edition
biochemistry, 3rd edition
clinical epidemiology and biostatistics
genetics
hematology
histology and cell biology, 2nd edition
human developmental anatomy
immunology, 3rd edition
introduction to clinical medicine
microbiology and infectious diseases, 3rd edition
neuroanatomy
pathology, 3rd edition
pharmacology, 3rd edition
physiology, 3rd edition
radiographic anatomy

In the clinical sciences

medicine, 3rd edition
obstetrics and gynecology, 4th edition
pediatrics, 3rd edition
preventive medicine and public health, 2nd edition
psychiatry, 3rd edition
surgery, 3rd edition

In the exam series

review for USMLE Step 1, 3rd edition
review for USMLE Step 2
geriatrics

The National Medical Series for Independent Study

3rd edition

microbiology and infectious diseases

EDITOR

Gabriel Virella, M.D., Ph.D.

Professor
Department of Microbiology and Immunology
Medical University of South Carolina
Charleston, South Carolina

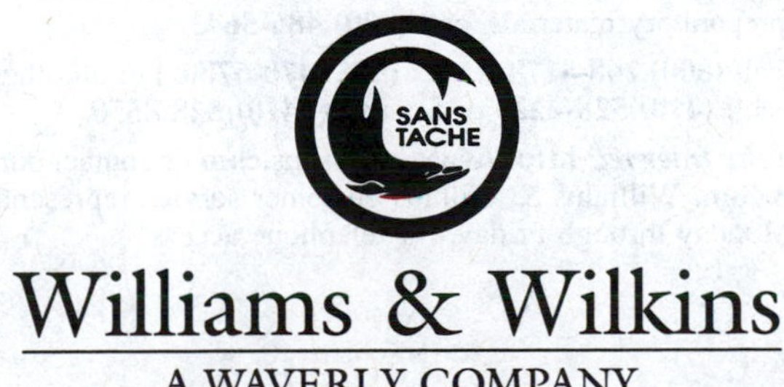

BALTIMORE • PHILADELPHIA • LONDON • PARIS • BANGKOK
BUENOS AIRES • HONG KONG • MUNICH • SYDNEY • TOKYO • WROCLAW

Editor: Elizabeth A. Nieginski
Managing Editor: Amy G. Dinkel
Development Editor: Melanie Cann
Production Coordinator: Cindy Park
Illustration Planner: Cindy Park
Cover Designer: Cathy Cotter
Typesetter: Maryland Composition
Printer: Port City Press
Binder: Port City Press

351 West Camden Street
Baltimore, Maryland 21201-2436 USA
Rose Tree Corporate Center
1400 North Providence Road
Building II, Suite 5026
Media, Pennsylvania 19063-2043 USA

Accurate indications, adverse reactions and dosage schedules for drugs are provided in this book, but it is possible that they may change. The reader is urged to review the package information data of the manufacturers of the medications mentioned.

Printed in the United States of America

First Edition,

Library of Congress Cataloging-in-Publication Data

Microbiology and infectious diseases.—3rd ed. / [edited by] Gabriel T. Virella.
p. cm.—(The National medical series for independent study)
Rev. ed. of: Microbiology / David T. Kingsbury, Gerald E. Wagner. 2nd ed. c1990.
Includes index.
ISBN 0-683-06235-2
1. Medical microbiology—Examinations, questions, etc. 2. Medical microbiology—Outlines, syllabi, etc. I. Virella, Gabriel, 1943– II. Kingsbury, David T. Microbiology. III. Series.
[DNLM: 1. Microbiology—examination questions. 2. Microbiology—outlines. QW 18.2 M622 1996]
QR46.K54 1996
616′.01′076—dc20
DNLM/DLC
for Library of Congress 96-5707
CIP

The publishers have made every effort to trace the copyright holders for borrowed material. If they have inadvertently overlooked any, they will be pleased to make the necessary arrangements at the first opportunity.

Call our customer service department at **(800) 638-0672** for catalog information or fax orders to **(800) 447-8438.** For other book services, including chapter reprints and large quantity sales, ask for the Special Sales department.

To purchase additional copies of this book or for information concerning American College of Sports Medicine certification and suggested preparatory materials, call **(800) 486-5643.**

Canadian customers should call **(800) 268-4178,** or fax **(905) 470-6780.** For all other calls originating outside of the United States, please call **(410) 528-4223** or fax us at **(410) 528-8550.**

Visit Williams & Wilkins on the Internet: **http://www.wwilkins.com** or contact our customer service department at **custserv@wwilkins.com.** Williams & Wilkins customer service representatives are available from 8:30 am to 6:00 pm, EST, Monday through Friday, for telephone access.

97 98 99
1 2 3 4 5 6 7 8 9 10

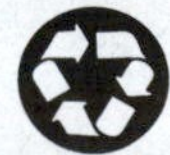

Dedication

This book is dedicated to my parents, wife, and daughters, and to the many students I have been privileged to teach during my twenty-one years at the Medical University of South Carolina.

G. V.

Contents

Contributors xvii
Preface xix
Acknowledgments xxi

Part I Basic Bacteriology

1 Overview **3**
I. Medical microbiology 3
II. Classes of pathogenic microorganisms 4

2 Bacterial Structure, Physiology, and Classification **7**
I. Bacterial structure 7
II. Bacterial physiology 12
III. Bacterial classification 18

3 Bacterial Genetics **21**
I. Bacterial genetic material 21
II. Bacterial mutation 22
III. Mutation repair mechanisms 23
IV. Mutation suppression 27
V. DNA transfer between bacteria 28
VI. Genetic basis of bacterial pathogenicity 34
VII. Operons 35

4 Antibacterial Agents **41**
I. General considerations 41
II. Classification 43

5 Bacterial Resistance to Antibacterial Agents **53**
I. Introduction 53
II. Acquisition of bacterial resistance 53
III. Mechanisms of bacterial resistance 54
IV. Bacterial resistance according to drug class 57
V. Antibiotic susceptibility testing 58

6 **Disinfection and Sterilization** 61
I. Definitions 61
II. Chemical antimicrobial agents 61
III. Physical antimicrobial agents 62

7 **Bacterial Virulence Factors** 65
I. Introduction 65
II. Capsules 65
III. Adhesins 65
IV. Invasiveness 66
V. Exoenzymes 66
VI. Toxins 67

Part II Immunity and Infection

8 **Anti-Infectious Host Defenses** 73
I. General considerations 73
II. Nonspecific defense mechanisms 73
III. Antibody-mediated (humoral) immunity 74
IV. Cell-mediated immunity (CMI) 76
V. Evasion of the immune response 78

9 **Immunoprophylaxis** 83
I. Introduction 83
II. History 83
III. Types of vaccines 84
IV. Vaccines as immunotherapeutic agents 86
V. Immunization schedules 87

Part III Clinical Bacteriology

10 **Laboratory Diagnosis of Bacterial Infections** 91
I. Introduction 91
II. Microscopic examination of patient specimens 91
III. Detection of pathogen-specific macromolecules 92
IV. Culture and isolation of microorganisms 93
V. Serologic testing 95

11 **Normal Flora** 97
I. Introduction 97
II. Role of normal flora 97
III. Normal flora as pathogens 97
IV. Anatomic location of normal flora 98

12 **Gram-Positive Cocci: Staphylococci and Streptococci** 101
I. Staphylococci 101
II. Streptococci 105

13 **Gram-Positive Rods: *Corynebacteria, Listeria, Clostridium,* and *Bacillus*** **113**
I. Introduction 113
II. *Corynebacterium diphtheriae* 113
III. *Listeria monocytogenes* 116
IV. *Clostridium* 118
V. *Bacillus* 123

14 **Gram-Negative Cocci: *Neisseria* and *Moraxella*** **125**
I. *Neisseria* 125
II. *Moraxella* 132

15 **Gram-Negative Rods I: *Haemophilus* and *Bordetella*** **133**
I. *Haemophilus* 133
II. *Bordetella* 136

16 **Gram-Negative Rods II: Enterobacteriaceae and Other Enteropathogenic Gram-Negative Rods** **141**
I. Introduction 141
II. Enterobacteriaceae 141
III. Vibrionaceae 151
IV. *Campylobacter* and *Helicobacter* 155

17 **Gram-Negative Rods III: Opportunistic and Zoonotic Bacteria** **159**
I. Opportunistic bacteria 159
II. Zoonotic bacteria 162

18 **Mycobacteria** **167**
I. Introduction 167
II. *Mycobacterium tuberculosis* 168
III. Mycobacteria other than tuberculosis (MOTT) 171
IV. *Mycobacterium leprae* 173

19 **Spirochetes** **175**
I. Introduction 175
II. *Treponema* 175
III. *Borrelia* 180
IV. *Leptospira* 183

20 **Legionellaceae, Mycoplasmataceae, Actinomycetaceae, and Related Organisms** **185**
I. Legionellaceae 185
II. Mycoplasmataceae 187
III. Actinomycetaceae 189

21 **Intracellular Bacteria: Chlamydiae, Rickettsiaceae, and Bartonellaceae** 193
I. Introduction 193
II. Chlamydiae 193
III. Rickettsiaceae 198
IV. Bartonellaceae 201

Part IV Basic Virology

22 **General Characteristics and Classification of Viruses** 205
I. General characteristics 205
II. Viral structure 205
III. Nomenclature and classification 208

23 **Viral Replication** 211
I. Relationship between the virus and the host cell 211
II. Stages of viral replication 211
III. Replication cycle of major human DNA viruses 216
IV. Replication cycle of major human RNA viruses 219

24 **Viral Genetics** 225
I. Viral genomes 225
II. Viral mutation 225
III. Interactions between viruses 226
IV. The role of genetic variation in the evolution of viruses 231

25 **Interferons and Antiviral Agents** 233
I. Introduction 233
II. Classes of antiviral agents 233
III. Resistance to antiviral agents 239

26 **Viral Infections: Epidemiology, Pathogenesis, and Pathology** 241
I. Epidemiology 241
II. Pathogenesis 243
III. Pathology 247

27 **DNA Tumor Viruses and Retroviruses** 251
I. Introduction 251
II. DNA tumor viruses 252
III. Retroviruses 256
IV. Two-hit theory of malignant transformation 260

28 **Viruses and the Immune System** 263
I. Introduction 263
II. Antibody-mediated (humoral) immunity 263

III. Cell-mediated immunity (CMI) 264
IV. Pathologic consequences of the antiviral immune response 265
V. Evasion of the immune response 266

Part V Clinical Virology

29 Diagnosis of Viral Infections 271
I. Culture and isolation 271
II. Serology 273
III. DNA hybridization 274

30 DNA Viruses I: Herpesviruses 277
I. Introduction 277
II. Herpes simplex virus (HSV) 277
III. Varicella-zoster virus 279
IV. Epstein-Barr virus 280
V. Cytomegalovirus (CMV) 281
VI. Human herpesvirus-6 (HHV-6, HBLV) 283

31 DNA Viruses II: Papovaviruses 285
I. Introduction 285
II. Papillomaviruses 285
III. Polyomaviruses 286

32 DNA Viruses III: Adenoviruses, Poxviruses, and Parvoviruses 289
I. Adenoviruses 289
II. Poxviruses 290
III. Parvoviruses 291

33 RNA Viruses I: Picornaviruses 293
I. Overview 293
II. Enteroviruses 293
III. Rhinoviruses 297

34 RNA Viruses II: Arboviruses and Rubella Virus 299
I. Overview 299
II. Arboviruses 299
III. Rubella virus 302

35 RNA Viruses III: Orthomyxoviruses 305
I. General characteristics 305
II. Epidemiology 305
III. Pathogenesis and clinical disease 306
IV. Diagnosis 306
V. Treatment 307
VI. Complications 307
VII. Prevention 307

36 **RNA Viruses IV: Paramyxoviruses** 309
I. Introduction 309
II. Parainfluenza viruses 309
III. Mumps virus 310
IV. Measles (rubeola) virus 311
V. Respiratory syncytial virus 313

37 **RNA Viruses V: Other RNA Viruses** 315
I. Rhabdoviruses 315
II. Coronaviruses 317
III. Caliciviruses 317
IV. Filoviruses 318
V. Arenaviruses 319
VI. Bunyaviruses 319
VII. Reoviruses 320

38 **Hepatitis Viruses** 323
I. Introduction 323
II. Hepatitis A virus (HAV) 323
III. Hepatitis B virus (HBV) 324
IV. Hepatitis C virus (HCV) 329
V. Hepatitis D virus (HDV, Delta virus) 330
VI. Hepatitis E virus (HEV) 331
VII. Other hepatitis viruses 332

Part VI Mycology

39 **Overview of Mycology** 335
I. Characteristics and classification of fungi 335
II. Morphology 335
III. Structure 335
IV. Pathogenesis 336
V. Epidemiology 337

40 **Diagnosis and Treatment of Fungal Diseases** 339
I. Diagnosis 339
II. Antifungal therapy 340

41 **Dermatophytes and Filamentous Fungi** 343
I. Cutaneous mycoses 343
II. Subcutaneous mycoses 344
III. Mycoses caused by other filamentous fungi 345

42 **Yeasts and Dimorphic Fungi** 347
I. Infections caused by yeasts 347
II. Infections caused by dimorphic fungi 349

43 **Opportunistic Mycoses** 357

I. Etiology 357
II. Predisposing conditions 357
III. Clinical disease 358
IV. Diagnosis 359
V. Treatment 359

Part VII Parasitology

44 **Diagnosis and Treatment of Parasitic Infections** 363

I. Overview 363
II. Diagnosis of parasitic infections 363
III. Treatment of parasitic infections 365

45 **Medical Protozoology** 371

I. Introduction 371
II. Amoebae 371
III. Flagellates 374
IV. Ciliates 381
V. Sporozoans 382
VI. *Pneumocystis carinii* 387

46 **Medical Helminthology** 389

I. Nematodes (roundworms) 389
II. Cestodes (tapeworms) 399
III. Trematodes (flatworms, flukes) 402

Part VIII Major Infectious Diseases

47 **Bacteremia and Sepsis** 409

I. Introduction 410
II. Diagnosis of bacteremia 411
III. Treatment of bacteremia and sepsis 412
IV. Bacteremic infections and sepsis 412

48 **Pneumonia** 419

I. Introduction 419
II. Bacterial pneumonia 420
III. Viral pneumonia 423
IV. Fungal pneumonia 425

49 **Meningitis and Encephalitis** 429

I. Introduction 429
II. Bacterial meningitis 429
III. Aseptic meningitis 434
IV. Viral encephalitis 439

50 Degenerative Brain Diseases Caused by Viruses and Unconventional Agents 441

I. Introduction 441
II. Subacute sclerosing panencephalitis (SSPE) 442
III. Progressive multifocal leukoencephalopathy (PML) 443
IV. Degenerative retroviral diseases of the CNS 444
V. Degenerative disease caused by unconventional agents 445

51 Urinary Tract Infections 449

I. Introduction 449
II. Infections of the urethra, bladder, and renal pelvis 449
III. Prostatitis 452

52 Gastroenteritis and Food Poisoning 455

I. Introduction 456
II. Infectious diarrhea and gastroenteritis 456
III. Food poisoning 459
IV. Viral diarrhea 460
V. Parasitic diarrhea 461

53 Infections Caused by Anaerobic Bacteria 465

I. General characteristics of anaerobic bacteria 465
II. Anaerobic infections 466

54 Sexually Transmitted Diseases 473

I. Introduction 473
II. Epidemiology 473
III. Approach to the patient 474
IV. Laboratory diagnosis 476
V. Treatment 477
VI. Prevention 477
VII. Complications 478

55 Viral Hepatitis 481

I. Introduction 481
II. Acute viral hepatitis 484
III. Chronic viral hepatitis 486

56 Viral Exanthematic Diseases 489

I. Introduction 490
II. Acute viral disease with maculopapular rash 491
III. Acute viral disease with vesicular rash 493
IV. Acute viral disease with urticarial lesions 496
V. Acute viral disease with petechial or purpuric lesions 496
VI. Acute viral disease associated with erythema multiforme and Stevens-Johnson syndrome 497

57 HIV and AIDS 501
I. Introduction 501
II. The human immunodeficiency viruses 502
III. Epidemiology 503
IV. Pathogenesis 504
V. Clinical stages of HIV infection 508
VI. Diagnosis 510
VII. Treatment 511
VIII. Immunoprophylaxis 514

Summary Tables 517
Summary of the Major Bacteria 518
Major Pathogenic Bacteria Organized by Type of Disease 522
Summary of the Major DNA Viruses 523
Summary of the Major RNA Viruses 524
Summary of the Major Pathogenic Fungi 526
Summary of the Major Human Pathogenic Parasites 528
Pathogens Involved in Infections at Different Ages 529

Comprehensive Exam 531

Index 557

Contributors

Salvatore Arrigo, Ph.D.
Assistant Professor
Department of Microbiology and Immunology
Medical University of South Carolina
Charleston, South Carolina

Victor Del Bene, M.D.
Professor of Medicine
Associate Dean for Students
College of Medicine
Medical University of South Carolina
Charleston, South Carolina

Edwin A. Brown, M.D.
Assistant Professor
Infectious Diseases Division
Department of Medicine
Medical University of South Carolina
Charleston, South Carolina

Arthur Di Salvo, M.D.
Director, Nevada State Health Laboratory
Reno, Nevada

Walton L. Ector, M.D.
Associate Professor
Director of Pediatrics
Director, Pediatric Primary Care Unit
Medical University of South Carolina
Charleston, South Carolina

Edmund Farrar, M.D.
Professor Emeritus of Medicine
Former Director of the Infectious Diseases Division and Professor of Microbiology
Medical University of South Carolina
Charleston, South Carolina

Sandra Fowler, M.D.
Assistant Professor
Department of Pediatrics
Medical University of South Carolina
Charleston, South Carolina

Robert M. Galbraith, M.D., M.B.A., F.A.C.P.
Director, Medical School Liaison
Department of Academic Support Services
National Board of Medical Examiners
Philadelphia, Pennsylvania
Former Chairman, Department of Microbiology and Immunology
Medical University of South Carolina
Charleston, South Carolina

Jean-Michel Goust, M.D.
Professor
Department of Microbiology and Immunology
University of South Carolina
Charleston, South Carolina

Thomas B. Higerd, Ph.D.
Professor
Department of Microbiology and Immunology
Medical University of South Carolina
Charleston, South Carolina

Eric R. James, Ph.D.
Associate Professor
Department of Ophthalmology
Medical University of South Carolina
Charleston, South Carolina

George M. Johnson, M.D.
Associate Professor
Department of Pediatrics
Medical University of South Carolina
Charleston, South Carolina

David T. Kingsbury, Ph.D.
Professor
Department of Microbiology
George Washington University Medical Center
Washington, D.C.

John Manos, M.D.
Professor and Vice Chairman
Director of Microbiology
Department of Pathology and Laboratory Medicine
Medical University of South Carolina
Charleston, South Carolina

John Sanders, M.D., M.P.H.
Assistant Professor
Infectious Diseases Division
Department of Medicine
Medical University of South Carolina
Charleston, South Carolina

Michael G. Schmidt, Ph.D.
Associate Professor
Department of Microbiology and Immunology
Medical University of South Carolina
Charleston, South Carolina

Lisa L. Steed, Ph.D.
Assistant Professor Department of Pathology and Laboratory Medicine
Assistant Director of Clinical Microbiology
Medical University of South Carolina
Charleston, South Carolina

Gabriel Virella, M.D., Ph.D.
Professor
Department of Microbiology and Immunology
Medical University of South Carolina
Charleston, South Carolina

Gerald E. Wagner, Ph.D.
Professor of Microbiology
St. George's University School of Medicine
St. George's, Grenada
West Indies

Preface

After 21 years of teaching, it has become clear to me that medical students need two types of textbooks: the comprehensive textbook, to use as a reference and source of clarification, and a simpler textbook containing essential facts and concepts likely to be taught everywhere, presented in a format that facilitates independent study. It was with this latter goal in mind that the third edition of *NMS Microbiology and Infectious Diseases* was developed. We have tried to limit the factual information to that we consider essential for a 21st century physician. We have made an effort to emphasize general concepts and mechanisms, and to illustrate the clinical relevance of basic science. The Infectious Diseases section has been rewritten with a new perspective reflective of the introduction of case-based learning components in many medical microbiology courses. Finally, the comprehensive exam that concludes the book has been prepared according to the stated desire of the National Board of Medical Examiners to test the student's ability to apply concepts and use a base of knowledge to solve questions based on clinical or experimental vignettes. All of us who labored in the preparation of this third edition did it with the hope that the unique features of this book will help the reader learn more effectively, with a better understanding of concepts and principles, and with a better appreciation of the importance of knowing the scientific principles that form a foundation for the practice of medicine.

Gabriel Virella

Acknowledgments

This book would not have been written without the collaboration of many generations of students who have given us their feedback and encouraged us to persist in our efforts to develop a text that would satisfy both faculty expectations and student needs. Some went beyond the call of duty by providing us with materials such as tables and diagrams. We wish to especially recognize Troy Marlow for his assistance in reviewing many of the book's chapters and for providing review diagrams, and Kent Jenkins for his mycology tables. Ms. Debra Dreger had a key role in the early stages, encouraging us to go ahead with the project and introduce new features, such as the cases that are interspersed throughout the clinical chapters. Ms. Melanie Cann and her team did an awesome job as editors, simplifying, clarifying, and ensuring consistency throughout the text. Finally, we wish to recognize the help of Ms. Alva Mullins, who has given us her unwavering support for many years, support that allows us to embark on ventures that always turn out to be more complex than anticipated.

PART I

BASIC BACTERIOLOGY

Chapter 1

Overview

David T. Kingsbury
Thomas B. Higerd
Michael G. Schmidt

I. MEDICAL MICROBIOLOGY is the study of interactions between humans and the microorganisms with which they coexist.

A. Microorganisms may be grouped according to the nature of their interactions with humans.

1. **Commensal organisms** routinely colonize body surfaces without doing harm and are often referred to as **normal microbial flora.** *Escherichia coli* is a commensal organism.
2. **Pathogens** damage the human host either by direct invasion and injury (e.g., *Shigella* species) or by the production of harmful toxic products (e.g., *Clostridium* species).
3. **Opportunistic organisms** are usually found in the environment or as part of the normal flora. In normal individuals, they are harmless, but they may cause severe disease in immunocompromised patients or if they penetrate a territory from which they are usually excluded (as a result, for example, of trauma or surgery).
4. **Zoonotic organisms** usually cause disease in vertebrates other than humans, but may be acquired through contact with infected animals or animal products.

B. Interaction with the host. The pathogenic potential of many organisms is variable. It is influenced by both the intrinsic properties of the microorganism and the state of health of the human host.

1. **Host defenses** and **natural immunity** refer to a multicomponent system of protective mechanisms that prevent entry of microorganisms into normally sterile areas and limit the spread of those invaders that overcome the first line of defense.
   - a. These mechanisms may be weakened by a variety of insults, including direct physical trauma, systemic disease, drugs, and toxins.
   - b. When normal defenses are impaired, the person loses the ability to limit the injury caused by microorganisms, even by those with low intrinsic virulence. In compromised hosts, infections are the usual cause of death.
2. **Microbial virulence** is the relative intrinsic ability of a microorganism to cause disease. All the factors that contribute to microbial pathogenesis are generically known as **virulence factors** (see Chapter 7).
   - a. **Adhesins (colonization factors)** are proteins associated with the outer layers of the bacterium. These factors usually determine adhesion to mucosal cells, an essential step for colonization of the host.
   - b. **Capsules,** usually formed of polysaccharides, inhibit phagocytosis or protect against digestion after the bacterium has been ingested by a phagocytic cell.
   - c. **Endotoxins,** chemically composed of lipid and polysaccharide moieties, are integral components of the cell wall of Gram-negative bacteria. Endotoxins are released as bacterial cells die, and may cause septic shock.
   - d. **Exotoxins** are toxic proteins secreted by bacteria. They are often the sole virulence factor of a given microorganism and may be responsible for the major clinical manifestation of infection (e.g., enterotoxins cause diarrhea, neurotoxins cause paralysis and other neurologic symptoms).
   - e. **Exoenzymes** are considered virulence factors when they **degrade cellular material** or **destroy antibiotics.**

C. Historical significance. Much of modern scientific medicine is a direct result of the development of medical microbiology.

1. The **germ theory of disease** (i.e., the recognition that a specific etiologic agent is responsible for a particular constellation of symptoms) is an outgrowth of enhanced understanding of infectious diseases.
2. **Koch postulates.** In the nineteenth century, Robert Koch developed a set of methodological principles for establishing a specific microbial etiology.
   a. The following principles remain important guidelines in medical research:
      (1) The organism occurs in every case of the disease in question and under circumstances that can account for the pathologic changes and clinical course of the disease.
      (2) The organism occurs in no other disease as a fortuitous and nonpathogenic parasite.
      (3) After being fully isolated from the body and repeatedly grown in pure culture, the organism can induce the same disease in another host.
   b. These postulates have provided an important conceptual model for studying the underlying pathology of infectious diseases. However, the model is not perfect; its conditions may not be met when a pathogen cannot be cultured *in vitro* or when the agent is not pathogenic to commonly available laboratory animals.

II. CLASSES OF PATHOGENIC MICROORGANISMS.

Pathogens vary in size and biologic complexity. Some are able to extract sufficient nutrients from an inanimate environment and, hence, may be cultured on artificial media. Others are incapable of growth outside living host cells and are referred to as obligate intracellular parasites. Pathogens are divided into four major groups.

A. Viruses are the smallest infectious agents. They are too small to be seen with a light microscope and are unable to perform any of the usual metabolic and reproductive functions characteristic of living organisms.

1. **Reproduction.** Viruses are **obligate intracellular parasites** that depend entirely on the host cell's synthetic machinery for reproduction.
   a. After binding to and entering the host cell, a mammalian virus sheds its coat and releases viral nucleic acid into the cell.
   b. During replication, the virus takes advantage of host cellular enzymes and protein-synthesizing structures to replicate.

TABLE 1-1. Distinguishing Characteristics of Procaryotes and Eukaryotes

Procaryotes	Eucaryotes
Size: 1–10 μm	Size: 10–100 μm
No nuclear membrane	Nuclear membrane
Single chromosome	Multiple chromosomes
No DNA-associated histones	Histones associated with DNA
Binary fission	Mitotic division
Lack membranous compartments	Have membranous compartments
Peptidoglycan cell wall	Chitin or cellulose wall (when present)
Steroids absent	Steroids may be present
70S ribosomes	80S ribosomes
Anaerobic respiration possible	No anaerobic respiration*
No tissue differentiation	Usually differentiated in tissues
Nitrogen fixation possible	Nitrogen fixation not possible

* Except for some yeasts

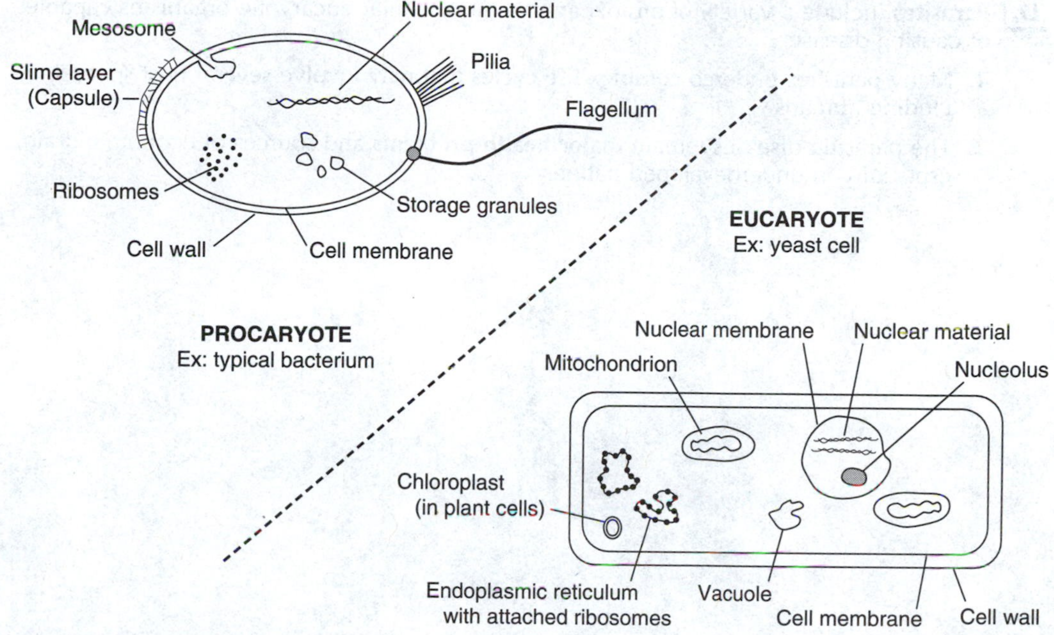

FIGURE 1-1. Major structural differences between procaryotic and eurcaryotic cells.

c. After the progeny particles are properly assembled in the cell, they are released, wherein additional cells may be infected, initiating a new cycle of virus replication.

2. Viruses **contain only one type of nucleic acid,** either DNA or RNA, but not both.

B. **Bacteria** are larger and more complex than viruses. Most bacteria are visible under the light microscope.

1. **Prokaryotes.** Bacteria are true living organisms that belong to the kingdom Procaryotae, which includes true bacteria and blue-green algae. The major distinguishing characteristics of prokaryotic organisms are summarized in Table 1-1 and illustrated in Figure 1-1.
2. Unlike viruses, bacteria **possess both DNA and RNA.**
3. Bacteria reproduce by an asexual process known as **binary fission.**
4. **Most pathogenic bacteria are capable of independent growth** and, thus, may be cultured on artificial media. Some bacteria, however, lack the ability to produce important metabolites, which must be provided exogenously. Exogenous sources include culture media, neighboring bacteria, and infected cells (when the bacteria are able to survive as intracellular parasites).

C. **Fungi** are larger than bacteria and have a more complex cell structure.

1. **Eukaryotes.** As eucaryotic organisms, the genetic material of fungi is separated from the cytoplasm by a nuclear membrane.
2. **Reproduction.** Some fungi reproduce by **budding** (yeasts), whereas others grow by developing tube-like structures known as hyphae and forming **specialized reproductive structures** (i.e., conidia and spores).
3. Most pathogenic fungi exist in nature as environmental **saprophytes,** and human infection does not appear to be necessary for their life cycle. On the other hand, *Candida,* a medically important yeast, is often found as part of the normal intestinal flora.

D. **Parasites** include a variety of protozoan and multicellular eucaryotic organisms capable of causing disease.

1. Many parasites undergo **complex life cycles** that may involve several host species, including humans.
2. The parasitic diseases remain **major health problems** and sources of economic drain, especially in underdeveloped nations.

Chapter 2

Bacterial Structure, Physiology, and Classification

Thomas B. Higerd
David T. Kingsbury
Michael G. Schmidt

I. BACTERIAL STRUCTURE (Figure 2-1)

A. Cell envelope

1. **Components.** Most bacterial cells have a cell envelope consisting of a cell wall and an underlying cytoplasmic membrane.
   a. **Cell wall.** The rigid cell wall, which provides protection and imparts shape to most bacterial cells, is entirely absent in a few unusual bacteria (e.g., Mycoplasmas).
      (1) **Peptidoglycan (murein)** is the principal structural component of the cell wall (Figure 2-2). This compound is found in both Gram-positive and Gram-negative organisms, although it is more abundant in Gram-positive bacteria.
         (a) **Peptidoglycan structure** [see also II C 5 e (2)]. Peptidoglycan polymers consist of repeating disaccharides formed by **N-acetylglucosamine** and **N-acetylmuramic acid.** The N-acetylmuramic acid links the disaccharides to an oligopeptide chain consisting of **four amino acids.**
            (i) Several of the amino acids are found only in bacterial cell walls (e.g., mesodiaminopimelic acid and the D-isomers of glutamic acid and alanine).
            (ii) **Lysozyme** hydrolyzes peptidoglycan by cleaving the glycosyl bonds between N-acetylmuramic acid and the N-acetylglucosamine (see Figure 2-2).
         (b) **Peptidoglycan crosslinking** involves the formation of a peptide bond between the terminal residue of a peptide side chain (usually D-alanine) with the penultimate residue of an adjoining side chain (L-lysine or mesodiaminopimelic acid). Unique to *Staphylococcus aureus* is the intercalation of a pentaglycine bridge unit between the two peptide side chains (Figure 2-3).
      (2) **Autolysins.** All bacterial cell walls have associated autolysins, enzymes that dissolve the peptidoglycan layer. This activity is essential for cell wall growth, cell septation, sporulation, and achieving competency for transformation.
   b. **Cytoplasmic membrane.** The cytoplasmic membrane (also referred to as the **cell membrane** or **plasma membrane)** is the physical and metabolic barrier between the interior and exterior of the bacterial cell.
      (1) The cytoplasmic membrane exhibits a well-defined **selective permeability.**
      (2) The **bacterial electron transport system,** the principal energy system, is located in the cytoplasmic membrane.
      (3) **Mesosomes** are complex invaginations of the cytoplasmic membrane seen in many, but not all, bacteria. Their function is not well established.

2. **Gram-positive versus Gram-negative bacteria**
   a. **Gram-positive bacteria** have a simpler but thicker cell wall consisting primarily of multiple layers of peptidoglycan with teichoic acid polymers dispersed throughout.
   b. **Gram-negative bacteria** have a cell wall that is thinner than that of Gram-positive bacteria, with a bimolecular layer of peptidoglycan and no teichoic acids (Figure 2-4).
      (1) An additional membrane, the **outer membrane,** lies above the peptidoglycan layer. The outer membrane is much thicker than the single peptidoglycan layer.

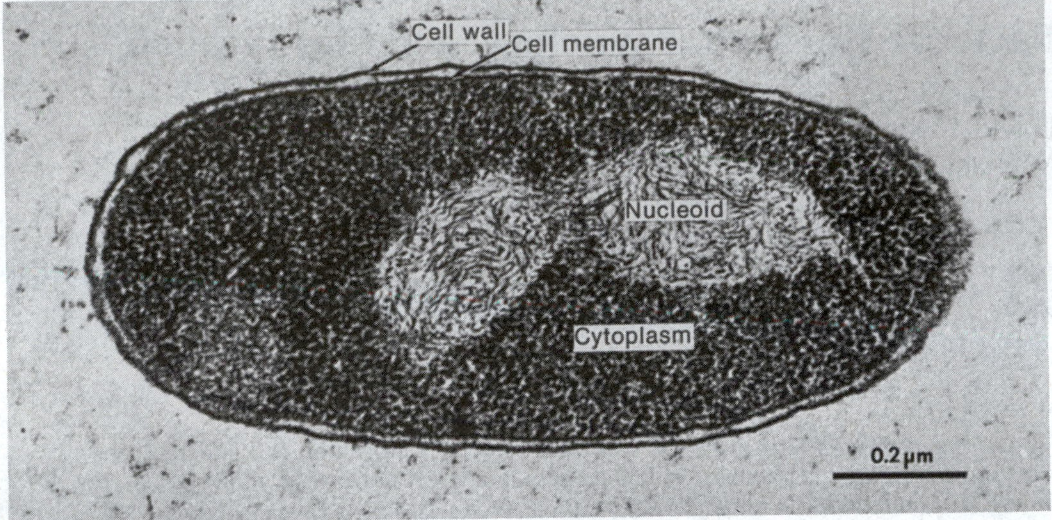

FIGURE 2-1. Electron microphotograph showing the structural organization common to all bacterial cells. (Reprinted with permission from Cota-Robles EH, Ringo DL: The structure of the bacterial cell. In *Infectious Diseases and Medical Microbiology,* 2nd ed. Edited by Braude AI, et al. Philadelphia, WB Saunders, 1986, p 2.)

(2) The outer membrane is composed of a **lipid bilayer, proteins,** and **lipopolysaccharide (LPS, endotoxin).**

- **(a)** The **lipid bilayer** is attached to the peptidoglycan by lipoproteins that cross the periplasmic space.
- **(b)** The **proteins** include **porins,** which form transmembrane channels involved in the transport of ions and hydrophilic compounds from the extracellular compartment to the periplasm.
- **(c)** **LPS** is composed of a lipid portion (lipid A), a polysaccharide-rich core, and a polysaccharide side chain (Figure 2-5).
  - **(i)** The **polysaccharide portion** of LPS is antigenic and is designated as the **O antigen.**
  - **(ii)** The **lipid portion** is **heat-stable** and responsible for the biologic effects of **endotoxin** (see Chapter 7).

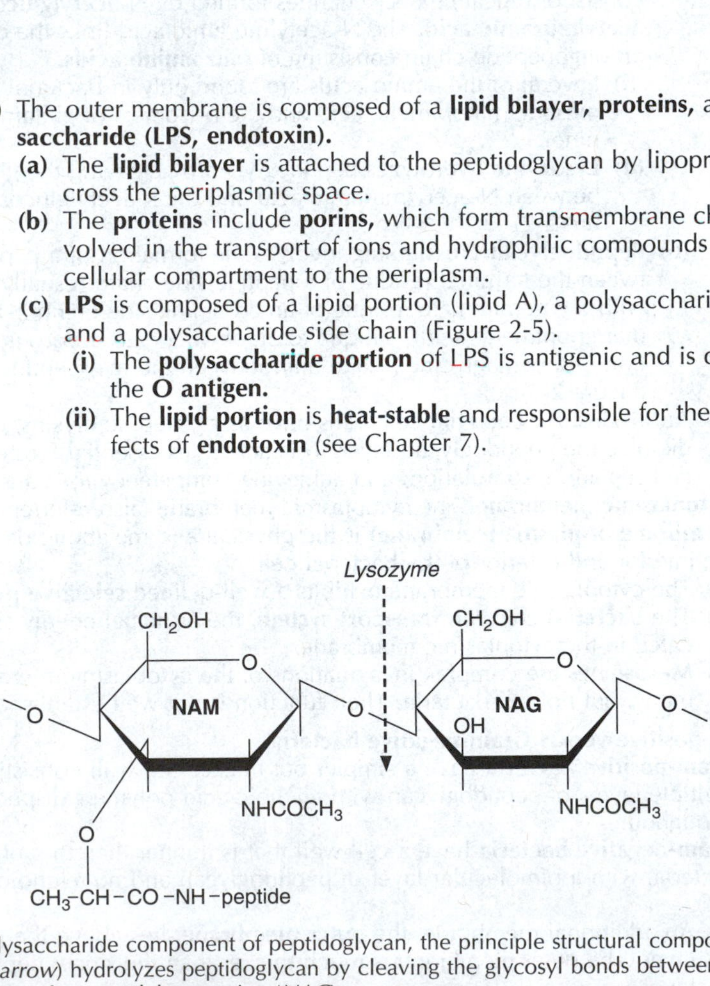

FIGURE 2-2. Polysaccharide component of peptidoglycan, the principle structural component of the cell wall. Lysozyme (*arrow*) hydrolyzes peptidoglycan by cleaving the glycosyl bonds between N-acetylmuramic acid (*NAM*) and N-acetylglucosamine (*NAG*).

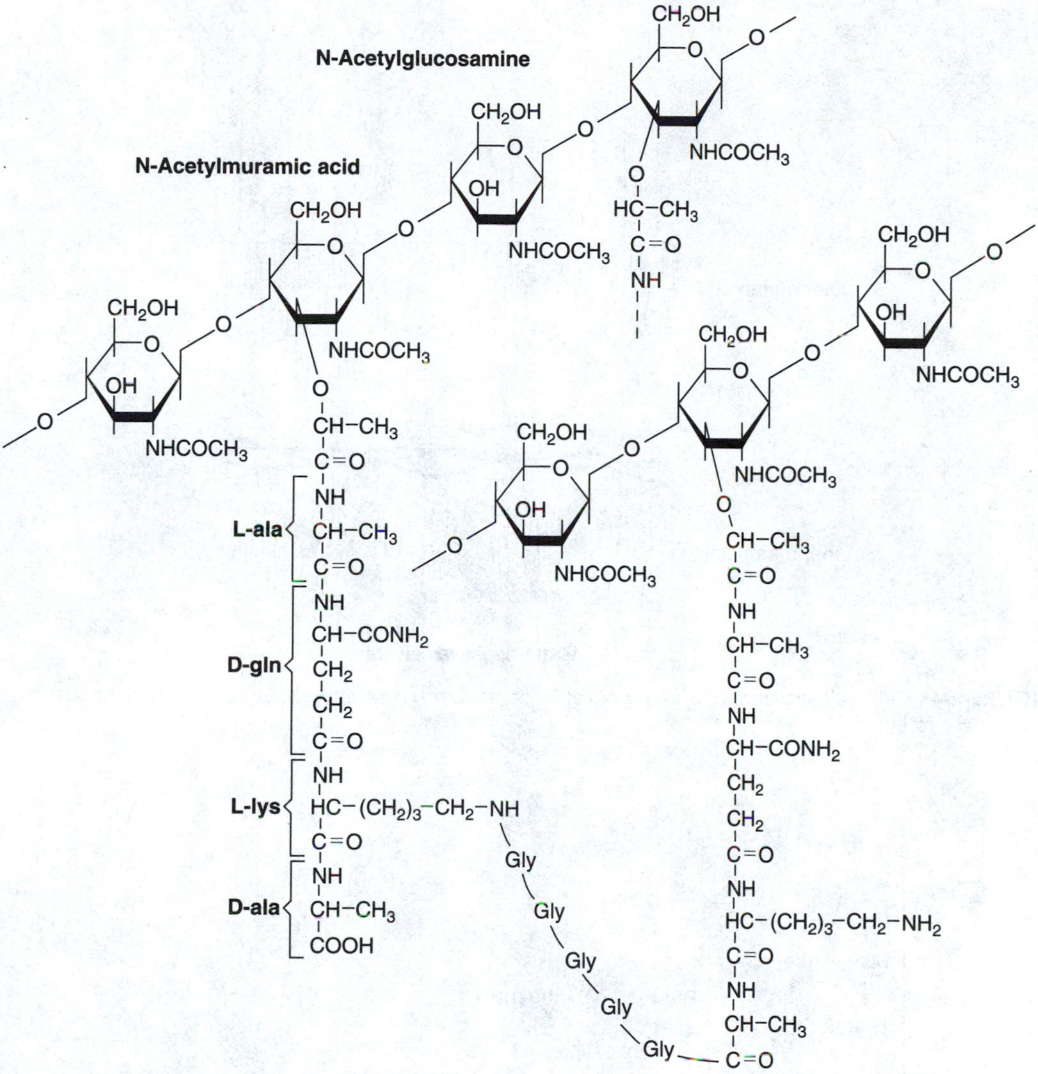

FIGURE 2-3. *Staphylococcus aureus* peptidoglycan. (Redrawn with permission from Moat AG, Foster JW: *Microbial Physiology,* 2nd ed. New York, John Wiley, 1988, p 7.)

3. **Removal of the cell wall,** which protects the delicate underlying cytoplasmic membrane and maintains the high intracellular levels of metabolites, results in bacterial lysis.
   a. **Gram-positive bacteria.** Complete removal of the bacteria cell wall of a Gram-positive bacterium results in the formation of **protoplasts,** which are constituted by the cytoplasmic membrane and the bacterial contents. Protoplasts require an isotonic medium in order to assume a spherical configuration; they cannot maintain integrity when placed in a hypo- or hypertonic medium.
   b. **Gram-negative bacteria.** The complexity of the Gram-negative cell wall results in innate resistance to enzymatic destruction of the cell wall. Cells with damaged cell walls become **spheroplasts** (i.e., they assume a spherical shape) even in a nonisosmotic medium (i.e., they are resistant to differences in osmotic pressure between the extracellular and intracellular compartments).
   c. **Wall-less organisms (L-forms)** may emerge during antibiotic therapy. These aberrant organisms can cause persistent infection, resisting the effects of antibiotics whose mechanism of action involves interference with cell wall formation.

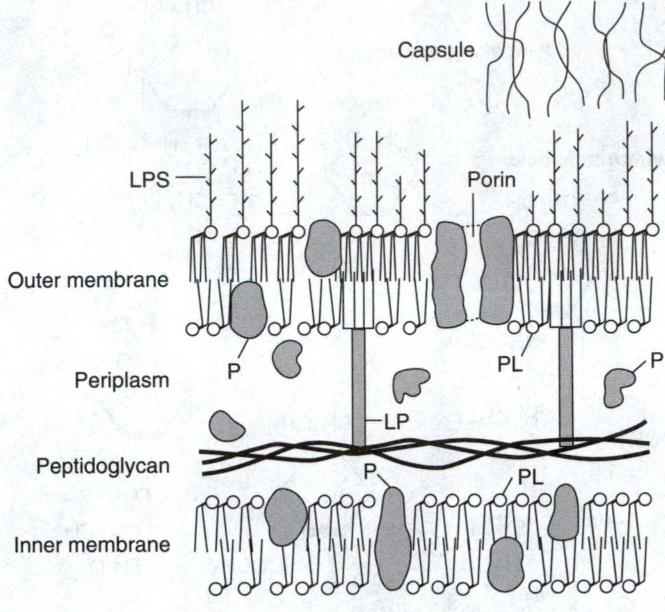

FIGURE 2-4. Cell wall structure of a Gram-negative bacterium. *LP* = lipoprotein; *LPS* = lipopolysaccharide; *P* = protein.

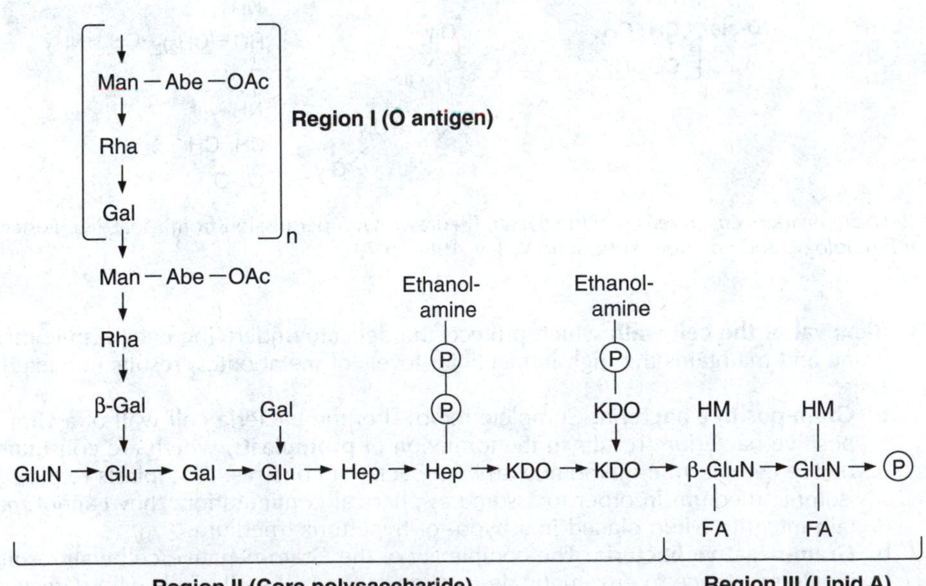

FIGURE 2-5. Bacterial lipopolysaccharide (LPS). *Arrows* indicate that the sugars are attached with their reducing group toward the lipid A region. *Abe* = abequose; *Ac* = acetyl; *FA* = fatty acid; *Gal* = D-galactose; *Glu* = D-glucose; *GluN* = N-acetyl-D-glucosamine; *Hep* = L-glycero-D-manno-heptose; *HM* = β-hydroxymyristic acid; *KDO* = 2-keto-3-deoxyoctonic acid; *Man* = D-mannose; *n* = repeating units; *P* = phosphate group; *Rha* = rhamnose. (Redrawn with permission from Moat AG, Foster JW: *Microbial Physiology*, 2nd ed. New York, John Wiley, 1988, p 73.)

B. Cytoplasmic components. The cytoplasm of most bacteria contains DNA, ribosomes, and storage granules. The variety of organelles seen in eucaryotic cells is missing in bacteria, because the cytoplasmic membrane performs many complex functions carried out by these organelles.

1. **DNA**
   - **a.** The bacterial cell lacks a nuclear membrane; instead, the DNA is concentrated in the cytoplasm as a **nucleoid.**
     - **(1)** The nucleoid consists of one double-stranded, circular, covalently closed, super-coiled DNA molecule that represents 2%–3% of the cell's dry weight (greater than 10% of the cell volume).
     - **(2)** In the case of *Escherichia coli,* the nucleoid codes for approximately 4000 different proteins.
   - **b.** In many bacteria, a small portion of the DNA persists as extrachromosomal elements referred to as **plasmids,** which are also circular but are much smaller than bacterial chromosomes. Plasmids encode variable numbers of genes and often determine virulent behavior (see Chapter 3 I B).

2. **Ribosomes** are complex globular structures composed of several RNA molecules and many associated proteins; they function as the active centers for protein synthesis.
   - **a.** Bacterial ribosomes are approximately 20 nm in diameter, and their coefficient of sedimentation is 70 Svedberg units (S). They are composed of **two subunits,** one with a sedimentation coefficient of **50S,** and the other with a sedimentation coefficient of **30S.**
   - **b.** The antibacterials **streptomycin, tetracycline,** and **chloramphenicol** inhibit protein synthesis by blocking some of the metabolic processes carried out by bacterial ribosomes (see Chapter 4 II D).

3. **Storage granules** temporarily hold excess metabolites. Their presence and amount vary with the species of bacteria and its metabolic activity.

C. External structures. Capsules, flagella, and pili are found outside the cell envelope.

1. **Capsules** surround many bacterial cells, including several pathogenic species. Bacterial capsules lack the well-ordered structure found in the bacterial cell wall.
   - **a.** Most bacterial capsules are composed of **complex polysaccharides.** Polysaccharidic bacterial capsules can be microscopically visualized using the Quellung (swelling) reaction.
     - **(1)** An antiserum specific for the capsule in question is added to the culture.
     - **(2)** The binding of the antibody to the capsule changes its light diffracting properties, causing the capsule to appear swollen when viewed through an optical microscope under adequate lighting conditions.
   - **b.** Some virulent bacteria (e.g., *Bacillus anthracis*) have a **polypeptide capsule** composed of D-glutamic acid. D-amino acids are resistant to proteolytic enzymes, enabling capsules to prevent phagocytosis (see Chapter 7).

2. **Flagella** are present on many bacteria and are responsible for the motility demonstrated by certain species.
   - **a. Structural components.** Bacterial flagella are composed exclusively of **flagellin** and are driven by the rotary action of a swivel-like **basal hook.**
   - **b. Distribution**
     - **(1) Peritrichous flagella** are distributed over the surface of the bacterium.
     - **(2) Monotrichus flagellum.** Some bacteria have only a single flagellum.
     - **(3) Polar flagella** are bundled at one or both ends of the bacterium.
   - **c. Genetic control of motility.** The genetic control of motility is complex. In the case of *Escherichia coli,* 3% of the genome (approximately 50 genes) are involved, most of which code for the proteins that form the locomotor apparatus, and the remainder of which code for the proteins and enzymes that are involved in transducing chemical stimuli.
   - **d. Phase variation.** Flagellin is immunogenic and some bacteria have developed a system of antigenic variation that allows them to switch between types of flagella (see Chapter 8).

3. **Pili** are protein fibers that cover the entire surface of Gram-negative bacteria.
   a. **Common pili (fimbriae).** Many Gram-negative bacteria have long, slender pili that originate at the cell membrane and extend through the cell wall.
      (1) Common pili are composed of a single protein type; the molecules form a helical filament.
      (2) Common pili appear to play a role in **bacterial adherence to mucosal surfaces,** which is usually an essential step in colonization and infection of a host.
   b. **Sex (F) pili** are pili that are specifically involved in **bacterial conjugation** (see Chapter 3 V A). They are few in number per bacterial cell and are usually coded by plasmids.

II. BACTERIAL PHYSIOLOGY

A. Nutritional requirements.
Bacteria grow best in an environment that meets their nutritional requirements.

1. **Carbon** is required by all bacteria for growth.
   a. **Autotrophs** use **carbon dioxide** as the sole source of carbon.
   b. **Heterotrophs** require more complex organic compounds, such as **carbohydrates** and **amino acids.**

2. **Inorganic ions.** Phosphate, potassium, magnesium, nitrogen, sulfur, and numerous trace metals are essential for bacterial growth. **Halophilic bacteria** require high concentrations of sodium for optimal growth.

3. **Organic nutrients** are required in different amounts by different species of bacteria.
   a. **Carbohydrates** are used by **organotrophic bacteria** as electron donors (i.e., as an energy source) and as the initial source of carbon skeletons for many biosynthetic pathways.
   b. **Amino acids** and, in some cases, **short-chain polypeptides** are absolutely essential to many bacteria.
   c. **Vitamins, purines,** and **pyrimidines** may also be needed for growth. The requirements for specific growth factors may change as a consequence of mutation. **Auxotrophs** can only grow in an environment supplemented with a particular growth factor that is not required by the wild strain (**prototroph**).

4. **Electron donors,** such as **ammonia, nitrites,** and **hydrogen sulfide,** serve as sources of energy.
   a. **Litotrophic bacteria** use **reduced inorganic compounds** as their energy source.
   b. **Heterotrophic bacteria** use **reduced organic compounds.**

5. **Electron acceptors** become reduced and play an essential role in respiration and fermentation.
   a. **Oxygen** serves as the terminal electron acceptor in **aerobic respiration.**
   b. **Pyruvate, lactate,** and **other organic compounds** are products of the terminal electron acceptance in **fermentation.**

6. **Oxygen**
   a. **Requirements.** Bacteria can be divided into five groups on the basis of their oxygen requirements.
      (1) **Obligate aerobes.** The growth of aerobic bacteria in a nutrient-rich medium is restricted by limited availability of oxygen.
      (2) **Obligate anaerobes.** Conversely, the growth of strict anaerobes may be inhibited by an oxygen tension as low as 10^{-5} atmospheres (atm).
      (3) **Facultative anaerobes** are able to use both molecular oxygen and organic compounds as terminal electron acceptors.
      (4) **Microaerophilic bacteria** grow best under increased carbon dioxide tension (i.e., decreased oxygen tension), as obtained in a candle jar.

(5) **Aerotolerant bacteria** can survive (but not grow) for a short period of time in the presence of atmospheric oxygen.

b. The **tolerance to oxygen** is related to the ability of the bacterium to detoxify superoxide and hydrogen peroxide, produced as by-products of aerobic respiration.

(1) **Superoxide dismutase,** which converts superoxide (the most toxic metabolite) into hydrogen peroxide, is present in aerobic and aerotolerant bacteria.

(2) **Catalase,** which converts hydrogen peroxide into water and oxygen, is also present in all aerobic bacteria but is lacking in aerotolerant organisms. Strict anaerobes lack both enzymes.

B. Energy metabolism. Energy used by bacteria primarily is produced by fermentative and/or respiratory metabolic pathways. The expression of genes necessary for the utilization of substrates or for the synthesis of critical compounds is tightly regulated to satisfy the bacterium's needs without consuming unnecessary energy (see Chapter 3 VI A).

1. **Fermentative metabolism** uses organic compounds as both the electron donors and electron acceptors.

a. **Glycolytic (Embden-Meyerhof) pathway.** The major glucose utilization pathway used by most aerobic and anaerobic bacteria is the glycolytic pathway. The feedback-sensitive (rate-limiting) enzyme is **fructose-6-phosphate dehydrogenase (phosphofructokinase).** This pathway produces a net yield of **two moles of adenosine triphosphate (ATP) per mole of glucose.**

(1) **Phase I glycolysis.** Glucose is converted to fructose-6-phosphate and, eventually, into pyruvate (two moles of pyruvate per mole of glucose).

(2) **Phase II glycolysis.** Bacteria use pyruvate in secondary metabolic processes to oxidize the reduced form of nicotinamide-adenine dinucleotide (NADH) produced during phase I glycolysis.

(a) **Homolactic fermentation,** characteristic of many streptococci and lactobacilli, is the simplest secondary process. In this process, pyruvate is converted to lactate.

(b) **Alcoholic fermentation.** Pyruvate is converted to carbon dioxide and ethanol.

(c) **Propionic fermentation.** Pyruvate is converted to oxaloacetate following the addition of a carbon dioxide molecule; the oxaloacetate is then converted to propionic acid.

(d) **Mixed acid fermentation,** common among most members of the Enterobacteriaceae, results in the production of lactate, acetate, and formate via several similar pathways. Often the end products are carbon dioxide, hydrogen, and ethanol.

b. **Entner-Doudoroff pathway.** The Entner-Duodoroff pathway is the major hexose-degrading pathway in organisms that lack phosphofructokinase (e.g., members of the Pseudomonas genus).

(1) This pathway degrades glucose into **glyceraldehyde-3-phosphate** and **pyruvate.**

(2) For each molecule of glucose, only **one pyruvate molecule** and **one ATP molecule are generated.**

c. **Pentose phosphate shunt (phosphogluconate pathway, hexose monophosphate shunt)**

(1) This pathway generates glucose 6-phosphate, which is oxidized into 6-phosphogluconate. This oxidation is coupled to the reduction of nicotinamide-adenine dinucleotide phosphate (NADP).

(2) Only one ATP molecule is generated per glucose molecule by this shunt. However, this pathway generates C4 and C5 compounds necessary for the synthesis of different bacterial products.

2. **Respiratory metabolism.** In **aerobic respiration,** the most common type of respiration for human pathogens and commensals, pyruvate formed by the Embden-Meyerhof pathway is converted to carbon dioxide via acetylcoenzyme A (acetyl-CoA) and the tricarboxylic acid (TCA) cycle.

a. The respiration process is facilitated by the **electron transport system,** a system whereby electrons move through a series of reversible electron carriers with successively higher oxidation–reduction potentials. These electron acceptors are embedded in the bacterial membrane and include NADH, reduced nicotinamide-adenine dinucleotide phosphate (NADPH), and oxygen.
   (1) The major elements of the electron transport system are cytochromes (hemoproteins), flavoproteins, and ubiquinones (e.g., coenzyme Q).
   (2) In the three stages of the electron transport sequence, energy is used to extrude a pair of protons (H^+) across an insulating membrane, thus creating an **electrochemical gradient** (i.e., a proton motive force).
   (3) The return of the protons through the membrane reverses the activity of adenosine triphosphatase (ATPase) and is referred to as **oxidative phosphorylation.**

b. Complete respiration results in **38 molecules of ATP produced for 1 molecule of glucose,** a much higher energy yield than that of fermentation.

3. **Autotrophic metabolism** uses a variety of inorganic sources for energy and reducing power.
   a. In **photosynthesis,** bacteria use energy from light to convert carbon dioxide to triose phosphate, which is then converted to other cell constituents.
   b. In **anaerobic respiration,** bacteria use inorganic substrates (e.g., nitrogen) as terminal electron acceptors in place of oxygen.

C. Biosynthetic pathways. The enormous diversity in the nutritional requirements of bacteria stems from their wide range of biosynthetic capabilities.

1. **Pathways.** Bacteria use various catabolic **bidirectional (amphibolic)** pathways for biosynthesis, including **glycolysis, pyruvate oxidation,** and the **TCA cycle.** The glyoxylate bypass of the TCA cycle allows bacteria to use acetate as a precursor for a variety of 4-carbon dicarboxylic acids, which can also be used for biosynthetic purposes.

2. **Amino acid biosynthesis** can be conveniently categorized based on points of origin in the amphibolic pathways.
   a. **Glutamate family.** Glutamate and glutamine are formed from reductive amination of α-ketoglutarate and serve as the carbon skeletons for proline and arginine.
   b. **Aspartate family.** Aspartate is synthesized by transamination of oxaloacetate, gives rise to asparagine, and can be reduced to lysine, methionine, threonine, and isoleucine.
   c. **Pyruvate family.** Alanine, valine, isoleucine, and leucine are formed from the initial transamination of pyruvate.
   d. **Serine family.** Serine, glycine, and cysteine are derived from 3-P-glycerate; glycine results from the transfer of the 1-carbon fragment to tetrahydrofolate.
   e. **Histidine** is synthesized from the 5-carbon backbone of phosphoribosyl pyrophosphate (PRPP). Histidine is unique in that its carboxyl group is not present on the starting compound; instead, it is formed later.
   f. **Aromatic amino acids.** Tyrosine, phenylalanine, and tryptophan are derived from shikimic acid.

3. **Nucleotide biosynthesis** in bacteria is identical to that in animal tissue.
   a. **Purine nucleotides** are built on the ribose-P chain from PRPP, glycine, and carbon and nitrogen.
   b. **Pyrimidine nucleotides** are formed via a series of carboxyl-containing intermediates, starting with carbamyl phosphate. Ribose-P is added late in the sequence.

4. **Macromolecule biosynthesis.** The principal macromolecules—**DNA, RNA,** and **protein**—are polymers of the nucleotide and amino acid building blocks.
   a. These macromolecules are synthesized via a highly regulated system in the **cell cytoplasm.**
   b. The sequence of information transfer for macromolecular synthesis involves **replication (DNA to DNA), transcription (DNA to RNA),** and **translation (RNA to protein).**
      (1) DNA acts as the template necessary for synthesis of both DNA and RNA.

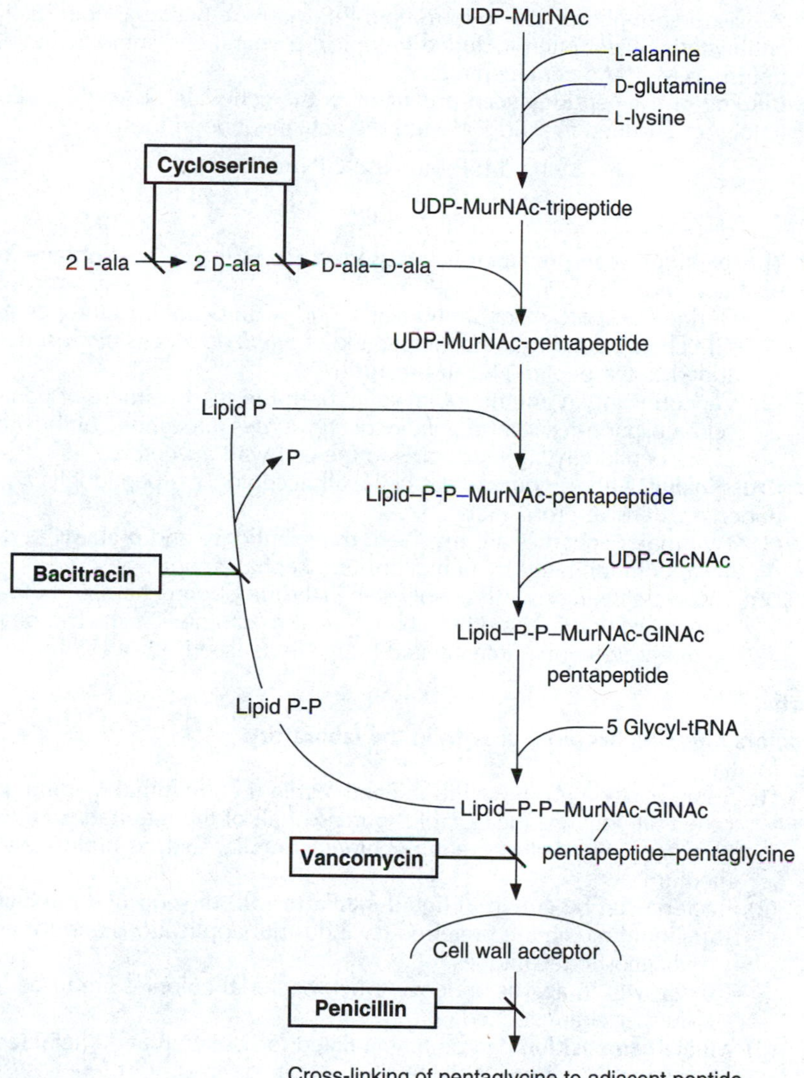

FIGURE 2-6. Biosynthesis of peptidoglycan by *Staphylococcus aureus.* Sites of action of antimicrobials that interfere with cell wall biosynthesis are indicated.

(2) RNA serves as the template for protein synthesis and provides the core of ribosomes on which the proteins are synthesized.

5. **Peptidoglycan biosynthesis** can be divided into five stages (Figure 2-6).
   a. **Synthesis of UDP-N-acetylmuramic acid (UDP-Mur-NAc).** UDP-Mur-NAc, the starting point, derives from UDP-N-acetylglucosamine. An enolpyruvic acid group is transferred from phosphoenopyruvic acid and is reduced by NADPH to form a lactic acid ether (muramic acid).
   b. **Addition of peptides.** First, a tripeptide constituted by alanine, glutamine, and lysine is added to UDP-Mur-NAc to form **UDP-MurNAc-tripeptide,** and then a dimer of D-alanine is added to form **UDP-MurNAc-pentapeptide.**
      (1) The D-alanine dimer is derived from two L-alanine molecules via an enzymatic reaction involving a D-alanine racemase and a D-alanyl-D-alanine synthetase.
      (2) These two enzymes are inhibited by cycloserine, an antimycobacterial drug.
   c. **Association with lipid P.** The UDP-MurNAc-pentapeptide associates with lipid P

(C_{55} isoprenol phosphate) to form lipid-P-P-MurNAc-pentapeptide. Bacitracin, an antibacterial agent often included in topical preparations, inhibits the binding of lipid P to MurNAc-pentapeptide.

d. Binding of the peptidoglycan precursor to the cell wall. N-Acetyl glucosamine (GlcNAc) is added to lipid-P-P-MurNAc-pentapeptide to form

lipid-P-P-MurNAc-GlNAc
|
pentapeptide

This peptidoglycan precursor is transported across the cell membrane to a cell wall acceptor.

(1) During transport, extra amino acids (bridge units, such as the pentaglycine side chain added to the pentapeptide of *Staphylococcus aureus*) may be added to the peptidoglycan precursor.

(2) Vancomycin, an antimicrobial agent useful in the treatment of penicillin- and cephalosporin-resistant *Staphylococcus aureus* infections, inhibits the binding of the peptidoglycan precursors to the cell wall acceptors.

e. Crosslinking. After binding to the cell wall acceptor, the peptidoglycan subunits undergo extensive crosslinking.

(1) Two major enzymes are involved: **transpeptidase** and **D-alanyl carboxypeptidase,** both inhibited by penicillins and cephalosporins.

(2) The crosslinking usually involves the L-lysine of one chain and the penultimate D-alanine in the other (the terminal D-alanine is lost). The binding can be direct or involve intercalated bridge units [see I A 1 a (1) (b)].

D. Growth

1. Factors affecting bacterial growth in the laboratory

a. Media

(1) Some bacteria grow well in **defined media** (i.e., minimal medium with glucose that contains measurable sources of all of the required nutritional elements), whereas others require **complex media,** such as brain–heart infusion medium.

(2) Bacteria can be grown in **liquid media (broth)** or **semisolid medium (agar).**

(a) Liquid media are preferred for industrial applications and for automated diagnostic techniques.

(b) Growth in agar is preferred when bacterial colonies are to be isolated or further characterized.

(3) Media composition can be manipulated for isolation and characterization of bacteria (see Chapter 10 IV B 2).

(4) Some bacteria cannot be grown *in vitro* (e.g., *Treponema pallidum, Mycobacterium leprae*).

b. Temperature. The optimal temperature for growth of some human pathogens is rather unique and can be a simple way to select those organisms. For example, *Campylobacter* species grow best at 42°C, a temperature that is excessive for the growth of most other human pathogens.

(1) Mesophilic bacteria grow best at temperatures ranging from 20°C–40°C. Most human pathogens are mesophilic.

(2) Thermophilic bacteria grow best at 50°C–60°C.

(3) Psychrophilic bacteria grow best at temperatures ranging from 0°C–10°C.

2. Measurement of bacterial growth is easiest to perform when the bacteria are grown in a liquid medium. The following techniques can be used:

a. Determination of weight per unit volume, by centrifuging a known volume of broth and determining the mass of the pellet (wet weight)

b. Turbidimetric assays, which are based on the fact that a bacterial suspension scatters light proportionally to the number of bacteria, following Lambert-Beer's law

c. Microscopic counting using a **Petroff-Hauser chamber,** similar in principle to the chambers used to count blood cells

d. Electronic counting using a **Coulter counter,** which takes advantage of the negative charge inherent to all microorganisms

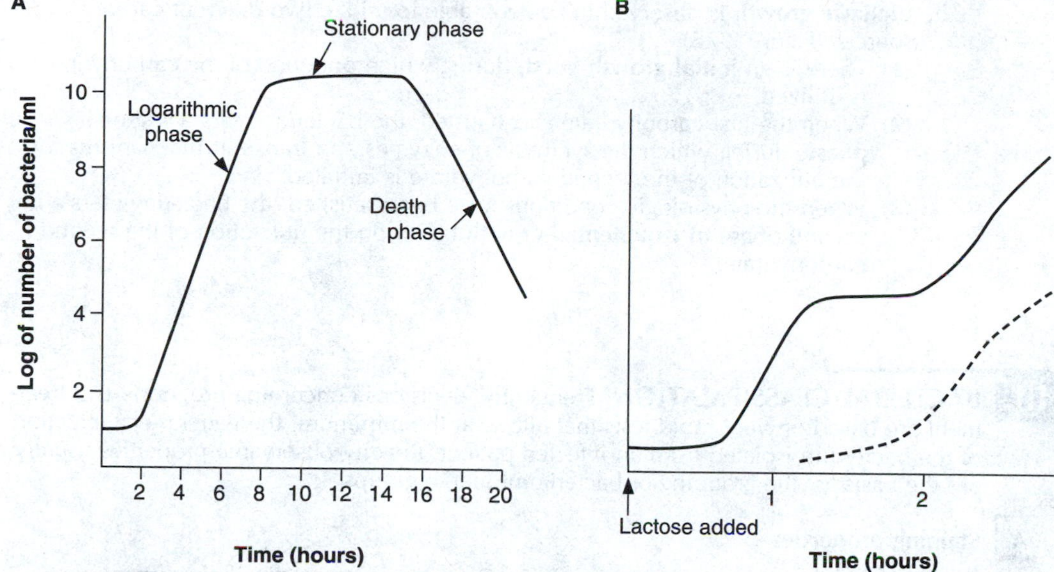

FIGURE 2-7. (*A*) Bacterial growth curve. (*B*) Biphasic growth curve of an organism that may use both glucose and lactose as energy sources. The *bold line* represents the optical density of the suspension, which is indicative of the number of bacteria present in the culture. The *dashed line* represents the breakdown of substrate, which is indicative of the relative activity of β-galactosidase.

3. **Bacterial growth curves.** Bacterial growth is regulated by the nutritional environment.
   a. **Growth cycle.** During typical bacterial growth, bacterial cells divide by binary fission and their mass and number increase in an exponential manner. Bacterial growth in culture can be separated into at least four distinct phases relative to the introduction of the bacteria to the medium (Figure 2-7A).
      (1) **Lag phase.** This is a period of intense physiologic adjustment involving the induction of new enzymes and the synthesis and assembly of ribosomes.
      (2) **Logarithmic (exponential) phase.** This phase is characterized by maximal rates of cell division. The generation time (i.e., the time required for doubling the number of bacteria) during the logarithmic phase is constant for a given bacterial species grown under the same set of conditions, but varies among species. For example, the generation time may be as brief as 14 minutes (for *Pseudomonas*) or as long as 24 hours (for *Mycobacterium tuberculosis*).
      (3) **Stationary phase.** During this period, the availability of essential nutrients becomes a limiting factor, and there is a balance between cell growth and division and cell death. Two genera of bacteria, *Bacillus* and *Clostridium,* are capable of undergoing **sporulation,** a model of prokaryote cell differentiation that is activated when the bacteria are placed under limiting nutritional conditions.
         (a) Each vegetative cell forms a single, dormant **endospore** that is resistant to heat, radiation, drying, and chemicals (including 70% ethanol). **Calcium dipicolinate** represents 10%–15% of the spore total mass and is responsible for the spore's ability to withstand heat.
         (b) The process of sporulation begins immediately after nutrient deprivation and is completed in approximately 8 hours. No external nutritional or energy sources are required.
         (c) The spore is released when the parent cell undergoes lysis and remains dormant until environmental conditions are once again favorable.
      (4) **Decline or death phase.** During this phase, bacterial cells undergo lysis, which reduces the number of viable cells.

b. **Biphasic growth** is observed in bacteria able to utilize two different carbon sources (Figure 2-7B).
   (1) There is an **initial growth burst,** during which only one of the carbohydrates is utilized.
   (2) When the first carbohydrate is exhausted, the bacteria enters a **stationary phase,** during which the synthesis of enzymes and transport mechanisms for the utilization of the second carbohydrate is initiated.
   (3) When the physiologic conditions have been satisfied, the bacteria enters a **second phase of exponential growth** based on the utilization of the second carbohydrate.

III. BACTERIAL CLASSIFICATION.

Frequently, decisions concerning prognosis and treatment are based on very rapid tests that allow, at the minimum, the general classification of the bacterium isolated from an infected patient. Readily observable properties usually are the basis for the grouping of bacteria into large groups.

A. Staining properties

1. **Gram staining,** the most common criterion for grouping medically important bacteria, is a simple differential staining technique that employs **crystal violet** (an aniline dye) as the primary stain and **safranin** (a red dye) as a counter-stain. The exact molecular basis for the Gram stain reaction is not understood, but the structure and integrity of the cell wall appear to be important factors.
   a. **Gram-positive bacteria** appear dark blue to purple because they retain the crystal violet and resist alcohol decoloration. Old colonies and heavy smears may show uneven staining as a result of variable uptake or retention of dyes.
   b. **Gram-negative bacteria** appear dark pink or red because they are decolorized completely by ethanol and they take up saffranin, the counter-stain.
2. **Acid-fast staining** is mainly used to identify *Mycobacterium* species, which are difficult to stain by the Gram stain. Other filamentous bacteria, such as some *Nocardia* species, are also stainable by this technique.
   a. The **Ziehl-Neelsen stain** is the most commonly employed acid-fast staining technique.
      (1) First, the sample is immersed in hot carbolfuchsin, which stains red. The sample is then destained with acid-alcohol, and counter-stained with methylene blue. Under the light microscope, the bacteria appear bright red against a light blue background.
      (2) The basis for the staining is the presence of unique fatty acids (e.g., mycolic acid) in the cell wall. Mycobacteria are rich in these fatty acids; therefore they retain the carbolfuchsin and are considered "acid-fast."
   b. Variations such as the **Kynuon stain** identify parasites, such as *Cryptosporidium.*

B. Morphologic features

1. **Shape.** Bacteria exist in three basic shapes.
   a. **Rods.** Cylindrical cells are referred to as **bacilli.**
   b. **Spheres.** Spherical cells are referred to as **cocci.**
   c. **Spirals.** The spirilla, vibrios, and spirochetes are examples of spiral bacteria.
2. **Arrangement.** Bacteria are found as single cells or in regular groups of two or more cells.

C. Metabolic activity

1. **Oxygen requirements**
   a. **Aerobic bacteria** employ molecular oxygen as the terminal electron acceptor during respiration. Most of them have a membrane-bound cytochrome C oxidase that plays a major role in the electron transport chain. The activity of this enzyme is

easy to test with the **oxidase test.** A colorless substrate (N,N′-dimethyl-p-phenylene-diamine) becomes purple following reduction.

b. **Anaerobic bacteria** do not use molecular oxygen as a terminal electron acceptor. These bacteria obtain their energy either by **fermentation,** in which organic compounds serve as terminal electron acceptors, or by **anaerobic respiration,** using an electron acceptor other than molecular oxygen (e.g., nitrate).

c. **Facultative bacteria** can generate energy either by respiration or by fermentation, depending on the environmental circumstances.

2. **Carbohydrate utilization.** Often bacteria can be identified by the variety of carbohydrate substrates they use as energy sources. For example, enterics are subclassified in two large groups depending on their ability to ferment lactose.

3. **Enzyme production**
   a. **Oxidase,** which transfers hydrogen directly from a substrate to oxygen, is present in some important pathogenic species but not in others.
   b. **Proteolytic (toxic) enzymes** are usually detected by gelatin liquefaction.
      (1) **Hemolysins** cause variable degrees of red blood cell lysis and are easy to detect when the organism can be grown in blood agar.
         (a) **Alpha hemolysins** lyse but do not dissolve red cell membranes.
         (b) **Beta hemolysins** lyse and dissolve red cell membranes.
      (2) **Coagulase** causes clotting of blood plasma.

D. **Serologic reactivity** is determined by using specific antisera that are directed against antigenic determinants.

1. **Antigenic determinants** can be:
   a. **Genus-specific** or shared by closely related members of a given species
   b. **Species-specific**
   c. **Specific for subgroups (serotypes)** within a species

2. **Serotyping** is usually carried out by **agglutination** techniques that entail mixing a drop of antiserum with a drop of a bacterial suspension. A positive reaction results in clumping of the bacterial suspension.

E. **Genetic relatedness** provides the best basis for the phylogenetic scheme of bacterial classification. Classification based on genetic relatedness is established by:

1. The ability to exchange genetic information (i.e., via transformation or conjugation), which is only possible between related organisms

2. The nucleotide base composition (i.e., G-C:A-T ratio)

3. Nucleic acid homology among bacteria, which can be determined by hybridization studies

4. Nucleic acid sequences, which provide the gold standard for determining "relatedness" among species

Chapter 3

Bacterial Genetics

Michael G. Schmidt

I. BACTERIAL GENETIC MATERIAL

A. Chromosomes

1. Bacteria have **one unique chromosome** that can encode up to 4000 separate genes necessary for bacterial maintenance and propagation.
2. Two to four copies of the chromosome are present in each cell, depending on the stage of replication.
3. A typical bacterial chromosome has a molecular weight of 10^{10} [5×10^6 base pairs (bp)].

B. **Plasmids** are extra chromosomal DNA molecules with a molecular weight of 10^6–10^8 that may encode from 40–50 genes. Plasmids play an important part in terms of the bacteria's genetic constitution, often determining important characteristics such as the ability to produce exotoxins or enzymes capable of inactivating antibacterial agents.

1. **Conjugative plasmids** are transferred from bacterium to bacterium (usually members of the same species or of very closely related species) through conjugation (see VA).
   - **a.** These plasmids are common in Gram-negative bacilli and are relatively large (25–150 million daltons).
   - **b.** Large plasmids are usually present at 1–2 copies per cell; their replication is closely linked to the replication of the bacterial chromosome.
2. **Nonconjugative plasmids,** common in Gram-positive cocci as well as in some Gram-negative organisms (e.g., *Haemophilus influenzae, Neisseria gonorrhoeae*) are usually small (1–10 million daltons).
   - **a.** Small plasmids may be present at more than 30 copies per cell; distribution to progeny during cell division is ensured by the large number present.
   - **b.** Nonconjugative plasmids can also be transferred ("mobilized") from cell to cell when the same bacterium carries both conjugative and nonconjugative plasmids. Once conjugation is established, the donor can transfer nonconjugative plasmids.

C. **Transposable genetic elements** are DNA units capable of mediating their own transfer from one chromosome to another, from one location to another on the same chromosome, or between chromosomes and plasmids. Transposition relies on the ability of the transposable element to synthesize its own specific recombination enzyme (transposase).

1. **Insertion sequences (IS elements)** are the simplest type of transposable element (Figure 3-1A). They are approximately 1000 bp in length and encode the enzymes necessary for site-specific recombination and the enzymes that control the frequency of transposition.
   - **a.** Transposition involves site-specific recognition of the ends of the IS elements by the transposases and the selection of a new area into which a new copy of the IS element is inserted. The original copy remains at the original site. Because of the duplication of the IS element, transposition is sometimes called **replicative recombination** (i.e., the molecular mechanism of transposition results in the direct repeats that precede and follow the IS element).
   - **b.** Transposition occurs infrequently (once every 10^5–10^7 generations).

A. IS Element

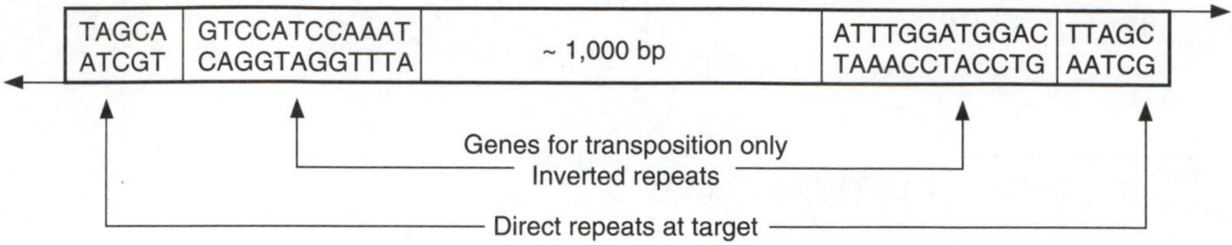

B. Transposon

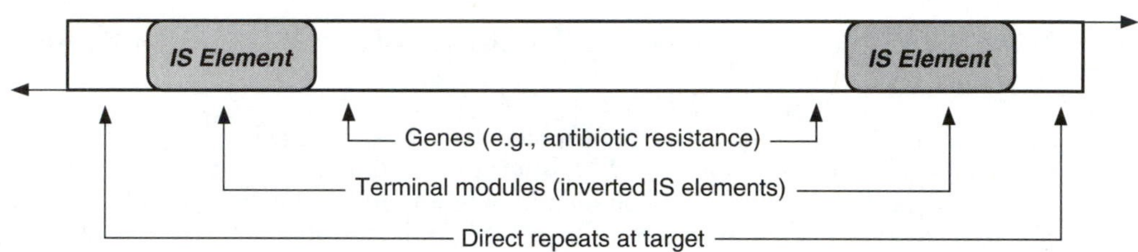

FIGURE 3-1. (*A*) Insertion sequence (IS element). (*B*) Transposon. (Modified with permission from Neidhart FC: The bacterial cell: genetic determinants of growth, survival, and colonization. (In *Medical Microbiology,* 2nd ed. Edited by Sherris JC. New York, Elsevier, 1990, pp 65–66.)

2. **Transposons** contain a DNA segment coding for specific genes flanked by two IS elements (Figure 3-1B). Each transposon usually encodes a gene that confers important characteristics to the organism, such as resistance to multiple antibacterial agents.
   a. Transposons are **self-integrating** DNA fragments (i.e., they do not require classic recombination systems). Therefore, they can integrate into DNA almost at random. Transposons can also insert into plasmids and flip-flop between plasmids and chromosomes.
   b. Because classic recombination requiring DNA homology is not a necessity for transposon integration, transposons have the potential to propagate among bacterial species.

II. BACTERIAL MUTATION

A. Origins

1. **Spontaneous mutations** result from **replication errors, genetic mispairing,** or **DNA changes** that cause replication errors and mispairing. Spontaneous mutations may cause genetic variation that is **advantageous** or **disadvantageous.**
   a. **Rate of occurrence.** The approximate rate of occurrence is once every 10^6–10^7 cells.
      (1) If one million organisms are plated on antibiotic-containing agar, one colony of antibiotic-resistant bacteria can be expected to survive as a result of a spontaneous mutation.
      (2) Although on an individual basis, the rate of mutation within a population of bacteria seems insignificant, one must remember that bacterial populations

are huge and replicate rapidly; therefore, the rates of mutation, when considered from the perspective of a population, are significant.

b. **Reversion mutations** reverse a spontaneous mutation, restoring the original genetic makeup. These mutations are observed once every 10^7–10^8 cells (i.e., they are at least ten times more rare than a forward spontaneous mutation.) Reversion mutations are rarer events because they need to affect a specific (previously mutated) DNA point.

2. **Experimentally induced mutations**

a. **Chemical mutagenesis.** Some chemicals significantly increase the mutation rate to rates as high as 1 mutation per 10^3–10^4 cells.

b. **Radiation mutagenesis** is caused by exposure to ultraviolet light and usually results in thymine dimers (see II B 3).

B. Types. Mutations can be classified according to nucleotide changes, additions, deletions, or distortions.

1. **Single-base (point) mutations** (Figure 3-2) involve the replacement of a nucleotide in the coding sequence.

a. **Same sense (silent) mutations** occur when, because of the redundancy of the genetic code, the resulting triplet codes for the same amino acid is the original triplet.

b. **Missense mutations** occur when the mutant base changes the coding sequence so that a different amino acid is produced. The resulting protein may be functional or not, depending on the importance of the area affected by the mutation.

2. **Frameshift mutations** occur when a nucleotide is added to or deleted from the coding sequence, resulting in a shift of the reading frame.

a. **Missense mutations** occur as described in II B 1 b.

b. **Nonsense mutations** occur when the mutation introduces a termination codon into the sequence, causing premature transcription termination. These mutations result in either a lack of protein synthesis or the synthesis of a very short, nonfunctional proteins.

3. **Helix distortion mutations** occur when ultraviolet radiation induces dimerization of adjacent nucleotides, particularly thymines. The resulting cyclobutane ring distorts the symmetry of the DNA and prevents faithful replication.

C. Detection. The detection of mutated bacteria in the laboratory requires the ability to screen for a property that is unique to the mutant strain. Common end points used to study bacterial mutations include:

1. The ability to grow in the presence of an antibiotic to which the bacteria is usually susceptible

2. Reversion of auxotrophy (i.e., the ability of mutants of an auxotrophic organism to survive in media not supplemented with the nutrient that the auxotrophic strain requires)

III. MUTATION REPAIR MECHANISMS.

Mutations caused by radiation, chemicals, and other mechanisms would cause the extinction of affected bacterial populations were it not for the cell's ability to repair damaged DNA.

A. Light repair is used to control helical distortion such as that caused by ultraviolet dimerization.

1. **Process. Photolyase,** a photo-reactivating enzyme, cleaves the thymine dimer and restores integrity to the adjacent thymines (Figure 3-3). The energy for the repair is provided by visible light.

2. Light repair is considered an **error-free** mechanism.

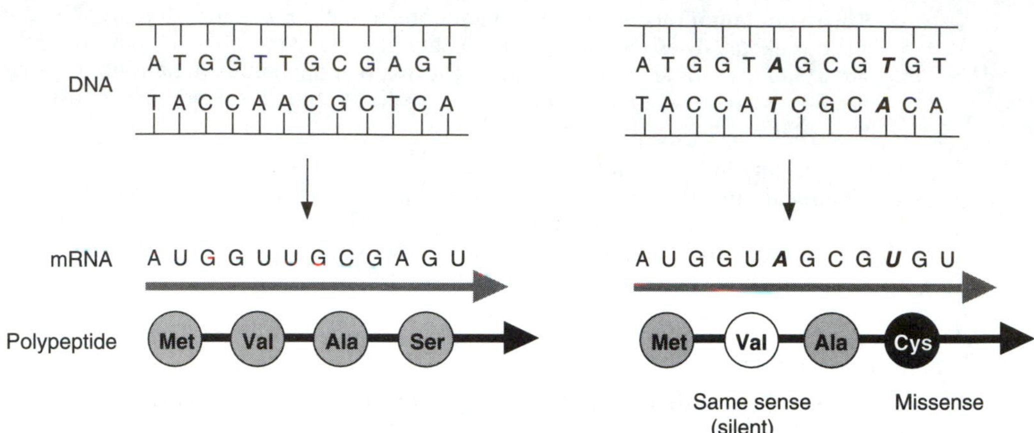

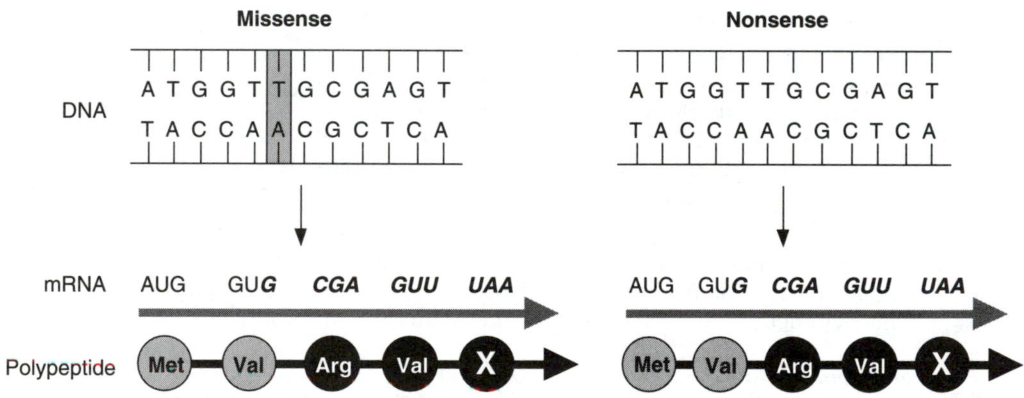

FIGURE 3-2. Types of bacterial mutations. (*1*) Normal transcription and translation. The DNA nucleotide bases, adenine (*A*), guanine (*G*), thymine (*T*), and cystosine (*C*) act as templates for mRNA. [In RNA, thymine is replaced by uracil (*U*)]. Ribosomes then translate the information coded by the mRNA into a polypeptide chain. In this example, *Met* = methionine, *Val* = valine, *Ala* = alanine, and *Ser* = serine. (*2*) Single base (point) mutations. The first mutation in this example results in a same-sense, or silent, mutation because the resultant amino acid, valine will occur whether the code is GUU (as in *1*) or GUA (as in *2*). The second mutation produces a missense mutation because the resulting triplet, UGU, codes for cysteine (*Cys*) instead of serine. (*3*) Frameshift mutations. A missense mutation occurs when a shift in the reading frame distorts the triplet coding pattern. In this example, the T-A nucleotide pair is deleted, which throws off the reading frame of the coding sequence. The first affected triplet is GUU, which changes to GUG. However, both GUU (as in *1*) and GUG will produce valine. The next triplet in the sequence is CGA instead of GCG; therefore, arginine (*Arg*) is produced instead of alanine (*Ala*). Each subsequent triplet is also affected. A nonsense mutation occurs when the mutation generates a premature termination codon.

B. **Dark repair** is also used to repair helical distortion. The simplest dark repair mechanism is the **nucleotide excision repair** system

1. **Process** (Figure 3-4)
   a. An **endonuclease** encoded by three genes, *uvrA, uvrB,* and *uvrC (uvrABC nuclease)* recognizes the distorted helix, binds to the abnormal area, becomes activated, and cleaves the DNA on both sides of the dimer.

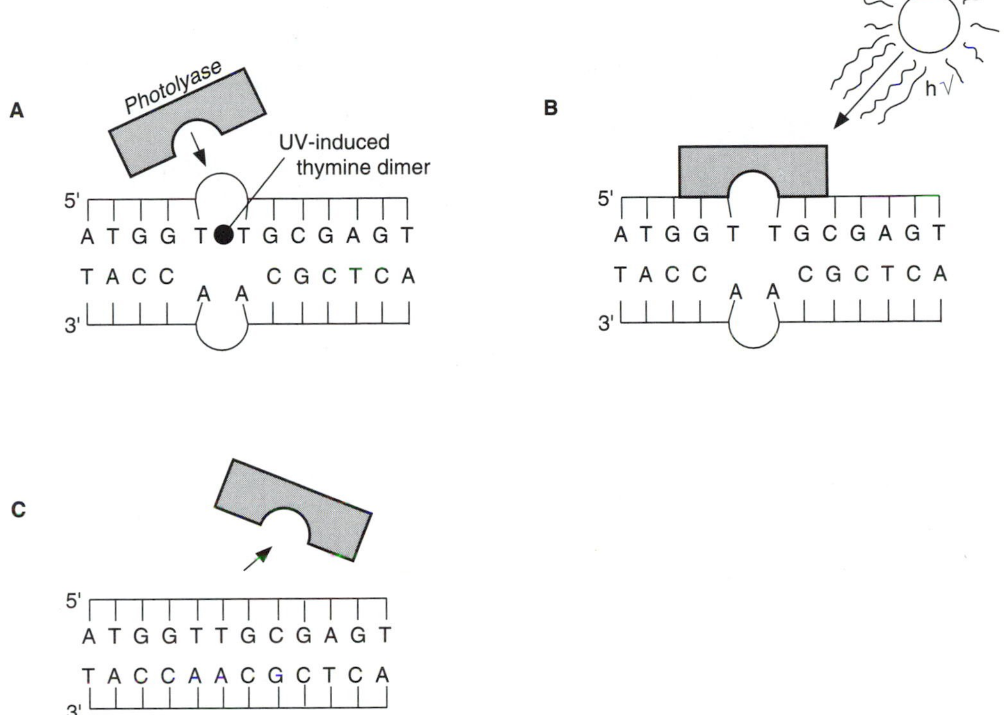

FIGURE 3-3. Light repair. Intrastrand dimers may be removed by photolyase, a bacterial enzyme that obtains its energy from a quantum of visible light. *UV* = ultraviolet.

- **b.** An **exonuclease** digests the thymines dimer, goes a little distance beyond, and stops, forming a gap in the DNA strand that is typically 12–13 nucleotides long.
- **c. DNA polymerase I** (the **repair enzyme**) enters the gap and resynthesizes the missing nucleotides on the basis of the remaining strand of DNA. Because the repair is based on a normal template, this system is largely **error-free**.
- **d.** A **ligase** seals the new DNA strand to complete the repair.

2. All living organisms studied, including humans, have repair systems similar to the nucleotide excision repair system of bacteria. In mammals, repair mechanisms are involved in copyediting DNA during replication and in eliminating spontaneously occurring mutations, such as those induced by ultraviolet irradiation.
   - **a.** The loss of these mechanisms is believed to play a crucial role in the pathogenesis of malignancies and in aging.
   - **b.** Xeroderma pigmentosum, a hereditary condition, is characterized by an increased incidence of skin cancer, which often develops in children under 10 years of age. The genetic basis for this disease is a lack of a functional nucleotide excision repair pathway.

C. DNA glycosylase-mediated repair. The DNA glycosylase system, an alternative to the *uvrABC*-mediated form of excision repair, is most often used to repair mutagen-damaged DNA.

1. The cell has a variety of DNA glycosylases that recognize alterations in the DNA resulting from alkylation, deamination, or ring-opening reactions. DNA glycosylases cleave the N-glycosidic bond that connects the damaged base to the sugar–phosphate backbone, leaving an apurinic or apyrimidinic site.
2. The absence of a base is recognized by an endonuclease, which cleaves the DNA

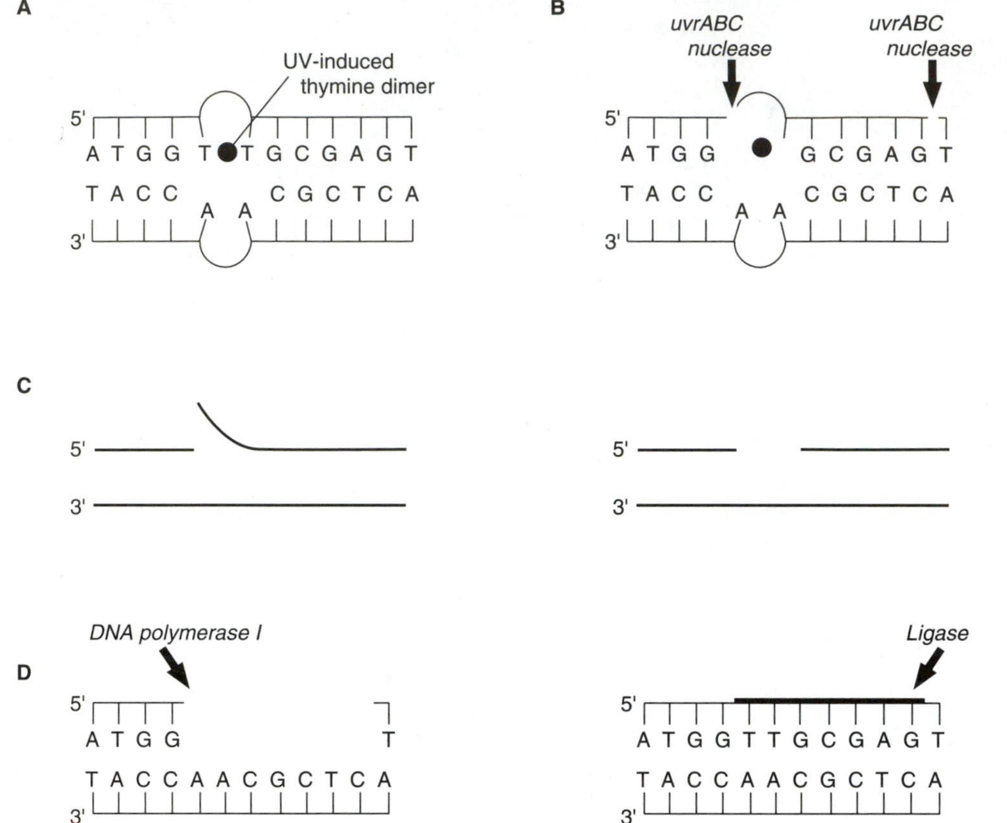

FIGURE 3-4. Nucleotide excision repair. (*A*) Mutated strand. (*B*) An endonuclease, *uvrABC,* cleaves the DNA on both sides of the dimer. (*C*) An exonuclease digests the thymine dimer and continues a short way, forming a gap that is approximately 12–13 nucleotides long. (*D*) DNA polymerase enters the gap and resynthesizes the missing nucleotides on the basis of the intact strand of DNA. A ligase seals the DNA gap to complete the error-free repair.

strand nearby. The fragment is released and the gap is filled in a sequence of events similar to that observed in *uvrABC*-mediated repair. Like *uvrABC*-mediated repair, DNA glycosylase-mediated repair is **error-free**.

D. **Post-replication recombination repair** is used when a helical distortion occurs immediately adjacent to the replication fork.

1. The DNA replication systems of bacteria do not recognize helical distortion (e.g., as caused by thymine dimers). DNA polymerase will replicate the abnormal strand to the point where the thymine dimer is, skip over the thymine dimer, initiate replication again, and then finish the strand. The other strand will be replicated without a problem. In other words, one of the pairs of chromosomes is normal, while the other has as a thymine dimer in a strand and a gap opposite it. Transmission of the defective DNA strand to a daughter cell would be lethal, because removal of the thymine dimer by the excision system would result in a lethal double-stranded break in the chromosome.
2. To avoid this problem, the cell performs post-replication (recombination) repair.
   a. Incomplete replication of the genetic material inhibits cell division, so that the cell contains both copies of the chromosome.
   b. Repair of the incomplete chromosome is accomplished by splicing the abnormal region in the abnormal chromosome and the complementary normal strand in

the neighboring normal chromosome. The normal segment is then displaced to fill the gap opposite to the thymine dimer in the abnormal copy. Specialized proteins, **recombinase A *(recA)*** and **recombinase BCD *(recBC),*** facilitate the incorporation and transfer of the homologous segment from the neighboring chromosome.

(1) **RecA** (molecular weight-38,000) is a multifunctional protein synthesized in an inactive form. Activation requires the binding of single-stranded segments of DNA to the *recA* protein.
   (a) *RecA* acts as a DNA helicase and as a DNA synaptase. It also serves as a specific intracellular protease involved in the control of at least two major regulons (SOS and lysogenic 1) within *E. coli.*
   (b) Mutations within the *recA* gene can reduce the frequency of recombination more than 1000-fold.

(2) ***RecBCD* nuclease (exonuclease V)** is coded by three separate genes—*recB, recC,* and *recD*—whose products form a multifunctional enzyme. Two activities of ***recBCD*** critical to recombination have been described:
   (a) The *RecBCD* nuclease transiently denatures the duplex DNA through the consumption of adenosine triphosphate (ATP) that is, it acts as a DNA helicase. The helicase is specific to DNA that contains either a short single-stranded gap or an end. Denaturation of the duplex provides a region of single-strand DNA (i.e., a binding site for *RecA*).
   (b) *RecBCD* nuclease is also responsible for the endonucleotydic cleavage of DNA after it passes the octanucleotide sequence 5′-GCTGGTGG-3′.

c. Following splicing, the thymidine dimer is excised and repaired by the **nucleotide excision repair system** using the recombinant strand as template, and the gap in the donor strand is filled using the same system. Post-replication repair is also considered to be **error-free** because it incorporates an identical piece of genetic information into the damaged chromosome.

E. **SOS repair** is the only mechanism available if duplex DNA receives multiple hits of ultraviolet light, producing overlapping thymine dimers. Overlapping dimers render excision or post-replication repair ineffective because the gaps in the second strand overlap those in the first.

1. The thymine dimers are excised by uvrABC nuclease and the resulting gaps are randomly filled with nucleotides.
2. Once the gaps have been filled, excision repair can be performed. Whether or not the repair is effective depends on what nucleotide sequences were replaced in the "repaired gaps." Because of its randomness, this repair mechanism is **error-prone,** more often than not resulting in non-coding sequences or sequences coding for abnormal, nonfunctional proteins.
3. In mammalian cells, error-prone repair is mediated by the *recA* protein. *RecA* binds to the damaged DNA and modifies one of the DNA polymerases into a form with relaxed specificity, allowing the gap to be filled at random.

IV. MUTATION SUPPRESSION.

An initial mutation can be reversed by a second mutation, which may occur within the gene (intragenic) or in another gene (extragenic).

A. **Intragenic suppression** results from a second mutation that corrects the effects of the initial mutation. For example, a point mutation resulting in the synthesis of an aberrant protein with no biological activity can be corrected if a second point mutation codes for an amino acid that restores proper configuration and activity to the protein.

B. **Extragenic suppression** is the reversion of a mutation in one gene as a result of a mutation in a second gene. For example, if a mutation occurs within a tRNA gene that results in the recognition of a nonsense codon, extension of the growing polypeptide will continue when the altered tRNA is incorporated at the stop codon. The mutant tRNA generally functions at a lower rate, thereby enabling the majority of normal terminations to be recognized by the ribosome.

V. DNA TRANSFER BETWEEN BACTERIA.

DNA TRANSFER BETWEEN BACTERIA. Bacteria transfer DNA amongst themselves by three basic mechanisms: conjugation, transformation, and transduction (Figure 3-5).

A. Conjugation (see Figure 3-5) is the most frequently observed mechanism of DNA transfer. Its biological significance became obvious after the introduction of antibiotics. Antibiotic resistance may develop as the result of a mutation at a rate of 1 mutation every 10^6 cell divisions. However, once developed, the genetic information can be rapidly spread among similar bacteria through conjugation, because one in every three related bacteria may engage in this modality of gene transfer.

1. The **fertility (F) factor,** or **transfer factor,** is an extrachromosomal molecule that encodes the information necessary for conjugation.
   a. Conjugation involves two cell types: **donors,** which possess the F factor and are referred to as **F$^+$,** and **recipients,** which lack the F factor and are referred to as **F$^-$.**
   b. The F factor contains the genes for the specialized pilus, called a **sex pilus,** used in conjugation and for other surface structures involved in interactions with F$^-$ cells.
   c. The F factor is **self-transmissible**—once it is passed to an F$^-$ cell, the recipient cell becomes F$^+$ and is able to pass the fertility factor to another F$^-$ cell. This is the means by which bacteria acquire multiple resistance to antibacterial agents. For example, if an F$^-$ bacterium carrying a tetracycline-resistance (Tet^R) nonconjugative plasmid conjugates with another bacterium carrying a conjugative plasmid with an ampicillin resistance gene (Amp^R), the F$^-$ cell will become F$^+$ and will contain the two resistance plasmids. The plasmids can then recombine, and the result is a bacterium containing a conjugative plasmid with two resistance genes. This process can repeat itself, resulting in large conjugative plasmids carrying up to ten individual antibiotic resistance genes.
   d. Bacteria with the F factor in **plasmid form** are referred to as **F$^+$.**

2. **High-frequency recombinant (Hfr) cells.** When the plasmid containing the F factor is integrated into the bacterial chromosome, the cells are referred to as Hfr cells.
   a. **Plasmid integration.** When the chromosome and the F plasmid carry DNA sequences that allow mutual recognition, the two types of DNA can combine.
      (1) **Recognition.** The recognition sequence of the plasmid can only associate with a specific recognition sequence on the chromosome (IS elements). An endonuclease recognizes these sequences and cleaves both the plasmid receptor sequence and the chromosome sequence (Figure 3-6).
      (2) **Additive recombination (Campbell model).** The chromosome and plasmid molecules combine to form a large, circular DNA molecule consisting of the plasmid and the chromosomal DNA (see Figure 3-6).
         (a) The complete F factor is incorporated into the chromosome.
         (b) The F factor retains all of its functions when it is incorporated into the chromosomal DNA and is replicated along with the bacterial chromosome.
   b. **Hfr conjugation**
      (1) **Donors.** Hfr bacteria perform as donors during conjugation. The chromosomal DNA is replicated. One strand of the chromosome copy is transferred to the recipient F$^-$ cell, while the other strand remains in the Hfr cell. The donor remains unchanged genetically.
      (2) **Recipients.** F$^-$ cells receive chromosomal fragments, the size of which depends on the time conjugation is allowed to persist. The limiting factor for gene transfer is the stability of the bond between the sex pilus and the pilus

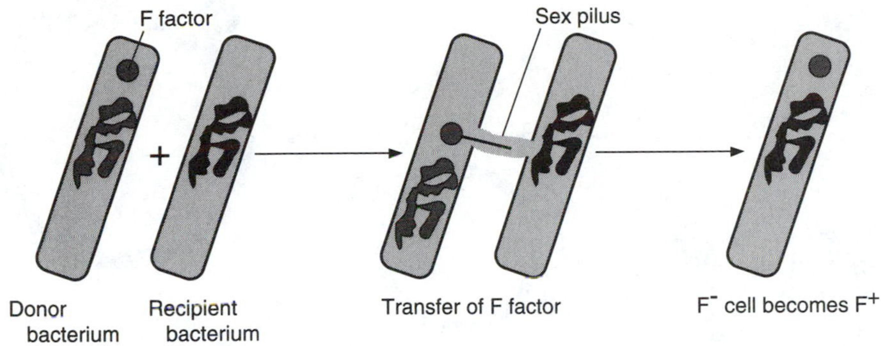

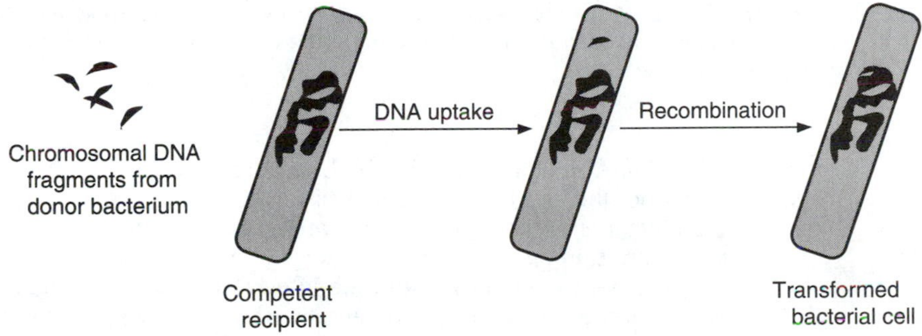

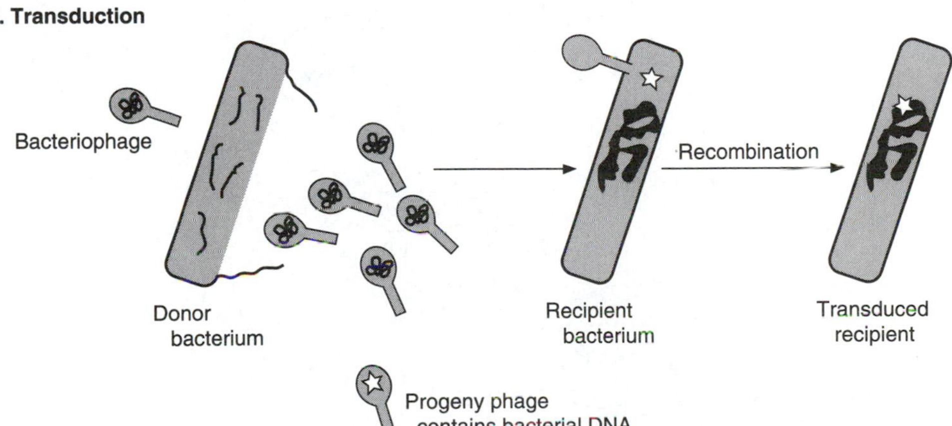

FIGURE 3-5. Mechanisms of bacterial DNA transfer. (*A*) Conjugation. (*B*) Transformation. (*C*) Transduction. (Modified with permission from Neidhart FC: The bacterial cell: genetic determinants of growth, survival, and colonization. In *Medical Microbiology*, 2nd ed. Edited by Sherris JC. New York, Elsevier, 1990, p 54.)

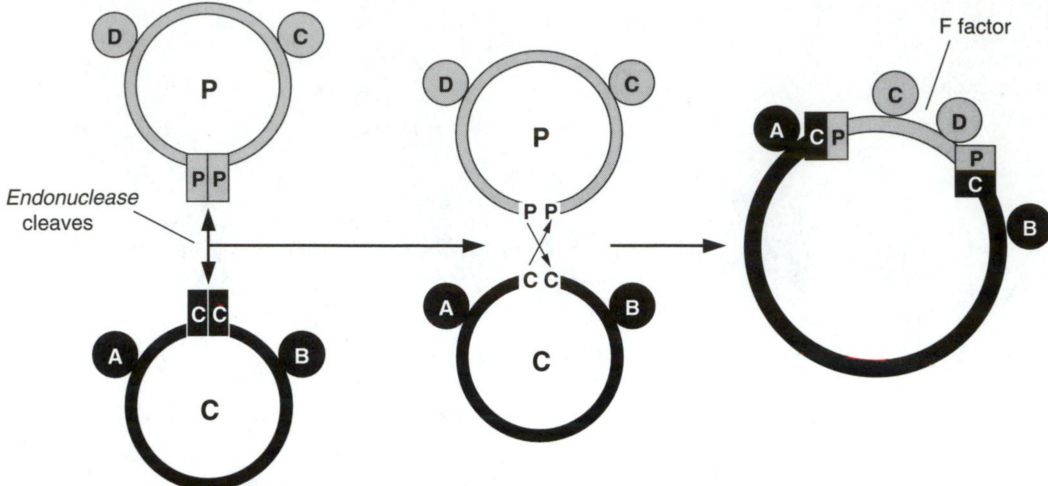

FIGURE 3-6. Campbell model for integration of plasmids into the bacterial chromosome (additive recombination). When the chromosome (*C*) and the F plasmid (*P*) carry complimentary recognition sequences on the DNA (*boxed PP* and *CC*), the two types of DNA can recombine. An endonuclease recognizes these sequences and cleaves both the plasmid sequence and the chromosome sequence. The plasmid and chromosome then recombine to form a larger, circular DNA molecule that contains both the plasmid and chromosomal DNA. The complete F factor is incorporated into the chromosome without losing any of its functions. *A, B, C,* and *D* = individual genes.

receptor (the OmpA protein). Usually, the bond breaks before the 2 hours needed to transfer the entire chromosome have passed.

(a) Once conjugation is initiated, chromosome material is transferred in a linear fashion, starting with the genes next to the origin of transfer. The origin of transfer usually lies within the integrated F plasmid (Figure 3-7).

(b) In a population of recipients, many acquire the first few genes to be transferred, but very few acquire all the genes. The last genetic material to be transferred is the portion of the plasmid containing the transfer

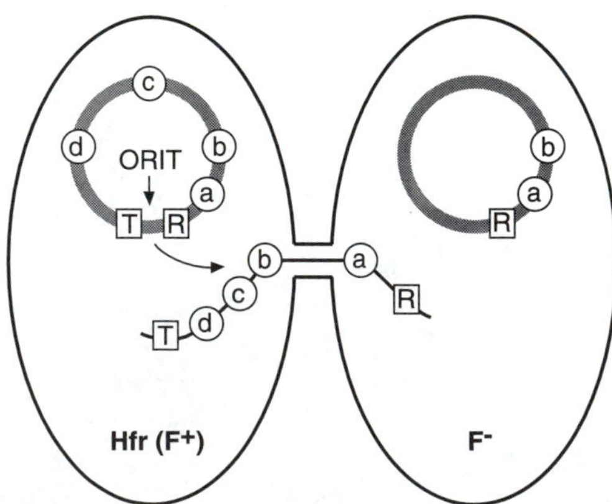

FIGURE 3-7. High-frequency recombinant (*Hfr*) conjugation. Hfr bacteria function as donors during conjugation. The chromosomal DNA is replicated. DNA transfer occurs in a linear manner and begins at the bifurcation of the F factor [i.e., the origin of transfer (*ORIT*)]. In this example, the first gene to be transferred would be *R* (an antibiotic resistance gene), followed by genes *a, b, c,* and *d.* If the entire chromosome is transferred, the last portion of genetic material to be transferred would be the F factor, or transfer gene (*T*). In *Escherichia coli,* this process takes 100 minutes. The bond between the sex pilus and the pilus receptor rarely lasts this long; therefore, most recipient cells do not receive the transfer gene (i.e., they remain F^-).

gene, which codes for the sex pilus. Because complete transmission is rare, the recipient cell of an Hfr conjugation usually remains F^-.

(3) In the laboratory, Hfr conjugation can be interrupted at specific times by vigorous shaking. Disruption of Hfr conjugation allows determination of the order of genes in the bacterial chromosome. Those near the origin of replication are transferred in a very short time; those far from the origin need progressively longer incubation for transfer. The time of incubation is directly related to the distance from the origin of replication.

3. F′ factors. The integration of an F factor into a chromosome is reversible; an endonuclease may recognize the DNA sequence of a chromosome–plasmid hybrid site and separate the two. Occasionally, this enzyme system makes a mistake. The DNA may be cut in the vicinity of the insertion point of the plasmid, but the resulting excised DNA will contain some adjacent chromosomal material in addition to the plasmid DNA. This hybrid molecule, an F factor plasmid with some chromosomal material, is called an F′ factor.

a. An F′ factor can conjugate. The recipient becomes F′, and the information passed across is part chromosome and part plasmid.

b. The bacterial gene carried on the F′ factor may duplicate a gene already existent in the recipient cell. If the two genes are slightly different (alleles), a situation of **functional diploidy** is created. Functional diploidy can also result from specialized transduction [see V C 2 b (2) (b)]). The creation of functional diploids allows the study of dominant and recessive relationships in bacterial genetics.

4. Requirements for conjugation

a. The **pilus receptor** needs to be expressed by the recipient bacteria. It must have **sufficient binding affinity for the sex pilus** to allow the formation of a stable bond between both.

b. The F factor must have an **origin of replication** in order to be recognized by the host replication machinery.

c. The F factor must be from a bacterium with a similar methylation pattern on its DNA to avoid degradation by endogenous restriction endonucleases.

d. Hfr conjugation requires almost perfect **homology.** The transfer on nonhomologous chromosomal material will not result in integration for two basic reasons:

(1) Restriction endonucleases quickly digest the nonhomologous DNA.

(2) Even if the restriction system were inactive, the piece of DNA entering the cell would not find an homologous region. Therefore, it would not be integrated or replicated. Homology is not a barrier to plasmid transfer, because plasmids self-replicate.

B. Transformation (see Figure 3-5). Dying bacteria are constantly releasing DNA, which can be taken up by other bacteria. As a rule, any "foreign" DNA that enters a bacterial cell is digested by restriction endonucleases. However, if some conditions are fulfilled, the DNA may become integrated. The transforming DNA may be chromosomal or plasmid in origin and may carry genes that "transform" the recipient bacterium. Thus, transformation can propagate genes coding for virulence factors among bacterial populations.

1. Regulation of transformation depends on two variables: the competence of the recipient bacterium and the qualities of the transforming DNA.

a. Competence is the ability of the bacterial cell to take up DNA and depends on the presence of proteins in the cell membrane that have a special affinity for DNA.

b. Qualities of the transforming DNA

(1) Homogeny

(a) In Gram-negative organisms, the specificity of the competence proteins is such that only homologous or very similar DNA will be taken up by a competent bacteria.

(b) In Gram-positive bacteria, the uptake is less restrictive, but if the DNA is not homologous it will not integrate fast enough and will be digested by endonucleases.

(2) **Double-strandedness** is required because one strand is degraded as the other strand is brought in. Degradation of one strand may provide the energy that is necessary for the entry of the surviving strand.

(3) **High molecular weight** (i.e., greater than 10^7) increases the chances of integration, which may take place even if portions of the DNA are attacked by endonucleases before integration is completed.

2. Process

a. Reversible association of DNA to the cell wall is mediated by an ionic interaction between DNA and the cell wall of a competent organism.

(1) This type of association occurs in bacteria all the time, but if the cell is not competent the association is tenuous and the DNA is released and adsorbed elsewhere.

(2) Artificial competence can be induced by treating bacteria with calcium chloride. Calcium chloride alters cell membrane permeability, enabling the uptake of DNA by cells that are normally incapable of DNA adsorption. Artificial competence allows transformation to be used as the basis for most recombinant DNA techniques.

b. Irreversible association of the DNA and the inner cell membrane is established following transport of the DNA through the cell wall.

c. Resistance **to extracellular DNAse** occurs as a consequence of conformational changes that take place after the DNA binds irreversibly to the cell membrane.

d. Entry of DNA into the cytoplasm. DNA enters the cytoplasm as a single strand.

e. Integration in the chromosomal DNA requires homology regions and involves displacement of one chromosomal strand, recombination of the invading strand, elimination of the remaining chromosomal segment, and duplication of the invading strand.

3. Applications to bacterial gene mapping. Transformation is a good chromosome mapping tool because transformed cells acquire different segments of DNA. By determining how frequently two given characteristics are simultaneously acquired (the closer the genes, the most likely that both will be included in the same DNA piece), an idea about the location of the corresponding genes in the chromosome is generated.

C. Transduction. In transduction, DNA is transferred from one cell to another by means of **bacterial viruses,** also known as **bacteriophages.**

1. Types of bacteriophage infection. Bacteriophages can interact with bacteria in two ways.

a. Virulent (lytic) infection eventually destroys the host bacterium (Figure 3-8).

(1) **Adsorption of the bacteriophage** to a bacterial cell is mediated by specific bacterial outer structures that act as receptors for the virus.

(2) **Injection of viral DNA.** Viral DNA is injected into the cytoplasm.

(3) Synthesis of phage proteins

(a) Viral DNA is transcribed by cellular RNA polymerase into mRNA, which in turn is translated by bacterial ribosomes into early proteins, including a viral RNA polymerase and proteins that may limit the expression of bacterial genes by a variety of mechanisms. The viral-specific RNA polymerase is necessary to transcribe late proteins, such as the structural proteins needed to assemble progeny phage particles.

(b) Some viruses digest the host cell chromosome for nucleotides to use in synthesizing their own nucleic acid.

(4) **Nucleic acid replication** is carried out by the newly synthesized viral DNA polymerase, which makes multiple copies of the viral nucleic acid.

(5) **Progeny assembly and release**

(a) The newly synthesized proteins form cytoplasmic pools of progeny "head" and "tail" precursors. Other pools contain progeny nucleic acid. Special affinity regions in the viral DNA induce the coalescence of head precursor units around nucleic acid aggregates (concatamers), forming DNA-containing heads. The full heads then attract tails, forming a func-

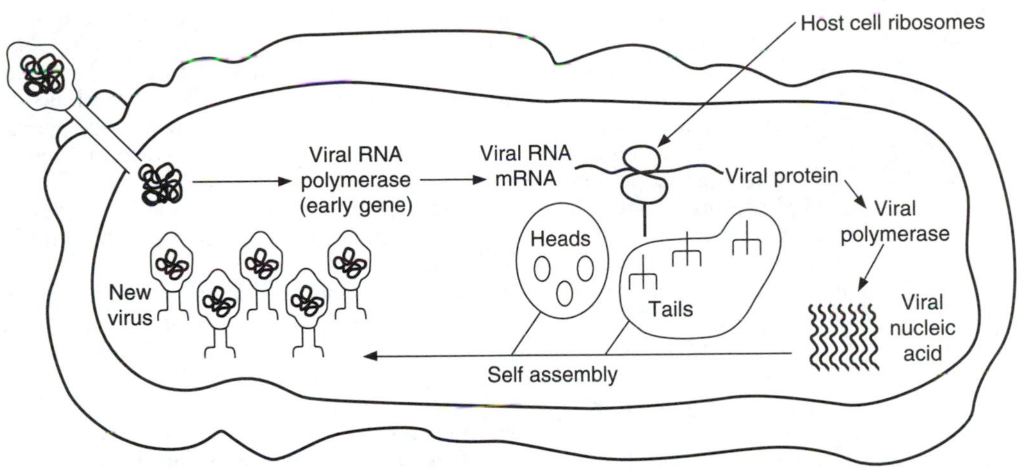

FIGURE 3-8. Virulent (lytic) infection by a bacteriophage. The bacteriophage injects its viral DNA into the bacterial cytoplasm. Cellular RNA polymerase transcribes viral DNA into viral mRNA, which is translated by bacterial ribosomes into viral RNA polymerase and other early proteins. The viral RNA polymerase makes multiple copies of the viral nucleic acid. Pools of progeny head and tail proteins form in the cytoplasm. These viral proteins combine with the nucleic acid to form progeny bacteriophages. Eventually, the progeny cause the host cell to rupture, releasing the new bacteriophages.

tional phage. The entire process, from adsorption to the appearance of newly synthesized virus, takes roughly 40 minutes.

(b) After sufficient progeny (10–200 from one injecting virus) have been synthesized, the host cell lyses, releasing the new virus to infect other cells.

b. Temperate (lysogenic) infection is characterized by the integration of viral DNA into the bacterial chromosome. For all practical purposes, the bacteria acquires a new set of genes: those of the integrated phages **(prophages).**

(1) Temperate bacteriophages are capable of infecting via the virulent mode, but virulent bacteriophages can only cause a virulent infection.

(a) Maintenance of the temperate infection depends on a protein repressor, synthesized by the viral DNA itself, which shuts off all the virulence functions of the bacteriophage.

(b) Conversion to a lytic life cycle occurs when synthesis of the protein repressor is suppressed. Under these circumstances, the integrated virus expresses all of its virulence functions, replicates, lyses, the cells, and may continue infecting in a virulent or a temperate fashion. In the laboratory, a temperate bacteriophage may convert to a lytic life cycle when the harboring bacteria is stressed by adverse conditions.

(2) There are several known examples of bacteria whose virulence factors (usually exotoxins or adhesins) are coded by lysogenic phages. In other words, the lysogenized bacteria is virulent, but the nonlysogenized counterpart is harmless.

2. Types of transduction

a. Generalized transduction (see Figure 3-5) results from a mistake in the assembly of DNA-filled phage heads. Instead of coalescing around a concatamer, the phage head coalesces around a segment of the bacterial chromosome or a segment of a plasmid. Once enough DNA is incorporated into the phage head, a viral endonuclease cuts the DNA, allowing the final assembly of a DNA-containing phage particle. The resulting phage is known as a generalized transducing particle.

(1) Properties of generalized transducing particles

(a) They carry all host DNA or plasmid DNA, but **no phage DNA.**

(b) They **cannot replicate.** When these viruses infect another host cell, they inject purely chromosomal DNA from their former hosts. They are no longer functional viruses, just vessels carrying a piece of bacterial DNA.

(c) The generalized transducing phages **can carry any part of the host chromosome** (hence their name), including genes that confer an evolutionary advantage on the recipient bacteria, such as antibiotic resistance genes. Plasmid transfer among staphylococcal species is believed to involve phage transduction.

(2) **Applications to bacterial gene mapping.** Generalized transduction can be used for mapping the bacterial chromosome, following the same principles involved in mapping by transformation.

b. **Specialized transduction** takes place when a prophage contained in a lysogenized bacterium replicates. Just as F′ plasmids are generated, a specialized transducing virus is generated when the cutting enzymes make a mistake. When this occurs, the DNA packed in the progeny particles contains small portions of the host genome, which are always very specific because they originate in the flank of the viral genome. (The viral genome is always inserted in a few specific locations where sufficient homology exists to allow recombination of phage and bacterial DNA.)

(1) **Properties of specialized transducing particles**

(a) When DNA is cleaved in the incorrect place, some of the viral DNA is sacrificed to make room for the chromosomal DNA. Viruses are limited by the size of their head as to how much genetic material they can carry. Therefore, a specialized transducing virus **cannot replicate,** just like a generalized transducing particle.

(b) Specialized transducing particles **carry hybrid DNA** (i.e., part phage DNA and part bacterial chromosome DNA). However, only some specific bacterial genes are carried by specialized transducing phages (i.e., those that are close to the site of phage integration). Specialized transduction can be a mechanism for transmission of virulence genes among bacteria, providing that those genes are located in close proximity to the integration points of prophages.

(2) **Integration of a specialized transducing phage**

(a) The recipient cell usually has a homologous copy of the chromosomal genes that the transducing phage carries on its genome. The hybrid prophage DNA interacts with the bacterial host DNA in the region where the homologous gene is located and becomes integrated on that same region.

(b) One possible result is diploidy, because insertion will result in coexistence of two copies of the same gene (one brought in by the virus, the other coexisting in the chromosome). Thus, specialized transduction is a good tool to study diploidy in bacteria.

(3) **Applications to bacterial gene mapping.** Specialized transduction is not a good mapping tool. One would have to isolate many thousands of different viruses all of which integrate at different sites to construct a complete bacterial chromosome map.

VI. GENETIC BASIS OF BACTERIAL PATHOGENICITY

A. Virulence Factors include adhesins, **capsules, toxins,** and enzymes.

1. Some virulence factors are structural units of the bacterium, are coded by chromosomal genes, and tend to be detected in the large majority of bacteria within a species. Capsules and enzymes, by and large, belong to this category.

2. Others are coded by plasmids and their distribution among members of a given bacterial species is variable. Most endotoxins and some surface adhesins are plasmid-coded.

B. Transmission of virulence genes among bacteria

1. **Lysogeny** has been well documented as a mechanism of transmission of virulence genes. The following are examples of this type of transmission:
   a. The *Corynebacterium diphtheriae* toxin is produced exclusively in bacteria lysogenized by a temperate bacteriophage that causes lysogenic conversion and provides the gene for toxin production (this may be a case of specialized transduction).
   b. Some lysogenized *Escherichia coli* produce a cytotoxin similar to the one classically produced by *Shigella dysenteriae.* The integrated prophage carries the gene coding for the Shiga-like toxin.

2. **Plasmid transmission** by conjugation is perhaps the most effective mechanism for transmission of virulence genes. Conjugation is induced by transfer factors which spread rapidly among a bacterial population.
   a. Transfer factors can carry virulence genes, or mobilize nonconjugative plasmids carrying the virulence genes.
   b. Plasmids carrying virulence genes can be classified as follows:
      (1) **Resistance plasmids** contain information for resistance to antibiotics. Often multiple genes determining resistance to multiple antibiotics are involved.
      (2) **Virulence plasmids** may code for exotoxins, adhesins, or invasion factors.
         (a) **Enterotoxin-coding plasmids** are present in enterotoxigenic *E. coli.* This organism causes profuse, watery diarrhea by synthesizing two toxins, **heat-labile toxin (LT)** and **heat-stable toxin (ST).**
         (b) **Adhesin-coding plasmids** are also present in enterotoxigenic *E. coli,* coding for specific pili known as colonization factors antigens (CFA).
         (c) **Invasiveness-coding plasmids** may determine local or systemic invasion.
            (i) The invasion plasmids of *S. dysenteriae,* for example, code for several proteins that determine mucosal cell invasion and direct propagation from cell to cell (see Chapter 7 IV A).
            (ii) The systemic invasiveness of some strains of *E. coli* is specified by a conjugative plasmid (Col-E) that codes for a bacteriocin and for an iron-binding protein (siderophore). This siderophore allows *E. coli* to scavenge iron from the blood.

VII. OPERONS.
Bacteria provide a useful model for the study of mechanisms controlling gene expression.

A. The Operon concept.
An operon is a functional genetic unit that regulates the expression of a gene or group of genes.

1. **General structure.** Usually, an operon includes a regulatory gene (R), a promoter region (P), an operator region (O), and several genes in sequence that are regulated by this particular operon (X, Y, Z).
   a. The **regulatory gene** codes for a protein known as a **repressor**—a DNA-binding protein that has high affinity for DNA in the area of the operator (see Figure 3-9A).
      (1) The repressor protein belongs to a large family of DNA-binding proteins that includes regulatory proteins and endonucleases. As DNA "breathes," by spontaneously opening and closing its double strand, DNA-binding proteins can "get a look" at the nucleotide sequences and will bind to DNA marked with some symmetrically arranged nucleotide sequence (e.g., a palindrome such as GGCCGGCC). **The longer the palindrome, the more specific the interaction with the binding protein.**
      (2) Restriction endonucleases have palindromic recognition sequences of four to eight nucleotides and can interact at multiple sites. **Highly specific** repressor proteins recognize longer palindromes that appear only once per genome.

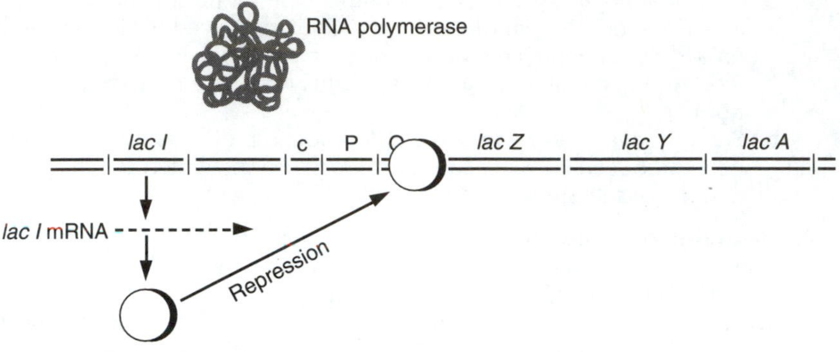
RNA polymerase
lac I
c
P
lac Z
lac Y
lac A
lac I mRNA
Repression
Repressor is made in an active state

B

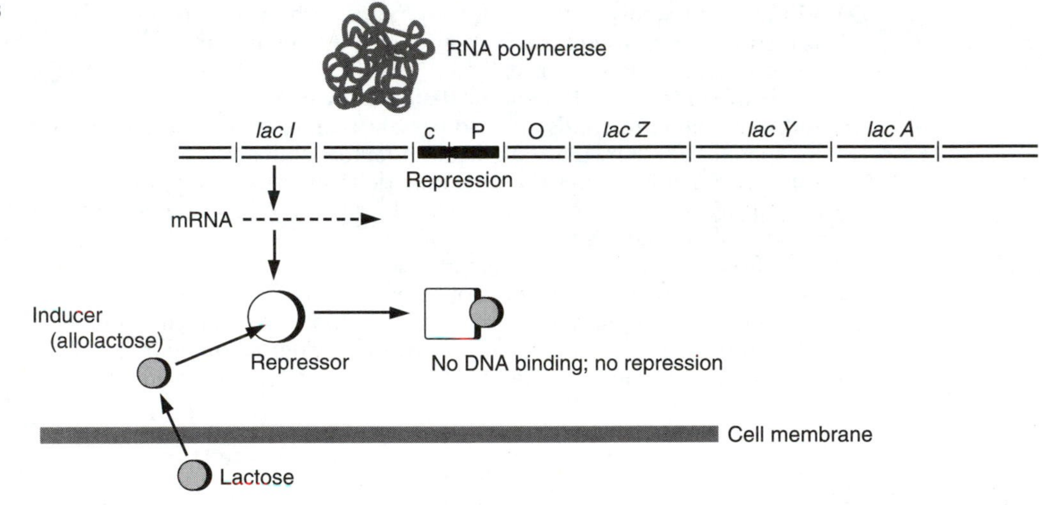
RNA polymerase
lac I
c
P
O
lac Z
lac Y
lac A
Repression
mRNA
Inducer
(allolactose)
Repressor
No DNA binding; no repression
Cell membrane
Lactose

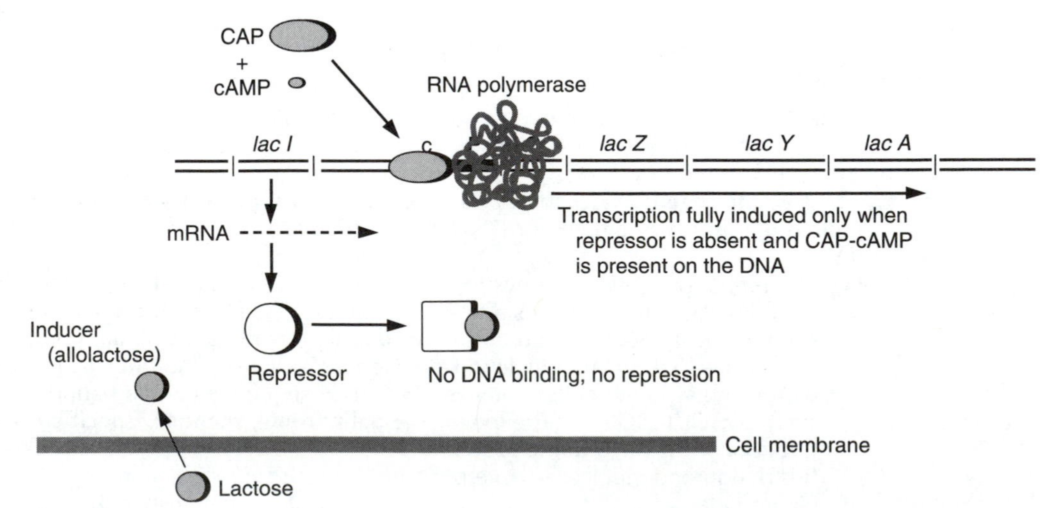
CAP
+
cAMP
RNA polymerase
lac I
c
lac Z
lac Y
lac A
Transcription fully induced only when
repressor is absent and CAP-cAMP
is present on the DNA
mRNA
Inducer
(allolactose)
Repressor
No DNA binding; no repression
Cell membrane
Lactose

b. The **promoter regions** of the operon contain sequences recognized by the RNA polymerase. The polymerase sigma factor confers specificity to the enzyme, allowing it to selectively bind to the promoter region.

(1) The sigma factor confers specificity and increases the affinity of RNA polymerase for the promoter.

(2) It initiates transcription and remains attached until the RNA polymerase enters the portion of the operon that encodes for the structural genes.

c. The **operator region** is where repressor proteins bind. It is located between the promoter and the structural genes. When a repressor protein is present, transcription is blocked. When the repressor protein is removed, the RNA polymerase gains access to the genes regulated by the operon.

2. Types

a. Inducible operons are **normally off** (i.e., normally the repressor is bound to the operator and little to no transcription takes place). Therefore, this type of operon is ideal for controlling the expression of genes coding for products that are not required at all times.

b. Repressible operons deal with the day-to-day functions of the cell (i.e., those that the cell would normally like to have on constantly. A good example would be an operon involved with the biosynthesis of an amino acid. The cell constantly needs amino acids and only at a time when it does not need them (very rarely) would the cell turn that operon off.

B. The *lac* operon (Lac-O) is the classic example of an inducible operon. The genes of this operon control the synthesis of the enzymes necessary to bring lactose into the cell, degrade it, and plug the breakdown products into the energy pathway.

1. No lactose requirement. When lactose is not required by the cell, the active repressor protein, synthesized by the gene *lacI*, binds to the operator region and blocks transcription, maintaining the operon in the "off" position (Figure 3-9A). The 21-bp palindrome in the operator region ensures specificity for the repressor protein.

2. Lactose requirement

a. Lactose is transported into the cell. β-galactosidase, which is always present in the cell in small amounts, isomerizes the lactose into allolactose (glucose-1,6-galactose), creating a gradient that favors the additional transport of lactose into the cell. Promoters are always "leaky," allowing minimal expression of the structural gene they control.

b. Lactose acts as the inducer for the Lac-O. The repressor protein, which has affinity for both the specific palindrome on the DNA and the allolactose, binds allolactose with higher affinity than it binds the DNA palindrome.

(1) The repressor–inducer complex changes the repressor's configuration and causes the repressor to lose its affinity for the DNA.

(2) Lactose not only causes preformed repressor protein to dissociate from DNA, it also associates with newly synthesized repressor protein, making it unavailable to block transcription.

FIGURE 3-9 The *lac* operon (Lac-O) controls the synthesis of enzymes necessary to use lactose as an energy source. (*A*) The Lac-O is an inducible operon. The regulatory gene (*lacI*) actively synthesizes the repressor protein, which binds to the operator region (*O*), maintaining the operon in the "off" position. RNA polymerase binds to the DNA in the promotor region (*P*); when the repressor protein is in place, transcription of the genes regulated by the operon (*lacZ, lacY, lacA*) is blocked. (*B*) Lactose acts as the inducer for Lac-O. Allolactose binds to the repressor protein, changing its conformation so that it cannot bind to the operator region. In principle, this should result in initiation of transcription, but active transcription requires the binding of an enhancer protein in the promotor region (catabolite repression). (*C*) Catabolite repression. A catabolite activator protein (*CAP*) binds to the promotor region in the presence of cyclic adenosine monophosphate (*cAMP*) and directs the RNA polymerase to the strand that should be used for transcription purposes. Transcription is now fully induced. (*A* and *B* modified with permission from Neidhart FC: The bacterial cell: genetic determinants of growth, survival, and colonization. In Medical Microbiology, 2nd ed. Edited by Sherris JC. New York, Elsevier, 1990, p 44.)

c. **Once the repressor stops binding to the operon, transcription can proceed** (Figure 3-9B).
   (1) ***LacY*** synthesizes a **permease** that promotes the active transport of large amounts of lactose as soon as the repressor protein loses its ability to block the operon. Within 30–60 seconds of the initial exposure to lactose, the cell is actively synthesizing permease to bring in large quantities of lactose.
   (2) ***LacZ*** synthesizes β-galactosidase. As mentioned earlier, this enzyme isomerizes lactose and, in doing so, creates a gradient that favors the additional transport of lactose. Isomerization is also an essential step in the metabolic processing of lactose. Thus, the operon not only codes for a protein that promotes the transport of large quantities of lactose into the cell, it also codes for the enzyme that degrades (metabolizes) lactose. Both ***LacZ*** and ***LacY*** are necessary to fulfill the purpose of the lactose operon (i.e., to promote the use of lactose as a source of energy).

d. **Depletion of lactose.** When lactose is no longer available to the bacteria, β-galactosidase will cleave the allolactose that is associated with the repressor. The repressor recovers its original configuration and binds to its homologous DNA palindrome in the operator region, terminating the expression of the operon.
   (1) The shut-off of the operon is not absolute. Small amounts of β-galactosidase are present in the bacterial cell at all times, and small amounts of lactose are transported into the cell at all times.
   (2) Other regulatory mechanisms (e.g., catabolite repression) ensure that the Lac-O) is not expressed until there is a need to use lactose as source of energy.

e. **Catabolite repression.** The ability to use lactose depends on the activation of the Lac-O, but a second level of control is exerted by catabolite repression, which involves a cyclic adenosine monophosphate (cAMP)-binding protein [catabolite activator protein (CAP)].
   (1) When bacteria are grown in a medium in which both lactose and glucose are available, a biphasic growth curve is observed (see Figure 2-8B). The initial growth reflects the preferential use of glucose as source of energy. Only after glucose is exhausted will the Lac-O be turned on and a second growth phase will be observed because of the utilization of lactose.
   (2) The preference for glucose utilization is based on the fact that glucose is brought into the cell by the PEP pathway, which phosphorylates it immediately. Therefore, the glucose that diffuses into the cytoplasm is already phosphorylated and can be immediately plugged into the energy pathways that produce ATP. Lactose, on the other hand, is transported into the cytoplasm as a complex molecule that has to be cleaved, then phosphorylated, and only then can be plugged into the energy pathways. Consequently, it is more economical for bacteria to use glucose.
      (a) Normally, when both glucose and lactose are available, the bacteria internalizes lactose at a much slower rate than glucose. However, it internalizes enough lactose to prevent the repressor from binding to DNA. In principle, this should result in initiation of transcription, but active transcription requires the binding of an enhancer protein (e.g., CAP) in the promoter region. The CAP binds to the promoter region in the presence of cAMP and may direct the RNA polymerase to the strand that should be used for transcription purposes (Figure 3-9C).
      (b) When glucose is being utilized as the source of energy, the levels of ATP in the cell are high. The ratio of ATP to other nucleotides (e.g., ADP) progressively increases as the other nucleotides become less available. cAMP levels decrease as the glucose is metabolized so that there is not enough cAMP available to bind to the CAP. In the absence of cAMP, CAP cannot interact with the upstream regulatory sequences and RNA polymerase is unable to initialize transcription.
      (c) As glucose is exhausted, the ATP levels decrease and the cAMP levels increase, enabling CAP to associate with the upstream regulatory sequences. The Lac-O is then actively transcribed.

C. The tryptophan operon is an example of a repressible operon.

1. Tryptophan is required by the cell under normal conditions, and the operon is normally **"on."** In this case, the regulatory gene codes for a repressor that is inactive.
2. **Excess intracellular tryptophan results in operon repression.** If tryptophan becomes available to the organism, there is no point in continuing to produce it. The controlling factor is designated as the **threshold level** of the product.
   - **a.** Assuming that the threshold level of tryptophan is the concentration necessary for normal cell proliferation, and assuming that the cell makes roughly that much, then in the presence of excess tryptophan (e.g., as a result of absorption from the medium), the threshold concentration will be exceeded. The excess tryptophan reacts with the inactive repressor, converting it into an active molecule that binds to the operator and inhibits transcription.
   - **b.** If the level of tryptophan starts to fall back down to the threshold, the repressor protein–tryptophan complex ceases to be present, the repression is relieved, and RNA polymerase becomes available to start transcribing mRNA.
3. **Attenuation.** A second level of control is also present in many aminoacid synthetic pathways.
   - **a.** When production of tryptophan mRNA begins, the RNA polymerase translates about 220 bases of mRNA (leader mRNA) and then pauses before completing transcription of the rest of the operon. Whether or not transcription proceeds depends on how large the intracellular pools of tryptophan charged and uncharged tRNA molecules are.
   - **b.** The remaining coding sequences of the mRNA are "looped" out around a repeating tryptophan coding sequence (six or seven contiguous tryptophan codons). As translation starts and the tryptophan codons are reached, the ribosomes call for a tRNA charged with tryptophan.
     - **(1)** If there are enough available, protein synthesis proceeds. As the ribosomes proceed through this loop, the mRNA assumes a transcriptional termination configuration resulting in the cessation of transcription.
     - **(2)** If there are not enough tryptophan-charged tRNA molecules available, an alternate loop is formed. This allows the polymerase to proceed into the structural genes, resulting in complete transcription of the tryptophan operon (Figure 3-17).

D. Mutations affecting inducible operons

1. **Mutations inactivating the regulatory gene** result in a lack of synthesis of the protein repressor, and the genes controlled by the operator will be expressed on a constant basis (i.e., the expression becomes **constitutive rather than inducible**).
2. **Mutations in the operator region** impair the binding of the repressor protein to the operator region (this region is usually short–24 or 25 nucleotides long in the case of the Lac-O—and 80%–90% of the operator corresponds to the palindrome that is necessary to recognize the repressor). If the affinity for the repressor protein is lost, the gene products of the operon will be constitutively expressed at a fairly constant rate.

Chapter 4

Antibacterial Agents

Victor Del Bene
John Manos
Gabriel Virella

I. GENERAL CONSIDERATIONS

A. Definitions

1. **Antibiotics versus antibacterial agents**
   a. An **antibiotic** is a substance produced by a microorganism that, in minute quantities, is able to inhibit other microorganisms. Therefore, this term is properly applied only to compounds directly derived from microorganisms.
   b. An **antibacterial agent** is any compound—natural, synthetic, or semisynthetic (i.e., chemically derived from natural substances)—that is clinically useful in the treatment of bacterial infections.

2. **Bacteriostatic versus bactericidal** (Figure 4-1)
   a. **Bacteriostatic agents** (e.g., sulfonamides, chloramphenicol) inhibit bacterial growth.
   b. **Bactericidal agents** (e.g., penicillin, streptomycin) significantly reduce the number of viable bacteria in the culture. Bactericidal agents generally kill only growing organisms; therefore, concurrent use of bactericidal and bacteriostatic agents is usually avoided because the latter interfere with bacterial growth. Nevertheless, this rule is often broken based on proven clinical experience with effective combinations.

3. **Narrow-spectrum versus broad-spectrum**
   a. **Narrow-spectrum antibacterial agents** are preferentially active against either Gram-negative bacteria or Gram-positive bacteria.
   b. **Broad-spectrum antibacterial agents** are active against both Gram-positive and Gram-negative bacteria.

B. General criteria for effective antibiotic action

1. **Microorganism.** A **unique** and **vital target** (e.g., a specific protein or nucleic acid) that is susceptible to a low concentration of the antibacterial agent must exist in the microorganism; this target must be sufficiently different from a related host target to minimize side effects.

2. **Antibacterial agent**
   a. The antibacterial agent must be able to penetrate the bacterial surface and reach the target in its active form.
   b. The antibacterial agent needs to reach the infected tissue. For example, the treatment of bacterial meningitis is difficult because many common antibacterial agents do not cross the blood–brain barrier effectively.
   c. Intracellular organisms present a special difficulty because many antibacterial agents do not seem to diffuse well into mammalian cells. Tetracyclines, however, are usually effective against intracellular bacteria.

3. **Host**
   a. **Intact immune system.** The immune system of the host must be able to collaborate effectively in the fight against the invading organism. The integrity of the phagocytic cell system is particularly important. Bacterial infections are exceedingly difficult to treat in neutropenic patients and those with primary or secondary immunodeficiencies.

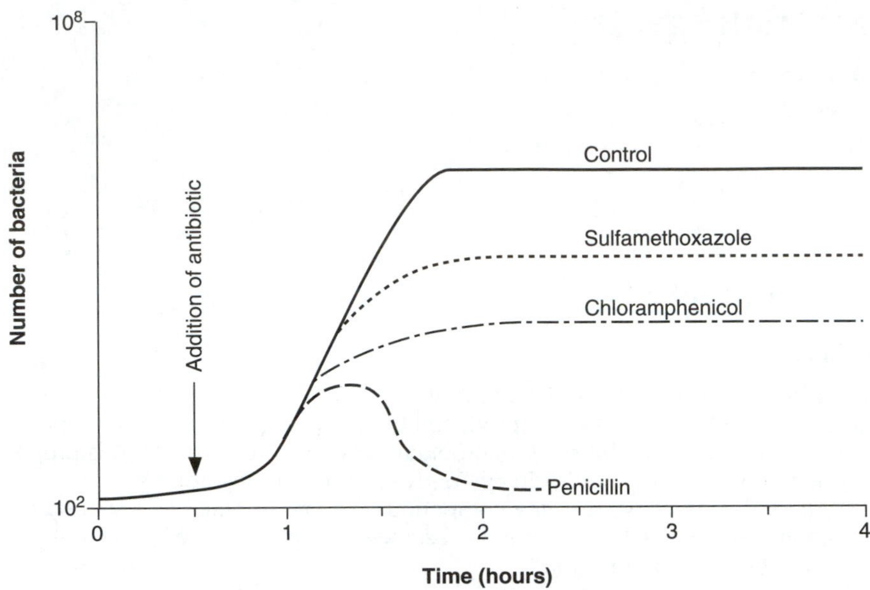

FIGURE 4-1. Bactericidal versus bacteriostatic agents. Penicillin, a bactericidal agent, kills growing organisms. Sulfamethoxazole and chloramphenicol, bacteriostatic agents, halt bacterial growth. The difference in the growth curves for sulfamethoxazole and chloramphenicol results from the different mechanisms of action of these drugs. Chloramphenicol inhibits protein synthesis and interferes with bacterial growth soon after it is added to the culture, whereas sulfamethoxazole interferes with the synthesis of nucleic acids. Its effects are delayed because the cells have a preformed pool that they can use before the antibacterial agent takes effect.

b. **Vascularization and drainage.** Impaired blood supply or drainage of the infected area usually diminishes the effectiveness of antibacterial agents.
   (1) Bacterial endocarditis, osteomyelitis, and abscesses are associated with minimal vascularization of the infected tissue.
   (2) Bronchiectasia, kidney stones, and gallbladder stones impair drainage of bronchial secretions, urine, and bile, respectively, and can give origin to bacterial infections that may be extremely difficult to treat unless the obstruction or anatomical abnormality is surgically removed.

C. General principles of effective antibacterial therapy. Observation of the following principles reduces selection of resistant strains, decreases the cost of therapy, and reduces toxicity to the patient.

1. **Use selectively.** Antibacterial treatment should be instituted only when necessary, for treatment of confirmed bacterial infections. The empirical use of broad-spectrum antibiotics increases, by selection, the prevalence of bacteria resistant to multiple antibiotics.
   a. The choice of antibacterial should be based on susceptibility tests (see Chapter 5 V), or if these are not available, on known epidemiological data showing the prevalence of resistant strains among bacteria isolated in that locale.
   b. When the infection is life-threatening or when early treatment is extremely important, treatment is initiated with empirically chosen broad-spectrum antibiotics. However, samples are collected prior to the initiation of therapy and sent for culture. Once the organism is identified and its antimicrobial susceptibility determined, a more appropriate specific therapy should replace the umbrella therapy.
   c. The prescription of potent, broad-spectrum antibacterials to patients who could be effectively treated with more common antibacterials leads to the rapid development of resistance and limits the number of agents available for use in hospitalized patients infected with organisms resistant to the more common antibacterial agents.

2. Institute promptly. When antibacterial therapy is deemed necessary, it should be promptly instituted.

a. Early treatment actively targets growing bacteria at a point when the bacterial population is relatively low, the majority are susceptible to bactericidal drugs, and abscesses have not had an opportunity to form.

b. Early treatment usually involves short-term therapy, which has the advantage of reducing the possibility of **superinfection** (i.e., infection with resistant strains as a result of alterations in the normal flora caused by prolonged treatment with broad-spectrum antibacterials).

4. Special situations

a. Infections of poorly vascularized tissues (e.g., endocarditis, osteomyelitis) should be treated with bactericidal antibacterial agents.

b. When abscesses have formed or the infection is associated with obstruction or foreign bodies, surgery is essential to correct the conditions that promote bacterial survival.

3. Follow through. Inadequate use of antibacterials, such as occurs with doses that are too low or when therapy is terminated prematurely, is a major factor contributing to the selection of resistant strains.

c. In immunocompromised patients, the choice, dosages, and route of administration of antibacterial agents need to be chosen carefully to increase the probabilities of success.

d. The treatment of infections caused by intracellular bacteria usually requires prolonged administration of appropriate antibacterials.

(1) All antiviral agents in use act intracellularly, because this is essential for proper interference with viral replication.

(2) In contrast, many antibacterial agents are not effective against intracellular organisms. Tetracyclines and chloramphenicol have been used with success in the treatment of some of these infections; more recently the fluoroquinolones have been found to accumulate and maintain their antibacterial activity in infected macrophages.

e. In all patients receiving broad-spectrum antibacterial agents, special attention needs to be given to signs and symptoms suggestive of superinfection, particularly antibiotic-associated colitis (see Chapter 12).

II. CLASSIFICATION.

The major antibacterial agents can be classified according to their mechanisms of action (Figure 4-2). Table 4-1 summarizes the mechanisms of action of the major antibacterials.

A. Antibacterial agents that inhibit cell wall synthesis

1. β-lactam antibacterial agents. Structurally, the most important feature of the penicillins, cephalosporins, carbapenems, and monobactams is the β-lactam ring. All β-lactam antibacterials are **bactericidal** and possess the same general mechanism of action.

a. Penicillins. Discovered by Fleming in the 1920s, the penicillins are true antibiotics—antibacterial compounds produced and released by molds of the genus *Penicillium.*

(1) Chemistry (Figure 4-3). All penicillins are derived from 6-aminopenicillanic acid, in which a β-lactam group is linked to a thiazolidine ring. The antibacterial and pharmacologic properties of the different penicillins depend on the side chains attached to the basic nucleus.

(2) Mechanism of action

(a) The **bacterial targets for penicillins** are known as **penicillin-binding proteins (PBPs).** There are several of these proteins (as many as seven different ones in *Escherichia coli*), some of which are better characterized than others.

(i) The major PBP is a **transpeptidase** involved in the D-alanyl-D-alanine

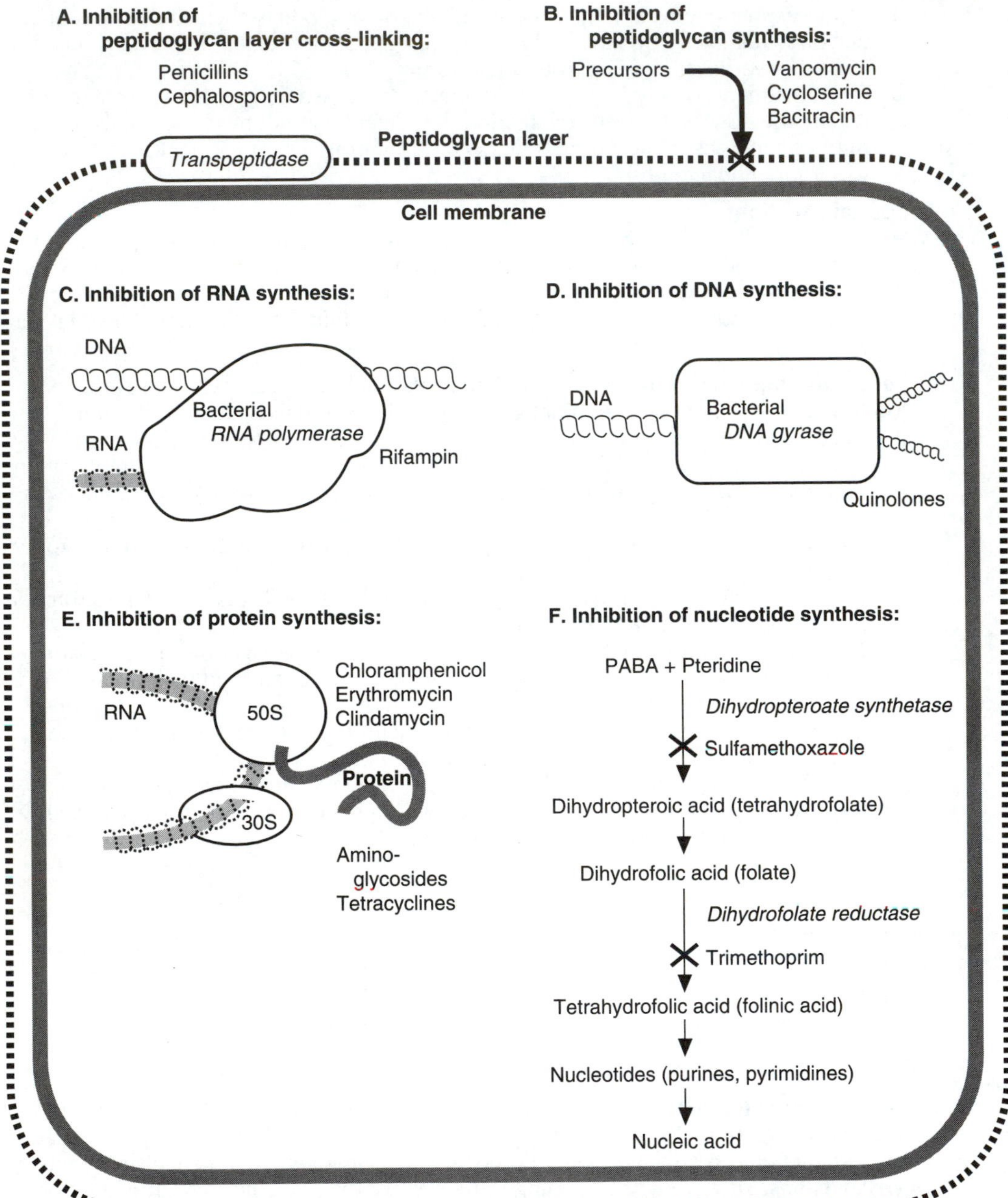

FIGURE 4-2. Classification of major antibiotics according to their points of action. (*A*) The penicillins and cephalosporins bind and inactivate transpeptidase, inhibiting peptidoglycan cross-linking. (*B*) Vancomycin, cycloserine, and bacitracin inhibit precursors for bacterial wall synthesis. (*C*) Rifampin inactivates DNA-dependent RNA polymerase. (*D*) The quinolones inhibit DNA gyrase. (*E*) Chloramphenicol and the macrolide antibiotics bind to the 50S subunit of the ribosome, inhibiting peptidyltransferase and leading to the premature termination of the peptide chains. Aminoglycosides and tetracyclines irreversibly bind to the 30S unit of the bacterial ribosome, inactivating initiation sites and rendering the bacteria incapable of synthesizing a peptide chain. (*F*) The sulfonamides and trimethoprim block the synthesis of dihydropteroate synthetase and dihyrofolate reductase, respectively, which leads to the inhibition of nucleotide synthesis. *PABA* = para-aminobenzoic acid, *X* = inhibits.

TABLE 4-1. Mechanisms of Action of Major Antibacterial Agents

Agent	Mechanism of Action
Penicillins and cephalosporins	Bind and inactivate transpeptidase and other enzymes involved in peptidoglycan cross-linking
Cycloserine	Inhibits incorporation of D-alanine in the nascent pentapeptide in the cytoplasm
Vancomycin	Inhibits polymerization of the peptidoglycan by binding to the D-alanyl-D-alanine peptide termini and interfering with transpeptidation
Bacitracin	Inhibits polymerization of the peptidogylcan by interfering with the recycling of the phosphorylated lipid carrier
Sulfonamides	Inhibit the synthesis of dihydropteroic acid
Trimethoprim	Prevents the formation of tetrahydrofolates
Quinolones	Inhibit DNA gyrase
Nitroimidazoles	Alkylate DNA
Rifampin	Inactivates DNA-dependent RNA polymerase
Aminoglycosides	Bind irreversibly to the ribosome, inhibiting peptide chain elongation; cause mRNA misreading
Tetracyclines	Inhibit the binding of tRNA to the 30S ribosomal unit
Chloramphenicol	Inhibits peptide bond formation
Erythromycin	Immobilizes peptidyl tRNA
Polymixins	Alter cell wall permeability

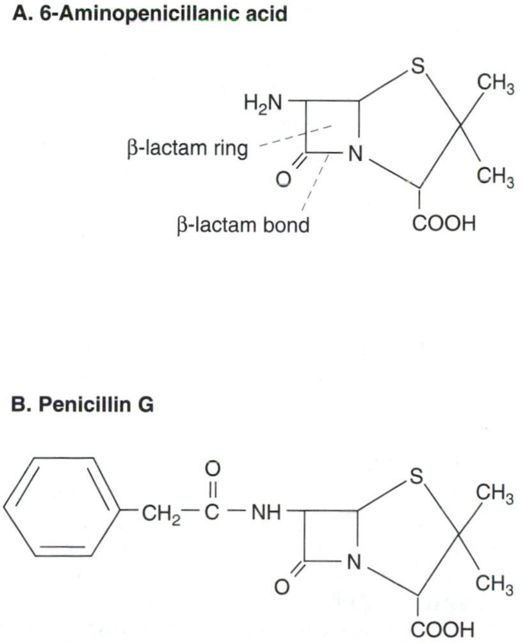

A. 6-Aminopenicillanic acid

B. Penicillin G

FIGURE 4-3. Basic chemical structure of the penicillins, (*A*) All penicillins are derivatives of 6-aminopenicillanic acid, which consists of a *β*-lactam ring and a thiazolidine ring. *β*-lactamases act at the *β*-lactam bond. The integrity of the *β*-lactam bond and the *β*-lactam ring is essential in order for antimicrobial activity to take place. (*B*) Penicillin G is the prototype penicillin.

cross-linking of peptidoglycan. Penicillins which are structurally homologous to D-alanyl-D-alanine, bind and inactivate the transpeptidase, inhibiting peptidoglycan cross-linking.

(ii) Other penicillin-binding proteins include **carboxypeptidases,** which also play a role in peptidoglycan cross-linking, and **autolytic enzymes,** which are involved in the normal turnover of cell wall material and separation of bacteria after cell division.

(b) The inactivation of transpeptidases and the activation of autolysins results in the rapid destruction of peptidoglycan and dissolution of the cell wall, which leads to **bacterial lysis.**

(3) Bacterial resistance. Some bacteria produce enzymes, known as ***β*-lactamases,** that inactivate *β*-lactams (see Chapter 5).

(4) Spectrum of activity

(a) Natural penicillins are **narrow-spectrum** antibiotics that are primarily active against **Gram-positive organisms** and most anaerobes. There are exceptions to these rules; *Treponema pallidum,* a Gram-negative organisms, is exquisitely susceptible to penicillin and *Bacteroides fragilis,* an anaerobe that produces a *β*-lactamase, is resistant.

(b) Semisynthetic *β*-lactamase–resistant penicillins have been designed so that the *β*-lactam ring is less accessible to bacterial penicillinases.

(i) Agents include **methicillin, oxacillin, cloxacillin, nafcillin,** and **dicloxacillin.**

(ii) Penicillinase-resistant penicillins are preferred for the treatment of ***Staphylococcus aureus* infections,** which have a high frequency of *β*-lactamase–positive isolates. Otherwise, these penicillins have the same spectrum of bacterial susceptibility as the natural penicillins.

(c) Extended-spectrum penicillins that are effective against a great variety of Gram-positive and Gram-negative bacteria have been obtained in the laboratory via manipulations of the 6-aminopenicillanic molecule.

(i) This group includes the aminopenicillins (e.g., **ampicillin, amoxycillin**) the carboxipenicillins (e.g., **carbenicillin, ticarcillin**) the ureidopenicillins (e.g., **azlocillin**) and the piperazine penicillins (e.g., **piperacillin**).

(ii) Some of these broad-spectrum penicillins, such as piperacillin, are active against some of the most difficult to treat Gram-negative organisms, especially *Pseudomonas.*

(iii) Broad-spectrum penicillins are **penicillinase susceptible.** The concurrent use of ***β*-lactamase inhibitors** (e.g., **clavulanic acid, sulbactam**) can reduce this susceptibility. *β*-lactamase inhibitors have *β*-lactam rings, but their antibacterial activity is negligible. These compounds bind to penicillinases with high affinity, blocking the binding sites of the enzymes and preventing the inactivation of penicillin and related antibacterial agents.

(5) Toxicity. Because the bacterial target of the penicillins are enzymes unique to bacteria, the penicillins, in general, have very limited toxicity. The most severe side effects are allergic reactions, which depend on individual predisposition.

b. Cephalosporins

(1) Chemistry. This important group of semisynthetic *β*-lactam antibacterial agents is derived from 6-aminopenicillanic acid; however, the thiazolidine ring is replaced by a dihydrothiazine ring (Figure 4-4).

(2) Classification. The cephalosporins are classified into **three generations** that roughly parallel their chronologic development.

(a) First-generation cephalosporins are available in oral and injectable forms. Preparations include **cefazolin, cephalexin,** and **cephalothin.**

(b) Second-generation cephalosporins are mostly injectables. Preparations include **cefamandole, cefaclor, cefoxitin,** and **cefuroxime.**

(c) Third-generation cephalosporins are also mostly injectables. Preparations include **cefotaxime** and **ceftriaxone.**

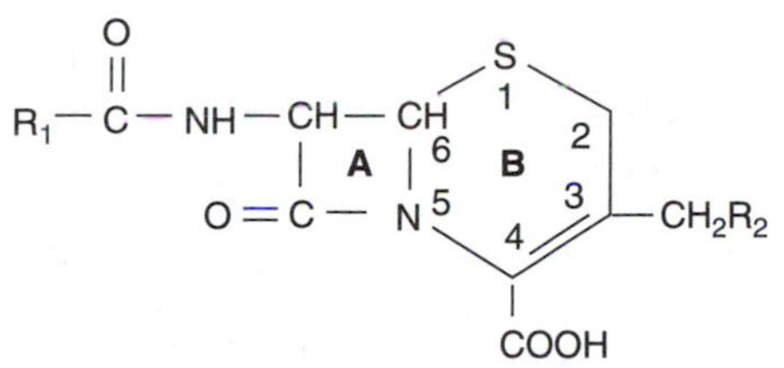

FIGURE 4-4. Basic chemical structure of the cephalosporins. The cephalosporins also are derived from 6-aminopenicillanic acid and possess a β-lactam ring *(A)*. The thiazolidine ring is replaced by a dihydrothiazine ring *(B)*. The side chains *(R_1, R_2)* are responsible for the specific pharmacologic properties of the cephalosporins.

(3) **Spectrum of activity.** Cephalosporins are active against a wide variety of bacteria and are considered broad-spectrum antibacterials.
- (a) Most cephalosporins are resistant to staphylococcal penicillinases.
- (b) Second- and third-generation cephalosporins are resistant to most β-lactamases produced by Gram-negative organisms.

(4) **Toxicity**
- (a) Because the structures of cephalosporin and penicillin are similar, 10%–15% of patients who are allergic to penicillin might also be allergic to cephalosporin.
- (b) The cephalosporins are more toxic than penicillin, and most are mildly **nephrotoxic.** Later-generation cephalosporins, however, are less nephrotoxic than early-generation cephalosporins.

c. **Other β-lactam antibacterial agents**

(1) **Carbapenems** (e.g., **imipenem**). A carbon replaces the sulfur in the thiazolidine ring of 6-aminopenicillanic acid. These agents have a very broad spectrum of activity—only *Listeria,* group D streptococci, *Pseudomonas,* and *Pasteurella multocida* are resistant.

(2) **Monobactams** (e.g., **aztreonam**) have a single monocyclic β-lactam nucleus and lack a thiazolidine ring. Monobactams are effective against a narrow spectrum of aerobic Gram-negative bacteria, including *Pseudomonas.*

2. **Other inhibitors of bacterial cell wall synthesis**

a. **Cycloserine** inhibits the incorporation of D-alanine into the UDP-MUrNAc-oligopeptide in the cytoplasm. Cycloserine is a rarely used, second-line antimycobacterial drug. It is ototoxic (particularly when administered parenterally) and should not be used unless absolutely necessary.

b. **Vancomycin** inhibits the polymerization of peptidoglycan by binding directly to the D-alanyl-D-alanine peptide termini and inhibiting cross-linking by the transpeptidase.

(1) **Spectrum of activity and administration.** Vancomycin is the antibiotic of choice for infections caused by **methicillin-resistant staphylococci** and **penicillinase-producing enterococci.** It must be given parenterally for treatment of systemic infections, because it is poorly absorbed by the intestinal mucosa, but it can be administered orally for the local treatment of intestinal infections (e.g., pseudomembranous colitis caused by *Clostridium difficile*).

(2) **Toxicity.** Vancomycin is more toxic than the penicillins. The main target of toxicity is the kidney.

c. **Bacitracin** inhibits the polymerization of peptidoglycan by interfering with the recycling of the phosphorylated lipid carrier. Bacitracin is nephrotoxic and ototoxic when administered parenterally; therefore, it is mainly used in topical ointments.

B. **Antibacterial agents that inhibit nucleotide synthesis**. One of the most important groups of antibacterial compounds are those that inhibit folinic acid synthesis by interfering with the metabolism of purines and pyrimidines.

1. **Sulfonamides**
   a. **Preparations.** Several sulfonamides have been developed over the years. Those still in use include **sulfadiazine** (short-acting), **sulfamethoxazole** and **sulfisoxazole** (medium-acting), and **sulfamethoxidiazine** (long-acting).
   (b) **Mechanism of action** (see Figure 4-2F). Sulfonamides are **bacteriostatic.**
      (1) These synthetic antibacterial agents, which are structurally similar to para-aminobenzoic acid (PABA), bind to dihydropteroate synthetase. As a result, the synthesis of dihydropteroic acid (tetrahydrofolate) and dihydrofolic acid (folate) are blocked.
      (2) In addition, sulfonamides are weak inhibitors of dihydrofolate reductase.
      (3) Because mammalian cells do not synthesize folic acid, the inhibition of these enzymes causes no side effects in humans.
   c. **Spectrum of activity.** The spectrum of affected bacteria is broad, and because these compounds are well absorbed in the intestinal tract, adequate systemic levels can be reached after oral administration.
   d. **Toxicity**
      (1) Sulfonamides are second only to penicillin in causing hypersensitivity, which is most often delayed and occurs following topical administration. For this reason, topical formulations of sulfonamides have been virtually abandoned, except in eye drop formulations.
      (2) High doses of sulfonamides may cause hematologic disorders and crystal formation in the urinary tract. Crystallization can be avoided by using combinations of sulfa drugs with different crystallization points, thereby preventing saturation and crystal formation by one particular type.

2. **Trimethoprim**, which is structurally similar to dihydrofolic acid, is bound by dihydrofolate reductase (see Figure 4-2F).

3. **Sulfamethoxazole–trimethoprim** is a strongly synergistic combination. Each one of the compounds, by itself, is bacteriostatic, but together, they are bactericidal. Sulfamethoxazole–trimethoprim is particularly useful in the treatment of genitourinary infections and bacterial gastroenteritis, and is also frequently used in the long-term prophylaxis of bacterial infections in immunocompromised individuals (e.g., prophylaxis of *Pneumocystis carinii* infections in HIV-infected individuals).

C. Antibacterial agents that inhibit nucleic acid synthesis

1. **DNA synthesis inhibitors**
   a. **Novobiocin,** the prototype for this group, interferes with DNA synthesis by inhibiting DNA gyrase. Of limited clinical use, it has been replaced by the quinolones, which have the same mechanism of action.
   b. **Quinolones** are also DNA gyrase inhibitors.
      (1) The first quinolone was **nalidixic acid,** a broad-spectrum antibacterial that is mainly used in the treatment of genitourinary infections. However, it is relatively toxic, often causing gastrointestinal and neurologic (mostly visual) symptoms.
      (2) The **fluoroquinolones** (e.g., **ofloxacin, ciprofloxacin, lomefloxacin**) are derivatives of nalidixic acid. These drugs, which can be administered orally and parenterally, are better tolerated and have a wider range of application than nalidixic acid because the development of resistant strains is rather infrequent.
   c. **Nitroimidazoles. Metronidazole,** the prototype of the nitroimidazoles, was introduced as an antiflagellate.
      (1) **Mechanism of action.** All sensitive organisms utilize low redox potential compounds (e.g., ferrodoxin) as electron acceptors. These compounds reduce the 5-nitro group of the imidazoles, producing metabolites, that apparently alkylate DNA and inhibit DNA synthesis.
      (2) **Spectrum of activity.** Nitroimidazoles are effective against *Trichomonas vaginalis, Giardia lamblia,* and *Entamoeba histolytica.* In addition, they are effective against obligate anaerobic bacteria.
      (3) **Toxicity.** Although the nitroimidazoles have mutagenic potential, their use in

humans has not been associated with evidence of increased incidence of any type of malignancy.

2. **RNA synthesis (transcription) inhibitors** such as **rifampin** inactivate DNA-dependent RNA polymerase. Rifampin is one of the first line anti-*Mycobacterium tuberculosis* agents and has been used in the treatment of leprosy. It is also used for the treatment of infections by *Legionella* and for chemoprophylaxis of patient contacts during outbreaks of meningitis resulting from *Neisseria meningitidis* or *Haemophilus influenzae.*

D. Antibacterial agents that inhibit protein synthesis

1. **Inhibitors of the 30S ribosomal unit**
   a. **Aminoglycosides**
      (1) **Mechanism of action.** Aminoglycosides inhibit protein synthesis by at least two mechanisms.
         (a) They bind irreversibly to the 30S unit of the bacterial ribosome, forming 30S–50S, which inactivates initiation sites and renders the bacteria unable to synthesize a peptide chain.
         (b) Streptomycin, and probably other aminoglycosides, distort the triplet coding of mRNA and cause mRNA misreading.
      (2) **Spectrum of activity.** The aminoglycosides are bactericidal and their spectrum of activity is broad, especially against Gram-negative organisms. All aminoglycosides are virtually nonabsorbed by the gastrointestinal tract, so they must be administered parenterally to achieve therapeutic blood levels.
         (a) **Preparations and therapeutic uses**
            (i) **Streptomycin,** the first to be developed, has been relegated to use as a second-line antimycobacterial agent, because of its marked ototoxicity. Streptomycin is only used when multidrug regimens are necessary and the bacteria have become resistant to less toxic antibacterial agents.
            (ii) **Neomycin** is mostly used as a topical antibiotic in ointments and in oral preparations. When given orally (e.g., to treat neonatal *Escherichia coli* diarrhea), neomycin is not absorbed; therefore, oral administration is also considered a form of local treatment.
            (iii) **Kanamycin** is primarily used to treat *M. tuberculosis* infections.
            (iv) **Gentamicin, tobramycin, amikacin,** and **netilmicin,** the newer aminoglycosides, are more commonly used because of their lower toxicity levels. Amikacin is more expensive but more effective than gentamicin; fewer bacterial strains are resistant to amikacin.
         (b) Aminoglycosides and β-lactams are synergistic when used in combination because both groups are bactericidal, but have independent mechanisms of action.
      (3) **Toxicity.** The structural differences between bacterial and mammalian ribosomes favors the preferential effect of these antibiotics against bacteria. However, they are relatively toxic, particularly to the nervous system and the kidney. In general, the therapeutic levels of aminoglycosides are so close to toxic levels that the serum concentrations of these drugs need to be closely monitored.
   b. **Tetracyclines** are either **short-acting** (e.g., tetracycline, oxytetracycline, chlortetracycline, demeclocycline, methacycline) or **long-acting** (e.g., doxycycline, minocycline). Long-acting tetracyclines require less frequent administration, which facilitates patient compliance.
      (1) **Chemistry.** Tetracyclines which are produced by organisms of the *Streptomyces* species, are composed of a four-ring hydronaphthacene nucleus (Figure 4-5).
      (2) **Mechanism of action.** Tetracyclines associate with the 30S unit of the bacterial ribosome, blocking the binding of tRNA to the ribosome–mRNA complex and stopping peptide elongation.
      (3) **Spectrum of activity.** Tetracyclines are broad-spectrum bacteriostatic agents.

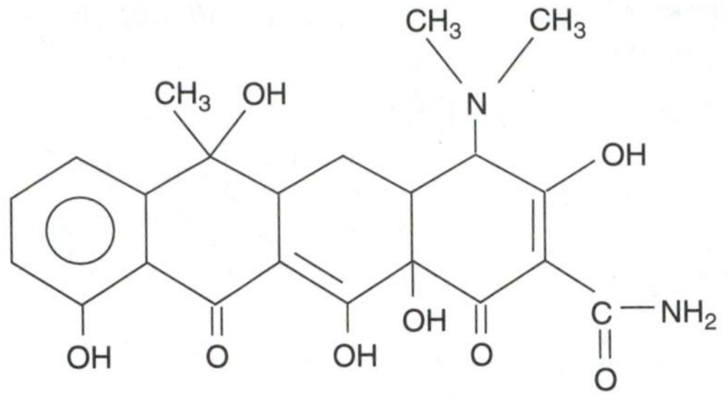

FIGURE 4-5. Basic structure of tetracycline.

(a) As a rule, they are effective in the treatment of infections caused by intracellular bacteria.
(b) They are also the recommended alternatives to penicillin in the treatment of syphilis and gonorrhea in patients allergic to penicillin.
(c) All tetracyclines are metabolized by the liver and are not excreted in the urine, therefore they are not useful for the treatment of urinary tract infections.

(4) **Toxicity.**
(a) The toxic effects of tetracyclines include **gastrointestinal upset** (any broad-spectrum antibiotic like tetracycline can lead to antibiotic-associated colitis) and **superinfections** (e.g., candidiasis, fungal infections) as a result of the loss of normal human flora.
(b) They can **stain developing teeth** yellow; therefore, they are contraindicated in pregnant women and children.
(c) Some patients show increased photosensitivity.

2. Inhibitors of the 50S ribosomal unit

a. **Chloramphenicol** was the first antimicrobial compound synthesized in the laboratory.
(1) **Chemistry.** Chloramphenicol is unique in that it contains nitrobenzene.
(2) **Mechanism of action.** It binds to the 50S subunit of the ribosome and inhibits the function of peptidyltransferase. Consequently, peptide bond formation is inhibited and peptide chains are prematurely terminated.
(3) **Spectrum of activity.** Chloramphenicol is an excellent broad-spectrum antibacterial, effective against **anaerobes.** It is one of the antibacterials of choice for the treatment of **typhoid fever, Rocky Mountain spotted fever,** and ***H. influenzae* meningitis.** In this last case, chloramphenicol is used because it penetrates the blood–brain barrier well and *H. influenzae* (as well as the other bacteria commonly causing meningitis) is usually susceptible.
(4) **Toxicity**
(a) **Gray baby syndrome.** Chloramphenicol is metabolized in the liver, where it is conjugated to glucocuronide. In newborns, who often do not have normal levels of glucuronyl transferase, chloramphenicol may accumulate in the blood until toxic levels are reached. Affected infants look gray (ashen); they experience seizures, heart failure, edema, and hepatomegaly and may die. When using chloramphenicol in infants, the dosage must be adjusted carefully.
(b) **Blood dyscrasias.** In adults, chloramphenicol can cause anemia, leukopenia, and thrombocytopenia, which may progress to aplastic anemia. Monitoring the dosage and the blood levels usually allows the physician to prevent irreversible pancytopenia from occurring. Some individuals, however, will develop an idiosyncratic aplastic anemia following a single dose of chloramphenicol (even when it is applied topically). Because of this serious adverse affect, the tendency is to avoid the use of chloramphenicol if there is a good alternative drug.

b. Macrolide antibiotics include **erythromycin, clarithromycin,** and **azithromycin.**

(1) Chemistry. Structurally, macrolide antibiotics are composed of a large lactone ring with attached sugar molecules.

(2) Mechanism of action. Macrolides bind to the ribosomal 50S unit, immobilize peptidyl tRNA, and cause premature peptide chain termination.

(3) Spectrum of activity. The spectrum of bacteria susceptible to macrolides is relatively narrow.

(a) Erythromycin is the drug of choice for *Legionella* and *Mycoplasma* and the alternate to penicillin to treat group A, β-hemolytic streptococcus and *Streptococcus pneumoniae* in patients allergic to penicillin.

(b) Clarithromycin is acid-stable and very useful to treat gastritis caused by *Helicobacter pylori.* It is also effective in the treatment of infections caused by *Mycobacterium avium-intracellulare.*

(c) Azithromycin is a very effective antichlamydial agent.

(4) Toxicity. The macrolides are metabolized by the liver and can be hepatotoxic.

c. Lincosamides include **lincomycin,** the prototype drug of this group, and **clindamycin,** a considerably more effective antibacterial agent for anaerobes. Clindamycin, however, is associated with profound disturbances of the intestinal flora, which may result in overgrowth of *C. difficile,* leading to antibiotic-associated diarrhea and pseudomembranous colitis.

Chapter 5

Bacterial Resistance to Antibacterial Agents

Victor Del Bene
John Manos
Gabriel Virella

I. INTRODUCTION

A. When antibiotics were first introduced in the 1940s and 1950s, it was expected that they would eradicate infectious disease. However, it soon became evident that some bacteria are **intrinsically resistant** to certain classes of antibiotics.

B. In the early 1960s, the appearance of penicillinase-producing *Staphylococci* marked the onset of **acquired resistance** to antibiotics. The same phenomenon was soon observed with Gram-negative bacteria. With time, it became obvious that **two basic mechanisms** accounted for the emergence of resistant strains:

1. Mutation
2. Transfer of resistance genes among bacteria, most often through plasmids

II. ACQUISITION OF BACTERIAL RESISTANCE

A. **Intrinsic resistance** is usually related to structural features (e.g., the permeability of the bacterial cell wall) and are usually determined by chromosomal genes. All strains of *Pseudomonas aeruginosa,* for example, are resistant to most antibiotics because the complex cell wall of this species limits penetration of antibacterials.

B. **Mutational resistance** usually results from a chromosomal mutation that renders the bacterium unable to interact with the antibacterial. For example:

1. The high level of resistance to streptomycin seen in *Mycobacterium tuberculosis* and *Streptococcus faecalis* is caused by a mutation that affects the specific streptomycin-binding protein of the 30S subunit of the ribosome.
2. Mutations in the porin proteins may result in impaired transport of antibiotics into the cell. This type of mutation is usually manifested as multiple resistance to antibiotics. The mechanism of resistance to aminoglycosides of *P. aeruginosa* also involves a mutational decrease in cell wall permeability.
3. Mutations in the penicillin-binding proteins (PBPs) of *Streptococcus pneumoniae* have resulted in penicillin resistance.
4. Mutations in DNA-dependent RNA polymerase have been demonstrated in rifampin-resistant *Mycobacterium tuberculosis* and *Neisseria meningitidis.*
5. Altered DNA gyrase is responsible for the resistance to quinolone exhibited by *Escherichia coli.*
6. Altered target enzymes are found in sulfonamide- or trimethoprim-resistant strains of many bacterial species.

C. **Acquisition of resistance genes** is most often plasmid-mediated [see Chapter 3 VI B 2 b (1)]. As discussed in Chapter 3 plasmids are self-replicating units of genetic material.

TABLE 5-1. Bacteria That Carry Resistance Plasmids

Enterobacteriaceae	Other Enteric Bacteria	Nonenteric Bacteria
Escherichia coli	*Pseudomonas aeruginosa*	*Haemophilus influenzae*
Shigella species	*Vibrio cholerae*	*Neisseria gonorrhoeae*
Salmonella species	*Bacteroides fragilis*	*Staphylococcus aureus*
Klebsiella	*Clostridium perfringens*	*Streptococcus* (group A)
Proteus species	*Streptococcus* (groups D and B)	
Serratia marcescens	*Aeromonas* species	
Enterobacter species		
Citrobacter freundii		

1. **Resistance (R) plasmids** which carry genes responsible for resistance to many different antibacterial agents, are carried by many different bacteria (Table 5-1).
   a. R plasmids usually contain one or more dominant genes that **code for the synthesis of a drug inactivating or drug-modifying enzyme.** Multiple resistance genes can be carried in transposons integrated into plasmids.
   b. Resistance plasmids are usually transmitted by conjugation (if they carry the F factor) or by mobilization by a conjugative plasmid. Rarely, plasmids or plasmid genes may be transmitted by transduction or transformation.
2. **Acquisition of "new" chromosomal genes** has been suggested as the mechanism involved in the acquisition of resistance to methicillin by staphylococci.
   a. A chromosomal gene (*mec*A) that codes for a PBP with low affinity for β-lactam antibacterials is shared by all methicillin-resistant *Staphylococcus aureus* (MRSA). This gene appears to be clonally derived from a single or a few "progenitor" strains.
   b. It is believed that the progenitors acquire the gene from an exogenous source, but once integrated, it remains stable and does not seem to be transmitted horizontally (i.e., from bacterium to bacterium).

III. MECHANISMS OF BACTERIAL RESISTANCE.

A variety of mechanisms of resistance have been acquired by bacteria, enabling them to resist the effects of antibacterials. Table 5-2 summarizes the most important mechanisms of resistance and the bacteria that have developed them.

A. Enzymatic inactivation of antibacterial agents. Bacteria may produce specific enzymes that inactivate or modify the drug either before or after it enters the bacterial cell. Enzyme production may be increased by mutations affecting the regulation of its expression or by amplification of the number of copies of the gene coding for its synthesis.

1. **β-lactamases** hydrolyze the β-lactam ring of penicillin G and many of the semisynthetic penicillins.
   a. In **Gram-positive bacteria,** β-lactamase is released from the cell.
      (1) Resistance occurs because the β-lactamase destroys the β-lactam antibacterial in the extracellular environment, and, as a consequence, the concentration of active drug in the extracellular environment falls.
      (2) Resistance is a **population phenomenon**—a large innoculum of organisms is much more resistant than a small one.
      (3) The β-lactamase gene is **inducible**—in the presence of the drug, a large amount of enzyme is produced.
   b. In **Gram-negative bacteria,** the outer membrane retards entry of the antibacterial into the cell and the β-lactamase is retained within the periplasmic space.
      (1) Each cell is responsible for its own protection—a more efficient mechanism

TABLE 5-2. Mechanisms of Resistance to Antibiotics

Antibiotic	Resistant bacteria	Genetic mechanism
I. Intrinsic resistance		
Antibiotic	**Resistant bacteria**	
β-lactams	*Pseudomonas, Enterobacter*	
Aminoglycosides	*Pseudomonas, Streptococcus faecalis, Serratia*	
Chloramphenicol, trimethoprim	*Pseudomonas*	
II. Alteration in the transport system, cell wall, or cell membrane		
A. Decreased uptake or increased removal		
Antibiotic	**Resistant bacteria**	**Genetic mechanism**
Tetracyclines	Enterobacteriaceae	Plasmid-mediated
Quinolones	*Escherichia coli*	Plasmid-mediated
B. Poor transport of enzymatically modified drug		
Aminoglycosides	Enterobacteriaceae, *Pseudomonas*	
Chloramphenicol	*Pseudomonas*	
III. Enzymatic inactivation of the drug		
A. β-lactamases		
Antibiotic	**Resistant bacteria**	**Genetic mechanism**
β-Lactams	*Staphylococcus aureus,* *Enterobacteriaceae, Haemophilus influenzae, Pseudomonas*	Plasmid-mediated
B. Chloramphenicol acetyltransferase		
Chloramphenicol	*S. aureus,* Enterobacteriaceae	Plasmid-mediated
C. Acetyltransferases, phosphorylases, nucleotidases		
Aminoglycosides	*S. aureus, Streptococcus, Pseudomonas,* Enterobacteriaceae	
IV. Target alteration		
A. Alteration of DNA gyrase		
Antibiotic	**Resistant bacteria**	**Genetic mechanism**
Quinolones	Enterobacteriaceae, Opportunistic Gram-negative organisms	Chromosomal mutation
B. Alteration of the β subunit of RNA polymerase		
Rifampin	Enterobacteriaceae	Chromosomal mutation
C. Alteration of the 50S ribosomal unit		
Erythromycin	*S. aureus, E. coli*	Plasmid-mediated
D. Alteration of the 30S ribosomal unit		
Streptomycin	Enterobacteriaceae	Chromosomal mutation

(continued)

TABLE 5-2. *(continued)*

E. Alteration of penicillin-binding proteins		
Penicillins	*Neisseria gonorrhoeae, Streptococcus pneumoniae*	
Cephalosporins	*S. faecalis, S. aureus,* *Enterobacteriaceae*	
Methicillin	*S. aureus*	
F. Synthesis of enzymes less sensitive to inhibitory drugs		
Sulfonamides	Enterobacteriaceae	Plasmid-mediated*
Trimethoprim	*S. aureus*	Plasmid-mediated†

* Code for an altered dihydropteroate synthetase
† Code for a drug-resistant dihydrofolate reductase

than that of Gram-positive bacteria. A small innoculum of bacteria may be almost as resistant as a large one.

(2) In most instances, enzymes are produced **constitutively** (i.e., even when the antibiotic is not present).

(3) The β-lactamases of Gram-negative bacteria have been classified into five groups according to a variety of characteristics. Some are active only against penicillins, others against cephalosporins, and others affect both. The genes responsible for their synthesis may be located in plasmids or in the bacterial chromosome. In most cases, the enzymes are constitutively expressed, but class I β-lactamases, active against cephalosporins, are inducible.

2. **Acetyltransferases, phosphorylases,** and **nucleotidases** modify aminoglycosides, rendering them incapable of binding to the ribosomal target.
   - **a.** The aminoglycoside-modifying enzymes are located at the surface of the cytoplasmic membrane.
   - **b.** Only those molecules of the drug that are in the process of being transported across the cytoplasmic membrane are modified. Thus, the concentration of drug in the extracellular environment is reduced only slightly (0.5%).
3. **Chloramphenicol acetyltransferase** has a mechanism of action similar to the aminoglycoside acetyltransferases.

B. Modification of cell wall permeability. Permeability is determined primarily by the nature of the cell wall. The cell wall usually is not a barrier in Gram-positive bacteria. In contrast, the cell wall in Gram-negative bacteria represents a barrier to many antibiotics—particularly those that have intracytoplasmic target molecules and are hydrophilic (e.g., most tetracyclines, aminoglycosides, erythromycin, clindamycin, sulfonamides). The degree of cell wall permeability varies among bacterial species and generally correlates with intrinsic resistance.

1. **Porins.** In Gram-negative bacteria, specific outer membrane proteins called porins provide entry for many hydrophilic antibiotics with molecular weights up to approximately 650 daltons. Mutations affecting porin structure may inhibit transport of multiple antibiotics.
2. **Lipopolysaccharide (LPS)** inhibits passage of hydrophobic (lipophilic) antibacterial agents through the cell wall. Thus rough mutants, which lack polysaccharide capsules and have minimal LPS in their cell walls, are more permeable to many antibiotics.
3. **Membrane transport proteins.** Mutations in membrane transport proteins appear to be responsible for resistance to tetracyclines, as a result of decreased transport into the cell.

4. **Electron transport.** The uptake of aminoglycosides depends primarily on electron transport to oxygen; thus, these agents are not effective against anaerobic bacteria or against facultative organisms in an anaerobic environment (e.g., an abscess). Primarily fermentative bacteria (e.g., streptococci) are also relatively resistant to aminoglycosides.

C. Alteration of target molecules. The target molecules may be located on the cytoplasmic membrane (e.g., PBPs) or inside the cytoplasmic membrane (e.g., ribosomes). In general, alteration of the target results in decreased affinity for the antibacterial compound. For example, the synthesis of an altered dihydropteroate synthetase with low affinity for sulfonamides or an abnormal dihydrofolate reductase resistant to the effect of trimethoprim results in resistance to these two antibacterial agents. The combination of a sulfonamide with trimethoprim reduces the frequency of resistant strains, but resistance to the combination is not uncommon.

D. Development of alternate pathways. In some cases, a mutant enzyme may bypass the synthetic block exerted by the antibiotic by using an alternative pathway. For example, vancomycin-resistant strains of enterococcus produce a D-alanine-D-lactate synthetase that results in the synthesis of a pentapeptide precursor with significantly less affinity for vancomycin. Of even more clinical significance is the possible emergence of staphylococci resistant to both methicillin and vancomycin. The acquisition of enterococcus resistance genes by staphylococci has been demonstrated, but whether the mechanisms of resistance of staphylococci and enterococci are identical has not yet been determined.

E. Active exclusion of the antimicrobial agent from the bacteria. Resistance to tetracyclines is mediated by the synthesis of new transport proteins that actively exclude tetracycline.

F. Development of tolerance. Impermeability of the outer membrane and inactivation of murein hydrolases (autolytic enzymes) renders an antibacterial agent bacteriostatic, as opposed to bactericidal. For example, some strains of *S. pneumoniae* "tolerate" penicillin to the point where the antibiotic effect is only bacteriostatic.

IV. BACTERIAL RESISTANCE ACCORDING TO DRUG CLASS.

Bacteria (of the same or different species) can achieve the same end by a variety of means (Table 5-3).

TABLE 5-3. Resistance Mechanisms According to Drug Class

Antibacterial Agent	Resistance Mechanisms
Penicillins and cephalosporins	Enzymatic inactivation (β-lactamase)
	Target modification (PCBs)
	Tolerance
Sulfonamides	Active exclusion via a plasmid-encoded transport system Target alteration (dihyropteroate reductase)
Aminoglycosides	Enzymatic inactivation (acetyltransferases, phosphorylases, nucleotidases)
	Target alteration (30S ribosomal unit)
	Decreased cell wall permeability
Tetracyclines	Active exclusion
Chloramphenicol	Enzymatic inactivation (acetyltransferase)
Macrolides	Target alteration (50S ribosomal unit)
Quinolones	Target alteration (DNA gyrase mutation)

PCBs = penicillin-binding proteins.

V. ANTIBIOTIC SUSCEPTIBILITY TESTING allows the choice of the best antibiotic with the narrowest spectrum and highest effectiveness against the isolated bacteria.

A. Minimal inhibitory concentration (MIC). The MIC is the lowest concentration of an antibiotic that will inhibit the growth of an organism.

1. **Clinical susceptibility.** A bacterium is considered clinically susceptible to a given antibiotic if a blood level 2–4 times the MIC can be attained with the usual dosages and no appreciable side effects.
   a. For example, if the MIC of an organism is 6 μg/ml and blood levels of 24 μg/ml can be safely reached, the organism is considered susceptible. When an organism is considered clinically susceptible to a given antimicrobial agent, its susceptibility is designated with an "S" on the laboratory report. In contrast, if the attainable blood level of the antimicrobial agent in question is only 10 μg/ml, the organism would be considered resistant ("R" on the report).
   b. The decision as to whether a given organism is clinically susceptible or not is based on a correlation between the antibiotic susceptibility *in vitro* and the *in vivo* attainable antibiotic concentrations. The safe attainable concentration for an antibiotic is based on the pharmacokinetics of the drug and its toxicity.
      (1) The attainable blood concentration used to predict clinical susceptibility is not the highest level that can be obtained, but the highest nontoxic concentration of antibiotic that can be safely obtained.
      (2) The attainable levels are average levels but may not reflect the actual levels reached in an individual patient (e.g., one with impaired absorption or impaired excretion may have lower or higher blood levels than expected).
   c. In some cases, the results of susceptibility testing may be misleading. For example, in the case of a urinary tract infection, the causative organism may be reported as "R" to a particular antibiotic based on the attainable blood levels. However, it may be known that the antibiotic in question is concentrated severalfold in its active form in the urine. In such a case, the antibiotic might be adequate for the treatment of the urinary infection.

2. **Methods for MIC determination**
   a. **Tube dilution**
      (1) **Procedure**
         (a) A series of tubes containing identical volumes of broth and doubling dilutions of a given antibiotic is prepared. An equal volume of a standardized suspension of the organism to be tested is added to the culture in each tube. (That is, the concentration of the organism is held constant and the amount of antibiotic varies.) The control tube does not contain antibiotic.
         (b) The suspensions are incubated overnight. In the tubes where the antibiotic concentration is below the inhibitory concentration, the bacterium will grow and the suspension will appear turbid. In the tubes where the antibiotic concentration is at or greater than the inhibitory level, the broth will remain clear. The lowest concentration of antibiotic that inhibits growth is the MIC (Figure 5-1).
      (2) To ensure reproducibility among laboratories, it is important to perform MIC assays with standard organisms (e.g., *S. aureus, E. coli, P. aeruginosa*) to verify that the results are consistent with those obtained by others.
      (3) MIC determination may be automated, based on **growth kinetics,** or semi-automated, using **microtiter plates** (i.e., prepared plates that have rows of different, prediluted antibiotics).
   b. **Kirby-Bauer technique.** The Kirby-Bauer methodology preceded the more modern semi-automated and automated methods used to determine antibiotic susceptibilities. This method is now used only for investigation or special purposes.
      (1) Broth culture of an isolated bacterium is spread into an agar plate and paper disks impregnated with known concentrations of different antibiotics are dropped on the surface of the seeded plate.
      (2) After adequate incubation to allow the growth of the seeded bacteria, clear

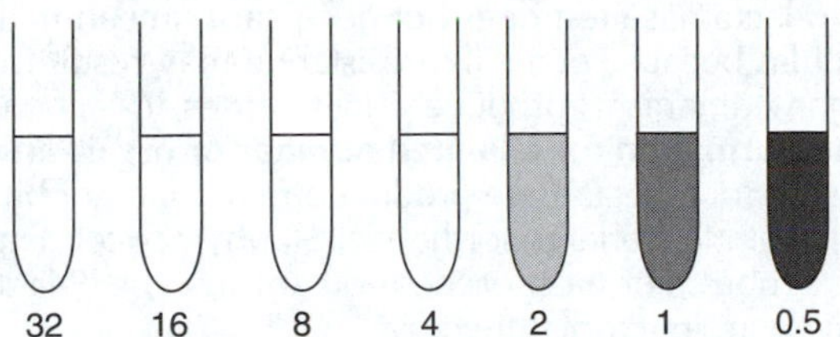

FIGURE 5-1. The tube method for determination of the minimal inhibitory concentration (MIC). The tubes contained identical volumes of a standardized suspension of the organism to be tested in broth and variable concentrations of a given antibiotic, as illustrated. No significant growth could be detected at antibiotic concentrations of 32, 16, 8, and 4 μg/ml, but there is visible growth at concentrations of 2, 1, and 0.5 μg/ml. The MIC is 4 μg/ml, the lowest concentration of antibiotic that inhibits growth.

areas where bacterial growth has been inhibited (i.e., **clear zones**) are seen around the disks. The concentration of antibiotic decreases as the distance from the antibiotic disk increases. As the concentration of antibiotic drops, it reaches a point where it cannot inhibit growth. This is called the **break point** and corresponds to the outer limit of the clear zone (Figure 5-2).

(a) The diameter of the clear zone is proportional to the susceptibility of the organism to each particular antibiotic. For a given antibiotic, the lower the MIC, the larger the clear zone.

(b) After the diameter is measured, a table is consulted that indicates whether the diameter corresponds to a susceptible or to a resistant strain. Basically, the cut-off to designate an isolate as susceptible is a diameter corresponding to at least twice the attainable blood level.

B. β-Lactamase tests

1. **Procedure.** An isolate can be tested directly for the production of β-lactamase using one of several methods. In the most commonly used method, the isolate is applied to a disk impregnated with a chromogenic cephalosporin (nitrocefin). If β-lactamase is produced, nitrocefin is hydrolyzed, resulting in a color change.

2. **Interpretation**
   a. A **positive** β-lactamase test indicates that the isolate is resistant to all β-lactamase–susceptible penicillins. This test does not indicate susceptibility or resistance to cephalosporins.

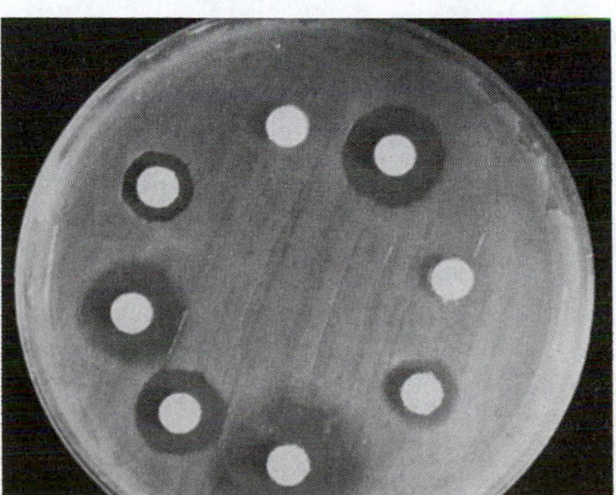

FIGURE 5-2. Kirby-Bauer disk diffusion test. The surface of an agar plate is seeded with a bacterial isolate and filter paper disks impregnated with different antimicrobial agents are dropped on the surface. Zones of growth inhibition (clear zones) are visible around some of the filter paper discs. The diameters are measured and compared to a table of values that indicate susceptibility or resistance to each antimicrobial agent.

b. A **negative** β-lactamase test does not necessarily mean that the isolate is susceptible to penicillin because penicillin resistance may result from altered PBPs.

c. Although many organisms produce β-lactamases, β-lactamase tests provide clinically **useful information for a limited number of organisms.** Organisms most commonly assessed for β-lactamase production are Haemophilus influenzae, Moraxella catarrhalis, Neisseria gonorrhoeae, Staphylococci, Enterococci, and Gram-negative anaerobes. For most of these organisms, the β-lactamase test result is sufficient to guide antimicrobial therapy.

Chapter 6

Disinfection and Sterilization

Michael G. Schmidt

I. DEFINITIONS (Table 6-1).

A. **Sterilization** is the **complete inactivation of all forms of microbial life.**

B. **Antiseptics** are compounds that are applied topically to human tissue. Antiseptics either inhibit the growth of microorganisms or they kill them, without adversely affecting the human tissue to which they are applied.

C. **Disinfectants** are compounds that kill microorganisms (except bacterial endospores). Because they may be harmful to human tissue, disinfectants are usually reserved for use on inanimate objects.

1. **High-level disinfectants** kill mycobacteria, viruses, and all but the most resistant spores.
2. **Low-level disinfectants** kill many vegetative bacteria and most viruses, but they are ineffective against mycobacteria.

II. CHEMICAL ANTIMICROBIAL AGENTS

A. **Surface active agents** disrupt the lipid bilayer by altering the orderly arrangement of proteins and lipids that compose the membrane.

1. **Cationic agents.** Positively-charged quaternary ammonium compounds disrupt the cell membrane by allowing the positively charged group to associate with the negatively charged phosphate groups of the phospholipids. The nonpolar residue penetrates the membrane, resulting in cell leakage. Examples include **Zephiran** (alkydimethylbenzyl ammonium chloride), **Triton K-12** (cetyldimethylbenzyl ammonium chloride), and **Ceepryn chloride** (cetylpyridinium chloride).
2. **Anionic agents** include soaps and fatty acids that dissociate in solution. In their soluble, negatively charged form, these agents associate with cell membrane lipids and disrupt the lipid bilayer.
   - **a.** These agents are most effective against Gram-positive organisms.
   - **b.** Examples include **Duponol LS** (sodium oleoyl sulfate) and **Triton W-30** (sodium salt of alkylphenoxyethyl sulfonate).
3. **Nonionic agents** include organic solvents such as phenolic compounds and alcohols. These compounds disrupt the cell membrane lipid bilayer.
   - **a.** **Phenolic compounds** are the active ingredient of domestic disinfectants (e.g., Lysol). **Hexachlorophene** is also a member of this group. Phenolic compounds are often used in conjunction with soaps and germicidal solutions.
   - **b.** **Alcohols** with disinfectant properties include **methanol, isopropyl alcohol,** and **ethanol.** The optimal concentration of ethanol for disinfectant purposes is 70%.

B. **Denaturing agents**

1. **Protein-denaturing compounds** may be either bases or acids. Extreme pH values alter the three-dimensional structure of the proteins, resulting in their denaturation. These compounds are primarily used as food preservatives and include benzoic acid, salicylic acid, acetic acid, lactic acid, and propionic acid.

TABLE 6-1. Terminology Used to Describe Disinfecting Agents

Term	Definition
Germicide	Agent (chemical or physical) that destroys most microorganisms, but not endospores, used on skin or inanimate objects
Sterilant	Chemical agent that destroys all microorganisms, including spores
Sporocide	Generally a chemical agent that destroys both bacterial (endo- and exo-) and fungal (mold) spores
Fungicide	Chemical agent that destroys fungi
Virucide	Chemical agent that destroys viruses
Bacteriostat	Chemical agent that inhibits the growth of bacteria
Sanitizer	An agent, usually a detergent, that reduces the numbers of bacteria to a safe level

2. **Heavy metals** (e.g., mercury, silver, arsenic) bind irreversibly to the sulfhydryl groups of proteins. Because the sulfhydryl groups are often at the active site of an enzyme, the binding of heavy metal results in enzyme inactivation, affecting vital chemical reactions required for bacterial survival.
   a. Examples include **merthiolate, mercurochrome,** and **silver nitrate** (which is highly bactericidal for gonococci).
   b. These compounds are toxic and are mostly used topically.
3. **Oxidizing agents** such as **hydrogen peroxide, sodium hypochlorite (bleach),** and **chlorine gas** affect both proteins and nucleic acids.
   a. Diluted (3%) hydrogen peroxide can be safely used for skin disinfection.
   b. Chlorine and its derivatives are commonly used for the disinfection of water and other inanimate objects.
4. **Alkylating agents** denature protein and nucleic acids by changing the oxidation state of the functional groups of those molecules. Included in this group are **formaldehyde, ethylene oxide,** and **glutaraldehyde,** commonly used for general decontamination and cold sterilization of surgical instruments and heat-sensitive materials (e.g., plastics).

III. PHYSICAL ANTIMICROBIAL AGENTS

A. **Heat** inactivates microorganisms by oxidizing intracellular components. In addition, heat denatures protein by causing the formation of large protein aggregates (coagulation). Heat may also cause breaks in nucleic acid.

1. Moist and dry heat are very effective means of sterilizing materials. The presence or absence of moisture along with the pressure determines the length of time and temperature necessary to inactive microorganisms.
   a. **Moist heat.** Steam sterilization is carried out in an **autoclave** in the presence of saturated steam under pressure for 15 minutes at a temperature of 121°C. Materials not suitable for sterilization in the presence of moist heat (e.g., viscous materials such as greases, lubricants, mineral oil, waxes, and powders) are often sterilized by dry heat.
   b. **Dry heat** is less efficient than moist heat; therefore, higher temperatures are required for a longer period of time. However, advantages of dry heat include the fact that it does not corrode metals (e.g., surgical instruments) or affect glass surfaces.
2. **Pasteurization** is a process using mild heat that reduces or destroys vegetative microorganisms to a level set by law. This process is used in the food industry.

B. **Radiation.** Electromagnetic energy of a specific wavelength can have profound, lethal effects on microorganisms.

1. Radiation ionizes cytoplasmic water, causing the formation of a variety of active compounds (e.g., hydrogen peroxide, superoxide) and hydroxyl radicals. These compounds and radicals have lethal denaturing effects on proteins and nucleic acids.
2. In general, shorter wavelengths, typical of ionizing radiation, are more strongly bactericidal. Sterilization doses are generally expressed in megarads, with a dose of 2.5 Mrad of ionizing radiation considered sufficient to insure sterilization.

C. **Ultrasonic energy** is also used to inactivate microorganisms. Sonic vibrations in the upper audible and ultrasonic range (20–1000 kc) disrupt cells.

D. **Filtration** is used to sterilize heat-labile (sensitive) liquids (e.g., culture media). A variety of filters, ranging in size from 14–0.023 μm, have been developed that exclude contaminating microorganisms while allowing the liquid to freely pass. The 0.22-μm size is used most commonly.

Chapter 7

Bacterial Virulence Factors

Victor Del Bene
Michael G. Schmidt

I. INTRODUCTION

A. Virulence factors are characteristics that enable bacteria to cause disease.

1. Pathogenic bacteria may have one or several virulence factors.
2. These factors may be common to all bacteria of a given genus or species, or they may be characteristic of special pathogenic strains.
   a. Virulence factors that are common to the genus or species appear to give the organism a survival advantage; they may have been selected during evolution.
   b. Those that are unique to some strains are usually acquired through mechanisms of genetic exchange (generally conjugation and transduction) and are not associated with specific survival advantage for the bacterium.

B. Applications to medicine. In addition to enabling scientists to understand the pathogenesis of disease, a knowledge of virulence factors can help prevent disease. For instance, many component vaccines are based on the use of modified virulence factors that lack toxic effects but retain immunogenicity. Recombinant bacteria lacking the genes responsible for the synthesis of the virulence factor have also been successfully used for **immunoprophylaxis.**

II. CAPSULES.

Located externally to the cell wall, capsules enable the bacterium to avoid or survive phagocytosis. Capsules are one of the most common virulence factors possessed by bacteria. In some bacteria, capsulated and encapsulated variants can be isolated; the capsulated are virulent and the encapsulated are harmless.

A. Composition. The capsule is a dense, well-defined **polymer layer** synthesized by enzymes in the bacterial cell wall. The polymer is most often a **polysaccharide.**

B. Production is **genetically determined.** The phenomenon of transduction was first defined when Avery observed that incubation of avirulent, nonencapsulated strains of *Streptococcus pneumoniae* with DNA extracted from virulent, encapsulated strains of the same organism resulted in the emergence of new virulent encapsulated strains. In other words, the ability to produce a capsule was transfected by the DNA of encapsulated strains.

C. Mechanisms by which capsules prevent phagocytosis are not completely understood. For example, *S. pneumoniae,* an organism that causes severe forms of pneumonia, as well as meningitis and other infections, has an antiphagocytic polysaccharide capsule.

1. The capsule may hinder the interaction between antibody and C3 bound to the bacterial outer membrane and their respective receptors on phagocytic cells.
2. Alternatively, the capsule may prevent C3b,Bb formation, thus limiting the activation of C3 via the alternative pathway.

III. ADHESINS.

Many bacteria depend on the ability to adhere to mucosal cells as a first step in causing disease. Without adhesion factors, many pharyngeal, intestinal, and urinary tract pathogens would be washed away before they could cause disease.

A. Types. Adhesion factors are **surface structures.**

1. **Pili.** In most cases, adhesion factors are **pili** [also designated as **fimbriae** and, in specific cases, as **colonization factor antigens (CFAs)].**

1. **Lipopolysaccharide (LPS) side chains (O antigens)** have also been implicated as playing a role in determining adhesion.

2. **M protein.** The ability of *Streptococcus pyogenes* to cause pharyngitis seems to be directly related to the production of M protein, the major virulence factor for this bacterium. The expression of M protein on the bacterial cell membrane mediates adherence of the bacterium to epithelial cells through poorly understood interactions.

B. Mechanism. Adhesion factors interact with cells and tissues depending on the expression of receptors for which they have affinity. Differences in tissue and organ tropism exhibited by bacteria that reach the systemic circulation reflect the different affinities of adhesion factors expressed by various bacteria.

IV. INVASIVENESS.

For many pathogens, the ability to invade the host cell is integral to the disease process.

A. The invasiveness of bacteria seems to be a multifactorial, complex process. For example, in the case of *Shigella,* a series of proteins known as **invasion plasmid antigens (Ipa)** and a protein called **Ics B (for intracellular spread)** expressed on the outer membrane play significant roles in the early stages of infection.

1. First, the Ipa permit the bacterium to bind to the luminal surface of intestinal mucosal M cells. Endocytosis and the rapid exit of the bacterium from the endosome into the cytoplasm follow.

2. In the cytoplasm, IcS B allows the bacterium to interact with cellular integrins. This interaction enables the bacterium to travel toward the cell membrane, which forms a protrusion and fuses with the cell membranes of adjacent cells, thereby allowing *Shigella* to diffuse from cell to cell.

B. The **pili** of *Neisseria gonorrhoeae* enable the organism to adhere to mucosal cells. In addition, they contain an **enzyme** that dissolves the mucosal cell lining, allowing *N. gonorrhoeae* to penetrate the submucosal tissues.

V. EXOENZYMES.

Many bacteria produce and secrete enzymes. These enzymes may play an important pathogenic role by a variety of mechanisms. For example:

A. Enzymes that break down collagen (i.e., collagenases, hyaluronidases) **and fibrin** (i.e., fibrinolysins) allow better penetration of bacteria into tissues.

B. Enzymes that break down cellular material include proteases and lecithinases. These enzymes are common to many of the *Clostridia.*

C. Enzymes that modify and inactivate antibiotics, such as β-lactamases, are one of the primary mechanisms of antibacterial resistance.

TABLE 7-1. Comparison of Endotoxin and Exotoxins

Characteristic	Endotoxin	Exotoxin
Source	Gram-negative bacteria	Gram-positive and Gram-negative bacteria
Chemical composition	Lipopolysaccharide	Protein
Toxic moiety	Lipid A	Active domain
Antigenic moiety	Lipopolysaccharide	Protein
Heat sensitivity	Stable	Labile
Species-specificity	No	Yes
Cellular release	Bacterial lysis	Active

VI. TOXINS.

TOXINS. Bacterial toxins can be classified into two broad categories. **Exotoxins** are proteins produced and released from the cell to cause toxicity, whereas **endotoxins** are part of the bacteria itself. Table 7-1 compares the main characteristics of each.

A. Exotoxins

Exotoxins can be common to all bacteria of a given genus (e.g., all isolates of *Clostridium tetani* produce tetanospasmin) or unique to pathogenic strains (e.g., diphtheria is caused only by toxin-producing strains of *Corynebacterium diphtheriae;* non-toxin producing strains are harmless). Table 7-2 summarizes the major bacterial exotoxins, their sources, and their effects.

1. **Genetics.** As a rule, toxins that are produced by all members of a genus or species of bacteria are encoded by chromosomal genes, whereas those that are not are encoded by transferable genetic elements (e.g., plasmids, lysogenic phages).
2. **Structure.** Most exotoxins have two structural domains: a **binding domain,** which binds to specific cellular receptors, and an **active domain,** which causes cell toxicity.
   a. The interaction between the binding domain and the receptor determines what tissues or cells are affected by the toxin.
   b. In some special cases, the toxin may exert its effects by blocking the binding of natural substrates to the same receptor. However, in most cases, once the binding site interacts with a receptor, the active site is cleaved and becomes internalized, causing toxic effects at the cellular level.
3. **Functional classification**
   a. **Enterotoxins** affect the **gastrointestinal tract** and include **heat-labile toxins (LT-I, LT-II), heat-stable toxin (ST),** and **cholera toxin.** These toxins are discussed in Chapter 16 II B 2 b and III A 2, respectively.
   b. **Neurotoxins** affect the nervous system and include **botulinum toxin** and **tetanus toxin (tetanospasmin).** These toxins are discussed in Chapter 13.
   c. **Cytotoxins** affect cells in a variety of tissues. Examples include **diphtheria toxin** (see Chapter 13) and **Pseudomonas toxin A.**
4. **Identification**
   a. The **ileal loop test** is used to determine if the virulence of a bacterium is associated with the production of an enterotoxin. Ligated loops of rabbit ileum are inoculated with the bacterium. If an enterotoxin is produced, accumulation of fluid in the lumen causes the loop to distend.
   b. **Cell culture tests.** Monolayers of sensitive cells, such as **Vero cells** or **Y-1 adrenal cells,** can be used to test for toxin production by determining the effects of a bacterium-free culture filtrate on the growth of the cell monolayer. If a toxin is contained in the medium, the monolayer will be disrupted.
   c. **Serologic tests (enzymoammunoassays).** Many bacterial exotoxins have been purified or produced through recombinant technology. Because the exotoxins are pro-

TABLE 7-2. Major Bacterial Exotoxins

Bacterium	Toxin	Bacterial Genetics	Effects	Mechanisms
Staphylococcus aureus	Enterotoxins (types A–E)	Lysogenized bacteria	Vomiting	Stimulates vomit center by binding to vagal brain receptors
	Exfoliatins		Scaled skin syndrome	Cytotoxic to dermal cells
	Toxic shock syndrome toxin 1		Shock	↑ IL-1, IL-6, TNF-α release
Streptococcus pyogenes	Pyrogenic (erythrogenic) exotoxin (types A–C)	Lysogenized bacteria	Rash of scarlet fever, fever, toxic shock	↑ IL-1, IL-6, TNF-α release, endothelial damage
Bordetella pertussis	Pertussis toxin	Chromosomal genes	Exaggerated responses to histamine and insulin, leukocytosis	↑ cAMP
Corynebacterium diphtheriae	Diphtheria toxin	Lysogenized bacteria	Cytotoxicity via inhibition of protein synthesis	Inactivation of EF-2
Escherichia coli	Enterotoxins (ST and LT)	Plasmid-coded	Diarrhea	↑ adenylate cyclase (LT); ↑ guanylate cyclase (ST)
	Shiga-like toxins (Verotoxins)	Lysogenized or transformed bacteria	Hemorrhagic colitis, hemolytic–uremic syndrome	Ribosomal inactivation; endothelial damage; ↑ IL-1, IL-6, TNF-α release
Shigella dysenteriae	Shiga toxin	Chromosomal genes	Bacterial dysentery, hemolytic–uremic syndrome	Ribosomal inactivation; endothelial damage; ↑ IL-1, IL-6, TNF-α release
Vibrio cholerae	Choleragen	Chromosomal genes	Life-threatening diarrhea	↑ adenylate cyclase
Pseudomonas aeruginosa	Exotoxin A	Chromosomal genes	Cytotoxicity	Inactivation of EF-2
Clostridium botulinum	Botulinum toxin	Lysogenized bacteria	Flacid paralysis	Blocks the release of acetylcholine from peripheral nerve junctions
Clostridium difficile	Toxins A and B	Chromosomal genes*	Enterocolitis	Disrupts the actin cytoskeleton; chemoattractant for neutrophils
Clostridium perfringens	α toxin	Chromosomal genes*	Gas gangrene; myonecrosis	Disrupts cell membranes
Clostridium tetani	Tetanospasmin	Plasmid-coded	Spastic paralysis	Inhibits the release of inhibitory neurotransmitters

cAMP = cyclic adenosine monophosphate; EF-2 = elongation factor 2; IL-1 = interleukin-1; IL-6 = interleukin-6; LT = heat-labile toxin; ST = heat-stable toxin; TNF-α = tumor necrosing factor-α.

* Strain variability in toxin production suggests that the chromosomal genes may be acquired by transformation or lysogenic phage infection.

teins, they are immunogenic and antisera can be produced to detect the presence of toxin, either in fecal material or in culture media.

d. Molecular techniques may allow detection of the DNA of toxin-producing bacteria in fecal material. This approach is still in its early stages of development.

B. **Endotoxins** are **lipopolysaccharides (LPS)** derived from Gram-negative bacterial cell walls. All Gram-negative bacteria have endotoxin in their outer membranes, but endotoxins of different bacteria vary in their potency and ability to cause characteristic symptoms.

1. Endotoxin is **not actively secreted;** rather, it is released as bacteria lyse.
2. **Sepsis and septic shock.** Endotoxins are primarily responsible for the development of

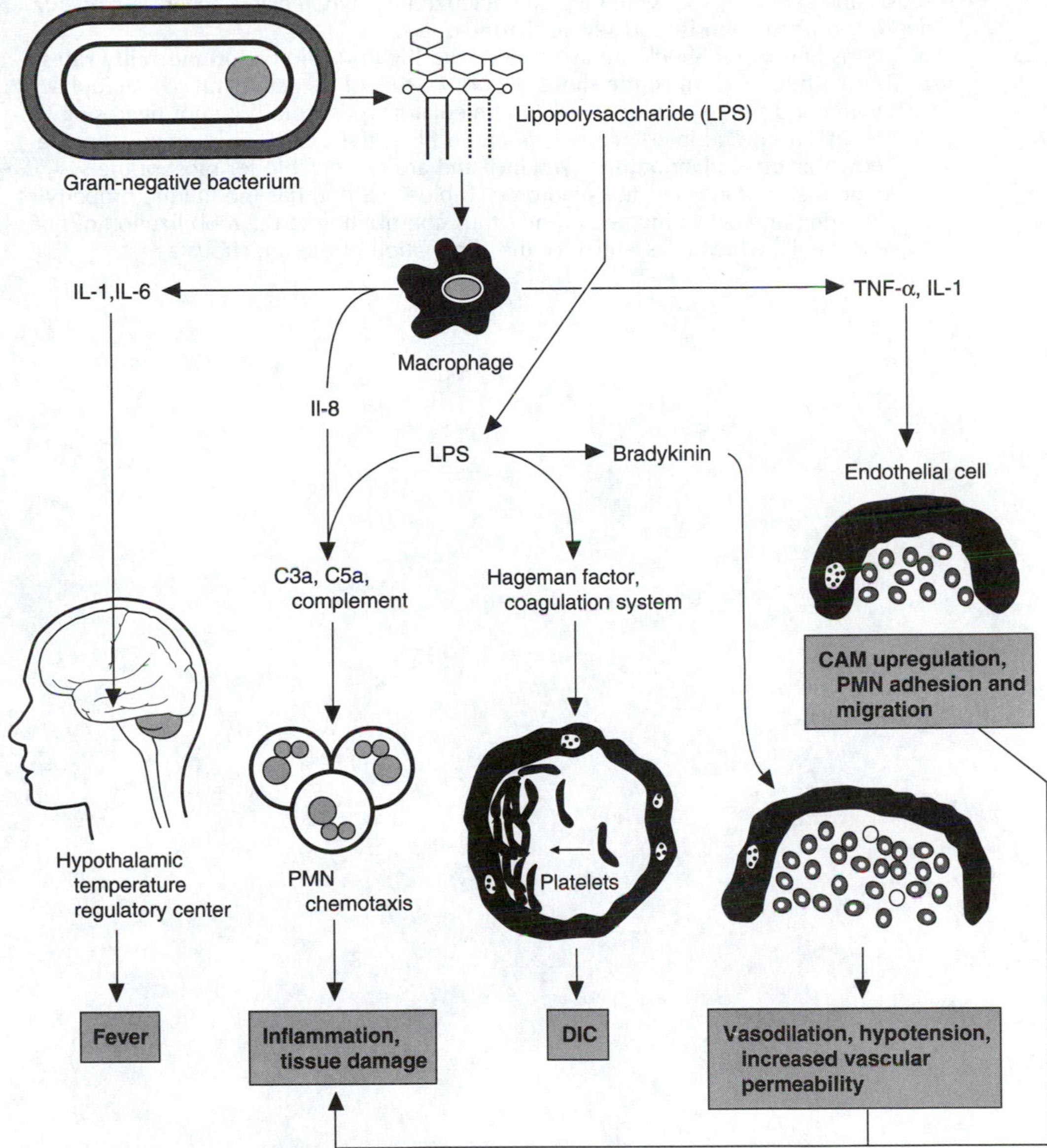

FIGURE 7-1. Pathogenesis of septic shock. *CAM* = cell adhesion molecule; *DIC* = disseminated intravascular coagulation; *IL-1* = interleukin-1; *IL-6* = interleukin-6; *IL-8* = interleukin-8; *PMN* = polymorphonuclear neutrophil; *TNF-α* = tumor necrosing factor-*α*.

TABLE 7-3. Properties of IL-1, IL-6, and TNF-*α*

Property	IL-1	TNF-*α*	IL-6
Pyrogen	+	+	+
Sleep inducer	+	+	−
Shock inducer	+	+	+
T cell activation	+	+	+
B cell activation	+	+	+
B cell differentiation	−	−	+

IL-1 = interleukin-1; IL-6 = interleukin-6; TNF-*α* = tumor necrosing factor.

sepsis and septic shock, which are characterized by hypotension, fever, leukopenia, depressed phagocytosis, and severe diarrhea.

a. Sepsis and septic shock are associated with **high morbidity and mortality rates.**

b. The **pathogenesis of septic shock** (Figure 7-1) involves activation of macrophages by LPS and the release of a variety of mediators, particularly tumor necrosing factor-α (TNF-α) and interleukins 1, 6, and 8 (IL-1, IL-6, IL-8). These mediators are known as **pro-inflammatory cytokines** and are responsible for most of the systemic manifestations of the syndrome (Table 7-3). IL-8 has the unique property of attracting and activating neutrophils, thus contributing to the mobilization of phagocytic cells which is essential for the elimination of the infectious agent.

PART II

IMMUNITY AND INFECTION

Chapter 8

Anti-Infectious Host Defenses

Gabriel Virella

I. GENERAL CONSIDERATIONS.

GENERAL CONSIDERATIONS. Humans (and most other vertebrates) have developed a complex system of specific and nonspecific mechanisms of protection against pathogenic microorganisms. These defense mechanisms also ensure a state of equilibrium with endogenous microbes, essential for maintenance of an infection-free status.

II. NONSPECIFIC DEFENSE MECHANISMS

NONSPECIFIC DEFENSE MECHANISMS play a most important role as a first line of defense (Table 8-1).

A. Local mechanisms

Local mechanisms (see Table 8-1). Although the importance of the nonspecific local mechanisms cannot be understressed, they will not be discussed further in this chapter.

B. Systemic mechanisms

1. **Fever** is induced by **cytokines,** particularly by **interleukin-1 (IL-1), tumor necrosis factor-α (TNF-α),** and **interleukin-6 (IL-6).**
   a. Microbes and their products activate macrophages and other cells, such as lymphocytes, to release cytokines.
   b. The cytokines stimulate the thermoregulatory center in the hypothalamus. The resultant increase in body temperature inhibits replication of the infectious agent.

2. **Production of interferons.** Interferons are a family of cytokines produced by a wide variety of cells, usually in response to viral infection.
   a. **Type I interferons [interferon-α (IFN-α)** and **interferon-β (IFN-β)]** are released by most nucleated cells and their release is triggered by the viral infection itself. Type I interferons block the synthesis of viral proteins in neighboring noninfected cells, thereby preventing viral replication.
   b. **Type II interferon [interferon-γ (IFN-γ, immune interferon)]** is released by activated T cells.
      (1) IFN-γ activates macrophages and natural killer (NK) cells and enhances their activity against infectious agents.
      (2) Opportunities for medical intervention have been increased by the production of recombinant cytokines, such as IFN-γ, which can induce significant clinical improvement in patients with phagocytic cell defects.

3. **Phagocytosis**
   a. **Two major cell types** are involved in phagocytosis: **polymorphonuclear leukocytes** (particularly neutrophils) and **macrophages.** Phagocytosis is enhanced by **opsonins** (see III A 1 b), but neutrophils are able to ingest unopsonized particles.
      (1) **Mannose receptors** on the neutrophil membrane allow neutrophils to recognize and ingest organisms with mannose-rich capsules, such as *Candida albicans* yeasts.
      (2) Many organisms activate complement by the **alternative pathway** and can then be recognized and ingested through C3b receptors.
      (3) Neutrophils are able to ingest a variety of inert particles through poorly characterized mechanisms.

TABLE 8-1. Nonspecific Defense Mechanisms

Local	Systemic
Physical integrity of skin and mucosae	
Lysozyme in tears, saliva, sweat, and other secretions	Fever
Gastric acidity	Interferon production
Flow of mucosal secretions in the respiratory tract	Phagocytosis
Intestinal transit	Natural killer cells
Urinary flow	

b. The importance of the role of neutrophils is proven by the high frequency of bacterial infections in neutropenic patients, particularly when the neutrophil count falls below 200/μl.

c. Because of the primary role that neutrophil phagocytosis has in the elimination of bacteria, neutrophil infiltrates and exudates and neutrophilia in the peripheral blood are classically associated with bacterial infections. The formation of neutrophil-rich purulent exudates is the basis for the generic description of classic bacterial infections as **pyogenic** (pus-generating).

4. **Natural killer (NK) cells** appear to play a role in the elimination of cells infected by viruses or intracellular bacteria. The recognition of the target is believed to result from differences in cell membrane composition, such as the increased glycoprotein content typical of viral-infected and viral-transformed cells.

III. ANTIBODY-MEDIATED (HUMORAL) IMMUNITY.

When the infectious agent is not quickly eliminated by nonspecific mechanisms, it proliferates and is eventually taken up by tissue macrophages in the regional lymphoid tissues, activating specific immune responses. One of the consequences is the synthesis of specific antibodies; the IgM isotype is produced first, followed by IgG, IgA, or both. While IgG is the predominant antibody in the circulation, IgA predominates on mucosal surfaces.

A. Protective mechanisms.

As soon as specific antibodies become available, they protect the organism against infection by several different mechanisms:

1. **Elimination of the infecting organism** can be achieved by three basic mechanisms: direct damage to the cell wall mediated by complement, promotion of phagocytosis, or recruitment of cytotoxic cells.

   a. **Complement-mediated lysis.** Complement-fixing antibodies (i.e., IgG, IgM) can promote the lysis of a microorganism through the activation of the complete sequence of complement, until insertion of the **membrane-attack complex (MAC)** on the cell membrane causes its disruption. The MAC is a complex formed by complement components 7 through 9. Insertion of the MAC on a cell membrane leads to osmotic lysis of the cell.

   (1) **Bacteria.** This mechanism appears to be very important to eliminate bacteria of the genus *Neisseria,* but in general bacteria are resistant to complement lysis because of their complex capsules.

   (2) **Viruses**

   (a) Enveloped viruses could lose their infectiousness if the integrity of the envelope was damaged as a consequence of complement activation, but whether antibodies are able to protect against viral infection by this mechanism has not been demonstrated.

   (b) Complement-fixing antibodies could also play a role in the elimination of viruses by destroying viral-infected cells. However, mammalian cells are highly resistant to complement-mediated lysis.

(3) **Parasites,** in general, are not affected directly by the complement system.

b. **Opsonization.** Antibodies promote phagocytosis through Fc or C3b receptors, or both. Phagocytic cells (neutrophils, macrophages) have FcRg, FcRa, and CR1 (C3b) receptors. Of these, FcRg and CR1 are most effective as mediators of opsonization under physiologic conditions.

(1) **Opsonins**

(a) **IgG antibodies** are the most effective opsonins, because they can promote phagocytosis in the presence or absence of complement. In contrast, **IgM antibodies** can only promote opsonization through C3b receptors, after activation of the complement system.

(b) **IgA** also functions as a weak opsonin.

(2) Killing through opsonization is probably the most important defense mechanism triggered by specific antibodies. It has been demonstrated to be **effective for the elimination of bacteria, fungi,** and **viruses;** however, phagocytosis of antibody- or complement-coated unicellular parasites has not been clearly demonstrated.

c. **Antibody-dependent cellular cytotoxicity (ADCC).** Antibodies of the IgG1, IgG3, and IgE isotypes can target infectious agents and cells modified as a consequence of intracellular infection, promoting their destruction via a variety of cells with Fc receptors:

(1) **Large granular lymphocytes (K cells)** are the most common effector cells in ADCC, particularly when the targets are virus-infected cells.

(2) **Eosinophils** play the principal role in cytotoxic reactions when parasitic infections are involved. Parasite killing is mostly mediated by the release of a **major basic protein** that has well documented toxic effects on parasites.

2. **Inhibition of attachment to mucosal cells. IgA,** the primary antibody in secretions of the respiratory and gastrointestinal tracts, imparts immunity to the mucosal surfaces. IgA prevents mucosal colonization, the first step in many infectious processes, by blocking, directly or indirectly, the interactions between microbial adhesion molecules or surface glycoproteins and the mucosal cell receptors.

3. **Toxin neutralization.** Many bacteria release exotoxins, which are often the major virulence factors responsible for human disease.

a. Antibodies to these toxins **prevent the binding of the toxins to their cellular receptors** by blocking the interaction between the toxin and its cellular receptor.

b. The toxin and antitoxin antibody form an immune complex, which is quickly removed from the circulation and degraded by phagocytic cells.

4. **Virus neutralization.** Viruses can be prevented from infecting their target cells (i.e., neutralized) by preformed antibodies that react with surface glycoproteins (e.g., capsid spikes or envelope glycoproteins).

a. It was originally believed that neutralization depended on blocking the interactions between viruses and their receptors. However, it has been proven that very few antibody molecules are required to neutralize a single viral particle (in some cases, a single antibody molecule is sufficient).

b. Most likely, neutralizing antibodies cause conformational changes in the viral capsid or envelope, impairing interaction with the cellular receptor or preventing the release of viral nucleic acid into the cell (if the particle is endocytosed).

B. Primary versus anamnestic responses

1. **Primary response.** Although antibodies are extremely effective as anti-infectious effector mechanisms, their protective role is somewhat limited by the time required between exposure to the infectious organism and synthesis of protective antibody, which for most primary immune responses is **approximately 1 week.**

2. **Anamnestic response.** If the relevant antibodies are present in the circulation, either as a result of vaccination, previous infection, or cross-reaction between different microorganisms, protection is most effective–- the microorganism or its toxins will be neutralized almost immediately and the infection will remain subclinical.

a. For protection against infections with very short incubation periods (such as influenza), it is essential to maintain protective levels of neutralizing antibody by means of frequent boosters.

b. For most infections, once immunologic memory has been acquired, antibody synthesis is sufficiently rapid to protect against subsequent exposures. Natural exposures act as natural booster doses, explaining the immunity for life associated with some common viral infections.

c. Cross-reactive antibodies. Circulating preformed antibodies may react with more than one microorganism when the microorganisms share similar antigenic determinants.

(1) Cross-reactive antibodies were historically designated **natural antibodies** because they were detectable prior to a known exposure to the infectious agent against which they appeared to be directed. Their anti-infectious protective role has been well documented in laboratory animals.

(2) Cross-reactive antibodies are often directed against polysaccharides, which have a similar structure across different microbial species, genera, and families.

IV. CELL-MEDIATED IMMUNITY (CMI)

IV. CELL-MEDIATED IMMUNITY (CMI) is essential for the elimination of intracellular pathogens, which are shielded from specific antibodies. The significance of CMI as a protective mechanism against intracellular infections is reflected in the frequency and severity of intracellular infections in patients with congenital CMI deficiencies.

A. Protective mechanisms. CMI may involve the killing of infected cells, as is the case in viral infections, or the activation of microbicidal mechanisms in the infected cells, as seems to be the case in infections with bacteria or unicellular parasites.

1. Cytotoxicity. Cytotoxic **T lymphocytes** are the main effector cells involved in the elimination of **virus-infected cells.**

a. Virus-infected cells express viral-derived peptides in association with their major histocompatibility complex (MHC) molecules. These peptides modify the self MHC molecules until they are recognized as non-self by the immune system. Cytotoxic T lymphocytes that recognize the modified MHC differentiate during the immune response and eventually destroy the infected cells.

b. Because of the involvement of T lymphocytes in the elimination of viral-infected cells, lymphocytic infiltration in the viral-infected tissues and lymphocytosis in the peripheral blood are indicative of a viral etiology for the infectious process.

2. Macrophage activation. In many cases of intracellular infection, the cells predominantly affected are tissue macrophages. A state of relative inactivity on the part of the macrophage, combined with mechanisms that allow the infectious agent to escape proteolytic digestion (e.g., capsules; see Chapter 7 II C) allow the infection to persist. Generalized stimulation of the reactions associated with intracellular killing is believed to be the mechanism leading to the elimination of **intracellular bacteria** and **parasites.**

a. Role of helper T lymphocytes. When helper T lymphocytes recognize microbial peptides associated with MHC-II molecules on the cell membranes of infected cells, they become activated and release a variety of cytokines. Of particular significance is the release of **IFN-γ,** which activates macrophages.

b. Activated macrophages produce higher concentrations of proteolytic enzymes and nitric oxide and have more energetic respiratory bursts after ingestion of opsonized particles. Intracellular organisms are effectively killed after activation of infected macrophages with IFN-γ.

B. TH_1 versus TH_2 responses. Differentiated helper T cells can be subclassified according to their functional properties.

1. T helper subsets

a. The **TH_1 subset** is predominantly involved in the potentiation of CMI. This subset releases primarily interleukin 2 (IL-2), IFN-γ, granulocyte-monocyte colony stimulating factor (GM-CSF), and tumor necrosis factor-β (TNF-β, lymphotoxin).

(1) IL-2 and IFN-γ activate macrophages, cytotoxic T lymphocytes, and NK cells.

(2) GM-CSF is an important promoter of cellular inflammation.

(3) TNF-β is directly toxic to altered cells.

b. The **TH_2 subset** primarily controls the magnitude and characteristics of the humoral immune response. This subset releases interleukins 4, 5, and 10.

(1) **IL-4** and **IL-5** are primarily involved in promoting the differentiation of activated B lymphocytes; therefore, they determine the magnitude of the response and the relative proportions of antibodies of different isotypes.

(2) **IL-10** down-regulates T lymphocytes and inflammatory cells in general.

2. The **regulation of TH_1 and TH_2 activity** is rather complex and involves macrophages and the two T helper subsets, which have regulatory effects on each other (Figure 8-1).

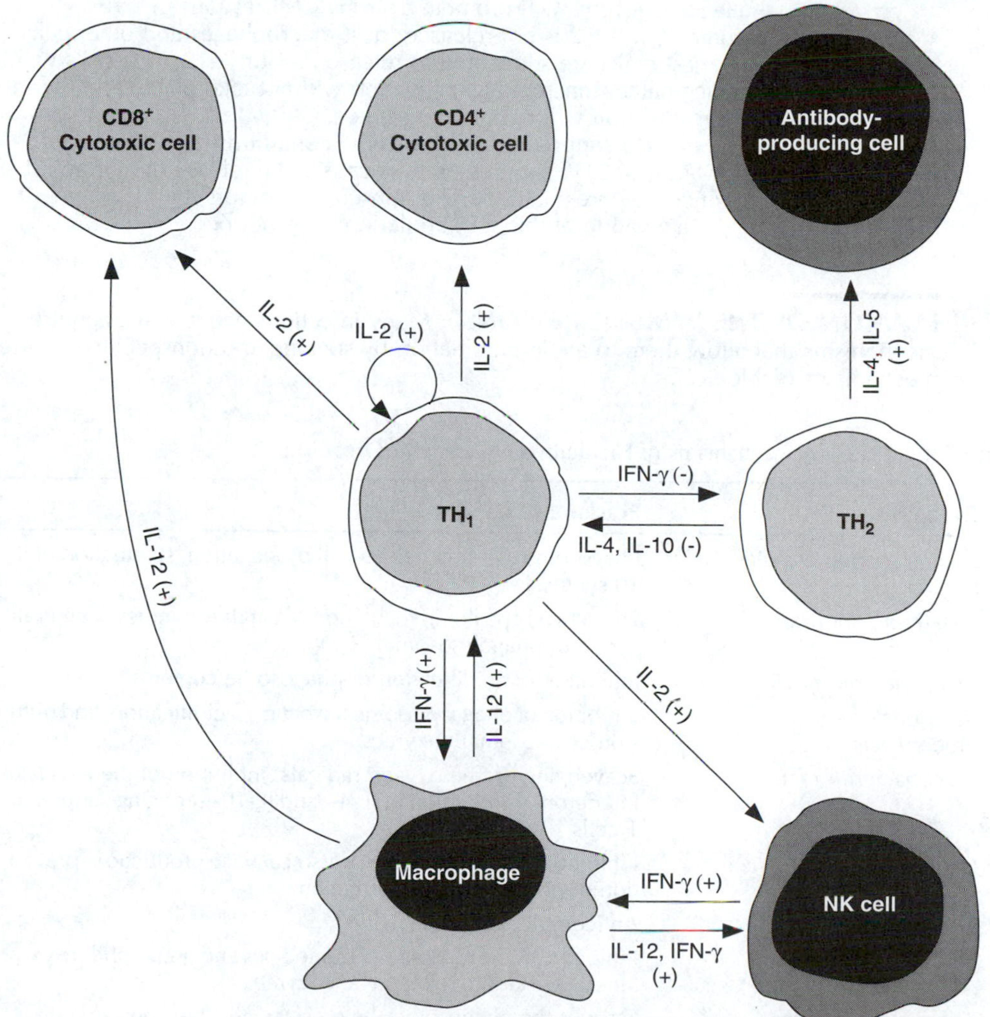

FIGURE 8-1. The regulation and effector functions of the TH_1 and TH_2 subsets of helper T lymphocytes. *IFN-α* = interferon-α; *IFN-γ* = interferon-γ; *IL-2, IL-4, IL-5, IL-10*, and *IL-12* = interleukins 2, 4, 5, 10, and 12 respectively; *NK* = natural killer; + = upregulates; - = downregulates.

a. Macrophages provide an activation signal to TH_1 cells through interleukin-12 (IL-12). Therefore, there is a mutual upregulatory circuit between these two types of cells.

b. TH_1 cells "turn off" TH_2 cells through the release of IFN-γ, while TH_2 cells "turn off" TH_1 cells by means of IL-4 and IL-10. Consequently, one of the subpopulations is always likely to predominate over the other one.

3. Determination of immune response. The effectiveness of a cell-mediated response required for the elimination of an intracellular infection depends on the dominance of an active TH_1 subpopulation. In many cases of persistent intracellular infection, the predominant immune response is TH_2-driven, as reflected by the synthesis of high concentrations of ineffective antibodies. Several factors may influence the final balance:

a. Antigen load. It is believed that a low antigen load favors TH_1 responses, whereas a high antigen load favors TH_2 responses.

b. Initial macrophage response. How microorganisms influence the pattern of cytokine synthesis by macrophages is unknown.

(1) If the initial infection is associated with IL-12 release, the differentiation of TH_1 lymphocytes will be potentiated and NK cell activity enhanced; at the same time, IL-12 down-regulates the differentiation of TH_2 cells. This sequence of events will promote a strong CMI response.

(2) In contrast, if IL-12 is not released, or if macrophages and other cells (e.g., mast cells) are stimulated to release IL-4 or IL-10, TH_1 cells will be downregulated, macrophage activation will not take place, and the intracellular infection will remain unchecked.

c. Activation of CD8 suppressor cells. In some conditions (e.g., lepromatous leprosy), activation of CD8 suppressor cells causes the release of IL-4 and IL-10, both of which downregulate the TH_1 subset. The factors that determine the preferential activation of this subpopulation have not been well defined.

V. EVASION OF THE IMMUNE RESPONSE.

Many infectious agents have acquired mechanisms that allow them to avoid elimination by specific and nonspecific defense mechanisms (Table 8-2).

TABLE 8-2. Evasion Mechanisms of Facultative Intracellular Organisms

Organism	Evasion Mechanism
Listeria monocytogenes	Phagosome evasion, cell-to-cell propagation, stimulation of IL-10 synthesis
Neisseria gonorrhoeae	Protective capsule, upregulation of catalase synthesis, neutralization of phagolysosomal H_2O_2
Mycobacterium avium	Inhibition of acidification of phagosome contents
Mycobacterium tuberculosis	Inhibition of phagolysosome formation, acidification, and diffusion of lysosomal enzymes
Mycobacterium leprae	Scavenging of free oxygen radicals, inhibition of the effects of interferon-γ; induction of IL-4– and IL-10–secreting suppressor T cells
Legionella pneumophila	Inhibition of the respiratory burst, catalase production, prevention of phagolysosome formation
Yersinia pestis	Anticomplementary activity
Leishmania	Inhibition of the response of monocytes and neutrophils to cytokines, resistant to proteolytic enzymes
Trypanosoma cruzi	Escapes the phagosomes before fusion of lysosomes
Toxoplasma gondii	Inhibition of phagolysosome formation

H_2O_2 = hydrogen peroxide; IL-4 = interleukin-4; IL-10 = interleukin-10.

A. **Antiphagocytic capsules** are frequently found in human pathogenic bacteria, both Gram-positive and Gram-negative, as well as in some yeasts. These capsules may prevent phagocytosis or they may protect ingested bacteria from proteolytic enzymes. The inhibition of phagocytosis may be related to:

1. **Charge effects** that repel phagocytic cells
2. **Poor immunogenicity** (polysaccharide capsules tend to be T-independent antigens that elicit immune responses in which IgM, a relatively ineffective opsonin, predominates)
3. **Anticomplementary activity** (see V B)

B. **Anticomplementary activity** has been characterized for bacterial capsules and outer proteins of some bacteria. For example:

1. **M protein,** found in group A *Streptococcus,* inactivates complement convertases, preventing activation of the alternative pathway.
2. **PLa protease** of *Yersinia pestis* cleaves C3 and probably C5a, reducing the release of this chemotactic fragment.

C. **Avoidance of intracellular digestion** is an escape mechanism shared by bacteria, viruses, and parasites.

1. The microorganism may secrete molecules that prevent the formation of functional phagolysosomes. This strategy allows the microorganism to survive inside phagosomes with low levels of antimicrobial compounds.
2. The microorganism may synthesize an outer coat or enzymes that protect it from proteolytic enzymes and free toxic radicals (e.g., superoxide radicals).
3. The microorganism may move rapidly from the phagosome into the cytoplasm, where it is protected from the respiratory burst and large concentrations of proteolytic enzymes.
4. The microorganism may synthesize compounds that neutralize the activating effects of IFN-γ.

D. **Direct cell-to-cell propagation** has been observed both with some intracellular bacteria (e.g., *Listeria*) and with a variety of viruses (e.g., herpes viruses, paramyxoviruses, human immunodeficiency virus). By moving directly from cell to cell, microorganisms are able to escape the effects of antiviral antibodies.

E. **Interference with the expression of MHC molecules** on the membranes of infected cells has been demonstrated with some intracellular organisms, particularly viruses. Interference with the expression of MHC molecules prevents or diminishes the recognition of infected cells by the immune system.

F. **Antigenic variation** has been characterized in bacteria (e.g., *Salmonella typhimurium, Borrelia recurrentis*), parasites (e.g., trypanosomes, *Giardia lamblia*), and viruses (e.g., HIV).

1. One of the major antigenic components in ***Salmonella typhimurium*** are the flagella. This bacteria has developed a system of antigenic variation, known as **phase variation,** that allows it to switch between different types of flagella (H1 and H2).
   a. The gene responsible for H2 flagellin synthesis is adjacent to a 970-bp promoter segment of DNA (*hin*), which can exist in two orientations (Figure 8-2).
   b. Included in the operon is a repressor gene (*rh1*), located 3′ to the H2 flagellin. The *rh1* gene encodes a protein that specifically represses the transcription of the H1 flagellin gene. Consequently, when the H2 gene is expressed, both H2 flagellin and the rh1 protein are synthesized; H1 flagellin is repressed and the phenotype of the bacterium is H2.

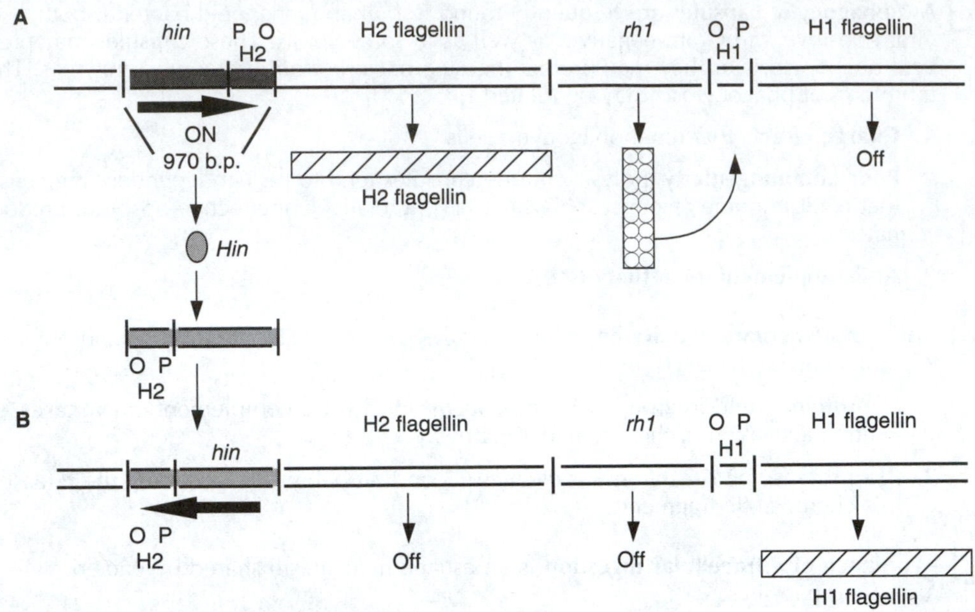

FIGURE 8-2. Control of flagellar phase variation in *Salmonella typhimurium.* Phase variation is the term used to describe a switch between two serological forms. (*A*) A promoter (*P*) and operator (*O*) immediately downstream of the H inversion gene (*hin*) are accessible and transcribed. As a result, H2 flagellin protein and the rh1 protein are produced and the H1 flagellin gene is repressed. (*B*) The orientation of the 970-base pair (bp) *hin* gene as well as the promoter and operator of the H2 flagellin gene have been inverted through the action of *Hin.* In the alternate orientation shown in panel *B*, the H2 flagellin as well as the repressor of the H1 flagellin gene (*rh1*) are off. Consequently, the operator of the H1 flagellin gene is open and the promoter is accessible to RNA polymerase, resulting in the synthesis of H1 flagellin.

c. On average, every 10^{-4} cell divisions the Hin protein is translated, resulting in the inversion of the promoter coding sequence. When the orientation of the promoter is inverted, it loses its function and the genes encoding for H2 flagellin and the repressor for the H1 gene (rh1 protein) are not expressed. Under these conditions, H1 flagellin is synthesized and the bacterium changes its phenotype accordingly.

2. Bacteria of the genus *Borrelia* change their antigenic membrane proteins by sequentially activating a pool of at least 26 genes that code for what is termed the **variable major proteins.** The genes of the pool are sequentially activated by duplicative transposition to an expression site, allowing the emergence of new mutants that can proliferate unchecked until antibodies are formed. The successive waves of bacteremia and fever correspond to the emergence of new mutants.

3. Sleeping sickness is caused by protozoa known as trypanosomes. Trypanosomes cause a chronic infection in spite of an energetic humoral immune response directed against the surface coat of the parasite, which consists mainly of a single glycoprotein.

a. The parasite is able to evade the immune response because only one of approximately 10^3 genes in the chromosome codes for the single protein. For every 10^6 or 10^7 trypanosome divisions, a mutation occurs that leads to the replacement of the active gene on the expression site with a previously silent gene. The new gene codes for an antigenically distinct glycoprotein that allows the mutant strain to proliferate unchecked for a period of time.

b. As antibodies emerge to the second glycoprotein, parasitemia declines, only to increase as soon as a new mutation occurs and a third glycoprotein is synthesized.

4. Malaria is caused by intracellular parasites known as plasmodia that primarily infect erythrocytes. One of the most severe forms of the disease is caused by *Plasmodium falciparum.*

a. The immune response of the host is directed against a parasite protein inserted in the membrane of parasite-infested erythrocytes. However, by periodically switching the gene that codes for that protein, *P. falciparum* manages to evade the immune response.
b. This ability to change antigenic determinants is why patients who appear to be cured often undergo relapses of the disease.

G. **Interference with the immune response** is a common mechanism of escape with many different variations.

1. **Interference with the inductive stages of the immune response.** Some intracellular bacteria and multicellular parasites interfere with the induction of CMI by disturbing immunoregulatory circuits.
2. **Interference with immune effector mechanisms**
   a. The synthesis of ineffective antibodies, known as **blocking factors,** prevents the recognition of the infectious agent by more effective effector systems. This mechanism is believed to be involved in the pathogenesis of meningococcal meningitis and of persistent viral infections. Sera from patients with meningitis contain large amounts of non–complement-fixing IgA antibodies that fail to show bactericidal activity.
   b. Schistosomes have multiple mechanisms of evasion, including stimulation of suppressor monocytes, down-regulation of surface protein expression, and adsorption of host proteins to their external surface. The last two mechanisms prevent proper recognition by antischistosomal antibodies.

Chapter 9

Immunoprophylaxis

Gabriel Virella

I. INTRODUCTION.

INTRODUCTION. Immunoprophylaxis is the active elicitation of immune responses with the aim of inducing protection against the subsequent development of an infectious disease. Together with improved sanitation, immunoprophylaxis has greatly contributed to a marked decrease in the frequency of infectious diseases, best exemplified by the worldwide eradication of smallpox.

II. HISTORY.

A. Lady Montagu. Variolation (i.e., the introduction of powdered smallpox scab material into healthy individuals via intradermal scarification) had been practiced in China as early as the 6th century B.C. and was introduced in Europe in the 1720s by Lady Montagu, who had observed the practice while living in Turkey. Variolation was a rather unreliable and accident-prone practice, but its introduction in England certainly constituted an important step toward the development of the first successful vaccine.

B. Jenner observed that milkmaids who had contracted a mild, pox-forming disease from infected cows were apparently immune to smallpox. As a consequence of these observations, Jenner introduced a cowpox vaccination in 1796. (The term **vaccination,** which refers to the intradermal scarification of material from cowpox lesions, is derived from the Latin word for cow, *vacca.*) Vaccination proved to be safer and more efficient than variolation.

C. Pasteur. The career of this illustrious French chemist was punctuated with brilliant triumphs in the area of immunoprophylaxis.

1. In 1879, he developed a vaccine that prevented fowl cholera using old cultures of cholera bacilli that had lost virulence.
2. In 1881, he introduced an attenuated vaccine that prevented anthrax in animals.
3. In 1885, he successfully immunized Joseph Meister against rabies using extracts of spinal cord from infected rabbits.

D. The discovery of diphtheria toxin by **Roux** and **Yersin** in the late 1890s was followed by the discovery of a chemical means of reducing the toxin's toxicity while preserving its immunogenicity. Soon thereafter, **Von Behring** and **Kitasato** used the attenuated toxins **(toxoids)** to produce antitoxins in horses, which were then used to protect patients from the infection **(passive immunization).** Tetanus and diphtheria toxoids, safe for human use and among the most effective vaccines available, were eventually developed and introduced for **active immunization.**

E. Calmette and **Guérin** developed a vaccine using an attenuated strain of *Mycobacterium bovis* to counteract tuberculosis in 1921.

F.

Sabin introduced an oral polio vaccine in the late 1950s that demonstrated once and for all the safety of mass immunizations with an attenuated virus.

III. TYPES OF VACCINES

A. Killed (inactivated) vaccines

1. **Bacterial.** Pertussis vaccine, prepared with killed *Bordetella pertussis,* the etiologic agent of whooping cough, is the prototypical killed vaccine. Other examples of killed bacterial vaccines include the typhoid vaccine prepared with acetone-inactivated *Salmonella typhi,* which is only 50%–70% effective, and the old cholera vaccines, also of limited effectiveness.

2. **Viral**
   a. The **influenza vaccine** is one of the most widely used inactivated viral vaccines. It contains one or two type A strains and one type B strain of influenza virus. Because of changes in the antigenic composition of the type A virus, the vaccine has to be reformulated annually to include the strains most likely to spread amongst the population (see Chapter 34).
   b. The killed **polio vaccine (Salk vaccine)** is prepared by mixing the three known types of poliovirus after inactivation with formalin. This effective vaccine has been used successfully for mass vaccination in several countries and is the preferred polio vaccine for immunocompromised children (see Chapter 33 II A 5).
   c. Killed **HIV vaccines** have been tested, both with preventative and therapeutic goals in mind. At this time, there has been no conclusive evidence supporting the efficacy of killed HIV vaccines as inducers of protective immunity. On the other hand, killed HIV vaccine is still being evaluated in HIV-infected patients to determine whether boosting immunity prior to the onset of AIDS can be beneficial (see chapter 57).

B. Attenuated (mutant) vaccines

1. **Bacterial.** As a consequence of recent developments in molecular genetics, attenuated bacterial strains are being developed for use in immunoprophylaxis. Usually the mutant strains lack the genes coding for critical virulence factors, but remain highly immunogenic.
   a. For example, a new **typhoid vaccine** has been developed based on the use of an attenuated strain that grows poorly and is virtually nonpathogenic. Vaccination with this strain induces protective immunity in 90% of patients.
   b. An experimental **vaccine for whooping cough** is based on genetically engineered *Bordetella* strains that contain mutant genes for the pertussis toxin. These genes code for molecules that are immunogenic but not toxic.

2. **Viral.** Attenuated viral vaccines, as noted in the introduction, were the first vaccines developed, well before viruses had been characterized.
   a. The **yellow fever vaccine,** introduced in the late 1930s, was developed using empirical approaches, although viruses had been roughly characterized by this time.
   b. **Sabin's oral polio vaccine** was the first attenuated viral vaccine successfully developed on a scientific basis, and the first to use the oral route for immunization. This vaccine is a mixture of attenuated strains of the three known types of poliovirus.
   c. Other attenuated viral vaccines in current use include vaccines against **mumps, rubella, measles,** and **chickenpox.**

C. Component vaccines

1. **Bacterial**
   a. **Polysaccharides** are used as vaccines against *Streptococcus pneumoniae, Neisseria meningitidis,* and *Haemophilus influenzae* type B. The main problems that arise with polysaccharide vaccines are related either to antigenic variation or to the poor immunogenicity of some polysaccharides.
   b. **Toxoids** are inactivated toxins that have lost their active site but have maintained their immunogenic determinants. Administration of the toxoid induces the produc-

tion of antibodies capable of neutralizing the toxins by blocking their adsorption to cellular receptors.

(1) Both **tetanus** and **diphtheria toxoids** are effective immunogens that induce long-lasting protection.

(2) Other toxoid vaccines are being tested. For example, ***Clostridium perfringens* type C toxoid** has been successfully used to prevent clostridial enteritis in New Guinea.

c. **Toxoid–polysaccharide conjugates.** In some cases (e.g., *H. influenzae* vaccine), immunogenicity is greatly enhanced if the polysaccharide is conjugated to a toxoid of known safety and immunogenicity, such as diphtheria toxoid.

(1) Although polysaccharides tend to elicit T-independent responses with little or no memory, the toxoid–polysaccharide conjugates behave in a sense like hapten-carrier conjugates. The response to both components is strong, T-dependent, and anamnestic, with memory provided by the carrier (toxoid).

(2) These hybrid vaccines are recommended for routine immunization of infants.

d. **Mixed component (acellular) vaccines** consist of inactivated toxin, a major determinant of clinical disease, and one or several adhesion factors, which mediate attachment to mucosal epithelial cells. Currently, several acellular vaccines are being evaluated for use against whooping cough (see Chapter 15).

2. **Viral.** The **hepatitis B vaccine** is the best example of a viral component vaccine. Originally, this vaccine was prepared with particles of the hepatitis virus outer coat protein **[hepatitis B surface antigen (HBsAg)]** isolated from the serum of chronic carriers. Currently, it is prepared with HBsAg produced by recombinant yeast cells transfected with plasmid constructs containing the gene coding for HBsAg flanked by promoter and terminator sequences. The transfected yeast cells produce large amounts of HBsAg, which is harvested by disrupting the recombinant yeast cells and purified by chromatography.

D. **Recombinant vaccines.** The ability to identify virulence mechanisms and manipulate bacterial and viral genomes has resulted in the emergence of a totally new class of vaccines, opening the door for multiple immunizations using a single construct. In recombinant vaccines, information coding for relevant antigens of unrelated viruses or bacteria is added to the genome of a carrier (vector) organism.

1. **Recombinant vaccinia viruses.** The vaccinia virus has a rather large genome, allowing the preparation of constructs carrying multiple genes. A major problem with the use of a recombinant vaccinia virus is the fact that this virus can be pathogenic in immunocompromised individuals.

2. **Attenuated bacteria** (e.g., *Salmonella*) are being investigated as vectors for recombinant vaccines. Constructs expressing hepatitis B nucleocapsid proteins or a nontoxic domain of the tetanus toxin have been tested in experimental animals and can induce double protection (i.e., against hepatitis B and tetanus).

3. **Insect viruses** (e.g., baculovirus) are also being considered as possible vectors. For example, a baculovirus expressing a nucleoprotein from a strain of influenza virus has been shown to induce protective cell-mediated immunity (CMI) in mice.

E. **Synthetic oligopeptide vaccines.** Development of synthetic vaccines focuses on the synthesis of peptide sequences corresponding to known epitopes recognized by neutralizing antibodies.

1. The use of synthetic peptides for vaccination has the advantages of easy manufacture and safety; however, this theoretically appealing concept meets with **two basic problems:**

a. It is questionable that a synthetic oligopeptide has the same tertiary configuration as the epitope expressed by the native antigen.

b. Small synthetic peptides are poorly immunogenic. This problem can be solved by injecting peptide–protein conjugates (e.g., tetanus toxoid) with a potent (but not toxic) adjuvant.

2. Currently, the use of peptide synthesis is being investigated as a way to develop vaccines against malaria and HIV.
   a. **Malaria.** Results obtained with a peptide-based vaccine against *Plasmodium falciparum* appear promising. A multirepeat region of the circumsporozoite protein, identified as the immunodominant B-cell epitope, is being used as a model for the vaccine.
   b. **HIV.** Considerable interest exists in the development of peptide vaccines against HIV. The principal neutralizing epitope of the virus is located on a variable domain, which precludes its successful use as the basis for a peptide vaccine. Efforts are underway to identify other epitopes that may induce protective cellular responses.

F. **DNA vaccines.** It has recently been reported that intramuscular injection of nonreplicating plasmid DNA encoding the hemagglutinin or nucleoprotein of the influenza virus elicits humoral and cellular protective reactions. It is not understood how DNA becomes expressed and its message translated into viral proteins, but the positive results obtained in this experiment have raised enormous interest in the scientific community.

IV. VACCINES AS IMMUNOTHERAPEUTIC AGENTS.

The use of vaccines to stimulate the immune system as therapy for chronic or latent infections is receiving considerable interest. Four areas of application have emerged:

TABLE 9-1. Recommended Schedule for Active Immunization of Healthy Infants and Children

Age	Recommended Immunization(s)	Comments
Birth	HepB	
2 months	DTP, OPV, HepB, HiB*	Can be initiated at 4 weeks of age in areas of high endemicity or during epidemics
4 months	DTP, OPV, HiB	2-month interval desired for OPV to avoid interference from previous dose
6 months	DTP, HiB	
6–18 months	HepB, OPV	
12–15 months	HiB†, MMR Varicella-Zoster virus‡	MMR vaccine is preferable to individual vaccines; tuberculin test is also indicated at this age
15–18 months	DTP or DTaP	
4–6 years	DTP or DtaP, OPV	At or before school entry
11–12 years	MMR Varicella-Zoster virus‡‡	MMR should be given at entry to middle school or junior high school unless two doses were given after the first birthday
14–16 years	Tetanus toxoid booster	Repeat every 10 years

Updated from the 1994 edition of the *Report of the Committee on Infectious Diseases* published by the American Academy of Pediatrics.

DTaP = diphtheria–tetanus–acellular pertussis vaccine; DTP = diphtheria–tetanus–pertussis vaccine; HepB = hepatitis B vaccine; HiB = conjugated *Haemophilus influenzae* vaccine; MMR = measles–mumps–rubella vaccine; OPV = oral polio vaccine.

* HiB is *Haemophilus influenzae* phosphoribosylribitol phosphate (PRP) conjugated with diphtheria toxoid or some other adequate carrier protein.

† The 12–15-month administration of HiB may not be necessary, depending on the actual vaccine used.

‡ To all children, from 12–18 months of age.

‡‡ To unvaccinated children without history of chickenpox.

A. Herpes virus infections, in which vaccination seems to reduce the rate of recurrence

B. Leprosy, in which administration of bacille Calmette-Guérin (BCG) seems to potentiate the effects of chemotherapy

C. Tuberculosis, in which a new vaccine made of killed *Mycobacterium vaccae* seems to potentiate the effects of antibacterial agents, even in patients resistant to therapy

D. HIV infection, in which vaccination with killed HIV may alter the TH_1:TH_2 balance in favor of TH_1 cells, which are more effective mediators of anti-HIV responses

V. IMMUNIZATION SCHEDULES.

Table 9-1 summarizes the recommended schedule for active immunization of normal infants and children.

PART III

CLINICAL BACTERIOLOGY

Chapter 10

Laboratory Diagnosis of Bacterial Infections

Lisa L. Steed
Gabriel Virella

I. INTRODUCTION. In order to properly execute antibacterial therapy, it is necessary to definitively identify the causative organism.

II. MICROSCOPIC EXAMINATION OF PATIENT SPECIMENS. Direct techniques, such as those that follow, provide clinically useful information within 4 hours of specimen receipt.

A. Staining is the classic approach to rapid diagnosis. The requirements are relatively simple: an adequate specimen, glass slides, staining and destaining solutions, and a microscope. Precise identification of the pathogen is usually not possible, but the morphologic and staining properties of the visualized organism reduce the list of probable etiologies and provide a more solid basis for empirical antimicrobial therapy.

1. **Common stains** include **Gram stain** (see Chapter 2 III A 1), **acid-fast stain** (see Chapter 2 A 2), **iodine stain,** and **Giemsa stain.**
2. **Fluorescent dyes (fluorochromes),** which cause microorganisms to brilliantly fluoresce against a dark background when examined under a fluorescent microscope, are useful for quickly scanning patient specimens for yeast and bacteria. Microbes stained with fluorochromes are more easily seen than traditionally-stained organisms, which may be the same color as host cells and organic debris.
   a. **Commonly used fluorochromes**
      (1) **Acridine orange,** which binds nucleic acid in bacteria and yeast
      (2) **Auramine rhodamine,** which binds mycolic acid in mycobacterial cell walls
      (3) **Calcofluor white,** which binds cellulose in fungal cell walls
   b. If necessary, acridine orange- and auramine rhodamine-stained slides can be counter-stained with Gram stain or with an acid-fast stain.

B. Darkfield examination employs a microscope that illuminates the object over a dark background. The light that reaches the eye is scattered from the object on the microscope stage, while directly transmitted light is excluded by a darkfield condenser. This method allows visualization of unstained organisms.

1. **Uses.** This technique is used extensively to identify **spirochetes,** which are too thin to be seen by staining.
2. **Limitations** of this test include the need for experienced personnel to perform the test and the need for a darkfield microscope. For these reasons, darkfield examination is available only at county and state health departments.

C. Direct immunofluorescence. Fluorescein-labeled monoclonal or polyclonal antibodies against specific microbial antigens are added to a tissue or cell suspension, enabling the detection of specific microorganisms.

1. **Uses.** Direct immunofluorescence is used commonly to detect *Legionella pneumophila* and *Bordetella pertussis* in respiratory specimens, *Chlamydia trachomatis* in genital and conjunctival specimens, and several viruses.
2. **Limitations.** Direct immunofluorescence is a relatively simple staining technique, but the price of reagents and the need for a fluorescent microscope and experienced personnel to read the stains are limiting factors.

III. DETECTION OF PATHOGEN-SPECIFIC MACROMOLECULES

A. Detection of bacterial antigens. The following techniques are generally as specific as direct immunofluorescence and can be extremely simple and rapid to perform.

1. **Enzyme immunoassay (EIA).** Most EIA tests use antibodies adsorbed or cross-linked to a solid phase (e.g., a microtiter plate, a bead, or a membrane) to capture antigen in a liquid specimen. (An extract of a more solid specimen may also be used.) After the antigen has been bound by the immobilized antibody, an enzyme-labeled antibody of the same specificity is added to the reaction mixture, forming a "sandwich." Addition of a chromogenic enzyme substrate produces a visible end product if the first antibody has successfully captured the antigen.
   a. **Streptococcal pharyngitis.** EIA kits are available for the diagnosis of streptococcal pharyngitis. Such kits, which employ a pharyngeal swab, require 5–10 minutes to perform and is easy to use with minimal training; their sensitivity and specificity can be excellent (greater than 95%).
   b. Other EIA tests are used to detect *C. trachomatis, Clostridium difficile* toxins, and many viruses. Most of these tests require 10 minutes to 3 hours to perform.

2. **Particle agglutination**
   a. **Technique.** The reaction of soluble antigens with antibody-coated particles results in the cross-linking of the particles into easily visible aggregates. The Fc regions of IgG antibodies are bound by latex beads or by protein A in killed *Staphylococcus aureus,* so that the Fab regions remain available to recognize and bind antigens.
   b. **Clinical applications**
      (1) **Bacterial meningitis.** Latex agglutination test kits have been developed for the diagnosis of meningitis.
         (a) The kit consists of five bottles, each of which contains a suspension of latex particles coated with antibodies against one of the five most common causes of bacterial meningitis. A drop of cerebrospinal fluid (CSF) is mixed with a drop of each latex suspension; agglutination of one of the mixtures indicates the identity of the infecting agent in the patient from whom the CSF was obtained.
         (b) The sensitivity of the latex agglutination test for diagnosis of bacterial meningitis is equivalent to that of a well-executed Gram stain of the CSF sediment. However, latex agglutination may be useful in patients who have been partially treated with antibiotics and thus may have a falsely negative Gram stain.
      (2) Many agglutination tests are used for rapid **identification of organisms grown in culture.**

B. Detection of nucleic acid sequences

1. **Nucleic acid probe tests**
   a. **Technique.** DNA encoding for a specific ribosomal gene sequence is isolated and denatured to the single-stranded state to construct a complementary DNA (cDNA) that is used as a probe to detect ribosomal RNA (rRNA) in specimens. An instrument that measures chemiluminescence emitted by a molecule attached to the cDNA is used to detect the probe–target hybrid.
   b. **Limitations.** The major limitations of DNA hybridization are the need for expensive instrumentation and the cost of reagents. To reduce cost, it is necessary to test specimens in batches (rather than individually as they arrive in the laboratory). Thus, nucleic acid probe testing is unlikely to be available in physicians' offices.
   c. **Clinical applications.** Nucleic acid probe tests permit the rapid identification of bacteria in patient specimens or in cultures of microorganisms where isolation is problematic, such as *Neisseria gonorrhoeae* and *C. trachomatis* cultures. Sensitivity and specificity depend on the incidence of *N. gonorrhoeae* or *C. trachomatis* in the patient population being tested and the quality of the specimens collected.

2. Polymerase chain reaction (PCR)

a. Technique

(1) Two short DNA **primers** specific for the flanking regions of the DNA segment one wishes to identify, microbial DNA (which may or may not contain the target sequence), a heat-resistant polymerase (taq polymerase), and free nucleotides are mixed together. The primers and nucleotides are present in excess.

(2) The reaction mixture is put into a thermocycler, which raises and lowers the temperature to permit and regulate the three steps of PCR.

(a) First, the microbial DNA is denatured into single strands during a heat cycle with temperatures between 90°C and 95°C.

(b) As the mixture cools to approximately 50°C, the primers will anneal wherever they complement the target DNA strands. Their presence in large numbers ensures that hybridization with primers will take precedence over hybridization with the homologous strand.

(c) As the temperature rises to 72°C, the taq polymerase adds exogenous nucleotides to the primers, which have hybridized with each original DNA strand. Elongation, the addition of nucleotides in both the 5′ and 3′ direction, results in the duplication of the target sequence in each chromosome (i.e., four copies are obtained from the original two).

(3) Typically, this process is repeated as many as thirty times to produce millions of copies of the chosen section of target organism DNA. PCR is sensitive enough to detect one microorganism in a patient specimen.

b. Limitations. The sensitivity of PCR is one of the test's major limitations, because contamination with microbial DNA from the environment can lead to false-positive results. Other limitations include high equipment and reagent costs and the need for technical expertise.

c. Clinical applications. Only one assay is commercially available, a PCR-based test for ***C. trachomatis.*** However, if practical problems are solved, the exceptional sensitivity of PCR may prove invaluable in the diagnosis of many infectious diseases.

IV. CULTURE AND ISOLATION OF MICROORGANISMS.

Bacterial culture describes the isolation of bacterial strains from patient specimens and the identification of those strains by a combination of characteristics (e.g., growth, biochemical profile, reactivity with specific antisera). Cultures require a minimum of 18 hours of incubation before preliminary results are available; however, they should always be attempted, particularly when the patient is severely ill, when the diagnosis is not clear, or when a highly contagious agent is suspected. In addition, bacterial culture is currently the only practical approach for determining antibiotic susceptibilities.

A. Specimen collection

1. Factors to consider prior to collecting a specimen for culture include the method of testing for the target organism, the geographic location (including the possibility of foreign or domestic travel), the time of year, and the stage of the patient's illness. The stage of the patient's illness is an important consideration: there are more organisms present soon after the onset of symptoms (i.e., during the acute phase of the disease). Later in the disease course, when fewer organisms are present, serologic testing, rather than culture, may be the preferred technique for identifying the etiology of the disease.

2. Specimens should be chosen according to the highest likelihood of positive yield. For example, in a patient with pneumonia, a properly collected sputum sample

TABLE 10-1. Suggested Specimens for Culture (Major Infectious Diseases)

Suspected Disease	Specimen
Pharyngitis	Throat swab*
Pneumonia	Sputum, bronchoalveolar lavage fluid, pleural fluid, blood
Endocarditis	Blood
Upper urinary tract infection	Urine, blood
Lower urinary tract infection	Urine
Gastroenteritis, enterocolitis	Feces
Enteric fever	Feces, blood, bone marrow
Unexplained fever	Blood, urine, CSF
Osteomyelitis	Exudate, bone, blood
Meningitis	CSF, blood
Septic arthritis	Joint fluid, blood

CSF = cerebrospinal fluid.
* A calcium alginate swab should be used if diphtheria is suspected.

would be ideal. Table 10-1 summarizes ideal specimens for several common diseases.

3. **Specimens should always be collected before antimicrobial agents are administered** to avoid false-negative results.
4. **Collected specimens should be placed immediately in appropriate transport media,** chosen according to the bacteria considered to be most likely involved.
   a. If anaerobic organisms are suspected, aerobic and anaerobic transport vials should be seeded.
   b. Some organisms (e.g., *N. gonorrhoeae, B. pertussis*) should be inoculated onto media at the patient's side because they are extremely environmentally sensitive.

B. **Culture media.** Table 10-2 summarizes the culture medium of choice for several common bacteria.

1. **General purpose media** include **blood agar** and **chocolate agar.** Most organisms will grow on these two media; therefore, these agars are inoculated with all specimens except stools. Characteristics that can be determined from growth on blood and chocolate agars include colonial morphology, pigmentation, and red blood cell hemolysis (blood agar only).
   a. **Blood agar** contains intact sheep red blood cells.
   b. **Chocolate agar** contains red blood cells lysed by gentle heating, which releases nicotinamide adenine nucleotide (NAD, factor V) and hemin (factor X). A few organisms (e.g., *H. influenzae*) require these growth factors and are easily isolated on chocolate agar but not on blood agar.
2. **Special media**
   a. **Enrichment (nutrient) media** enhances the growth of desired organisms, rather than excluding undesirable one. **Chocolate agar** is an example of enrichment media.
   b. **Selective media** contain substances that inhibit the growth of bacteria other than the targeted organism(s). For example, **Thayer-Martin agar** (chocolate agar plus antibiotics) inhibits the growth of organisms normally found in the genitourinary tract, allowing *N. gonorrhoeae* to be isolated.
   c. **Differential media** allow the definition of specific biochemical properties of the target bacteria. For example, **MacConkey agar** grows most, but not all, Gram-negative bacilli and allows the classification of those that grow into lactose fermenters and lactose non-fermenters.
   d. **Anaerobic media** are nutritionally enriched and prereduced of molecular oxygen to enhance recovery of anaerobes from patient specimens.

TABLE 10-2. Culture Media for Common Bacteria

Medium	Type	Use	Crucial Components
Sheep blood agar	General purpose	Most medically significant bacteria	Sheep blood
Chocolate agar	General purpose, enrichment	Most medically significant bacteria plus *Haemophilus influenzae, Neisseria meningitidis**	Lysed sheep blood, hemoglobin
MacConkey agar	Selective (Gram-negative bacilli), differential (lactose fermenters)	Enterobacteriaceae	Crystal violet and bile salts to inhibit Gram-positive bacteria; neutral red as an indicator of lactose fermentation
Sheep blood agar with colistin and nalidixic acid	Selective	Gram-positive organisms	Colistin and nalidixic acid to inhibit Gram-negative bacteria
Thayer-Martin agar	Selective	*Neisseria gonorrhoeae*	Hemoglobin to enhance growth; four antimicrobial agents to inhibit contaminants
Charcoal yeast extract agar	Enrichment	*Legionella*	Charcoal, buffering agents, and three antimicrobial agents
Löwenstein-Jensen agar	Enrichment, selective	*Mycobacterium tuberculosis*	Eggs to enhance growth; malachite green inhibits contaminants

* All *Neisseria* species grow well on chocolate agar, but Thayer-Martin agar is preferred when specimens are likely to contain contaminating normal flora (vaginal exudates).

C. Identification. Bacteria can often be identified presumptively by growth characteristics on media and the results of biochemical tests. Most organisms require a battery of biochemical tests for identification purposes (e.g., carbohydrate utilization, indole production, urease production, phenylalanine deamination, nitrate reduction).

1. Media that allow determination of these properties are inoculated with a bacterial isolate and incubated for 18–24 hours.
   a. Identity of an isolate is established by consulting biochemical profile tables that list the reactions of different genera and species.
   b. End products of fermentative metabolism can be identified by gas–liquid chromatography, which reveals patterns characteristic of different genera or species.
2. Comparisons of characteristic chromatographic profiles of fermentative end products and cell wall fatty acids are used to identify anaerobic bacteria and mycobacteria, respectively.

D. Antimicrobial susceptibility testing. Culturing the organism provides an isolate that can be tested for susceptibility to antimicrobial agents. Isolation of organisms in pure culture is essential to determine antimicrobial agent susceptibilities.

V. SEROLOGIC TESTING is based on antibody detection in the host.

A. General considerations

1. In general, the diagnosis of an infectious disease based on the detection of specific antibody by serological tests has **two major limitations:**

a. Early in the evolution of the disease, the antibody titers may be undetectable, which nullifies the possibility of an early diagnosis.
b. If the serologic assay shows a raised antibody titer, it is often difficult to decide how that titer correlates with the patient's disease.

2. **Clinical applications.** There are several instances when the diagnosis of an infectious disease relies on serologic assays:
   a. When the agent is difficult to isolate (e.g., viral infections, Mycoplasma infections, syphilis)
   b. When the infection is deep-seated (e.g., brucellosis, tularemia, streptococcal osteomyelitis, pneumonia)
   c. To document prior infections (e.g., rheumatic fever, glomerulonephritis)

3. **Interpretation.** As a rule, proper diagnosis using a serologic assay requires the collection of **two blood specimens:** one during the acute phase of the disease and a second 2–3 weeks later (i.e., during convalescence). A significant increase in titer (i.e., fourfold or greater) between the two specimens, which are tested at the same time, is good evidence for exposure to the bacteria against which the antibodies are directed.

B. **Complement fixation tests** are the classic approach to infectious disease serologies. Complex in execution and control, many bacterial complement fixation tests have been replaced by EIAs and immunofluorescence. However, classic complement fixation tests are still very much in use for some fungal infections, many viral infections, and Q fever (caused by *Coxiella burnetii*).

C. **Flocculation tests** are based on the visual detection of large aggregates that form when a suspension of particulate antigen reacts with specific antibody present in the patient's serum. Classic flocculation tests include the **Venereal Disease Research Laboratory (VDRL)** and the **rapid plasma reagin (RPR)** tests for syphilis.

D. **Indirect immunofluorescence tests** use a fluorescein-labeled anti-human antibody to detect specific human antibodies bound to a known organism.

1. The **fluorescent treponemal antibody absorption** test **(FTA-ABS)** is widely used to confirm the results of the less specific screening assays, such as the VDRL or RPR tests discussed in V C.
2. Other commercially available indirect fluorescent antibody test kits are available for the detection of *L. pneumophila, Borrelia burgdorferi, Mycoplasma pneumoniae,* several rickettsiae, and a variety of viruses either in direct patient specimens or after cultivation. Limitations of this technique are the same as those of direct immunofluorescence testing (see II C).

E. **Immunodiffusion assays,** which are primarily used to detect fungal antibodies, have limited application to the diagnosis of bacterial infections.

Chapter 11

Normal Flora

Victor Del Bene

I. INTRODUCTION.

INTRODUCTION. Microscopic organisms are found in many areas of the human body. Generally, these organisms exist in harmony with their healthy carrier (i.e., they do not cause disease).

A. It is calculated that the population of normal bacterial flora in an adult is approximately 10^{14} bacterial cells. Most of these bacteria are anaerobic or facultative anaerobic organisms.

B. Certain yeasts (e.g., *Candida* species) are also part of the normal flora, but viruses and parasites are always considered pathogens.

C. In any given anatomical site where normal flora are found, one organism will always predominate. This balance between microbes tends to be stable in a given individual; it may vary with age, when antibacterial agents are given, or when there is a disruption of normal anatomic or physiologic function.

II. ROLE OF NORMAL FLORA

A. Infection resistance

1. **Occupation of binding sites.** The occupancy of binding sites on the surface of human body cells by harmless commensal bacteria prevents the attachment of pathogens to the same sites.
2. **Mucin secretion.** Many bacteria secrete mucins. In doing so, they lay down a mucous "blanket" that prevents attachment of pathogenic organisms.
3. **Secretion of noxious substances.** Normal flora secrete metabolic products that may be noxious to pathogenic bacteria. For example, the normal flora of the gut secrete a short-chain fatty acid that is inhibitory to *Salmonella* (i.e., an organism that causes enteritis). This mechanism is so effective that an oral inoculum of 10^6 *Salmonella* organisms is usually necessary to cause enteritis in a normal individual; however, if the normal flora is disturbed by the ingestion of antibiotics (even in small amounts), an oral inoculum of only 10^1 or 10^2 *Salmonella* organisms may be sufficient to cause enteritis.

B. Stimulation of the immune system. Normal flora, especially Gram-negative rods, are **strong immunogens.** Because of cross-reactivity between related bacteria, the antibodies produced in response to commensal organisms confer protection to the host from many pathogenic organisms.

C. Nutrient source. Members of the normal flora provide vitamin K, a cofactor essential for the synthesis of clotting factors II, VII, X, and XI. Without this contribution from the normal flora, the human clotting system would be grossly ineffective.

D. Stimulation of epithelial turnover. Without normal flora, the gut is atonic and thin.

III. NORMAL FLORA AS PATHOGENS

A. Opportunistic infection by organisms considered part of the normal flora is a common problem under certain conditions.

1. **Immunocompromised status.** If a patient is immunocompromised, either as a result of congenital defects, disease, or therapy, a wide variety of ordinarily harmless microorganisms can cause severe infections. A good example is the prevalence of mucosal candidiasis in AIDS patients.

2. **Antibacterial therapy.** Administration of broad-spectrum antibiotics can disturb the equilibrium of the normal flora, creating favorable circumstances for the overgrowth of pathogenic organisms or leading to the selection of antibiotic-resistant strains. Antibiotic-associated colitis caused by *Clostridium difficile* and mucosal infections caused by yeasts often follow antibiotic administration and disturbance of the normal flora.

3. **Penetrating trauma,** accidental or surgical, can facilitate the invasion of tissues by normal flora. Postoperative abdominal abscesses and posttraumatic peritonitis are common examples of infections acquired when the normal flora disseminate from their normal habitat.

B. Tissue invasion. Occasionally, products produced by bacteria that are part of the normal flora may lead to local tissue invasion. For example, *Streptococcus mutans,* a part of the normal flora in the oral cavity, causes dental caries by producing gelatinous deposits that allow acid-producing bacteria to adhere to the tooth enamel. The acid demineralizes the enamel, leading to the formation of caries.

C. Bacterial translocation is the passage of viable bacteria from the gastrointestinal tract through the epithelial mucosa into the splanchnic and systemic circulation.

1. **Predisposing factors**
   a. Translocation occurs primarily in situations of **splanchnic ischemia,** which can occur secondary to hemorrhagic shock or major burns.
   b. **Conditions that alter the normal flora of the gastrointestinal tract** (e.g., antibiotic administration) or that **slow intestinal transit** (e.g., total parenteral nutrition, administration of opiates) favor translocation.
   c. **Prematurity.** Newborns (particularly premature infants) seem prone to translocation. Abnormal permeability of the intestinal mucosa may be a contributing factor.
   d. Translocation is also common in critically ill patients that have reached the **preagonal stage.**

2. **Mechanism.** The mechanism responsible for translocation has not been clearly identified, but the prognosis in these patients once bacteremia develops is very poor.

IV. ANATOMIC LOCATION OF NORMAL FLORA.
The microorganisms that comprise the normal flora vary throughout the body (Figure 11-1).

A. Skin. There are approximately 10^4–10^5 organisms/cm^2 of skin, mostly Gram-positive anaerobes. In the hair follicles, the concentration of organisms is 10^5–10^6 organisms/cm^2, mostly anaerobes. The follicular bacteria repopulate the surface of the skin after bathing.

1. **Distribution**
   a. Larger numbers of organisms are found in moist areas than in dry areas.
   b. The density of microorganisms below the waist is greater than that above the waist, because bacteria are shed from the gastrointestinal and genitourinary tracts and spread from the perineal region.

2. **Type**
   a. The bacteria that exist on the skin are primarily Gram-positive.
      (1) ***Staphylococcus epidermidis*** is found in 85%–100% of normal humans.
      (2) ***Staphylococcus aureus*** is carried by 5%–25% of normal individuals.

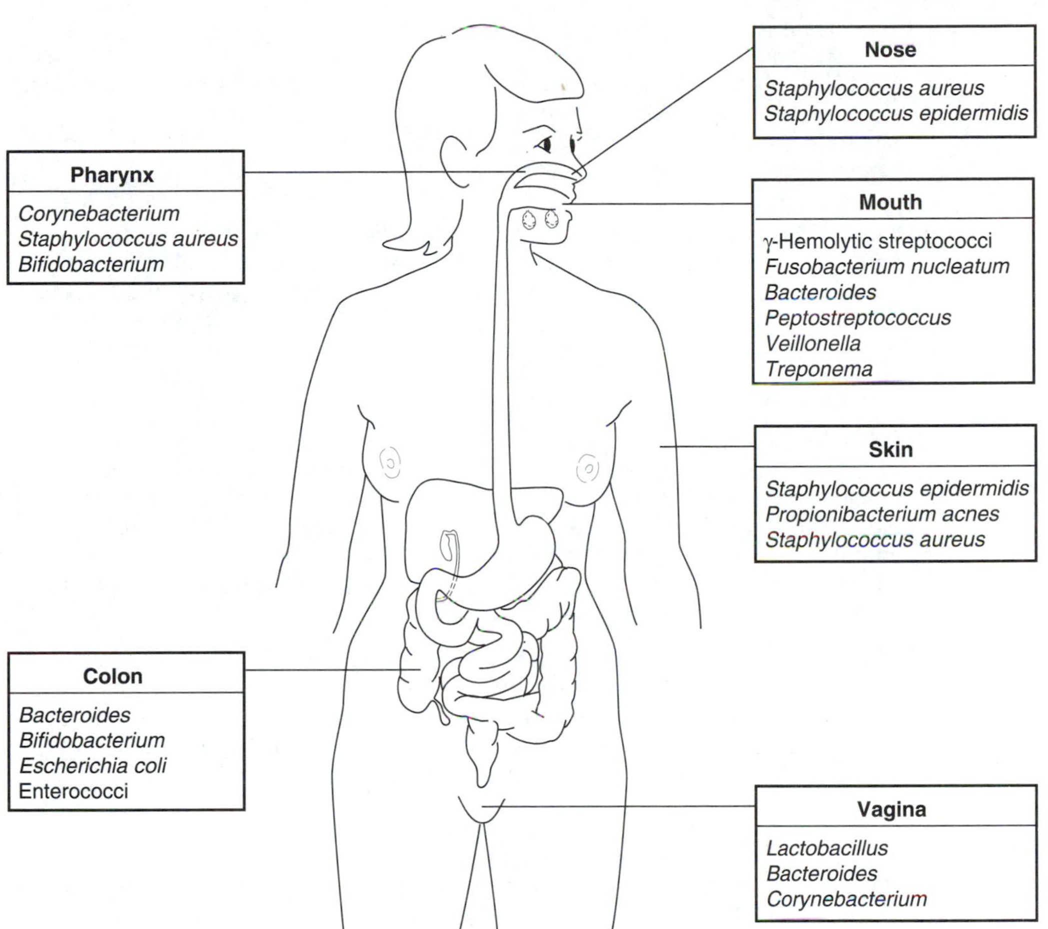

FIGURE 11-1. Most common normal flora by anatomical location.

(3) ***Propionibacterium*** is normal flora in 45%–100% of teenagers. Overgrowth of *Propionibacterium* is one of the causes of acne.

(4) **Fungi** are usually found under the nails and between the toes.

b. In elderly individuals, the Gram-positive organisms tend to be replaced by **yeasts** such as *Candida albicans.*

B. Oral cavity and upper respiratory tract

1. Oral cavity

a. Neonates

(1) **Vaginal delivery.** The predominant bacterial species in the normal oral flora of a baby born through the vaginal canal is ***Lactobacillus,*** a Gram-positive bacillus.

(2) **Cesarean section.** If the baby is born by cesarean section, the type of oral flora that the baby develops depends on whether it is breast-fed or bottle-fed.

(a) **Breast-fed babies** acquire Gram-positive cocci from the mother's skin.

(b) **Bottle-fed babies** have predominantly Gram-negative bacilli.

b. **Children.** When tooth development begins, the oral flora once again becomes predominantly Gram-positive and anaerobic bacteria establish themselves between the teeth and gums, where the oxygen concentration is low.

c. **Young to middle-aged adults**

(1) **Gingivodental sulcus.** The flora of the gingivodental sulcus is mostly anaerobic. Commonly found organisms include ***Streptococcus*** species, ***Peptostrepto-***

coccus species, ***Veillonella*** species, ***Fusobacterium*** species, ***Bacteroides*** species, and ***Treponema*** species.

(2) **Saliva.** *Streptococcus* species, the major bacterial species in tissues adjacent to the buccal epithelium, are found in saliva.

d. **Elderly adults.** The oral flora reverts to predominantly Gram-negative rods as teeth are lost.

2. **Upper respiratory tract**
   a. **Nose. *Staphylococcus aureus*** and ***S. epidermidis*** predominate in the anterior nares. The predilection of *S. aureus* for the anterior nares is probably a consequence of the fact that *S. aureus* grows best at temperatures between 30°C and 37°C.
   b. **Nasopharynx. *Corynebacterium*** species predominate in the nasopharynx.

C. Gastrointestinal tract

1. **Stomach.** The average concentration of organisms in the stomach is approximately 10^3; most ingested organisms are killed by the acidic environment of the stomach.
   a. Notable exceptions are ***Mycobacterium tuberculosis*** and ***Helicobacter pylori,*** both of which resist the acidity of the stomach. However, only *H. pylori* has been identified as a gastric pathogen.
   b. Achlorhydric individuals are more likely to develop bacterial gastritis and gastroenteritis.

2. **Upper small intestine.** Peristaltic motility and the rapid transit of intestinal contents contribute to this portion of the small intestine's low bacterial count.

3. **Lower small intestine, colon, and feces**
   a. **Lower small intestine.** Motility is considerably slower in the lower portion of the intestine; therefore, the bacterial count is higher.
   b. **Colon.** The concentration of organisms in the colon can be as high as 10^{11}, more than at any other anatomical site in the human host. Anaerobic bacteria represent more than 90% of the flora.
      (1) ***Bacteroides*** species are the predominant species in the colon in two-thirds of the population.
      (2) ***Bifidobacterium*** species predominate in the remaining third.
      (3) ***Clostridium perfringens*** is present in smaller numbers, but can be found in virtually every normal individual.
      (4) **Facultative organisms** (e.g., *Escherichia coli,* enterococci) and **yeasts** (e.g., *C. albicans*) constitute the remainder of the normal flora of the colon.
   c. **Feces.** All bacteria found in fecal matter are anaerobic.

D. Urogenital tract

1. **Urethra.** Urethral flora are not abundant— 10^3–10^4 organisms in the distal urethra, less in the proximal urethra—and most of the organisms are Gram-positive bacteria. The male urethra, because of its length, is more likely to be relatively sterile and effectively prevents the entry of bacteria into the bladder.

2. **Vagina.** Vaginal flora are usually rich in anaerobic bacteria.
   a. **Premenopausal women.** During the reproductive years, the most numerous species is ***Lactobacillus.*** These organisms, which generate lactic acid as a by-product of fermentative metabolism, help maintain an acidic environment in the vagina.
      (1) The low pH of vaginal secretions inhibits the growth of other types of microorganisms.
      (2) A woman is likely to get vaginitis following antibiotic therapy because the antibiotics lower the normal concentration of *Lactobacillus,* increasing the pH of the vagina, favoring the multiplication of yeast and other bacteria. Yeast overgrowth is a particular problem because they are unresponsive to antibiotics.
   b. **Postmenopausal women** show a predominance of Gram-negative bacilli in the vaginal canal.

Chapter 12

Gram-Positive Cocci: Staphylococci and Streptococci

Thomas B. Higerd
Sandra Fowler

I. STAPHYLOCOCCI

A. General properties (Table 12-1). Staphylococci (from the Greek *staphyle,* bunch of grapes) owe their name to the fact that they appear to be **clustered** as a result of division in many planes during replication (Figure 12-1).

B. Classification. There are three medically important species in this group. Table 12-2 summarizes differences among these species.

1. ***Staphylococcus aureus*** is responsible for most staphylococcal infections in humans.
2. ***S. epidermidis*** often causes opportunistic infections in debilitated or immunocompromised patients.
3. ***S. saprophyticus,*** another opportunistic organism, may cause urinary tract infections in women.

C. Structure

1. **Cell wall teichoic acid.** The cell wall of *S. aureus* is composed of ribitol teichoic acid, whereas that of *S. epidermidis* is composed of a glycerol teichoic acid.
2. **Peptidoglycan.** *S. aureus* peptidoglycan is unique because of the pentaglycine bridges linking the tetrapeptides attached to muramic acid residues (see Figure 2-3). This pentaglycine bridge is the biochemical basis for sensitivity to lysostaphin, an enzyme produced by *S. staphylolyticus* that destroys staphylococci.

D. Determinants of pathogenicity. Staphylococci cause illness in a variety of ways, ranging from invasion and abscess formation to the release of exotoxins.

1. **Exotoxins**
   a. **Pyrogenic exotoxins**
      (1) **Mechanism of action**
         (a) The pyrogenic exotoxins interact with both major histocompatibility complex (MHC)-II molecules on macrophages and specific types of variable regions of the b chain on T lymphocyte receptors. The interaction is not antigen-specific (i.e., it has significant functional consequences for large numbers of T lymphocytes); therefore, these exotoxins are often referred to as **"superantigens."**
         (b) Activation of T cells and macrophages may be direct (by exotoxins) or indirect [by T-cell lymphokines such as γ-interferon (γ-IFN)] and causes the release of large amounts of interleukin-1 (IL-1), tumor necrosis factor-α (TNF-α), and interleukin-6 (IL-6). These cytokines induce fever, capillary leakage, circulatory collapse and shock.

TABLE 12-1. General Characteristics of Staphylococci

Clustered Gram-positive cocci
Catalase positive
Prefer aerobic conditions but may behave as facultative anaerobes
Grow in the presence of 7.5% sodium chloride

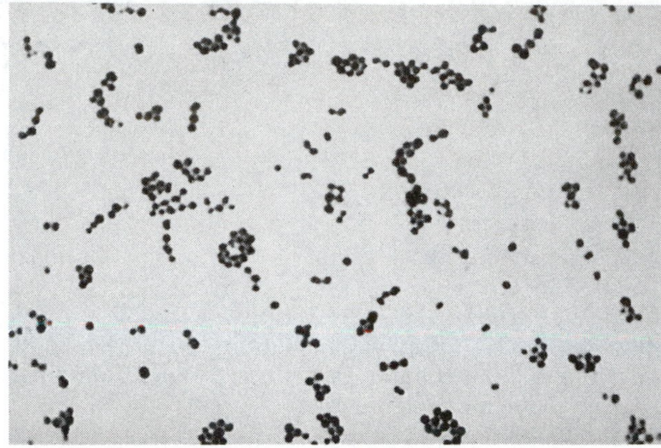

FIGURE 12-1. *Staphylococcus aureus* are Gram-positive cocci that occur in clusters.

(2) **Types.** A single *S. aureus* isolate can produce several pyrogenic exotoxins.

(a) **Enterotoxins.** Approximately 33% of all *S. aureus* strains produce enterotoxins, heat-stable proteins resistant to digestive enzymes. The production of some enterotoxins is determined by lysogenic phages. Enterotoxins A through F have been identified.

(i) **Enterotoxin A** is the best characterized of this group of toxins and is responsible for the majority of food poisoning cases in the United States. This toxin induces diarrhea and stimulates the vomit reflex through neural receptors in the upper gastrointestinal tract.

(ii) **Enterotoxins B through F** are structurally and functionally similar to enterotoxin A.

(b) **Toxic shock syndrome toxin-1 (TSST-1)** is produced by isolates from patients with toxic shock syndrome (TSS). TSST-1 is a pyrogenic exotoxin that causes fever, multiple organ dysfunction, and shock. In addition, it is nearly identical to enterotoxin F.

b. **Leukocidin** kills polymorphonuclear leukocytes and macrophages.

c. **Exfoliatins** cleave the stratum corneum, causing separation and loss of the most superficial layers of the epidermis.

(1) Two similar exfoliatins have been characterized, one coded by a chromosomal gene and the other coded by a plasmid.

(2) These toxins are immunogenic; antibodies have been detected in recovering patients.

2. **Hemolysins** (α, β, γ, and δ) lyse erythrocytes. **α-Hemolysin** is believed to facilitate the tissue destruction associated with staphylococcal growth.

3. **Protein A** is a surface protein that is covalently bound to the peptidoglycan layer of more than 90% of *S. aureus* isolates.

TABLE 12-2. Differentiating Characteristics of Staphylococci

Characteristic	*S. aureus*	*S. epidermidis*	*S. saprophyticus*
Color of colonies	Yellow to white	White	White to pale gray
Hemolysis	+	±	–
Coagulase production	Yes	No	No
Mannitol fermentation	Yes	No	Yes
Novobiocin sensitivity	Sensitive	Sensitive	Resistant

a. **Mechanism of action.** Protein A binds to the Fc portion of IgG, preventing specific antibodies from binding to the bacteria and hindering Fc-mediated opsonization. However, complement is activated by the protein A-bound immunoglobulins, which can contribute to a vigorous inflammatory reaction.

b. If *S. aureus* reaches the blood stream, both protein A-bound immunoglobulins and exposed peptidoglycan can induce massive complement activation, contributing to the pathogenesis of septic shock syndrome.

4. **Enzymes.** Staphylococci produce **β-lactamase (penicillinase), fibrinolysin (staphylokinase), DNase, phospholipase, hyaluronidase,** and many other enzymes.

E. **Clinical disease** is primarily associated with *S. aureus.*

1. **Superficial infections** occur most frequently and are characterized by intense suppuration, local tissue necrosis, and the formation of a pus-filled local abscess.
   a. **Pyoderma (impetigo)** is a highly communicable superficial skin infection.
      (1) **Etiology.** Pyoderma is often caused by phage type 71 *S. aureus,* but may also be caused by *S. epidermidis* and by streptococci.
      (2) **Clinical presentation.** Pyoderma is characterized by vesicles of variable size filled with clear or yellowish fluid. As the infection progresses, scabs form over the vesicles. Impetigo is seen most often on the extremities following infection of previous mosquito bites or skin trauma.
   b. **Folliculitis, furuncles (boils),** and **sties** result from infection of the hair follicles.
      (1) **Folliculitis,** the most limited infection, may be caused by *S. aureus, S. epidermidis,* or *Pseudomonas aeruginosa.* The variety caused by *P. aeruginosa* is referred to as whirlpool folliculitis.
      (2) **Furuncles** are more extensive and may require drainage. **Sties** are small furuncles on the eyelids.
   c. **Abscesses** and **carbuncles** (i.e., multiple, interconnected abscesses involving hair follicles, sebaceous glands, and surrounding tissues, and often found on the back of the neck) are more serious. Because these infections can be a source of bacteremia, treatment entails aggressive antimicrobial therapy and surgical debridement.

2. **Deep infections**
   a. **Osteomyelitis.** *S. aureus* is the most common bacterial cause of acute osteomyelitis, particularly in children. The organism usually reaches the bone via hematogenous dissemination from a distant infection site.
   b. **Pneumonia,** often associated with the formation of lung abscesses, is most often seen in debilitated patients, as a complication of viral influenza, or following aspiration of foreign matter.
   c. **Acute endocarditis,** which is characterized by localized pockets of bacterial growth on heart valves, may occur in intravenous drug abusers or following valve replacement surgery. *S. epidermidis* is the most frequent cause of early prosthetic valve endocarditis, whereas late prosthetic valve endocarditis (i.e., endocarditis occurring more than 2 months after surgery) is usually caused by viridans group streptococci.
   d. **Arthritis, bacteremia, septicemia,** and **deep organ** (e.g., **brain, kidney, lung) abscesses** may be caused by *S. aureus. S. epidermidis* and *S. saprophyticus* are being isolated with increasing frequency from patients with urinary tract infections and bacteremia.

3. **Staphylococcal toxin diseases**
   a. **Scalded skin syndrome** is the cutaneous manifestation of an infection with an exfoliatin-producing strain of *S. aureus.* This illness most frequently involves infants and children younger than 5 years of age.
      (1) Exfoliatin causes the formation of numerous large blisters at sites that are often distant from the original infection. The blisters eventually rupture, exposing the dermis.
      (2) Milder clinical expressions of infections with exfoliatin-producing strains include bullous impetigo and staphylococcal scarlet fever.
         (a) **Bullous impetigo** is characterized by the development of a few large, localized blisters that may rupture. Cultures from these lesions reveal *S. aureus.*

(b) **Staphylococcal scarlet fever** is characterized by a nondesquamative, erythematous rash, similar to that seen in streptococcal scarlet fever [see II B 2 a (8)]. However, unlike the streptococcal disease, the staphylococcal rash rarely involves the tongue and palate.

b. Staphylococcal food poisoning is characterized by explosive vomiting and diarrhea that occurs 1–5 hours after the ingestion of contaminated food (e.g., meat, cream-filled pastries, mayonnaise-containing salads).

(1) *S. aureus* grows well in food, but the ingestion of viable *S. aureus* is not necessary because the disease is caused by heat- and protease-stable enterotoxins.

(2) The disease is self-limiting; with proper hydration, complete recovery occurs within 24–48 hours.

c. TSS is clinically defined as a febrile illness that may progress to organ failure and death. The syndrome is characterized by vomiting, diarrhea, an erythematous skin rash, muscle pain, and hypotension.

(1) **Predisposing factors.** TSS was first described in women using high-absorbency tampons. *In vitro,* the toxin is produced when oxygen is available; some investigators believe that the woven texture of high-absorbency tampons could predispose to the production of the toxin by maintaining pockets of air. It should be noted, however, that men and children are also susceptible.

(2) **Etiology**

(a) **Strains producing TSST-1** are responsible for most of the cases of TSS associated with the use of tampons. However, **any of the pyrogenic exotoxins** can induce TSS if they reach the systemic circulation (e.g., via a deep tissue infection).

(b) Ingested enterotoxins that cause food poisoning do not lead to the development of systemic symptoms.

F. Epidemiology

1. *S. aureus* is a relatively hardy microorganism that **colonizes the skin and mucous membranes of approximately 30% of normal humans.** The **anterior nares** is the most commonly populated site.

2. **Human-to-human transmission** is most common.
   a. *S. aureus* is one of the major causes of **nosocomial infection.** Newborns and debilitated individuals are at increased risk.
   b. Staphylococcal food poisoning often involves **contamination of food by food handlers** carrying enterotoxin-producing strains of *S. aureus.*

3. **Phage typing** can be used to trace the source of *S. aureus* infections. Isolates of *S. aureus* can be identified by their pattern of sensitivity to a battery of bacteriophages. This technique is useful to trace carriers in hospital settings and to conduct epidemiological studies in the community (e.g., in cases of food poisoning).

G. Laboratory diagnosis

1. **Microscopic examination.** Visualization of clusters of Gram-positive cocci in the patient's specimen is strongly suggestive of infection by staphylococci.

2. **Culture.** Staphylococci grow rapidly on rich media under aerobic conditions; they can grow anaerobically and can actually grow under conditions that are usually inhibitory to other bacteria (e.g., 7.5% sodium chloride or 40% bile).
   a. Blood agar is preferred for the isolation of staphylococci from samples with little or no microbial contamination.
   b. When the samples are likely to have other contaminant organisms, selective media are required. Media containing 7%–10% sodium chloride, polymyxin, or 40% bile will allow staphylococcal growth while preventing the growth of many other organisms.
   c. Mannitol salt agar is selective (salt prevents the growth of most bacteria) and differential for staphylococci: *S. aureus* ferments mannitol, whereas *S. epidermidis* does not.

TABLE 12-3. General Characteristics of Streptococci

Gram-positive cocci that form chains
Catalase negative
Mostly facultative aerobes; some strict anaerobes
Grow best in blood agar, which provides catalase and allows aerobic growth

3. **Identification.** Once *S. aureus* has grown in culture, it can be quickly differentiated from other staphylococci by the **coagulase test.** Coagulase is an enzyme produced by *S. aureus* that activates thrombin and causes clotting of plasma. Hence, if a suspension of *S. aureus* is mixed with a drop of plasma, fibrin clots form almost immediately.

H. Treatment

1. **Indications.** Antibacterial treatment is indicated both for superficial and deep infections. However, **deep infections** require more intensive, prolonged chemotherapy.
2. **Agents.** Although originally susceptible, most isolates are now resistant to penicillin G.
   a. Empirical therapy of *S. aureus* infections should be initiated with a **penicillinase-resistant penicillin** (e.g., methicillin, oxacillin, nafcillin) or with a **first-generation cephalosporin** (e.g., cephalexin).
   a. **Vancomycin** is the drug of choice for methicillin-resistant staphylococci.
   b. **Cephalosporins, erythromycin,** or **clindamycin** may be used in patients who are allergic to penicillin.

I. Control and prevention.

Suppressing the carrier state population and implementing diligent aseptic practices are the most effective measures of infection control. No vaccine is available.

II. STREPTOCOCCI.

The genus *Streptococcus* includes a large number of species, some of which are frank pathogens, and others that are members of the normal flora of the oropharynx and gastrointestinal tract. Diseases associated with streptococci range from dental plaque and trivial skin infections to life-threatening complications such as necrotizing fasciitis, toxic shock, rheumatic fever, and glomerulonephritis.

A. Introduction

1. **General properties** (Table 12-3). Streptococci form **linear chains** of varying length (Figure 12-2).

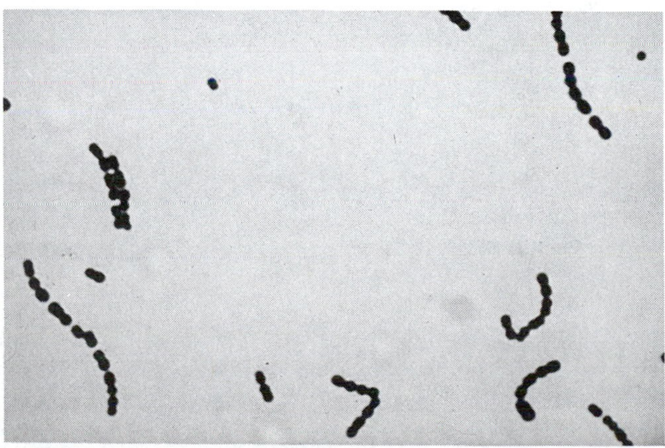

FIGURE 12-2. *Streptococcus pyogenes* are Gram-positive cocci that form chains.

2. Classification

a. Hemolysis pattern. The first system for classification of streptococci was based on the **type of hemolysis** the organism exhibited on blood agar.

(1) α-Hemolytic streptococci exhibit **incomplete hemolysis,** which imparts a green appearance to the hemoglobin. These species are called **viridans** (from the Latin *viridis,* green). Most streptococci in this group lack a polysaccharide capsule; *Streptococcus pneumoniae* is a notable exception.

(2) β-Hemolytic streptococci exhibit **complete hemolysis,** which produces a clear zone in the agar. β-Hemolytic streptococci account for the majority of streptococcal diseases, although not all β-hemolytic streptococci are pathogenic.

(3) γ-Hemolytic streptococci are **nonhemolytic.** The streptococci included in this group are usually not pathogenic.

b. Lancefield system. Determination of the antigenicity of a streptococcal cell wall carbohydrate called the **C substance** (or, in the case of group D streptococci, a glycerol teichoic acid component of the cell membrane) allows grouping of streptococci into groups A through R.

(1) Species can be grouped on the basis of antigenic differences of the cell wall proteins (e.g., **M protein, R protein, T protein).**

(2) Serious human pathogens fall into groups A, B, C, D, and G.

3. Determinants of pathogenicity. Pathogenic streptococci tend to produce a **hyaluronic acid capsule** and a surface protein called an **M protein.** The general characteristics of the main pathogenic groups are summarized in Table 12-4.

4. Laboratory diagnosis. Isolation and identification of the causative organism is important because many of the clinical diseases associated with streptococcal infections are indistinguishable from diseases caused by other bacterial or viral infections. Preliminary identification relies on the type of hemolysis, analysis of biochemical characteristics and sensitivity to special compounds, and serotyping of isolated organisms (Table 12-5).

a. Fluorescein-labeled antibodies specific to the antigenic groups of streptococci or antibodies directed to the capsular polysaccharide of *S. pneumoniae* are used to serotype isolated organisms.

b. Rapid diagnostic enzyme immunoassay (EIA) kits have been introduced for the di-

TABLE 12-4. Main Pathogenic Streptococci

Species	Lancefield Group	Subtypes	Characteristics
S. pyogenes	Group A	>80 M protein subtypes	β-Hemolytic Highly pathogenic
S. agalactiae	Group B	5 Capsular types	β-Hemolytic Pathogenic for neonates
Enterococci, including *S. faecalis* and *S. faecium*	Group D	...	*α, β,* or γ-hemolytic Grow in 6.5% sodium chloride Opportunistic
Viridans streptococci	Cannot be classified	...	α-Hemolytic Associated with dental caries and endocarditis
S. pneumoniae	Cannot be classified	80 Capsular types	Mostly α-hemolytic Bile soluble, optochin sensitive Highly pathogenic

TABLE 12-5. Differentiating Characteristics of Streptococci

Characteristic	Group A	Group B	Viridans Streptococci	Enterococci	*Streptococcus pneumoniae*
Hemolytic pattern	β	β	α	α, β, or γ	α
Growth in 6.5% NaCl	–	–	–	+	–
Bacitracin sensitivity	+	–	–	–	–
Bile solubility	–	–	–	–	+
Optochin sensitivity	–	–	–	–	+

NaCl = sodium chloride.

agnosis of streptococcal pharyngitis (see Chapter 10 III A 1 a). These kits use an immobilized anti-group A streptococcus antibody to capture the bacteria for the sample.

B. Group A streptococci (*S. pyogenes*)

1. Determinants of pathogenicity

a. Proteins

(1) **M protein** is the major virulence factor of group A, β-hemolytic streptococci.

(a) The M protein has **antiphagocytic** and **anticomplement properties.** It is also cytotoxic for neutrophils (in the presence of serum).

(b) The M protein is **strongly immunogenic** and antibodies against type-specific M protein are protective. However, because there are more than 80 antigenic types, development of a general vaccine is not feasible.

(2) **Protein F (fibronectin-binding protein)** is an adhesion factor that, together with protein M, enables group A streptococci to bind to pharyngeal epithelial cells.

(3) **Protein G** binds IgG through the Fc region (which is the wrong orientation for opsonization) and may hinder antibody binding, thus preventing effective phagocytosis.

b. Hyaluronic capsule. The capsule is not immunogenic (probably because bacterial hyaluronic acid is similar, if not identical, to human hyaluronic acid) but has antiphagocytic properties. Group C streptococci also produce hyaluronic acid capsules.

c. C substance and **cytoplasmic membrane antigens** are believed to play a pathogenic role in the nonsuppurative sequelae of streptococcal infections. These molecules are structurally similar to human tissue antigens, particularly those of the heart, kidneys, and joints. Consequently, an immune response directed against group A *Streptococcus* may became auto-reactive and contribute to the development of endocarditis, glomerulonephritis, or arthritis.

d. Exotoxins

(1) **Erythrogenic toxins** are only produced by lysogenized strains (i.e., bacteria carrying an integrated phage). These toxins act directly on the hypothalamus to exert their pyrogenic properties, and they cause the rash characteristic of scarlet fever.

(2) **Exotoxin A,** which is closely related to erythrogenic toxin and perhaps to TSST-1, is a superantigen responsible for the systemic manifestations of group A *Streptococcus* infection.

(3) **Exotoxin B,** a cysteine protease, is responsible for tissue destruction in patients with necrotizing fasciitis.

(4) **Cardiohepatic toxin** causes heart and liver failure.

e. Hemolysins

(1) **Streptolysin O.** This oxygen-labile protein is responsible for the area of complete hemolysis seen around group A streptococcus colonies. It is also believed to be toxic to leukocytes. Streptolysin O is **strongly immunogenic;** the ti-

tration of antistreptolysin O antibodies is used diagnostically as an indicator of prior or recent streptococcal infection.

(2) **Streptolysin S** is oxygen-stable and nonimmunogenic. However, like streptolysin O, streptolysin S is hemolytic and cytotoxic.

f. **Spreading factors** are enzymes that help streptococci to invade tissues by dissolving clots and destroying connective tissues. Proteins in this group include **hyaluronidase, proteinases, streptokinase,** and **nucleases** (e.g., **streptodornase,** a deoxyribonuclease). Most of those enzymes are immunogenic and the quantification of antibodies formed against them is used diagnostically to determine whether a patient has been infected in the recent past with group A *Streptococcus.*

2. **Primary infections** are generally **suppurative** (i.e., characterized by pus formation). M protein-producing strains of group A streptococci are most often responsible.

a. **Diseases caused by group A streptococci**

(1) **Pharyngitis.** Group A streptococci are the most common bacterial cause of pharyngitis and tonsillitis. (Viruses are more often involved in pharyngitis than bacteria.) Symptoms of a streptococcal throat infection include malaise, fever, headache, and a sore throat. A white exudate is visible in the pharynx, the tonsils are enlarged and erythematous, and swollen anterior cervical nodes may be present. Preschool children may complain of a headache and abdominal pain instead of a sore throat.

(2) **Pyoderma** and **impetigo** (see I E 1 a) may also be caused by group A streptococci. Spread of the infection to the deep tissues can lead to lymphadenitis, cellulitis, and erysipelas, and may require treatment with systemic antibiotics.

(3) **Erysipelas,** spreading infections of the skin or mucous membranes, are usually seen on the face.

(4) **Cellulitis** is an inflammation of skin and underlying connective tissue.

(5) **Puerperal fever** is infection of the uterus that occurs following childbirth.

(6) **Necrotizing fasciitis** is characterized by extensive fascial and subcutaneous tissue necrosis, and seems to be favored by several factors, including concurrent infection with other bacteria (particularly anaerobes), delayed or inappropriate treatment, and host debilitation. The streptococci involved secrete **exotoxin B.**

(7) **Otitis media, sinusitis, mastoiditis, bacteremia,** and **pneumonia** are less common suppurative infections caused by group A streptococci.

(8) **Scarlet fever**

(a) **Etiology.** Scarlet fever is caused by strains producing one of two closely related erythrogenic toxins. It can accompany pharyngitis or a streptococcal skin infection.

(b) **Clinical presentation.** A fine, papular, red rash disseminated over the whole body (sometimes described as a "sandpaper rash") and "strawberry tongue" are accompanied by fever.

(i) Unlike petechial rashes, the skin rash associated with scarlet fever blanches when pressure is applied.

(ii) After the fever subsides, peeling of the skin of the hands and feet may occur.

(9) **Streptococcal toxic shock syndrome.** Infrequently, streptococcal infections can cause systemic toxicity, which is similar to the toxic shock syndrome induced by staphylococci and may lead to death. The strains involved in systemic toxicity appear to be lysogenized with a toxin-coding phage and elaborate **pyrogenic exotoxin A,** which has superantigenic properties similar to those of TSST-1.

b. **Epidemiology.** Streptococcal infections are rare in children younger than 3 years of age. Infections are most frequent in school-age children because transmission is facilitated by crowding in closed environments.

c. **Treatment**

(1) All strains of group A β-hemolytic streptococci are susceptible to **penicillin.** Penicillin needs to be taken for 10 full days for pharyngitis, despite the fact that most symptoms are alleviated after 2–3 days of therapy. Extended therapy is necessary because large numbers of streptococci persist in the pharynx,

TABLE 12-6. Jones Criteria

Major	Minor
Carditis	Fever
Polyarthritis	Arthralgia
Chorea	Prolonged P-R interval
Subcutaneous nodules*	Increased erythrocyte sedimentation rate
Erythema marginatum	History of rheumatic fever

* Usually occurring on extensor surfaces.

even after 3–4 days of treatment, and effective treatment prevents development of rheumatic fever.

(2) **Erythromycin** is the drug of choice in patients who are allergic to penicillin.

(3) **Cephalosporins** may also be used.

3. **Nonsuppurative sequelae** may follow primary infection by group A streptococci and presumably result from cross-reactive autoimmunity triggered by the host's response to the microbe or to tissue damage inflicted by streptococcal toxins and extracellular factors. Attempts to isolate streptococcal organisms are usually unsuccessful.

a. **Rheumatic fever** follows a streptococcal throat infection and is characterized by **carditis,** which may affect the myocardium or the heart valves, **arthritis,** which usually affects large joints, and neurologic symptoms, particularly **chorea,** which is characterized by uncontrolled, involuntary movements.

(1) **Epidemiology.** Rheumatic fever is most prevalent in children and adolescents. Proper treatment of streptococcal pharyngitis has reduced the incidence of rheumatic fever to the point that it is infrequently diagnosed in the United States.

(2) **Diagnosis** is based on the Jones criteria (Table 12-6) and serologic evidence of a previous streptococcal infection (e.g., an elevated titer of antistreptolysin O or anti-DNAase B antibodies). The fulfillment of either two major criteria or two minor criteria and one major criterion is necessary.

(3) **Treatment** involves administration of **nonsteroidal anti-inflammatory drugs** (e.g., aspirin) to alleviate joint pain.

(4) **Prevention of recurrences.** A significant number of patients are left with cardiac valvular disease that can be aggravated by a recurrence of rheumatic fever. These patients require **prophylactic penicillin** for the rest of their lives.

b. **Acute poststreptococcal glomerulonephritis** usually follows cutaneous infections, but may follow pharyngeal infections as well. Kidney damage was originally believed to be secondary to the deposition of immune complexes. However, because patients have no evidence of active infection, it seems more likely that the formation of antigen–antibody complexes *in situ* (involving antigens in the basement membrane of the glomerulus of the kidney and cross-reactive antistreptococcal antibodies) may be responsible. The occurrence of poststreptococcal glomerulonephritis is not prevented by proper antibiotic therapy of skin infections.

(1) **Clinical presentation.** Symptoms and signs include facial edema, dark urine (hematuria), and hypertension.

(2) **Diagnosis.** Serology shows increased antibody titers to streptococcal enzymes and low levels of serum C3, reflecting the activation of complement by immune complexes deposited or formed in peripheral organs or tissues.

c. **Erythema nodosum,** which is believed to be a manifestation of hypersensitivity to the peptidoglycan of the bacterial cell wall, is characterized by small red nodules under the surface of the skin.

C. **Group B streptococci** (e.g., ***S. agalactiae***) are often isolated from the nasopharynx, oral cavity, intestinal tract, and vagina of healthy individuals. Group B streptococci are found in the urogenital region in 5%–50% of pregnant women.

1. **Clinical disease.** Group B streptococci are a significant cause of **neonatal infections,** acquired during passage through the birth canal.
   a. Group B streptococci are the most common bacterial cause of life-threatening disease of newborns in the United States. One percent of babies born to infected mothers become ill, and the fatality rate ranges from 20%–80%.
   b. In the first week of life, **bacteremia** and **pneumonia** are the most frequent presentations; between the first and eighth weeks, **meningitis** and **bacteremia** are the most frequent manifestations.

2. **Treatment. Ampicillin** is the drug of choice.

3. **Control and prevention.** Pregnant women carrying group B streptococcus and those who have other risk factors associated with neonatal infection should receive prophylactic antibiotics prior to delivery to reduce the risk of transmission.

D. **Group D streptococci (enterococci)** include ***S. faecalis*** and ***S. faecium***. These organisms are commonly found as normal flora in the intestinal tract as well as in the oral cavity. They are opportunistic pathogens that can cause urinary tract infections in debilitated or immunosuppressed patients. Enterococci can also be involved in bacterial endocarditis.

E. **Viridans streptococci** (i.e., ***S. mitis,*** *S. salivarious, S. sanguis, S. mutans*) are α-hemolytic and can be found in the oropharynx of healthy individuals.

1. **General properties.** These bacteria are **microaerophilic** and **require protein-rich medium** for growth. They **lack group-specific cell wall antigens;** therefore, they can not be included in the Lancefield classification scheme.

2. **Clinical disease.** Viridans streptococci are associated with **dental caries** and **subacute bacterial endocarditis,** which often occurs following dental manipulation. A transient bacteremia is associated with dental work, creating favorable conditions for colonization of heart valves (particularly abnormal or previously damaged valves). Therefore, patients with rheumatic fever or congenital heart disease are at increased risk for subacute bacterial endocarditis.

F. ***Streptococcus pneumoniae*** **(pneumococcus)**

1. **General properties** (Table 12-7)
   a. **Morphology.** The morphology of *S. pneumoniae* is distinctive in that the cocci are **ovoid** or **lancet-shaped** and are often **seen in pairs** on Gram-stained samples (Figure 12-3).
   b. **Growth characteristics.** As a catalase-negative facultative aerobe, *S. pneumoniae* **grows best under increased carbon dioxide tension,** such as that obtained in a candle jar. The organism also grows well in blood agar, which contains catalase and supports the growth of *S. pneumoniae* under aerobic conditions.

2. **Classification.** *S. pneumoniae* **lacks group-specific cell wall antigens;** therefore, it cannot be classified using the Lancefield system.

3. **Virulence factors**
   a. **Polysaccharide capsule.** Some strains of *S. pneumoniae* produce a large polysaccharide capsule, which has **antiphagocytic** properties. Colonies may appear

TABLE 12-7. General Characteristics of *Streptococcus pneumoniae*

Paired Gram-positive cocci
Catalase negative
α-Hemolytic
Bile-soluble
Optochin-sensitive

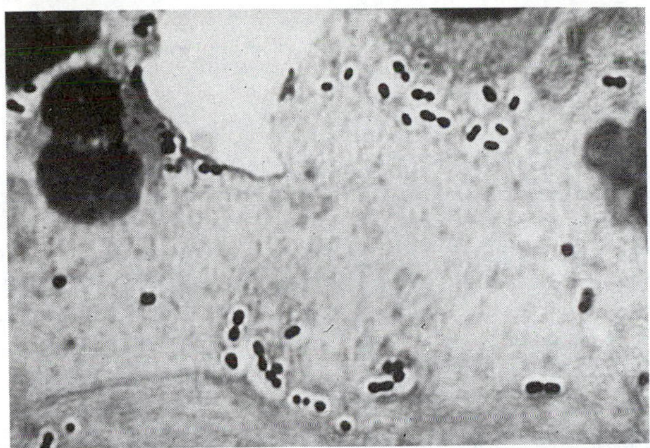

FIGURE 12-3. *Streptococcus pneumoniae* appear in pairs, and the individual cells are ovoid or lancet-shaped. This pairing was the basis for the organism's original designation, *Diplococcus pneumoniae.* The clear area surrounding the pairs of cells is the large polysaccharide capsule.

smooth or **rough,** depending on the presence or absence of capsules. Only capsulated strains are pathogenic.

(1) Capsule production is **encoded by a chromosomal gene.** DNA from a smooth strain can confer the ability to produce a capsule to a rough strain—this is a classic example of **transformation** (see Chapter 3 V B).

(2) Antigenic differences among polysaccharide capsules resulting from variations in the chemical composition of the polysaccharide have allowed the identification of at least **83 serotypes.**

b. IgA protease. *S. pneumoniae* produces an IgA protease that inactivates secretory IgA antibodies.

4. Clinical disease. *S. pneumoniae* is the leading cause of **bacterial pneumonia** in adults and children. Other infections frequently caused by *S. pneumoniae* include **otitis media, meningitis, sinusitis,** and **bronchitis.**

a. Predisposing factors

(1) An **impaired immune response** predisposes individuals to serious pneumococcal infections.

(2) **Viral induced-immunosuppression** and **viral-induced tissue alterations** may contribute to the increased frequency of pneumococcal pneumonia following a viral infection of the respiratory tract.

(3) **Loss of splenic function** consequent to splenectomy, sickle sell anemia, or congenital asplenia predisposes to systemic spread of capsulated bacteria, including *S. pneumoniae.*

b. Postinfectious sequelae. *S. pneumoniae* infections are not associated with postinfectious sequelae (other than those that may be caused by irreversible tissue damage resulting from inflammation associated with the acute infection.)

5. Epidemiology. *S. pneumoniae* is a human pathogen (i.e., there are no animal reservoirs). **Person-to-person contact** is essential for transmission, which is usually mediated by inhalation of contaminated droplets.

6. Laboratory diagnosis

a. Rapid diagnostic tests are most useful for the diagnosis of meningitis (see Chapter 10 III A 2 a).

b. Culture and isolation

(1) In a febrile patient with clinical symptoms and a chest x-ray suggestive of pneumonia (particularly when the x-ray shows a lobar consolidating pneumonia), it is important to obtain an adequate **sputum sample** and two or three **venous blood samples** collected from different sites.

(2) The sputum should be Gram-stained and cultured; the blood should be cul-

tured. Detection of Gram-positive diplococci in the sputum sample of a patient with appropriate clinical signs is considered presumptive evidence of pneumococcal pneumonia.

c. **Confirmation**

(1) **Optochin sensitivity testing.** Pneumococci are inhibited by optochin, a quinine derivative; α-hemolytic streptococci are not.

(2) **Bile solubility testing.** Pneumococci are soluble in bile; α-hemolytic streptococci are not.

(3) **Serologic testing** has the additional advantage of allowing determination of the isolate's serological type. One of the simpler techniques is the **Quellung reaction:** the interaction of capsular polysaccharide and the corresponding antibody changes the optical properties of the capsule, causing it to appear swollen under the microscope.

7. **Treatment**

a. **Penicillin** has been the drug of choice for many years, but resistant strains (carrying penicillin-binding proteins with lowered affinity for penicillin) are being isolated with increasing frequency. Therefore, antibiotic susceptibility testing is indicated in cases of severe infections, such as meningitis and bacteremia.

b. **Third generation cephalosporins** (e.g., ceftriaxone) are gaining acceptance as the initial treatment for severe pneumococcal infections because even strains with intermediate degrees of resistance to penicillin can be susceptible to these agents. However, strains highly resistant to penicillin are being isolated with increased frequency, and those are also resistant to cephalosporins. Some groups recommend treating patients with *S. pneumoniae* meningitis with **vancomycin** (± rifampin) pending the results of susceptibility tests.

c. **Vancomycin** is the drug of choice for highly resistant strains of *S. pneumoniae.*

8. **Control and prevention. Polyvalent vaccine,** made from the capsular polysaccharides of 23 serological groups, is recommended for high-risk individuals.

a. The value of this procedure is limited in immunocompromised patients, who constitute a significant percentage of people in the high-risk category.

b. An additional problem with the vaccine is its low immunogenicity (a problem common to all polysaccharide vaccines). On the basis of the positive results obtained with the conjugate *Haemophilus* vaccines, a conjugate vaccine made of pneumococcal polysaccharide and a bacterial toxoid is currently being evaluated.

Chapter 13

Gram-Positive Rods: *Corynebacteria, Listeria, Clostridium,* and *Bacillus*

John Manos
Michael G. Schmidt
Victor Del Bene

I. INTRODUCTION. The Gram-positive rods can be classified as either non-spore forming or spore-forming. Although *Clostridium* and *Bacillus* are both spore-forming, *Clostridium* are anaerobic and *Bacillus* are aerobic.

II. *CORYNEBACTERIUM DIPHTHERIAE.* The genus *Corynebacterium* includes several species, most of them members of the normal flora of the skin, nasopharynx, oropharynx, urogenital tract, and gastrointestinal tract. These species are collectively known as **diphtheroids.** *C. diphtheriae* is the only pathogenic species.

A. General characteristics. The defining characteristics of *C. diphtheriae* are summarized in Table 13-1.

1. The **club-like appearance,** which is responsible for the name of the genus (from the Greek *koryne,* club) is evident in Figure 13-1.
2. C. diphtheriae grows well in blood agar, but cultures in Loeffler agar and Tindale agar (which contains potassium tellurite) are more informative.
   - **a. Loeffler's agar** enhances the formation of metachromatic granules.
   - **b. Tinsdale's agar** is selective, inhibits other bacteria, and allows differentiation from other *Corynebacterium* species by colony morphology.

B. Determinants of pathogenicity. *C. diphtheriae* is not an invasive organism; systemic symptoms are attributable to production of an **exotoxin.** Nontoxigenic *C. diphtheriae* do not cause systemic disease.

1. **Synthesis.** Only strains of *C. diphtheriae* that have been lysogenized with a bacteriophage carrying the *tox* gene produce diphtheria toxin.
   - **a.** Toxin synthesis is activated as the bacterial population enters the death phase, but lytic growth of the phage is not necessary for release of the toxin.
   - **b.** Toxin synthesis is regulated by the availability of iron. It peaks when the concentration of iron in the culture medium is very low.
2. **Structure.** The toxin is a protein with two moieties.
   - **a. Fraction B,** the **binding** moiety, mediates attachment of the toxin to cells (via a receptor for an epidermal growth factor that is expressed by many different cell types) and transport of the toxin into cells.
   - **b. Fraction A**, the **active** moiety, is responsible for the biologic properties of the toxin.
3. **Mechanism of action.** Fraction A catalyzes the transfer of an adenosine triphosphate (ADP) ribose from cytoplasmic nicotinamide-adenine dinucleotide (NAD) to the elongation factor-2 (EF-2). The ribosylation of EF-2 blocks polypeptide chain elongation.
   - **a.** Unmodified EF-2 forms a complex with guanosine triphosphate (GTP) and tRNA, which binds to mRNA with more or less affinity, depending on proper pairing. Proper pairing allows the incorporation of the amino acid bound to the tRNA into the nascent polypeptide chain, but the reaction depends on the dissociation of the GTP–EF-2 complex.

TABLE 13-1. Defining Characteristics of *Corynebacterium diphtheriae*

Pleomorphic Gram-positive rods, often with clubbed ends, arranged in pairs and trios
May contain intracellular metachromatic granules (polyphosphate)
Noncapsulated, nonmotile
Catalase-positive, oxidase-positive, facultative, grows best under aerobic conditions

b. Dissociation of the complex is caused by the hydrolysis of bound GTP to guanosine diphosphate (GDP) + P by the EF-2 itself and is activated by codon recognition. The ribosylation of EF-2 results in loss of GTP hydrolytic activity, and as a consequence, the GTP–EF-2–tRNA–mRNA complexes do not dissociate and polypeptide chain elongation is blocked.

C. Pathogenesis and clinical disease

1. **Pathogenesis.** Although *C. diphtheriae* can cause skin infections, in western countries (including the United States), the infection is usually localized to the oropharynx.
   a. Following infection, the bacilli grow on mucous membranes (or in skin abrasions). After a **2- to 6-day incubation period,** those strains that are toxigenic begin producing toxin.
   b. Locally, the toxin causes epithelial destruction, which leads to the formation of a **pseudomembrane** over the tonsils, uvula, soft palate, or pharyngeal wall. The pseudomembrane is composed of fibrin, granulocytes, necrotic epithelium, lymphocytes, and *C. diphtheriae* colonies.
   c. The exotoxin is absorbed into the systemic circulation, where it causes **myocarditis** and **peripheral neuropathy.** The neuropathy, which is usually reversible, is caused by demyelination.

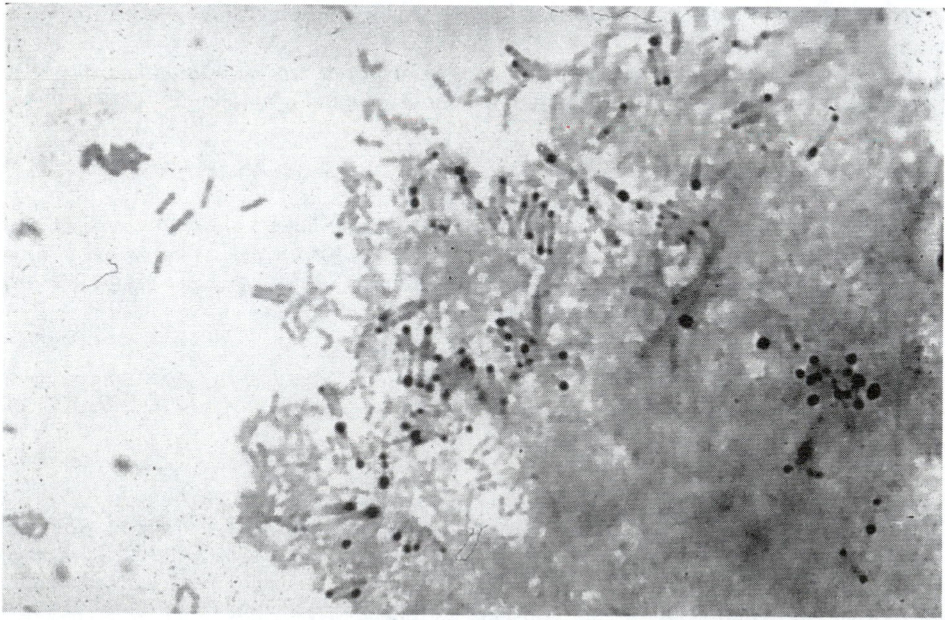

FIGURE 13-1. A smear of a colony of *Corynebacterium diphtheriae,* grown in Loeffler medium and stained with Albert stain. *C. diphtheriae* organisms appear as slender, straight or curved rods with characteristic terminal black (volutin) granules. Note that the rods often appear to form the letters V, L, and Y. Some authors describe these groups as resembling "Chinese characters."

2. **Clinical presentation**
   a. The **initial symptoms** are suggestive of pharyngitis or tonsillitis.
      (1) The pseudomembrane that forms is typically grayish, but may appear green or black.
      (2) The clinical presentation depends on the location and extent of the infection.
         (a) **Anterior nasal diphtheria** is usually not very severe.
         (b) **Tonsillar diphtheria** causes a sore throat.
         (c) **Pharyngeal diphtheria** is associated with a more extensive pseudomembrane, which can obstruct the airway and cause suffocation.
   b. **Advanced signs** include arrhythmia and difficulties with movement of the extremities, speech, swallowing, and vision.

D. Epidemiology

1. **Transmission.** *C. diphtheriae*, a very contagious organism, is transmitted via intimate contact. **Aerosolized nasopharyngeal secretions** are the most common means of transmission.
   a. Children are most often affected.
   b. There are no animal reservoirs for this organism.
2. **Incidence**
   a. Morbidity before mass immunization of children varied, depending on the extent of major outbreaks (which tended to occur every 10 years or so). In the United States, from 1920 to 1975, morbidity rates declined from a high of 200 cases/100,000 to approximately 0.002 cases/100,000.
   b. Since the onset of mass immunization efforts in the 1940s, no major outbreaks have been recorded. The total number of cases per year reported in the United States after 1980 has varied between five and zero—in 1992, three cases were reported, and no cases were reported in 1993.
   c. Because immunity declines with age (because of lack of exposure to the disease and inadequate immunization), some outbreaks have been reported in developed countries of late.
      (1) An outbreak of diphtheria in the Russian Federation started in 1990 and, as of 1994, approximately 80,000 cases were reported. Seventy-two percent of the affected patients were older than 14 years of age. One of the factors contributing to this epidemic was a marked decline in the percentage of children receiving the full immunization with diphtheria toxoid.
      (2) In the United States, it is estimated that less that 50% of young children are properly immunized. In addition, the percentage of protected adults is estimated to vary between 30% and 60%. Thus, a resurgence of this disease is highly possible.

E. Diagnosis

1. The initial diagnosis is based on clinical presentation. **Differential diagnoses** include infectious mononucleosis, streptococcal pharyngitis, and leukemia with agranulocytosis.
2. Confirmation usually involves **culture and isolation** of toxin-producing *C. diphtheriae.* The production of toxin by *C. diphtheriae* can be established by means of **Elek's test.**
   a. Elek's test is a double-diffusion test performed directly on the surface of an agar plate. A filter paper strip is impregnated with antiserum to the toxin. If the strain is a toxin-producing strain, precipitation of the toxin with the antitoxin antibodies will form a precipitin line.
   b. This test is too slow to be used as a basis for therapeutic decisions. Its main value is to confirm a diagnosis. Confirmation is important for epidemiologic reasons because diphtheria is a disease of mandatory notification.

F. Treatment entails **suppression of bacterial growth, neutralization of the toxin,** and **supportive measures.** The patient should be admitted to a hospital and isolated.

1. **Penicillin** is the antibiotic of choice.
2. **Diphtheria antitoxin** in dosages proportional to the severity of the infection (20,000 U in a mild case; 100,000 U in a severe case) is administered intramuscularly to neutralize the toxin.
   a. The antitoxin is produced in horses and can cause serum sickness.
   b. Mortality rates, as high as 50% prior to the introduction of the antitoxin, declined to approximately 15% after its introduction.
3. **Supportive measures** should be used as indicated (e.g., tracheotomy for airway obstruction, full cardiovascular support in cases of myocarditis).

G. Control and prevention

1. **Vaccination with diphtheria toxoid** will effectively prevent diphtheria. Diphtheria toxoid is included in the **diphtheria–pertussis–tetanus (DPT) vaccine.**
   a. The first DPT shot is administered at 2 months of age.
   b. Boosters are given prior to entering school and every 10 years thereafter.
2. **Establishment of immune status**
   a. Lack of reaction following the Schick test, which involves the intradermal injection of a very small amount of toxin, indicates that the individual is able to neutralize the injected toxin.
   b. Enzymoimmunoassay will reveal a level of antibody greater than 0.15 U/ml.

III. *LISTERIA MONOCYTOGENES* is widely distributed in nature and in a variety of animal reservoirs. In humans, it behaves as an opportunistic agent, producing infection in the very young and in immunocompromised adults.

A. General characteristics.

The defining characteristics of *L. monocytogenes* are summarized in Table 13-2.

B. Determinants of pathogenicity.

L. monocytogenes is a **facultative intracellular** parasite.

1. **Internalin** is a membrane protein produced by *L. monocytogenes* that may facilitate ingestion of the organism by a variety of cells (e.g., macrophages,endothelial cells). Once internalized, *L. monocytogenes* can escape the phagocytic vesicle and multiply in the cytoplasm.
2. **Listeriolysin O,** a hemolytic protein, is responsible for the disruption of the phagolysosome membrane. It is considered a major virulence factor for this species.
3. **Phospholipases** may facilitate the dissolution of cell membranes, allowing *L. monocytogenes* to spread to uninfected cells. This form of **cell-to-cell spread** is an effective escape mechanism that keeps the organism sequestered from antibodies produced by the infected host.

TABLE 13-2. Defining Characteristics of *Listeria monocytogenes*

Small, pleomorphic Gram-positive rods
Motile
Catalase-positive
Growth occurs on a wide variety of common media; produces a very narrow zone of β-hemolysis on sheep blood agar
Microaerophilic
Grows over a wide range of temperatures (5–40°C, optimal 37°C)

a. The intracellular progeny bind and polymerize actin fibrils, enabling them to move toward the cytoplasmic membrane.
b. Protrusions on the membrane of infected cells fuse with the membranes of neighboring cells, allowing *Listeria* to penetrate the uninfected cells.

C. Pathogenesis and clinical disease

1. **Pathogenesis.** In humans, *L. monocytogenes* behaves as an opportunistic agent, producing infection in the very young and in immunocompromised adults. The gastrointestinal tract is the major portal of entry for *L. monocytogenes.*
   a. Normal microbial flora modulates *Listeria* colonization of the gut and subsequent penetration of the intestinal epithelial barrier.
   b. In humans, the usual cellular response in cases of disseminated bacterial infection is a polymorphonuclear leukocytosis with microabscess formation. However, because of a surface component of *L. monocytogenes* that has the ability to mobilize monocytes into the blood stream and infected sites, monocytosis may be striking. This marked monocytosis seen in some cases of listeriosis is the origin of the species designation (i.e., *monocytogenes*).
2. **Clinical disease.** Listeriosis is associated with a wide variety of clinical syndromes. *L. monocytogenes* exhibits tropism for the fetus and placenta of most animals and for the central nervous system (CNS) of primates.
   a. **Neonatal listeriosis** is characterized by the development of **meningitis** during the first 3 weeks of life. Fulminant neonatal listeriosis is associated with mortality rates of 54%–90%.
   b. **Adult listeriosis.** Presentations range from a mild influenza-like illness to fulminant listeriosis.
      (1) **Meningitis** accounts for 55% of the infections. Listeriosis is the leading cause of meningitis in cancer patients and renal transplant recipients.
      (2) **Bacteremia** is detected in 25% of patients.
      (3) **Endocarditis** occurs in 7% of patients.

D. Epidemiology.

Listeriosis is typically sporadic in occurrence and worldwide in distribution. *L. monocytogenes* is widely distributed in nature and in a variety of animal reservoirs.

1. **Transmission**
   a. Listeriosis of the newborn can be contracted during **vaginal delivery,** in which case the infection is usually localized to the CNS, or by **transplacental transmission,** in which case the infection is widely disseminated and granulomatous foci may be found in the liver, spleen, lungs, and CNS.
   b. **Food** is the most common vehicle for transmission of human listeriosis in both adults and neonates. Common sources include unpasteurized milk and raw vegetables.
2. The **overall mortality rate** is 30% (60% in cancer patients).

E. Diagnosis

Diagnosis requires culture and isolation of the organism. Growth at low temperatures is used to distinguish the organism from clinical isolates containing mixed flora.

F. Treatment.

Treatment. Beta-lactam antibiotics are the drugs of choice.

G. Immunity

1. The eventual elimination of *L. monocytogenes* from infected macrophages depends on a **cell-mediated** immune response, probably directed against epitopes expressed in association with major histocompatibility complex (MHC)-II molecules on the membranes of infected cells. The effectiveness of the immune response depends on whether TH_1 cells predominate over TH_2 cells.
   (a) Activated TH_1 lymphocytes and natural killer (NK) cells release interferon-γ (IFN-γ), which activates macrophages. Activated macrophages effectively kill intracellular *Listeria* and release interleukin-12 (IL-12), which further promotes TH_1 and NK differentiation and activation.

(b) TH_2 cells secrete interleukin-4 (IL-4) and interleukin-5 (IL-5), which facilitate the development of humoral responses. Humoral responses are inefficient against intracellular organisms.

2. Immunity is apparently **long-lasting.** No second clinical infections with *Listeria* have been observed in patients cured of proved listeriosis.

IV. *CLOSTRIDIUM.*

The genus *Clostridium* includes over 60 species. The most common pathogens are *C. perfringens, C. difficile, C. botulinum,* and *C. tetani.* The defining characteristics of clostridia are summarized in Table 13-3.

A. *C. perfringens*

1. **Determinants of pathogenicity.** *C. perfringens* produces 12 exotoxins and an enterotoxin. Five types of this organism (A through E) can be differentiated according to toxin repertoire.
   a. **Exotoxins.** The **major exotoxins** are **α-toxin, β-toxin, ϵ-toxin,** and **τ-toxin.**
      (1) **α-Toxin,** a **lecithinase,** is the primary toxin. It is common to all types of *C. perfringens,* but it is produced in the largest amounts by type A.
         (a) This toxin hydrolyzes lecithin and sphingomyelin.
         (b) Disruption of cell and mitochondrial membrane phospholipids produces the *in vivo* effects of α-toxin.
      (2) **All of these toxins are lethal to laboratory animals.**
   b. **Enterotoxin** is produced during sporulation. It inhibits glucose transport, causes protein loss, and damages the epithelium.

2. **Pathogenesis and clinical disease**
   a. **Skin and soft tissue infections**
      (1) **Pathogenesis**
         (a) **Exogenous contamination** of wounds may occur (e.g., from soil, water, or sewage).
         (b) **Endogenous contamination.** *C. perfringens* is part of the normal flora of the gastrointestinal and female genital tracts. Most infections are secondary to abdominal surgery or trauma, which allow contamination of tissues with fecal material or genital tract secretions.
      (2) **Clinical disease**
         (a) **Suppurative infections** and **abscesses** are often seen in the gallbladder, uterus, fallopian tubes, and abdomen.
         (b) **Localized cellulitis** may occur (e.g., in a diabetic stump following amputation).
         (c) **Enteritis necroticans,** usually caused by the β toxin of type C *C. perfringens,* is a severe necrotizing disease of the small intestine in which an acutely ulcerative process denudes the gut. It is frequently fatal.
         (d) **Gas gangrene (myonecrosis)** occurs in contaminated deep wounds and is the most serious type of soft tissue infection caused by *C. perfringens.* This type of gangrene is characterized by necrosis and a foul smell.
   b. **Food poisoning** is usually caused by the ingestion of meat dishes (e.g., stews, soups, gravy) contaminated by *C. perfringens,* type A spores.

TABLE 13-3. Defining Characteristics of *Clostridium*

Gram-positive rods
Spore-forming
Motile (except for *C. perfringens*)
Obligate anaerobes

(1) **Pathogenesis.** The spores resist boiling for variable periods of time but start germinating as the temperature drops below 75°C (e.g., when they reach the gastrointestinal tract). Release of the heat-labile enterotoxin upon sporulation occurs primarily in the ileum and large intestine.

(2) **Clinical disease.** The disease is usually self-limiting and is characterized by the onset of diarrhea within 18 hours of ingestion.

3. **Diagnosis**
   a. **Soft tissue infections.** Culture from a site other than the natural habitat of the organism is considered diagnostic.
   b. **Food poisoning.** In a suspected case of *C. perfringens* food poisoning, the diagnosis cannot be based on identification of bacteria in the feces because *C. perfringens* is a normal commensal. Some physicians rely on bacterial counts: a count lower than 10^3 bacteria/g of fecal material is characteristic of normal flora, whereas counts greater than or equal to 10^6 bacteria/g of fecal material are characteristic of food poisoning.

4. **Treatment**
   a. **Soft tissue infections**
      (1) **Postsurgical infections** require immediate treatment. Penicillins are the drugs of choice for *C. perfringens* infections, but they are usually used in association with broad-spectrum antibiotics because therapy is initiated before the precise nature of the infection is known.
      (2) **Gas gangrene.** The treatment of gas gangrene involves **debridement** to remove dead tissue, and administration of one of the **penicillins,** which may help accelerate recovery. Exposure to **hyperbaric oxygen** has been recommended on the basis that the procedure may inhibit the growth of *C. perfringens* and the release of toxins.
   b. **Food poisoning.** Treatment of food poisoning is essentially supportive.

B. *C. difficile*

1. **Determinants of pathogenicity.** Noninvasive *C. difficile* produce cytotoxins. The two best characterized are **cytotoxins A** and **B.** These heat- and acid-labile proteins attach to the intestinal epithelial cells at the microvilli level, causing cell death and denudation of the mucosa.

2. **Pathogenesis and clinical disease**
   a. **Pathogenesis.** Administration of broad-spectrum antibiotics (e.g., clindamycin, ampicillin, cephalosporins) is often associated with gastrointestinal symptoms (e.g., nausea, discomfort, diarrhea).
      (1) **Antibiotic-associated diarrhea** is usually associated with imbalance of the normal intestinal flora and, in most cases, will subside after therapy is discontinued. However, it can also promote the overgrowth of antibiotic-resistant microbial species, particularly *C. difficile.* Other organisms can also cause diarrhea in patients receiving broad-spectrum antibiotics.
      (2) In severe cases, a **pseudomembranous (necrotizing) colitis** develops as a consequence of the release of cytotoxins by noninvasive *C. difficile* in the colon.
   b. **Clinical presentation**
      (1) **Antibiotic-associated *C. difficile* diarrhea** is watery and profuse, sometimes bloody. Leukocytes are found in the stools of 50% of patients, and leukocytosis is common. The patient often experiences colicky abdominal pain ("cramps") and temperatures of 39°C or higher.
      (2) **Pseudomembranous colitis** is a life-threatening complication of severe disease. Exudates composed of fibrin, mucin, and polymorphonuclear leukocytes attach to the mucosal surface. These exudates have a membrane-like appearance when viewed via colonoscopy.

3. **Epidemiology**
   a. **Nosocomial infections.** Infection of hospitalized patients with *C. difficile* can result from overgrowth of the patient's own intestinal flora, or the organism may be acquired from the environment.

(1) Colonization of normal individuals is estimated at 3%, but this percentage jumps to 20% after a few days of hospitalization.
(2) Healthcare providers play an important role in transmission, which can be minimized by careful hand washing and the use of sterile gloves.

b. Individuals older than 50 years of age are more likely to develop clinical symptoms.

4. **Diagnosis.** Antibiotic-associated *C. difficile* diarrhea is suggested when a patient receiving broad-spectrum antibiotics develops severe diarrhea with constitutional symptoms. Confirmation of the diagnosis is more problematic, and several approaches (not mutually exclusive) are used:
   a. **Colonoscopy** is used to visualize the typical mucosal lesions associated with pseudomembranous colitis.
   b. **Culture and isolation** of *C. difficile* followed by **identification of the secreted exotoxins** is probably the most definitive method, but it takes several days.
   c. **Detection of toxins in fecal material.** Enzyme immunoassays (EIAs) for the detection of toxins A and B in fecal material have been developed and appear to be both adequately specific and sensitive.

5. **Treatment**
   a. For very mild cases, **discontinuing the offending antibiotic** may be sufficient.
   b. For mild to moderate cases, **oral metronidazole** or **vancomycin,** given orally, are recommended. Metronidazole is preferable because it is less expensive.
   c. For severe cases, intravenous metronidazole or oral vancomycin are recommended.

C. *C. botulinum*

1. **Determinants of pathogenicity.** The toxin produced by *C. botulinum* is generically designated as **botulin;** however, the various strains of *C. botulinum* actually produce eight toxins **(A, B, C_a, C_b, D, E, F,** and **G).**
   a. These toxins are **structurally homologous**—an active (A) region and a binding (B) region can be defined in all of them.
   b. Generally, a given strain produces only one toxin. Human pathogenic strains most frequently produce toxins A, B, or E.
      (1) **Toxins A through F** are **neurotoxins** that interfere with neurotransmission at the peripheral cholinergic synapses by preventing the release of acetylcholine (ACh), causing **flaccid paralysis.**
      (2) **Toxin G** is the only toxin with which no disease is associated.
   c. Although the toxins are **considered exotoxins,** they are only released when the bacterium undergoes autolysis. Some require partial digestion by proteolytic enzymes to become active.
   d. Botulin is **heat-sensitive,** but total inactivation requires **boiling for 20 minutes.**

2. **Pathogenesis and clinical disease**
   a. **Pathogenesis.** The active form of botulin toxin is absorbed in the small intestine and reaches the neuromuscular junctions through the circulation.
   b. **Clinical disease** is generically designated as **botulism.**
      (1) **Food poisoning** presents as a life-threatening paralytic illness in its most severe form. The paralysis is characterized as **descending;** it first affects the cranial nerves and progresses centripetally, usually symmetrically.
         (a) The **incubation time** is 12–36 hours following ingestion of contaminated food (usually home-canned vegetables preserved at an alkaline pH).
         (b) **Symptoms** include diplopia, dysphagia, paralytic ileum, urinary retention, lassitude, and, eventually, respiratory paralysis.
      (2) **Infant botulism** is the most common presentation of botulism today. Infants between 3 and 20 weeks of age are most commonly affected.
         (a) Feeding of **honey containing *Clostridium* spores** is believed to be involved. The toxin cannot be detected in serum but it is assumed that the symptoms are caused by the release of toxin into the intestine by proliferating *C. botulinum.* The lack of detection probably results from a combi-

nation of factors: low level synthesis or poor intestinal absorption and quick removal from the circulation by high affinity binding at the neuromuscular junctions.

(b) **Symptoms.** Affected children present with weakness and flaccid paralysis ("floppy infant" syndrome). Electromyographic studies show muscle conduction patterns typical of botulism.

(c) Some **protective immunity** must develop, because *C. botulinum* can be isolated from feces weeks after recovery from a clinical infection.

(3) **Wound botulism,** which has clinical symptoms identical to those of food poisoning, is caused by toxin released from infected wounds.

3. Epidemiology

a. Reservoirs. C. botulinum is **ubiquitous.**

(1) It is abundant in **soil** and **marine sediment.**

(2) In the United States, most isolates produce toxins A or B. Strains producing toxin A are prevalent in the western states, whereas strains producing toxin B predominate in the eastern states, and strains producing toxin E are usually found in fish products in Alaska.

b. Incidence

(1) **Food poisoning.** Twenty-five to thirty cases of food poisoning are reported yearly.

(2) **Infant botulism** is currently the most common presentation. Approximately 70 cases are reported annually.

4. Diagnosis is primarily by clinical presentation. Culture and isolation of *C. botulinum* take a few days.

5. Treatment

a. Supportive measures are most important. Ensuring proper pulmonary ventilation, using assisted respiration if necessary, is critical.

b. Penicillin is the antibiotic of choice, but its usefulness is limited (particularly when the disease is caused by the ingestion of preformed toxin).

c. Antitoxin. The use of a trivalent antitoxin (with antibodies to toxins A, B, and E) is controversial.

D. *C. tetani* (Figure 13-2)

1. Determinants of pathogenicity. *C. tetani* produces a potent neurotoxin, **tetanospasmin,** at the site of infection.The toxin inhibits the release of inhibitory transmitters, causing **spastic paralysis.**

2. Pathogenesis and clinical disease

a. Pathogenesis

(1) The usual mode of infection is by **penetrating trauma,** which provides an anaerobic environment for growth of the organism.

(2) The organism begins to elaborate toxin, which binds to peripheral nerve endings, is internalized, and travels via retrograde intraaxonal transport to the spinal cord, where it interferes with the activity of the inhibitory interneurons. The **incubation period** varies from a few days to as long as 3 weeks, depending on the site of injury and the dosage.

(a) A longer incubation time is usually related to injury sites farther from the CNS.

(b) Shorter incubation times are associated with more serious disease and with increased mortality rates.

b. Clinical disease

(1) **Local tetanus** is characterized by persistent spasm around the injury site. This is a mild form with a low mortality rate.

(2) **Cephalic tetanus** is associated with dysfunction of one or more of the cranial nerves, most commonly cranial nerve VII.

(3) **Generalized tetanus** is the most common form of tetanus. The spasm of potent muscles predominates over that of weak muscles, leading to the typical symptoms of **trismus (lockjaw), risus sardonicus,** and **opisthotonos.** Other

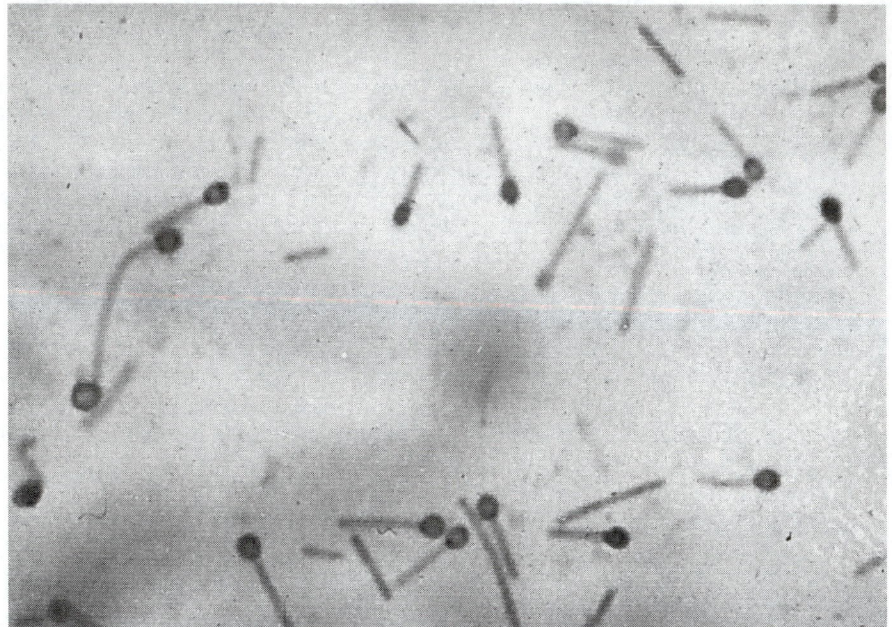

FIGURE 13-2. Gram stain of a smear of *Clostridium tetani.* The organism, a slender bacillus with a terminal spore, is often described as "drumstick-shaped" or "racket-shaped."

symptoms include seizures, tachycardia, arrhythmias, bacterial meningitis, hypocalcemia, and respiratory arrest.

3. **Epidemiology**
   a. **Reservoirs.** C. tetani is found in feces and soil.
   b. **Incidence**
      (1) Tetanus is prevalent in third-world countries.
      (2) Each year, 50–150 cases are reported in the United States; however, the actual number of cases may be twice as high because there is poor compliance with mandatory notification.
   c. **Fatality rates.** More than 50% of the infected individuals are over 60 years of age. On average, the fatality rate is 15%–30%, but infants and the elderly have greater fatality rates.
4. **Treatment** must be initiated based on a clinical diagnosis, because *C. tetani* is difficult to isolate and there is no time to wait for the results of bacteriological examinations.
   a. **Debridement.** Wounds should be debrided.
   b. **Tetanus immunoglobulin (TIG)** and **tetanus toxoid** should be administered to provide passive and long-lasting immunity, respectively. Table 13-4 contains treatment guidelines applicable to soil-contaminated wounds.
   c. **Penicillin** should be administered to terminate bacterial growth.
   d. **Supportive care** should be meticulous.
      (1) Respiratory support may be necessary.
      (2) The patient should be placed in a dark, quiet room because sudden noise can trigger spasmodic crises.
5. **Control and prevention.** Tetanus is a fully preventable disease. Prevention involves immunization with **tetanus toxoid** (chemically detoxified toxin).
   a. In infants, tetanus toxoid is administered in association with diphtheria toxoid and killed *Bordetella pertussis,* beginning at 6–8 weeks of age.
   b. Boosters should be administered at 6–12 months of age, preschool age, and every 10 years thereafter. (In adults, it is recommended to continue boosting with diphtheria and tetanus toxoids only.)

TABLE 13-4. Guidelines for Immunotherapy of Patients with Soil-contaminated Wounds

	Questionable		Over 10 years		Less than 10 years*	
Wound	**TT**	**TIG†**	**TT**	**TIG†**	**TT**	**TIG†**
Low risk	+	–	+	–	–	–
Tetanus-prone	+	+	+	–	+‡	–
Over 24 hours old	+	+	+	+	+	+

TIG = tetanus immune globulin; TT = tetanus toxoid.
* Since last booster.
† Dose is 250–500 U intramuscularly.
‡ If last booster shot was administered over 5 years previously.

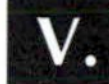

V. *BACILLUS.*

The genus *Bacillus* includes 48 recognized species. Of these, ***B. anthracis***, the cause of anthrax, is the most significant human pathogen. The defining characteristics of *Bacillus* are summarized in Table 13-5.

A. *B. anthracis*

1. **Determinants of pathogenicity**
   a. **Capsule.** In infected tissue (and special culture media), *B. anthracis* develops a unique capsule that is constituted by a high-molecular-weight polypeptide of D-glutamic acid.
   b. **Exotoxin.** *B. anthracis* produces an exotoxin that is comprised of three different proteins. The best characterized of the three is an adenylate cyclase, which is able to generate high levels of cyclic adenosine monophosphate (cAMP) once it is internalized by a susceptible cell. Toxicity is only manifest when the three proteins of the endotoxin are associated in a complex. The three proteins act synergistically to induce **cell death** and **edema.**
2. **Pathogenesis and clinical disease**
   a. **Pathogenesis.** Infection can be acquired through abrasions and cuts, by inhalation, or, rarely, by ingestion. After multiplying locally, the organisms disseminate throughout the body.
   b. **Clinical disease**
      (1) **Cutaneous anthrax** is the most usual clinical presentation.
         (a) Two to five days after infection, a small, painless papule develops. The papule evolves into a vesicle, which, when ruptured, releases a dark fluid and reveals a black eschar at the base with strong surrounding inflammation.
         (b) These papules are usually found on the hands, forearms, or head.
      (2) **Pulmonary anthrax** (**wool sorter's disease**) is acquired by inhalation of spores from infected animal products. Initially, the symptoms are influenza-like, but a serious pneumonia rapidly develops and is usually fatal.
      (3) **Gastrointestinal anthrax** is contracted by ingestion of contaminated food. Symptoms include nausea, vomiting, and diarrhea. Severe prostration, shock, and death may ensue.
      (4) **Bacteremia** and **secondary infections,** particularly **meningitis,** are complications of all three forms of the disease.

TABLE 13-5. Defining Characteristics of *Bacillus*

Gram-positive rods
Form oval, centrally located spores
Nonmotile
Mostly obligate aerobes, some facultative anaerobes

3. **Epidemiology.** *B. anthracis,* a soil microorganism that usually infects herbivores, can be transmitted to humans by infected animals and animal products. Therefore, anthrax can be considered a **zoonosis.**
   a. **Goat** and **sheep herds** are the most common source of contaminated materials. Anthrax foci exist in Louisiana, Oklahoma, Colorado, and California.
   b. Humans are contaminated by dealing with infected products (e.g., goat hair, wool, infected carcasses). Imported hides and ivory can also carry the spores.

4. **Diagnosis.** Identification of *B. anthracis* depends on a variety of biochemical properties. One distinctive feature is **penicillin susceptibility.**
   a. *B. anthracis* cultured on a penicillin-containing solid medium will assume a rounded morphology (i.e., the organisms will become **spheroplasts).**
   b. Because the spheroplasts form chains, *B. anthracis* cultures resemble a **string of pearls.**

5. **Treatment**
   a. **Penicillin** is the drug of choice.
   b. Incision and drainage of cutaneous lesions is contraindicated, because this approach might facilitate the spread of infection.

6. **Control and prevention**
   a. One of Louis Pasteur's major achievements was the development of a living spore vaccine, made from a noncapsulated strain. This vaccine is still used for herd vaccination.
   b. Nonliving vaccines are preferred for protection of humans at risk of occupational exposure.

B. ***B. cereus*** and ***B. subtilis*** are widely distributed in the environment and may cause human disease, particularly in immunocompromised individuals.

1. ***B. cereus***
   a. **Pathogenesis and clinical disease**
      (1) **Food poisoning.** *B. cereus* causes food poisoning, which can mimic both staphylococcal food poisoning (i.e., short incubation, nausea, and vomiting as the predominant symptoms) and clostridial food poisoning (i.e., a longer incubation, abdominal cramping, and diarrhea as the most prominent symptoms).
         (a) *B. cereus* is usually acquired by ingesting toxin-contaminated food (fried rice is a common source). The heat-resistant spores of *B. cereus* survive cooking, and if the cooked food is kept warm for a period of time (e.g., on a buffet table), *B. cereus* may germinate in the food and release an enterotoxin. In this situation, the intoxication will have a very short incubation period and will be clinically similar to staphylococcal food poisoning.
         (b) Alternatively, the spores may be ingested, germinate in the intestine, and release the toxin. In this case, the incubation period will be longer, and the disease will be similar to clostridial food poisoning.
      (2) **Systemic infection.** *B. cereus* can also cause systemic infections in immunocompromised patients.
   b. **Treatment**
      (1) **Food poisoning** is usually a self-limiting situation that requires supportive treatment only.
      (2) **Systemic infection.** For the treatment of systemic infections, the drug of choice is **clindamycin,** but aminoglycosides, tetracycline, and erythromycin are also effective. *B. cereus* is resistant to penicillin.

2. ***B. subtilis*** is fairly ubiquitous in the environment and is usually harmless, but it can infect the immunocompromised. For example, intravenous drug users may become infected from contaminated street heroin, leading to septicemia. **Penicillin** is the drug of choice.

Chapter 14

Gram-Negative Cocci: *Neisseria* and *Moraxella*

Edmund Farrar
Michael G. Schmidt
Gabriel Virella
Gerald E. Wagner

I. *NEISSERIA*

A. Introduction

1. **General characteristics** of the *Neisseria* genus are summarized in Table 14-1.
2. **Classification.** The genus *Neisseria* includes **two pathogenic species—*N. meningitidis*** (the meningococci) and ***N. gonorrhoeae*** (the gonococci)—as well as several nonpathogenic species. There are many approaches to species differentiation:
   - a. **Carbohydrate utilization patterns.** *N. meningitidis* produces acid from glucose and maltose, but not from sucrose, lactose, or fructose. *N. gonorrhoeae* uses only glucose.
   - b. **Serotyping** can be performed using species-specific antisera or monoclonal antibodies.
   - c. **Species-specific complementary DNA (cDNA) probes** can also be used to differentiate species.
3. **Epidemiology**
   - a. Pathogenic *Neisseria* have **no known animal reservoirs.**
   - b. Pathogenic *Neisseria* are **distributed worldwide.**
     - (1) *N. gonorrhoeae* is highly prevalent but usually causes mild infections with a low mortality rate.
     - (2) *N. meningitidis* is considerably less prevalent but causes life-threatening infections with a high mortality rate.
4. **Culture and isolation.** The isolation of *Neisseria* requires special attention.
   - a. *Neisseria* are sensitive to drying and must be plated immediately in fresh, moist medium.
     - (1) **Chocolate agar** is used to isolate *Neisseria* when it is likely to be the only, or predominant, bacterial species present in the specimen (as would be the case with blood, cerebrospinal fluid, or male urethral exudates).
     - (2) **Thayer-Martin** or **modified Thayer-Martin medium** (e.g., TransGrow) is used if the sample is contaminated with normal flora, as would be the case with specimens obtained from the pharynx, rectum, or cervix.
   - b. Care should be taken not to mistake nonpathogenic species, which may be isolated as members of the normal flora, with pathogenic ones upon initial isolation.

B. N. meningitidis, one of the most virulent human pathogens, is the etiologic agent of meningitis.

1. **Classification**
   - a. **Serogroups.** Meningococci can be grouped into nine serogroups according to antigenic differences in capsular polysaccharides.
     - (1) The serogroups are **A, B, C, X, Y, Z, 29e, L,** and **W-135.**
     - (2) Serogroups **A,B,C,** and **Y** are widespread and are **most frequently involved as human pathogens.**
   - b. **Serotypes.** Serogroups B and C are subdivided into serotypes according to outer membrane proteins. Serotype 2 is the most common isolate from human meningococcal disease caused by serogroups B and C. The type-2 antigens from both

TABLE 14-1. General Characteristics of the Genus *Neisseria*

Gram-negative cocci, ranging from 0.6–1.0 μm in diameter
Kidney bean-shaped, often seen as (diplococci)
Capsulated and piliated
Aerobic, oxidase-positive (most other cocci are oxidase negative)
Complex growth requirements; grow best on chocolate agar supplemented with solubilized starch under increased carbon dioxide tension at 37°C

groups are chemically and serologically identical, and they induce antibodies that are bactericidal in the presence of complement.

2. **Determinants of pathogenicity**
   a. **Adhesion factors.** Pili serve as adhesion factors for the oropharyngeal mucosa and probably mediate attachment to the meningeal tissues as well.
   b. **Capsule.** The capsular polysaccharide has antiphagocytic properties.
   c. **Lipopolysaccharide (LPS, endotoxin).** Indices of biologic activity show that *N. meningitidis* endotoxin is ten times more potent than most other endotoxins.
   d. **IgA proteases.** *N. meningitidis* produces IgA proteases, which cleave IgA at the hinge region. Many organisms that infect the mucosa (e.g., *Streptococcus pneumoniae, Haemophilus influenzae*) produce these enzymes, which are believed to protect bacteria against the effects of secretory IgA.
3. **Immunity**
   a. Complement-fixing IgM and IgG antibodies can promote bacterial elimination from circulation and tissues.
      (1) The full activation of the complement sequence, including the terminal components (C6 to C9), seems to be essential for the elimination of *Neisseria.* [Recall that these final components comprise the membrane attack complex (MAC), which causes bacterial cell lysis.]
      (2) Complement-deficient individuals (particularly those deficient in C5, C6, C8, or other components of the terminal sequence) are approximately 8000 times more susceptible to infections caused by *Neisseria* than normal individuals; however, the infections in MAC-deficient patients are not as severe as in normal controls. When the formation of MAC is impaired, the bacteria will not be eliminated, but neither will they be destroyed. Because the bacteria are unable to release endotoxin in large amounts, the infection is not as clinically severe.
   b. The capsular polysaccharides of some serotypes induce antibody formation, but the role of antibodies in immunity to meningococcal disease is not well established.
4. **Pathogenesis** (see Chapter 49 I B)
   a. *N. meningitidis* attaches to the cells of the nasopharynx following the inhalation of contaminated droplets.
   b. In a nonimmune, susceptible host, it invades locally, disseminates hematogenously, and reaches the meninges, its primary target tissue. (The bacterial component responsible for this strong affinity for the meninges has yet to be identified.)
   c. Once bacteria reach the meninges, they proliferate, causing inflammation.
5. **Clinical disease**
   a. A **febrile illness,** usually self-limiting, is the mildest form of meningococcal infection. A blood culture may reveal *Neisseria.*
   b. **Meningitis** (see also Chapter 49 I B). **Symptoms** include:
      (1) **Severe headache, fever** and a **stiff neck** (rare in infants)
      (2) **Vomiting**
      (3) **Neurologic signs** (e.g., cranial nerve palsies corresponding to inflammation of the basal meninges)
      (4) **Myalgias** and **athralgias**

(5) **Altered mental status** and **coma**

c. **Acute meningococcemia** is systemic infection with *N. meningitidis* leading to septic shock, widespread petechial or hemorrhagic skin lesions, disseminated intravascular coagulation (DIC), and death within 8–12 hours of the initial appearance of symptoms.

(1) Initial symptoms include a pinkish **rash** that progressively becomes darker and hemorrhagic.

(a) **Skin purpura.** The irregularly shaped petechiae will not blanch with pressure.

(b) **Necrosis** may require skin grafting.

(c) **Gangrene of the digits** may also occur.

(2) **Hypotension, multiple organ failure,** and **septic shock** develop rapidly following the release of endotoxin. Once a patient progresses to septic shock, the mortality rate is very high, even if adequate antibiotic and supportive therapy are instituted.

(a) Internal organs are affected in a variety of ways, including hemorrhage and ischemia. Postmortem examination often reveals tremendous hyperemia and hemorrhage on the brain surface, which can be associated with thrombosis and brain infarct. Pus may be seen in the subarachnoid space or at the base of brain.

(b) The **Waterhouse-Friderichsen syndrome** (fulminant meningococcemia of short evolution) is characterized by myocarditis and bilateral hemorrhagic destruction of the adrenals.

d. **Pharyngitis, pneumonia,** and **presentations usually associated with *N. gonorrhoeae*** [e.g., urethritis, chronic meningococcemia (characterized by low-grade fever, joint pain, and skin lesions)] may also occur.

6. **Epidemiology**

a. *Transmission. N. meningitidis* is transmitted by respiratory secretions and is highly contagious. The probability of isolating *N. meningitidis* from the nasopharynx is 500–800 times higher among **household contacts** of patients than in the general population; therefore, close contacts of patients are at increased risk of contracting meningococcal meningitis.

(1) **Carriers** harbor *Neisseria* in the nasopharynx but may be asymptomatic. The **carrier rate** varies from 3%–20% in nonepidemic areas to as high as 50%–95% during epidemics.

(2) **High transmission rates** are found in **day-care centers** and **military barracks.**

b. The **mortality rate** in untreated cases during epidemics is as high as 85%.

7. **Diagnosis** (see also Chapter 49 I B)

a. **Examination of the cerebrospinal fluid (CSF).** After ascertaining that the intracranial pressure is not too high, a spinal tap should be performed to obtain a CSF sample for evaluation. (Performing a spinal tap when the intracranial pressure is too high can cause herniation of the cerebellar amygdala and death.) Evaluation of CSF can serve two purposes:

(1) **Establishment of the diagnosis.** In cases of suspected meningitis, examination of the CSF is essential for establishing a proper diagnosis. A **CSF profile,** including glucose and protein determinations and a white blood cell count and differential, should be obtained. These parameters are nonspecific but valuable indicators (see Table 49-3).

(a) Leukocytosis with a predominance of neutrophils suggests active inflammation, which is usually associated with bacterial or fungal infections. In contrast, low white cell counts with lymphocyte predominance are suggestive of viral or mycobacterial infections.

(b) The CSF changes seen in bacterial meningitis include an elevated protein concentration and a low sugar concentration. Activated inflammatory cells release a variety of enzymes that cause tissue damage and increase protein concentration; at the same time, their metabolic activity leads to increased glucose utilization.

(2) **Establishment of a precise etiology.** To establish the precise etiology of a meningeal infection, it is necessary to identify a pathogen (or its products) in the

spinal fluid. It is important to perform the spinal tap **before** antibiotic therapy is initiated, otherwise false-negative results are likely.

(a) A **Gram stain** will not precisely identify the organism, but it will provide information about morphology and staining characteristics.

(b) **Culture.** Antibiotic susceptibility tests must be performed in order to determine the treatment protocol for the patient.

(c) **Rapid diagnostic tests,** based on the agglutination of latex particles coated with antibodies to the most common bacteria and fungi involved in meningitis, are more specific than the Gram stain. Although their sensitivity and speed of performance are equivalent to Gram staining, these tests fail to yield information concerning antibiotic susceptibility.

b. Blood cultures. In cases of suspected bacterial meningitis, blood cultures are obtained because the organisms most likely reached the meninges through the blood stream.

c. Other cultures

(1) In cases of suspected *N. meningitidis* infection, cultures from **nasopharyngeal secretions** are indicated.

(2) If the patient develops **skin lesions,** those can also be cultured.

(3) **Joint fluid, tracheal aspirate,** or **urethral exudate** may be examined by Gram stain and cultured, depending on the patient's symptoms.

8. Treatment

a. Antibacterial therapy should be instituted as soon as possible, and the antimicrobial agent should be effective for the bacteria most likely to be involved. The most important factors to consider are the spectrum of bacteria susceptible to the antimicrobial agent and the ability of the antimicrobial agent to gain access to the cerebrospinal space.

(1) **Penicillin G** is effective when large doses are administered intravenously. **Resistance to penicillin has not been reported for *N. meningitidis.*** However, because some other common bacteria that cause meningitis are beta-lactamase producers, beta-lactam antibiotics (other than second- and third-generation cephalosporins) should not be used before *N. meningitidis* has been identified as the causative agent.

(2) **Ceftriaxone** and other third-generation cephalosporins distribute to the CSF and, because of their broad spectrum, are effective against other bacteria often isolated from patients with meningitis. For these reasons, the third-generation cephalosporins are gaining acceptance as agents to be used for the initial, empirical treatment of meningitis.

(3) **Chloramphenicol,** which has excellent meningeal penetration, is an adequate choice for patients who are allergic to penicillin.

b. Corticosteroids. In spite of the best treatment, many survivors of bacterial meningitis are left with some degree of mental or neurologic impairment. It has been suggested that the administration of corticosteroids to reduce the inflammatory response may improve patient outcome.

9. Control and prevention. During epidemics, both chemoprophylaxis (for short-term protection) and immunization (for long-term protection) are indicated.

a. Chemoprophylaxis. Therapy with **rifampin** or **ciprofloxacin** is recommended for individuals with close patient contact (e.g., family members) because of their increased risk of infection. Day-care and medical personnel may also benefit from chemoprophylaxis in special cases.

b. Immunoprophylaxis

(1) A **vaccine** constituted by the **capsular polysaccharide of serotypes A** and **C** is available. Infants (e.g., children younger than 2 years of age) respond only to the serotype A polysaccharides.

(2) A **quadrivalent vaccine** (containing the polysaccharides of **serotypes A, C, Y,** and **W-135**) has recently been introduced.

(3) **Conjugate vaccines** made with A and C polysaccharides and a nontoxic mutant of diphtheria toxin are currently being evaluated with the hopes that these vaccines will be more immunogenic and effective, even in infants.

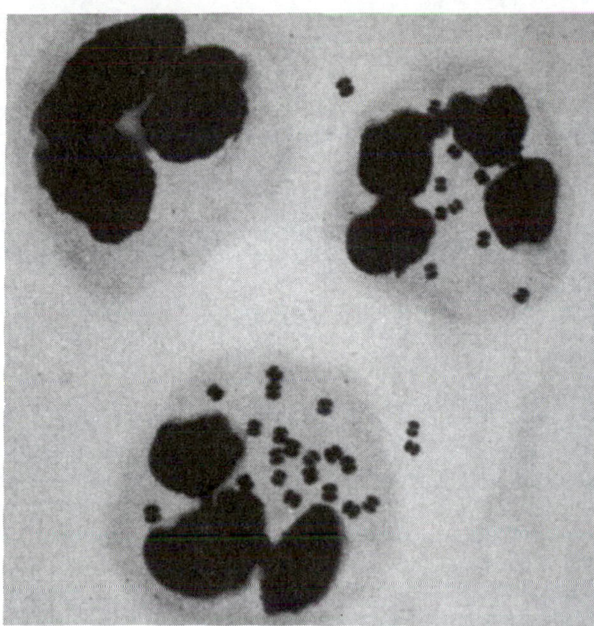

FIGURE 14-1. *Neisseria gonorrhoeae* are usually observed as Gram-negative diplococci inside inflammatory cells, particularly neutrophils. The individual cells typically are described as kidney bean-shaped.

C. *N. gonorrhoeae* (Figure 14-1)

1. **Classification**
   a. **Serotypes.** The outer membrane proteins are the basis for defining 16 gonococcal serotypes.
   b. **Auxotypes.** More than 30 auxotypes have been characterized. The most significant one is the AHU⁻ auxotype, which requires arginine, hypoxanthine, and uracil for growth and is associated with systemic infections.

2. **Determinants of pathogenicity**
   a. **Pili** are involved in bacterial adherence to host cells.
   b. **Outer membrane proteins**
      (1) **Outer membrane protein I** is associated with serum resistance, invasion, and disseminated infection.
      (2) **Outer membrane protein II** comprises a special set of membrane proteins, the **opacity (Opa) proteins.** These proteins, the primary virulence factors of *N. gonorrhoeae,* mediate attachment to mucosal cells and have antiphagocytic properties.
   c. **Capsule.** The capsule surrounding *N. gonorrhoeae* does not prevent phagocytosis, but it does seem to allow intracellular survival of ingested organisms.
   d. **Endotoxin,** which probably plays an important role in disseminated infection, is much less toxic than the endotoxin produced by *N. meningitidis.*
   e. **Peptidoglycan** has pro-inflammatory properties.
   f. **Enzymes**
      (1) **IgA protease** may help *N. gonorrhoeae* evade secretory IgA on mucosal surfaces.
      (2) **Beta-lactamase.** The synthesis of beta-lactamase is coded by a small nonconjugative plasmid, mobilized by a large conjugative plasmid. Transfer of genetic information by transformation is also possible, because *N. gonorrhoeae* remains competent throughout its growth cycle. In some urban areas, up to 30% of gonococci are penicillinase-producing gonococci, as a result of importation in the 1970s from the Far East, where such strains are extremely prevalent.

3. **Immunity.** Both the core region of gonococcal LPS and the outer membrane proteins are immunogenic. Antibodies directed against these bacterial components are bactericidal in the presence of complement. However, *N. gonorrhoeae* possesses **evasion mechanisms** that compromise the protective role of these antibodies.
   a. **Antigenic variation** (see Chapter 7 V F)
      (1) **Pili.** The variability of pili structure depends on the transfer of variable sequences from a large repertoire of silent loci to the expression locus. The large repertoire of pili sequences may be a result of transformation because, as noted previously, *Neisseria* remains in a state of competence for most of its growth cycle.
      (2) **Opa proteins.** The variability of Opa proteins is attributable to rapid switching between multiple genes scattered around the genome. Mutations caused by frameshifting may play a role.
   b. **Adhesion and invasion**
      (1) **Neutrophils.** The association of *N. gonorrhoeae* with neutrophils is obvious, even in Gram stains of exudates from infected patients. Adhesion to the membrane is mediated by Opa proteins; once attached, *Neisseria* tend to remain uningested. When ingested, this organism survives intracellularly by upregulating the synthesis of catalase and neutralizing toxic hydrogen peroxide produced in the phagolysosome.
      (2) **Epithelial cells.** Bacterial invasion of epithelial cells shields the organism from antibodies and phagocytic cells.
   c. **Anticomplementary activity.** Several of the bacterial proteins limit complement binding or prevent full activation of the complement system.

4. **Pathogenesis**
   a. **Adhesion.** *N. gonorrhoeae* adhere to the surface of epithelial cells, particularly those of the urethra, genital tract, rectum, and throat.
   b. **Invasion.** Eventually the bacteria invade the epithelial cells and penetrate the submucosal space, causing a suppurative infection.
   c. **Dissemination**
      (1) **Direct propagation.** Bacteria can spread from the initial focus of infection by direct propagation. For example, in men, the bacteria spread from the mucosa of the external portions of the urogenital tract to the prostate and epididymis, and in women, they spread to the paracervical glands, fallopian tubes, and possibly, the peritoneal cavity.
      (2) **Hematogenous spread.** Some strains of *N. gonorrhoeae* disseminate via the bloodstream (see I C 5 b).

5. **Clinical disease**
   a. **Local infection**
      (1) **Urethritis,** the predominant manifestation in men, is characterized by spontaneous purulent urethral discharge ("drip") and dysuria. Complications are rare, but spread of the infection may lead to epididymitis, prostatitis, or disseminated gonococcal infection (DGI; see I C 5 b).
      (2) **Cervicitis** is the predominant manifestation in women. Dysuria (as a result of associated urethritis) and dyspareunia are frequent symptoms. Results of the physical examination are often unremarkable, but mucopurulent cervicitis or urethral discharge may be evident. Complications include pelvic inflammatory disease (PID), anorectal gonorrhea, and DGI.
         (a) **Pelvic inflammatory disease (PID)** occurs in 10%–20% of women with endocervical gonorrhea and results from the direct propagation of bacteria through the genital tract.
            (i) **Symptoms** include lower abdominal pain and adnexal tenderness during pelvic examination.
            (ii) **Complications.** Acute salpingitis, tubo-ovarian abscess, or pelvic peritonitis may develop during the acute phase of the infection; complications of chronic infection include ectopic pregnancy, infertility, and chronic pelvic pain.
         (b) **Anorectal gonorrhea** is common in homosexual men and women with

gonococcal cervicitis (approximately 40% of women with gonococcal cervicitis have positive rectal cultures as well). Anorectal gonorrhea is usually asymptomatic but may cause proctitis.

(c) **DGI** is discussed in I C 5 b.

(4) **Neonatal ophthalmia (ophthalmia neonatorum)** presents as a conjunctivitis in the newborn. The infection is acquired during passage through an infected birth canal and can lead to blindness. Because prophylactic measures are now routinely practiced in hospitals, this disease has become rare.

(5) **Pharyngeal gonorrhea** is usually acquired by fellatio and is usually asymptomatic. Pharyngeal infection often responds poorly to treatment.

(6) **Perihepatitis (Fitz-Hugh–Curtis syndrome)** is gonococcal infection of the hepatic capsule and subcapsular space. The disease typically presents as right upper quadrant pain in young, sexually active, usually female, patients. Perihepatitis may be confused with hepatitis or cholecystitis.

b. **Disseminated infection. DGI** is estimated to occur in approximately 1% of cases of gonococcal infection and results from the hematogenous spread of the organism. Most common in women, 80% of cases follow asymptomatic local infection.

(1) **Factors predisposing to dissemination**

(a) **Host-dependent factors** include menses, pregnancy, and deficiency of certain complement components (C5, C6, C7, or C8).

(b) **Organism-dependent factors** have been under intensive investigation.

(i) Resistance to penicillin has been eliminated as a characteristic, because most strains recovered from patients with systemic infections are penicillin-sensitive.

(ii) Metabolic properties may be more relevant, as suggested by the fact that most recovered strains belong to the AHU^- auxotype. However, the correlation between these particular metabolic properties and dissemination remains unexplained.

(2) DGI has been associated with **septic arthritis, skin lesions,** and **tenosynovitis.** Rare complications include **endocarditis, meningitis,** and **osteomyelitis.**

6. **Epidemiology**

a. **Transmission.** *N. gonorrhoeae* is generally transmitted person-to-person via **sexual intercourse.** It may also be transmitted from mother to infant during **childbirth.** Rarely, it is acquired from **inanimate objects** (e.g., soiled towels).

b. **Incidence.** Gonorrhea is the most commonly diagnosed infectious disease in the United States. Although cases are grossly underreported; it is estimated that there are approximately three million new cases every year.

(1) Because gonococcal infections are frequently asymptomatic (90% of cases in women and 40% in men) and undiagnosed, spread of the disease is favored.

(2) *N. gonorrhoeae* is only weakly immunogenic and, as stated, has different serotypes. Therefore, patients in high-risk groups may have repeated gonococcal infections.

c. **High-risk groups.** The highest incidence is reported in adults between 20 and 24 years of age, particularly unmarried individuals of low socioeconomic status living in urban areas. Teenagers and male homosexuals are also at high risk.

7. **Diagnosis**

a. **Local disease**

(1) **Identification**

(a) **Gram-staining** of urethral or cervical exudates is the simplest and fastest approach to diagnosis. The demonstration of **intracellular Gram-negative diplococci in a symptomatic patient** is usually considered diagnostic. Unquestionably positive Gram stains are obtained in 90% of symptomatic men. In women, however, only 50%–60% of Gram stains are unquestionably positive because the presence of normal flora can confound interpretation.

(b) **Direct immunofluorescence** (using fluorescent anti-*N. gonorrhoeae* monoclonal antibodies) and **hybridization techniques** (using DNA or RNA probes) are also rapid means of diagnosis and they do not require living bacteria in the sample. These are very specific techniques, but considerably more expensive than a Gram stain.

(2) **Culture and isolation** is necessary to determine susceptibility to antimicrobial agents. Therefore, it is necessary to obtain samples for culture prior to administering antimicrobials.

(a) Culture of **cervical exudates** is positive in 80%–90% of cases.

(b) **Rectal cultures** are frequently positive in women with acute gonorrhea.

b. DGI

(1) **Blood cultures** are indicated in all suspected cases of disseminated infection.

(2) **Other areas and tissues** (e.g., skin lesions, joint fluid) can be examined and cultured depending on the lesions and patient's symptoms.

8. Treatment

a. Uncomplicated genital infection

(1) **Combination approach.** Uncomplicated genital infections can be treated empirically with a combination of drugs most likely to be effective against the three most common sexually-transmitted bacteria: *N. gonorrhoeae, Treponema pallidum,* and *Chlamydia trachomatis.*

(a) ***N. gonorrhoeae*** and ***T. pallidum***

(i) **Ceftriaxone** will eradicate *N. gonorrhoeae* and *T. pallidum* and is resistant to beta-lactamase (one in three isolates of *N. gonorrhoeae* is a beta-lactamase producer). A single **250-mg** dose is administered intramuscularly.

(ii) **Cefixime** is also effective and can be administered as a single oral dose.

(iii) **Fluoroquinolones** (e.g., **ciprofloxacin**) have also been used effectively as a single oral dose.

(b) ***C. trachomatis,*** which is not affected by beta-lactam antibiotics, responds to **doxycycline** and **azithromycin.**

(2) **Spectinomycin.** For patients allergic to beta-lactam drugs, a single dose of the aminoglycoside spectinomycin administered intramuscularly is the recommended alternative. This antibacterial compound has a sufficiently broad spectrum to cover the usual sexually transmitted bacteria.

b. **Gonococcal PID** can be treated with the same combination of drugs (i.e., a cephalosporin and a tetracycline), but the treatment should be continued for at least 48 hours after the patient improves. If the patient is hospitalized, the cephalosporin should be administered intravenously.

c. **DGI.** Patients with DGI should be hospitalized. **Ceftriaxone** or **cefotaxime** should be administered parenterally for at least 24–48 hours after the symptoms resolve. After the patient has been discharged from the hospital, **amoxicillin, cefixime,** or **ciprofloxacin** should be administered orally.

9. Control and prevention

a. **Follow-up cultures** should be performed to evaluate therapy. All sites cultured initially should be recultured 7 days after treatment.

b. **Treatment of contacts.** Contacts of a patient with a proven case of gonorrhea should be treated.

c. **Screening for other sexually transmitted diseases,** including syphilis and HIV, is indicated in all patients with a confirmed sexually transmitted disease.

II. *MORAXELLA.* *M. catarrhalis,* formerly called *Branhamella* or *Neisseria catarrhalis,* is a Gram-negative, oxidase-positive, aerobic diplococcus. This organism is ranked third behind *H. influenzae* and *S. pneumoniae* as a causative agent of **otitis media** and **sinusitis,** but these rankings are likely to change following the widespread adoption of the conjugate vaccines against *H. influenzae.*

Chapter 15

Gram Negative Rods I: *Haemophilus* and *Bordetella*

Gabriel Virella

I. HAEMOPHILUS.

HAEMOPHILUS. The genus *Haemophilus* (from the Greek *hemal,* blood, and *philos,* friendly) includes several human pathogenic species of which *H. influenzae* is the most important.

A. *H. influenzae*

1. **General properties.** The defining characteristics of *Haemophilus influenzae* are summarized in Table 15-1.
   a. **Growth requirements**
      (1) **Chocolate agar.** *H. influenzae* grows best in plates prepared by adding erythrocytes to melted agar at 80°C and incubated at 50°C for approximately 15 minutes.
         (a) The mild heating of erythrocytes causes the release of **factor X** [protoporphyrin IX (hematin), a precursor of hemin] and **factor V** [nicotinamide-adenine dinucleotide (NAD)]. Both of these factors are required for growth of *H. influenzae.*
         (b) Only freshly prepared chocolate agar plates support the growth of *H. influenzae* because factor V is labile.
      (2) **Blood agar**
         (a) Regular blood agar plates that contain intact red blood cells do not support growth of *H. influenzae* because the concentration of factor V is inadequate.
         (b) **Satellitism.** *H. influenzae* may grow on blood agar plates if *Staphylococcus aureus* is simultaneously seeded. Factor X is present in blood agar plates, and, with the addition of the feeder bacteria, there are two sources of NAD—NAD produced by the *S. aureus* itself and NAD released from red cells lysed by the α-hemolysin of *S. aureus.*
   b. **Colonies** may be **smooth** or **rough.**

2. **Classification.** There are **six major serotypes** (a to f) of *H. influenzae,* defined by antisera to capsular polysaccharides.
   a. Observation of the **Quellung reaction** is the classic approach to serotyping *H. influenzae.*
   b. With the availability of fluorescein-labeled antibodies to *H. influenzae,* **direct immunofluorescence** is often preferred for quick identification after culture and isolation.

3. **Determinants of pathogenicity**
   a. **Capsular polysaccharide**
      (1) The capsular polysaccharide of ***H. influenzae* type b** is constituted by **phosphoribosylribitol phosphate (PRP).** Capsular PRP has antiphagocytic properties and is the **prime virulence factor for *H. influenzae* type b.**
      (2) The capsular polysaccharide is constituted by other sugars in the other serotypes.
   b. **Membrane lipooligosaccharide.** The lipooligosaccharide of *H. influenzae* is similar to the lipopolysaccharide (LPS) of *Escherichia coli;* however, the lipooligosaccharide has a shorter and less variable sugar chain and the lipid A portion is less toxic than that of *E. coli.* Membrane lipooligosaccharide may play a role in bacterial attachment, invasiveness, and paralysis of the ciliated respiratory epithelium.

TABLE 15-1. Defining Characteristics of *Haemophilus influenzae*

Gram-negative, short-rod (coccobacillus)
Non–spore-forming
Nonmotile
Facultative anaerobe
Fastidious

c. **IgA protease** is believed to inactivate secretory antibodies.

4. **Pathogenesis and clinical disease**
   a. **Pathogenesis**
      (1) The usual **portal of entry** for all strains of *Haemophilus* is the **upper respiratory tract,** particularly the nasopharynx.
      (2) **Dissemination.** *H. influenzae* type b penetrates the nasopharyngeal epithelium and either disseminates hematogenously or spreads directly to the meninges. Direct propagation from the sinuses is suggested by the fact that *H. influenzae* is second only to *S. pneumoniae* as a cause of recurrent meningitis, especially in patients with head trauma, chronic otitis media, or cerebrospinal fluid (CSF) leak.
   b. **Clinical disease** (Table 15-2). *H. influenzae* can cause the following diseases.
      (1) **Meningitis** is most frequently seen in children between 6 months and 2 years of age, with unexplained prevalence among blacks. Nonimmunized patients with a history of head trauma, otitis media, hypogammaglobulinemia, or sickle cell anemia are particularly susceptible.
      (2) **Otitis media** and **sinusitis** are particularly prevalent in young children.
      (3) **Acute bacterial epiglottitis** tends to affect children between 2 and 5 years of age, and is more frequently observed in whites. Acute bacterial epiglottitis can cause respiratory obstruction and arrest.
      (4) **Cellulitis** often involves the face and neck. Infants younger than 2 years of age are most frequently affected; the disorder is rarely seen in older children or adults.
      (5) **Bacteremia.** Systemic infections are **always caused by capsulated strains.**
         (a) *H. influenzae* type b can cause bacteremia in children. The child is febrile but has no evidence of local disease. The organism may eventually disseminate to the joints and cause septic arthritis.

TABLE 15-2. Pathogenic Roles of Capsulated and Noncapsulated Strains of *Haemophilus influenzae*

Strains	Isolation Rate*	Principal Manifestations of Pathogenicity	Patient Profile
Noncapsulated	50%–80%	Bacterial pneumonia exacerbation of chronic bronchitis; otitis media, sinusitis, and conjunctivitis	Adults
Capsulated type b	2%–4%	Meningitis, epiglottitis, pneumonia, septic arthritis, cellulitis, osteitis, otitis media, pericarditis, bacteremia	Children
Capsulated, types a and c–f	1%–2%	Rarely incriminated as pathogens	...

* From upper respiratory tract.

(b) Type b may also cause bacteremia in immunocompromised adults.

(6) **Respiratory disease.** Noncapsulated, non-typeable strains are common colonizers of the respiratory tract.

(a) **Chronic bronchitis.** The role of *H. influenzae* as an etiologic agent in cases of chronic bronchitis is controversial.

(b) **Pneumonia.** *H. influenzae* can cause bacterial pneumonia in adults, particularly in debilitated individuals, chronic smokers, older patients, and chronic alcoholics. Clinically, it is difficult to distinguish bacterial pneumonia caused by *Haemophilus* from pneumococcal pneumonia, but *Haemophilus* is much less frequently involved.

5. **Epidemiology**

a. **Reservoirs.** *Haemophilus* is a **strictly human pathogen;** there is **no known animal reservoir.** Usually, human carriers are colonized by noncapsulated strains (60%–90% of healthy children and 35% of adults); however, 2% of normal children are asymptomatic carriers of capsulated *H. influenzae* type b.

b. **Transmission** is by **inhalation of infected droplets.** Close contact favors transmission.

c. **Incidence.** The frequency of invasive infection is **inversely related to age,** but infections during the first 2 months of life are rare because infants are protected by passively transferred maternal antibodies.

d. **Susceptibility.** Host-factors contributing to disease susceptibility include primary or secondary humoral immune deficiency, sickle cell disease, and chronic pulmonary infection. Splenectomy increases the risk for bacteremia.

6. **Laboratory diagnosis**

a. A **Gram-stain of sputum or CSF** will demonstrate a Gram-negative coccobacillus.

b. **Culture.** The same specimen should be cultured for isolation and identification of the organism. In patients with suspected bacteremia, especially febrile patients, a blood sample should be cultured as well.

c. **Particle agglutination tests.** In patients with suspected meningitis, rapid confirmation is essential. Tests that use latex particles coated with anti-*H. influenzae* type b antibody are most frequently used.

7. **Treatment**

a. **Empiric therapy.** In patients with suspected *H. influenzae* infection, therapy should be started immediately (particularly if the infection is life-threatening) even if antibiotic susceptibility has not yet been determined by culture. Either **ampicillin plus chloramphenicol** or a **third-generation cephalosporin** may be used for initial therapy in a patient with suspected H. influenzae infection.

b. **Ampicillin** or **amoxicillin** are the drugs of choice, but 30% of invasive strains are resistant to penicillins and ampicillin. Resistance, which is plasmid-mediated, involves beta-lactamases.

c. **Third-generation cephalosporins** and **chloramphenicol** are the drugs of choice in cases of penicillin resistance.

8 **Immunity and prophylaxis**

a. **Immunity.** Protection is mostly dependent on **humoral** immunity.

(1) Capsular polysaccharides and lipooligosaccharides are antigenic; anti-capsular antibody is the main protective antibody.

(2) Passive immunotherapy using antibody preparations enriched in IgM can be useful in very young children, who tend to respond poorly vaccination, or immunodeficient infants.

b. **Prophylaxis**

(1) **Immunoprophylaxis**

(a) The first vaccine introduced for prophylaxis of *H. influenzae* infections contained **purified PRP.** PRP is well-tolerated and induces a vigorous antibody response, but only in individuals older than 18 months of age. Prior to the introduction of the PRP vaccine, *H. influenzae* was a frequent cause of serious infections in children.

(b) The newer vaccines are **conjugates of PRP** and **immunogenic proteins** (e.g., tetanus toxoid) or **immunogenic polypeptides.** These conjugates, which are comparable to hapten-carrier conjugates, are able to induce a protective immune response in young infants. It is now recommended that all children be immunized with the PRP-toxoid (or equivalent preparations) starting at 2 months of age, following the same schedule as immunization with diphtheria–pertussis–tetanus (DPT).

(2) Chemoprophylaxis. Rifampin is used for chemoprophylaxis.

(a) Rifampin has been proposed as a means of **preventing or eradicating colonization in carriers,** but its use in this capacity is controversial because of the risk of inducing the emergence of rifampin-resistant strains.

(b) Rifampin is **recommended for chemoprophylaxis among close contacts of a child with confirmed bacterial meningitis** caused by either *H. influenzae* or *Neisseria meningitidis.*

B. ***H. parainfluenzae*** is differentiated from *H. influenzae* by the fact that it **does not require factor X for growth** (hence the designation *para*). Although its virulence is considerably lower than that of *H. influenzae,* it can be implicated in cases of pneumonia and endocarditis.

C. ***H. aegyptius,*** a variant of *H. influenzae,* causes an acute conjunctivitis of variable severity.

D. ***H. ducreyi*** causes **chancroid,** a venereal disease characterized by painful genital ulcers, edema, and regional lymphadenopathy. Chancroid is treated with sulfonamides or aminoglycosides.

II. *BORDETELLA.* ***B. pertussis,*** the causative organism of **whooping cough,** was isolated and described for the first time in 1906 by Bordet and Gengou.

A. General properties. The general characteristics of *B. pertussis* are summarized in Table 15-3.

B. Determinants of pathogenicity. The virulence factors of *B. pertussis* seem to be controlled by at least two sets of genes, which may act in tandem. It has been demonstrated *in vitro* that at 25°C, the genes coding for adhesins and pertussis toxin are inactive, but when the temperature is raised to 37°C, the genes are activated. Changes in external conditions (e.g., temperature, intracellular environment) may "turn off" the genes responsible

TABLE 15-3. Defining Characteristics of *Bordetella pertussis*

Gram-negative, short rod (coccobacillus)
Non–spore-forming
Hemolytic
Capsulated*
Strict aerobe
Fastidious†

* Fresh isolates from patients are usually smooth. Culture results in an irreversible change from smooth to rough, with loss of the ability to induce hemolysis and an accompanying loss of virulence.

† *B. pertussis* is sensitive to unsaturated fatty acids, sulfides, and peroxides. It is usually isolated on Bordet–Gengou medium, which contains potato starch, blood, and glycerol; the blood albumin plays an essential role by binding and neutralizing fatty acids. In other suitable culture media, the effects of unsaturated fatty acids, sulfides, and peroxides are neutralized by the addition of charcoal.

for virulence to allow survival and dissemination by carriers infected with the less virulent forms of *B. pertussis.*

1. **Adhesins.** Adherence of *B. pertussis* to ciliated epithelial cells is essential for the production of disease and is mediated by **capsular fimbriae** or **agglutinogens.** The most important adhesin, **filamentous hemagglutinin,** causes red blood cell agglutination as well.

2. **Toxins**
   a. **Pertussis toxin** is the major toxin produced by *B. pertussis.*
      (1) **Mechanism of action** (Figure 15-1). Pertussis toxin consists of an active (A) region and a binding (B) region. The A region is an adenosine diphosphate (ADP)-ribosyl transferase that transfers the ADP-ribosyl moiety from NAD to a membrane-bound regulatory guanosine triphosphate (GTP)-binding protein (G_i). This protein normally inhibits adenylate cyclase, but its activity is blocked by ribosylation. As a consequence of ribosylation, when adenylate cyclase is activated in response to stimulatory ligands (e.g., hormones, chemical mediators), it remains activated, resulting in increased cyclic adenosine monophosphate (cAMP) synthesis and a general hyperresponsiveness of the affected cells to a variety of stimuli.
      (2) **Effects** include:
         (a) Heightened sensitivity to histamine and serotonin with a corresponding increased susceptibility to anaphylaxis
         (b) Increased insulin synthesis, resulting in depressed blood sugar levels and inhibition of epinephrine-induced hyperglycemia
         (c) Leukocytosis, secondary to an alteration in the migration pattern of lymphocytes
            (i) The toxin may alter the lymphocyte cell membrane.
            (ii) Pertussis is a potent T cell mitogen, which could contribute to the accumulation of lymphocytes in the intravascular compartment.
         (d) Increased binding to the CR3 receptor of phagocytic cells, which may be associated with phagocytosis without activation of the superoxide burst
   b. **Adenylate cyclase-like toxin.** *B. pertussis* produces a toxin that has the properties of an adenylate cyclase. This toxin enters noninfected cells and causes intracellular increases in cAMP. It also inhibits chemotaxis and the superoxide burst in polymorphonuclear leukocytes, contributing to the intracellular survival of this organism.
   c. **Tracheal cytotoxin** damages the tracheal epithelium, causing the ensuing characteristic cough.
   d. **Endotoxin** does not seem to play a major pathogenic role.

C. Pathogenesis and clinical disease

1. **Pathogenesis.** *B. pertussis* is a local pathogen of the upper respiratory tract; most symptoms of whooping cough are directly related to mucosal destruction by this organism. Systemic effects are caused by either diffusion of pertussis toxin through the blood stream or cross-reactive immune reactions.

2. **Clinical disease** evolves in well defined phases:
   a. **Catharral phase.** After an incubation period of 7–14 days, the patient enters the catharral phase, characterized by a **low-grade fever, rhinorrhea,** and a **progressively worsening cough.**
   b. **Paroxysmal phase.** Severe paroxysmal **coughing episodes** that involve an initial spasmodic phase followed by a rapid inhalation of air (a "whoop") characterize this phase and have led to the designation of the disease as "whooping cough.". Patients may also exhibit a **leukemoid reaction,** characterized by **marked leukocytosis** (i.e., counts as high as 100,000/mm^3). The paroxysmal phase may last 6 weeks or longer; after 6 weeks, the patient is considered noninfectious, even if the cough persists.
   c. **Convalescence** lasts 1–3 weeks.

A

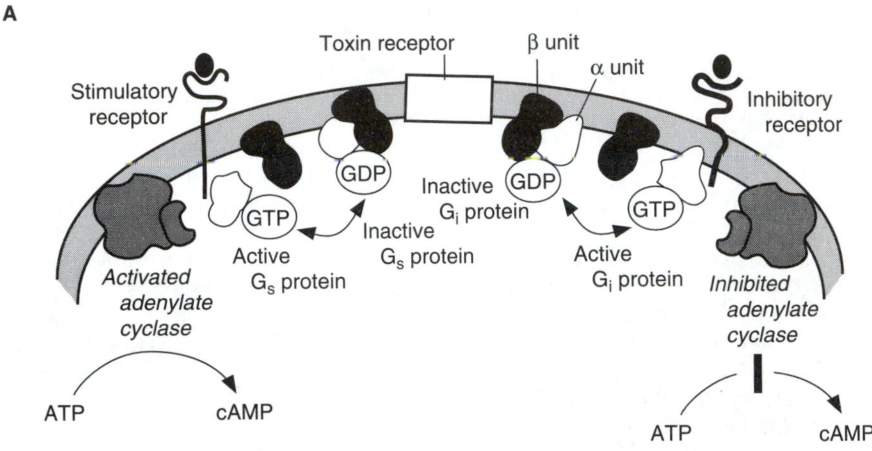

B

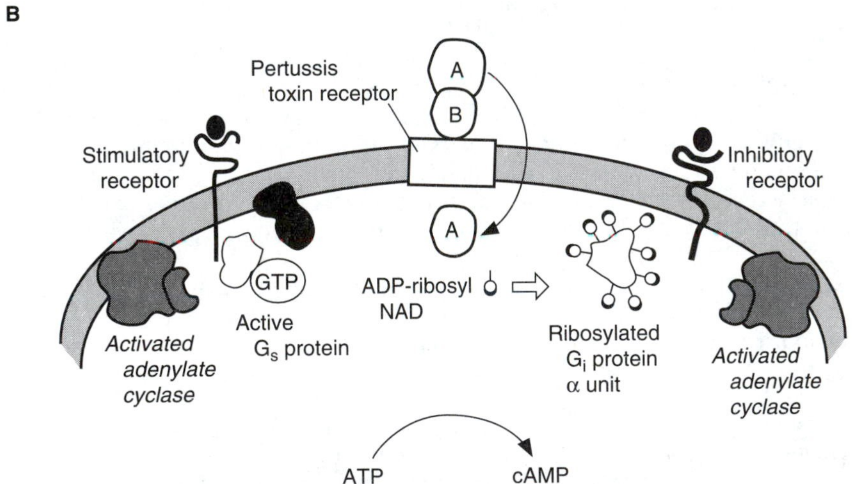

FIGURE 15-1. Mechanism of action of pertussis toxin. (*A*) The fine-tuning of cellular responses depends on the balance between activating and inhibitory signals. Different guanosine triphosphate (*GTP*)-binding proteins (G proteins) are able to transduce different types of signals from receptors that can be activated by the same ligand and often coexist in the same cell. In panel *A,* a cell is shown as carrying two receptors for the same ligand, one coupled to a G stimulatory protein (G_s), and the other to a G inhibitory protein (G_i). Under physiologic conditions, the degree and duration of the activation state of the cell will depend on the balance between the two types of receptors. (*B*) The active (*A*) region of pertussis toxin is an adenosine diphosphate (*ADP*) ribosyl transferase that transfers the ADP-ribosyl moiety from nicotinamide-adenine dinucleotide (*NAD*) to the G_i protein. Ribosylated G_i proteins are unable to bind and inactivate adenylate cyclase. As a result, a ligand able to bind to both types of receptors will always cause a state of activation, because of the inhibition of the G_i-mediated response. *ATP* = adenosine triphosphate; *cAMP* = cyclic adenosine monophosphate; *GDP* = guanosine diphosphate.

2. **Sequelae** may be **pulmonary** (e.g.,bronchitis or pneumonia caused by other organisms) or **neurologic** (e.g., encephalopathy). Rarely, the neurologic complications are observed following vaccination, generally only in children with antecedents of convulsive disorders (e.g., epileptic or febrile children).

D. Epidemiology

1. **Reservoir.** There is no animal reservoir of this strictly human pathogen.
2. **Transmission** is mostly **person-to-person** by inhalation of bacteria-containing droplets expelled by a coughing patient.
   a. Whooping cough is a **highly communicable** disease with attack rates of 90% in nonimmunized close contacts of patients.
   b. Patients are **most contagious during the early catharral phase** of the disease and should be isolated.
3. **Incidence.** Whooping cough is still a cause of significant morbidity and mortality in underdeveloped countries. There is concern about a resurgence of the disease in the United States and other western countries as a result of poor immunization practices stemming from concerns about the safety of the vaccine [see II G 2 a (2)]. During this decade, the rate of infection in the United States has been calculated as 1.1:100,000; in 1993, 5000 cases were diagnosed.
4. **Susceptibility.** The disease affects mostly infants and is particularly severe during the first 6 months of life. Morbidity and mortality rates are higher in girls.

E. Laboratory diagnosis

1. **Culture and isolation** of *B. pertussis* from adequate samples is necessary to confirm the diagnosis. Specimens for culture should be collected during the catarrhal phase on calcium alginate nasal swabs moistened with aqueous penicillin to facilitate access to the posterior nares and also to limit the growth of commensals. (Cotton inhibits the growth of *Bordetella*.)
2. **Direct immunofluorescence** permits **rapid diagnosis.** Smears of nasopharyngeal exudates are examined using fluorescein-labeled antibodies to *B. pertussis.*
3. **Enzyme immunoassay (EIA).** An EIA that detects pertussis-specific IgA has been suggested to be valuable in the diagnosis of acute infection. EIA is likely to be less useful for rapid identification of *B. pertussis* than indirect immunofluorescence; however, it may be very useful when the diagnostic hypothesis is considered during the paroxysmal phase, at which time the number of organisms in the oropharynx is low and their demonstration is difficult. Anti-*Bordetella* IgA antibodies arise only after natural infection, not after parenteral vaccination.

F. Therapy

1. **Supportive measures** are most important.
2. **Erythromycin** is considered the drug of choice. According to some authors, it causes more rapid elimination of *B. pertussis* from the oropharynx, reducing the period of communicability. It also has been suggested that erythromycin treatment shortens the catharral stage.

G. Immunity and prophylaxis

1. **Immunity.** After a clinical infection, patients acquire long-lasting immunity; second infections are rare.
   a. Protection is **species-specific;** infection by *B. pertussis* does not confer immunity to other species of *Bordetella* (i.e., *B. bronchiseptica, B. parapertussis),* which cause mild forms of whooping cough.
   b. Both pertussis toxin and the agglutinogens appear to elicit protective immunity. The protection appears to be mediated by both **humoral and cellular mechanisms.** The apparent lack of protection by maternal antibodies in the newborn suggests that cell-mediated mechanisms may play the most significant protective role.

(1) Work with experimental animals suggests that cell-mediated immunity (CMI) is essential to eliminate *B. pertussis* from the respiratory tract, and that the acellular vaccines are not effective inducers of this type of immunity.

(2) On the other hand, antitoxin-neutralizing antibodies were efficiently induced by both acellular and whole killed bacteria vaccines.

2. Immunoprophylaxis

a. The **classic vaccine** is prepared with killed encapsulated organisms and is usually incorporated in the DPT vaccine.

(1) When properly administered, starting at 2 months of age, it can effectively prevent the disease in infants younger than 1 year of age.

(2) There is debate about whether general vaccination is justified because of the risk of neurologic complications. It must be noted that the frequency of such complications is extremely low. Furthermore, although the disease usually runs a mild course, the fatality rate from the natural disease is considerably higher than the complication rate of the vaccine.

b. Several **acellular vaccines** are being evaluated. All of them contain inactivated pertussis toxin; in addition, they may contain one or several of the following components: filamentous hemagglutinin, a 69-kD membrane protein (pertactin), or fimbriae 2 and 3.

(1) Two of these preparations, one containing toxoid and hemagglutinin, the other containing all five components, have been approved for administration as a booster to properly immunized infants. Preliminary data suggest that these acellular vaccines may be equally effective for primary immunization.

(2) The main advantage of the acellular vaccines is the lower incidence of undesirable reactions (e.g., neurologic complications).

Chapter 16

Gram-Negative Rods II: Enterobacteriaceae and Other Enteropathogenic Gram-Negative Rods

Gabriel Virella
Michael G. Schmidt

I. INTRODUCTION.

INTRODUCTION. A variety of Gram-negative bacilli referred to as "enteropathogenic bacteria," "enteric bacilli," or simply "enterics," can be implicated in gastrointestinal infections. Occasionally, these bacteria are involved in extra-intestinal infections.

A. Taxonomic classification. Enteropathogenic bacteria usually belong to one of **three major groups: Enterobacteriaceae, Vibrionaceae,** and **Campylobacteriaceae** (Table 16-1).

1. **Enterobacteriaceae.** Most Gram-negative bacteria recovered from aerobic stool cultures belong to the family Enterobacteriaceae.
   - **a.** Most Enterobacteriaceae are ubiquitous, commensal organisms that exist in large numbers in the human large bowel but may also be found on the skin, in the oropharynx, and in water. **Most are opportunistic pathogens,** infecting the ill or debilitated. They are involved in wound infections, sepsis, urinary tract infections, secondary pneumonias, and iatrogenic and nosocomial infections.
   - **b.** Some Enterobacteriaceae (e.g., *Salmonella, Shigella*) are **true pathogens** that usually cause gastrointestinal infection.
2. **Vibrionaceae and campylobacteriaceae.** Other important gram-negative rods that cause gastrointestinal disease are *Vibrio, Campylobacter,* and *Helicobacter* species.

B. Pathologic classification. Intestinal pathogenic bacteria can be classified according to their degree of invasiveness and the type of gastrointestinal disease they cause (Table 16-2).

II. ENTEROBACTERIACEAE

A. General properties

1. **Features.** The features listed in Table 16-3 are common to most members of the Enterobacteriaceae family.
2. **Classification**
   - **a.** Currently, the most important criterion for bacteria classification is **genetic homology.** Thus, bacteria classified as Enterobacteriaceae have common structural, antigenic, and genetic characteristics.
   - **b.** Most Enterobacteriaceae are part of the normal intestinal flora or cause gastrointestinal disease, but some bacteria of this genus exist in the environment and may only exceptionally be involved as causative agents of gastroenteritis.
3. **Genetic exchange.** Gram-negative bacteria can conjugate and exchange genetic information.
   - **a.** Enterobacteriaceae, in particular, exchange genetic information among themselves frequently, predominantly by **conjugation** and **plasmid transmission,** but also by **transduction.** The genetic similarities among species of the Enterobacteriaceae family facilitate these processes.
   - **b.** Genetic exchange accounts for the **transmission of multiple resistance genes**

TABLE 16-1. Major Enteropathogenic Bacteria

Organism	Major Reservoirs	Major Clinical Diseases
Enterobacteriaceae		
Opportunistic organisms		
Escherichia coli (most strains)	Human GI tract, possibly animal carriers	Diarrhea, urinary tract infections, neonatal meningitis
Citrobacter, Enterobacter, Serratia, Klebsiella species	Human GI tract, environment	Pneumonia, septicemia, infection in immunocompromised or hospitalized patients
Proteus species	Environment	Urinary tract infections
Yersinia enterocolitica	Animal and human carriers	Enterocolitis
Pathogenic organisms		
E. coli (some strains)		
Enterotoxigenic (ETEC)	Human carriers	Traveler's diarrhea
Enterohemorrhagic (EHEC, VTEC)	Human carriers, possibly cattle	Diarrhea, hemorrhagic colitis, hemolytic-uremic syndrome
Enteroadherent (EAEC)	Human carriers	Diarrhea
Shigella dysenteriae, S. flexneri, S. boydii, S. sonnei	Human GI tract,	Dysentery, diarrhea
Salmonella typhi	Human GI tract	Typhoid fever, bacteremia
*Salmonella enteritidis**	Cattle, poultry	Gastroenteritis
Vibrionaceae		
Vibrio cholerae	Human GI tract	Profuse, watery diarrhea
Vibrio parahaemolyticus	Seawater, seafood	Watery diarrhea
Campylobacter* and *Helicobacter		
Campylobacter fetus, C. jejuni	Animals, human carriers	Diarrhea, septicemia
Helicobacter pylori	Unknown	Chronic gastritis, peptic ulcer, gastric cancer

EAEC = enteroadherent *E. coli;* EHEC = enterohemorrhagic; ETEC = enterotoxigenic *E. coli;* GI = gastrointestinal; VTEC = verotoxin-producing *E. coli.*

* *S. enteritidis* is subclassified into hundreds of serotypes.

among Enterobacteriaceae and for the **acquisition of genes coding for the synthesis of toxins and colonization factors,** important virulence factors for Enterobacteriaceae.

4. Determinants of pathogenicity

a. Major antigens

(1) K antigens (from the German *kapsel*) are associated with polysaccharide capsules.

(2) H antigens [from the german *hauch* (breath), a term originally used to de-

TABLE 16-2. Types of Enteric Infection

	Noninflammatory	Inflammatory	Invasive
Mechanism	Enterotoxin	Invasion, cytotoxin	Bacteremia
Location	Proximal small bowel	Colon	Distal small bowel*
Illness	Watery diarrhea	Dysentery	Entericoid fever
Stool leukocytes	None	Mostly neutrophils	Monocytes
Agents	*Vibrio cholerae* Enterotoxigenic *Escherichia coli* Enteropathogenic *E. coli*	*Shigella* sp Enteroinvasive *E. coli* Enterohemorrhagic *E. coli* *Salmonella enteritidis* *V. parahaemolyticus* *Campylobacter* species *Entomoeba histolytica*	*Salmonella typhi* *Yersinia enterocolitica*

* Portal of entry; the bacteria spreads systemically through the blood stream

scribe swarming colonies of flagellate bacteria] are **flagellar antigens** important for the serotyping of *Salmonella.*

(3) O antigens [from the German *ohne hauch* (without breath), a term originally applied to nonmotile, nonflagellate bacteria] are **somatic antigens.** Differences in the polysaccharide chain of the **lipopolysaccharide (LPS, endotoxin)** determine the type of O antigen.

b. Virulence factors

(1) Endotoxin (LPS) is composed of three parts: a **polysaccharide core, O (immunogenic) antigen,** and **lipid A.** Not all endotoxins are equally toxic; toxicity seems to depend on structural variations of lipid A.

(2) Exotoxins, such as the enterotoxins produced by *Escherichia coli,* the Shiga toxins, and the Shiga-like toxins (verotoxins, verocytotoxins), may be present.

(3) Adhesion colonization factors are involved in bacterial attachment to cells and tissues and in bacterial conjugation. **Fimbriae (pili)** usually play the role of adhesion factors, but the **O antigens** and **outer membrane proteins** may also be involved in bacterial adhesion.

(a) The **fimbrial antigens,** which were described before fimbriae were morphologically demonstrated, were originally thought to be part of the capsule. Hence, they were originally designated as K antigens.

(i) More recently, descriptive designations, such as **colonization factor antigens (CFAs),** have been assigned to specific fimbrial antigens related to intestinal colonization.

(ii) A different set of **P fimbrial antigens** is detected in *E. coli* strains that cause pyelonephritis.

TABLE 16-3. General Characteristics of Most Enterobacteriaceae

Gram-negative rods
Non–spore-forming
Facultative anaerobic
Grow in simple media
Ferment glucose and produce acid
Have peritrichous flagella and are motile
Possess a capsule

TABLE 16-4. Defining Characteristics of *Escherichia coli*

Ferments lactose on MacConkey agar
Produces gas when fermenting glucose
Produces indole when breaking down tryptophane
Often hemolytic (particularly urine isolates)

(b) Certain **O antigens** are associated with strains that infect the intestine and others with strains that infect the urinary tract.

(4) Capsules and other protective surface antigens are either antiphagocytic [as in the case of *E. coli* responsible for neonatal meningitis; see II B 2 (c), or they prevent destruction in the phagocyte (as in the case of *Salmonella*).

B. *Escherichia coli*

1. **General properties** (Table 16-4). *E. coli* and certain related bacteria (e.g., *Klebsiella, Enterobacter, Citrobacter*) form the group known as the **coliforms.** The presence of any of these bacteria in drinking water is considered evidence of fecal contamination and, thus, an unsafe water supply.

2. **Determinants of pathogenicity.** *E. coli* is a ubiquitous organism normally present in large numbers in the human large bowel, as part of the indigenous flora. Occasionally, strains of *E. coli* acquire virulence factors through genetic exchange.

   a. **Adhesion factors.** Many pathogenic strains of *E. coli* develop the ability to colonize the epithelial lining of the gastrointestinal and urinary tracts.

      (1) Strains of *E. coli* involved in lower urinary tract infections have specific O antigens that are thought to allow adhesion to the bladder epithelium.

      (2) Strains of *E. coli* involved in upper urinary tract infections have unique P fimbrial antigens that allow adhesion to the epithelia of the calyx and collecting ducts.

   b. **Enterotoxins** are implicated in many gastrointestinal disorders caused by pathogenic strains of *E. coli.*

      (1) The enterotoxigenic strains of *E. coli* (ETEC) produce two types of enterotoxins.

         (a) Heat-labile toxins (LT-I and LT-II are closely related to cholera toxin both structurally and functionally (see III A). These toxins, which are plasmid-coded, stimulate intestinal guanylate cyclase.

         (b) Heat-stable toxin (ST) is resistant to heat denaturation. This toxin binds to cellular guanylate cyclase and causes an increase in the intracellular levels of cyclic guanosine monophosphate (cGMP), which in turn deregulates ion transporters and causes effects similar to those of LT. The genes coding for LT are also carried by plasmids, when the same plasmid carries genes coding for LT, ST, and adhesion factors these genes appear to be part of a transposon.

      (2) Enterohemorrhagic (verotoxin-producing) *E. coli* (EHEC, VTEC). The most virulent uropathogenic strains of *E. coli* produce **hemolysins,** which have general cytotoxic properties.

   c. **Antiphagocytic capsule.** The K1 strain of *E. coli,* which is involved in 80% of cases of neonatal meningitis, has an antiphagocytic capsule.

      (1) The K1 sialic acid homopolymer capsule, which does not activate complement (and therefore, does not induce opsonization), seems to be antigenically cross-reactive with the human adhesion molecule N-CAM.

      (2) Newborns and infants are tolerant to N-CAM, which may explain their lack of reactivity against the K1 capsule determinants.

3. **Pathogenesis and clinical disease.** Virulent strains of *E. coli* predominantly cause gastroenteritis, urinary tract infections, and neonatal meningitis. Sporadically, *E. coli* may cause sepsis, secondary pneumonia, and iatrogenic and nosocomial infections.
   a. **Gastrointestinal disease**
      (1) **Three man "virulence types"** (virotypes) of pathogenic *E. coli* have been associated with gastrointestinal disease.
         (a) **ETEC** cause **traveler's diarrhea** and other types of diarrhea in patients of all ages. The diarrhea usually is rapid in onset, profuse, and self-limiting, but it can follow a more serious course in infants. The pathogenesis of diarrhea caused by ETEC strains has two main steps:
            (i) **Intestinal colonization** (mediated by CFA-I and CFA-II)
            (ii) **Hypersecretion of water and electrolytes** caused by ST or LT enterotoxins, or both.
         (b) **EHEC** can cause **common diarrhea, hemorrhagic colitis** (a unique type of self-limiting, profuse, bloody diarrhea), and the **hemolytic-uremic syndrome** (acute renal failure, thrombocytopenia, and microangiopathic hemolytic anemia).
            (i) **Serotype O157:H7** is commonly involved in the most severe forms of disease and has been shown to produce a **Shiga-like toxin,** also designated as **verotoxin** or **verocytotoxin** because it is cytotoxic to Vero cells in culture.
            (ii) Production of this toxin depends on lysogenic infection by bacteriophages carrying gene coding for toxin synthesis.
         (c) **Enteropathogenic *E. coli* (EPEC),** which cause diarrhea, affect mostly children and infants and are frequently isolated in developing countries. The pathogenesis of diarrhea caused by EPEC strains is not completely understood; however, it is known that EPEC strains adhere tightly to the surface of epithelial cells, destroying microvilli without overtly invading mucosal cells. The adherence properties seem to depend on a plasmid known as **EPEC adherence factor.**
      (2) **Rarer strains** of pathogenic *E. coli* have been isolated from infants and children with diarrhea, including:
         (a) **Enteroinvasive *E. coli* (EIEC, INVEC),** which resemble *Shigella* in their pathogenicity and general properties, but do not produce a Shiga-like toxin.
         (b) **Enteroaggregative *E. coli* (EAggEC)** produce a special type of fimbriae that may allow the bacteria to attach to the intestinal mucosa.
   b. **Urinary tract infection.** *E. coli* is the most common agent isolated from women with uncomplicated lower urinary tract infections.
   c. **Neonatal meningitis.** In neonates, *E. coli* is one of the two most important causes of bacterial meningitis, which can be acquired during birth or postnatally.

4. **Epidemiology**
   a. **Fecal-oral transmission.** *E. coli* usually is a human pathogen transmitted from person to person, typically by the fecal-oral route. Fecal-oral transmission probably explains the high frequency of transmission among infants in hospital nurseries.
   b. **Food-borne transmission.** Cases of severe gastroenteritis caused by *E. coli,* serotype O157:H7 have been traced to contaminated meat, and this particular type of *E. coli* can be isolated from cattle. Thus, from an epidemiological point of view, *E. coli* O157:H7 behaves as a zoonotic agent.
   c. **Endogenous source.** In the case of urinary tract infection, the source of *E. coli* usually is endogenous, contaminating the urinary tract from the perineum. In women, urinary tract infection often is associated with sexual activity, hence the term **"honeymoon cystitis".**

5. **Diagnosis.** The clinical picture, age of patient, and travel history are important in diagnosing an intestinal or extra-intestinal *E. coli* infection.
   a. **Clinical diagnosis.** In most cases of acute gastroenteritis, a clinical diagnosis will suffice and a laboratory (confirmatory) diagnosis need not be aggressively pursued.

b. Laboratory diagnosis

(1) General principles. Laboratory identification of *E. coli* is based on culture and isolation of organisms from adequate samples. The organism may then be identified using biochemical analysis or serologic tests, or both.

(a) Culture and isolation

(i) The **source of culture material** depends on the clinical symptoms.

- **Feces** are the best source of culture material when the patient is ill with gastroenteritis.
- **Infected tissue** may be more adequate when the bacteria are locally invasive.
- **Blood** is the best source from which to attempt isolation of systemically invasive bacteria (i.e., those causing bacteremia and sepsis).
- **Urine,** collected using the clean-catch method is preferred for investigation of urinary tract infections.

(ii) **Culture on differential media** helps to identify Enterobacteriaceae. Most grow on **MacConkey agar,** which contains lactose and a pH indicator. If lactose is fermented, acid will be generated and the colonies will turn pink. This allows some narrowing down of species; although *E. coli* usually ferments lactose, most true pathogens among the Enterobacteriaceae do not.

(b) **Biochemical analysis and serotyping.** Final identification of the species requires further biochemical analysis (e.g., glucose fermentation, sorbitol fermentation, production of indole and H_2S, oxidase reaction) and serotyping. Specific serotypes are indicated by the initial designating the type of antigen (i.e., O, K, H) and a number. For example, a complete phenotype would read: O111:K55:H3.

(2) Cases of extra-intestinal infection or epidemiological investigation of outbreaks of gastroenteritis may require varying degrees of laboratory investigation, including:

(a) Isolation

(b) Biochemical analysis

(c) Serotyping

(d) Testing for pathogenic factors, such as:

(i) Toxin production (classically tested by the ileal loop test but currently tested by enzymoimmunoassays)

(ii) Invasiveness (e.g., using the Sereny test)

(iii) Presence of CFAs (detected by agglutination tests with anti-CFA antibodies)

(e) Detection of antibodies to specific pathogens in retrospective studies

(3) Cases of severe disease or disease that fails to respond to conventional antibiotic therapy require culture and determination of antibiotic susceptibilities.

5. Treatment

a. Rehydration with electrolyte-rich liquids is essential when the diarrhea is profuse. In infants, children, and debilitated individuals, intravenous administration of fluids and electrolytes may be indicated.

b. Antibiotics are used in the very young, in patients with extra-intestinal infections, and in patients with chronic infections irrespective of their location. Trimethoprim–sulfamethoxazole is usually effective, but resistant strains are frequently isolated.

6. Control and prevention

a. Sanitation, particularly proper handling of raw sewage and strict control of water quality, plays an important role in preventing the spread of gastroenteritis-causing strains of *E. coli.*

b. Breast feeding may play an important protective role for the infant, because secretory IgA antibodies may be transferred from mother to infant via breast milk.

TABLE 16-5. Defining Characteristics of *Shigella* species

Nonmotile
Do not ferment lactose readily on MacConkey agar
Do not produce gas from fermentable carbohydrates
Do not produce H_2S from thiosulfate

c. **Chemoprophylaxis** with doxycycline or trimethoprim–sulfamethoxazole has been recommended for travelers visiting regions where traveler's diarrhea is prevalent.

C. *Shigella*

1. **General properties.** The defining characteristics of *Shigella* are listed in Table 16-5.
2. **Classification.** *Shigella* species have been grouped according to differences in somatic (O) antigens:
   a. Group **A. *(S. dysenteriae)***
   b. Group **B. *(S. flexneri)***
   c. Group **C *(S. boydii)***
   d. Group **D *(S. sonnei)***
3. **Determinants of pathogenicity.** Several virulence factors, some plasmid-determined and others encoded by chromosomal genes, seem to act synergistically to determine the pathogenicity of *Shigella* species (Table 16-6). Although all species share the properties of being invasive and causing mucosal cell death, the production of **Shiga toxin** is limited to ***S. dysenteriae* type 1**, which causes the most severe infections. It is currently believed that this toxin, which is only released when the bacteria die, causes the hemolytic-uremic syndrome by inducing vascular damage that is compounded by endotoxin.
4. **Pathogenesis and clinical disease.** *Shigella* is the agent of **bacterial dysentery *(shigellosis).*** It can also cause watery diarrhea.
   a. **Pathogenesis of bacterial dysentery** (Figure 16-1). The infection is limited to the colonic mucosa and submucosa. Systemic invasion through the blood stream does not occur in most cases.
   b. **Clinical disease.** Dysentery typically is characterized by **severe abdominal cramps** and **frequent, painful passage of low-volume stools containing blood and mucus.** The **hemolytic-uremic syndrome** can develop in cases of infection by *S. dysenteriae* type I, and may be attributable to the effects of Shiga toxin, which causes disseminated endothelial damage, leading to intravascular clotting, hemolysis, and renal failure.
5. **Epidemiology**
   a. *Shigella* is a **true human pathogen,** for which there is no animal reservoir. *Shi-*

TABLE 16-6. Determinants of *Shigella* species Pathogenicity

Virulence Factor	Mechanism of Action
Invasion plasmid antigens	Mediate attachment to, and penetration of, mucosal epithelial cells
	Mediate escape from phagocytic vesicles
Intercellular spread proteins	Mediate attachment to cytoskeleton proteins facilitate transfer of bacteria to adjacent cells through membrane protrusions
Shiga toxin*	Inactivates 60S ribosomal subunit of mammalian cell ribosomes, thus inhibiting protein synthesis

* Heat-labile, cytotoxic exotoxin produced by *S. dysenteriae*

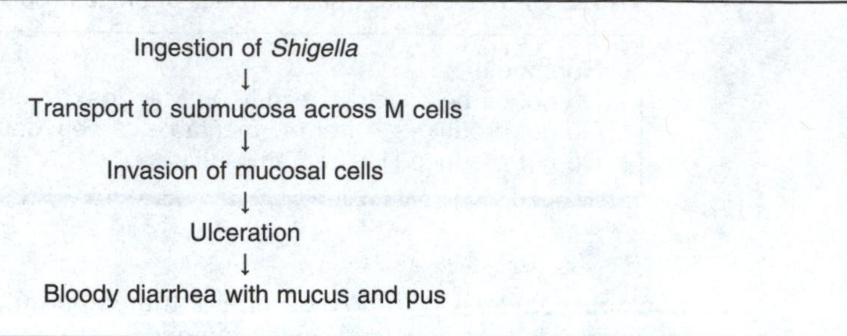

FIGURE 16-1. Pathogenesis of bacterial dysentery.

gella is transmitted by the **fecal-oral route** from person to person by direct contact (including sexual contact) or through contaminated food and water.

b. The different species of *Shigella* show predominance in different regions of the world. In the United States, *S. sonnei* predominates (70% of cases) followed by *S. flexneri*. In developing countries, *S. dysenteriae* and *S. boydii* predominate.

6. **Laboratory diagnosis.** To confirm the diagnosis, *Shigella* must be isolated from an adequate sample.
   a. **Sources of culture material** include **feces** or a **rectal swab** of a mucosal ulcer obtained through a sigmoidoscope. Swabs are preferred, but sigmoidoscopy is an uncomfortable procedure and may cause intestinal perforation.
   b. A **methylene blue stain of fecal leukocytes** indicates mucosal invasion (i.e., dysentery) but is not specific for shigellosis.
   c. A **Sereny test** can confirm the invasiveness of isolated *Shigella;* however, this test is not routinely used. A drop of invasive isolate deposited in the cornea of a guinea pig or a rabbit will produce severe keratoconjunctivitis followed by ulceration.

7. **Treatment**
   a. **Supportive therapy,** including fluid replacement, is essential for patients with shigellosis (particularly when it is associated with watery diarrhea).
   b. **Antibiotics** may be given, particularly to young patients, because they shorten the duration of disease and the carrier state, thus limiting secondary cases. Drugs of choice are **ampicillin** and **amoxicillin,** but resistant strains are relatively common; if the antibiotic susceptibility of the infecting strain is unknown, **trimethoprim–sulfamethoxazole** may be preferred, because resistance to this drug is less common.

8. **Control and prevention.** Sanitation and personal hygiene are the most effective means of controlling outbreaks of *Shigella,* because they interfere with the fecal-oral chain of transmission (feces, flies, and fingers).

D. *Salmonella*

1. **General properties.** The defining characteristics of *Salmonella* species are listed in Table 16-7.

2. **Classification.** Major species include *S. choleraesuis, S. typhi,* and *S. enteritidis. S. enteritidis* is subclassified into hundreds of serotypes.

TABLE 16-7. Defining Characteristics of *Salmonella* species

Do not ferment lactose on MacConkey agar
Produce gas when fermenting glucose
Produce H_2S from thioulfate

3. **Determinants of pathogenicity**
   a. **Endotoxin.** The *Salmonella* envelope contains LPS with an antigenic polysaccharide **(O antigen).**
   b. **Invasins,** proteins that mediate adherence to, and penetration of, intestinal epithelial cells, are important determinants of *Salmonella* pathogenicity.
   c. **Factors involved in resistance to phagocytosis** allow the bacteria to survive inside phagocytic cells. (*Salmonella* is a classic example of a **facultative intracellular organism.**)
      (1) Some of these factors (e.g., catalase, superoxide dismutase) neutralize active oxygen radicals.
      (2) Others neutralize defensins, small cationic proteins that facilitate bacterial killing by phagolysosomes.
   d. **Factors involved in resistance to acidic pH** may contribute to the ability of *Salmonella* to survive the acidity of the stomach and of the phagolysosome.
   e. **Vi *"Virulence"* antigen,** a special capsular polysaccharide of *S. typhi,* has antiphagocytic properties; however, its precise role as a virulence factor is unclear.
   f. **Other virulence factors** appear to exist. Based on work with attenuated strains of *S. typhi,* a series of genes that code for enzymes involved in the synthesis of aromatic amino acids (The AroA–D series) appears to be closely related to the virulence of invasive *S. typhi* and *S. typhimurium.*

4. **Pathogenesis and clinical disease**
   a. **Pathogenesis.** The portal of entry (small bowel epithelium) is common to all species. All virulent species apparently can survive gastric acidity and penetrate the intestinal epithelium and subepithelium, but only *S. typhi* is systemically invasive (Figure 16-2).
      (1) **Mucosal penetration,** mediated by *Salmonella* invasins, is followed by acute inflammation and ulceration.
      (2) **Mucosal inflammation** induces prostaglandin synthesis, activating adenyl cyclase and leading to fluid and electrolyte loss.
   b. **Clinical disease.** Different species and serotypes of *Salmonella* cause different diseases.
      (1) **Enterocolitis (salmonellosis)** is caused by *S. enteritidis* and *S. enteritidis typhimurium.*
         (a) **Characteristic symptoms** (diarrhea, fever, abdominal pain) develop after an 18- to 24-hour incubation period and usually are self-limited, lasting 2–5 days.
         (b) **Complications.** Dehydration and electrolyte imbalance are possible problems in the very young or old.
      (2) **Osteomyelitis** may be caused by *S. enteritidis* in patients with sickle cell anemia.
      (3) **Typhoid fever** (i.e., **systemic infection by *S. typhi***) affects humans exclusively.
         (a) **Characteristic symptoms**
            (i) **Symptoms** during the **first week** include **lethargy, malaise, fever, aches,** and **pains. Constipation** is the rule during this stage.
            (ii) In the **second week,** the organism reenters the circulation **(bacteremia),** producing high fever, tender abdomen, and, possibly, **rose-colored spots** on the skin. **Diarrhea** begins at the end of the second week or early in the third week.
         (b) **Complications.** The disease is self-limiting, but severe complications are possible (e.g., intestinal perforation, severe bleeding as a result of disseminated intravascular coagulation, thrombophlebitis, cholecystitis, pneumonia, abscess formation).

5. **Epidemiology**
   a. **Salmonellosis** is most often caused by **animal pathogens** that are easily transmitted to humans through contaminated food, particularly **poultry** and **eggs.**
   b. **Typhoid fever**
      (1) Typhoid fever is acquired via **fecal-oral transmission, contaminated water**

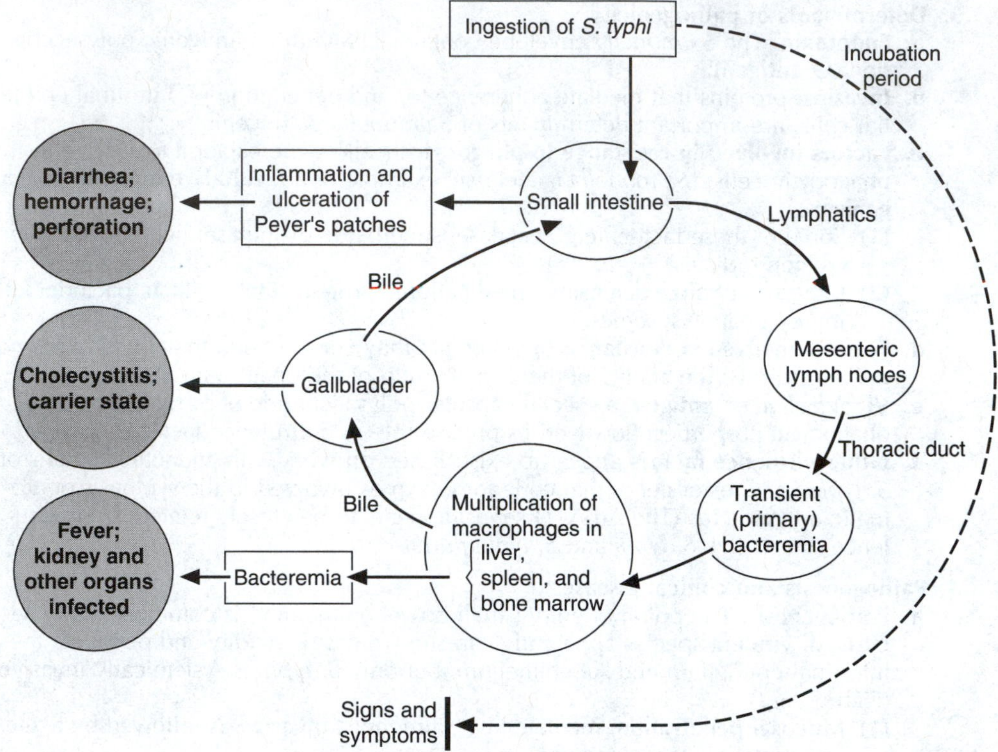

FIGURE 16-2. Pathogenesis of typhoid fever. *Salmonella typhi* invades the mucosa and regional lymph nodes without causing mucosal damage. From the lymph node, it spreads through the blood stream and is taken up by tissue macrophages, where the organism replicates. Those organisms that replicate in Kupffer cells can diffuse into the biliary spaces and gallbladder, reinfect the ileum, and cause enteric disease, including necrosis of Peyer's patches. (Redrawn with permission from Schaechter M, Medoff G, Eisenstein BI: *Mechanisms of Microbial Disease,* 2nd ed. Baltimore, Williams & Wilkins, 1993, p 274).

(e.g., following an earthquake or flood), or food processed by **asymptomatic chronic carriers** (usually older women with gallbladder disease, in whom the organism resides in gallstones or scars in the biliary tissue and is excreted in large numbers in the feces).

(2) The infection rate is approximately 25% with an infectious dose of 10^5 organisms and 95% with an infectious dose of 10^9 organisms.

6. Laboratory diagnosis. Culture and isolation are essential to confirm a diagnosis. Identification is based on biochemical characteristics and serology. The optimal culture sample varies with the presentation.

a. In a classic case of salmonellosis, a fecal sample is best.

b. If typhoid fever is suspected when the symptoms are characteristic of systemic disease, blood culture or a bone marrow aspirate is most likely to yield positive results. Later, with intestinal involvement, a swab of an ulcer obtained by sigmoidoscopy is indicated.

7. Treatment

a. Salmonellosis is usually treated supportively.

b. Typhoid fever

(1) Patients with typhoid fever. Chloramphenicol has traditionally been the drug of choice for patients with typhoid fever, despite the risks of blood dyscrasia associated with its use; **ampicillin** and **trimethoprim–sulfamethoxazole** are alternatives with less severe side effects. Recent trials suggest that **quinolones** (e.g., **norfloxacin, ciprofloxacin**) are as efficient as chloramphenicol, ampicillin, and trimethoprim-sulfamethoxazole for the treatment of patients with typhoid fever as well as chronic carriers, and these drugs have fewer serious side effects than chloramphenicol.

(2) Chronic carriers

(a) Antibiotics. Ampicillin has traditionally been the drug of choice for chronic carriers, but **quinolones** may be gaining favor.

(b) Surgical removal of the gallbladder is indicated in carriers with gallbladder disease.

8. Control and prevention

a. Salmonellosis is prevented mainly through **adequate sanitation** and **immunization** of domestic animals bred for human consumption. **Proper cooking of poultry products and meat** is important in reducing risk of infection. The indiscriminate use of antibiotics to promote growth of poultry and cattle should be avoided, as doing so favors the emergence of resistant strains.

b. Typhoid fever is controlled by **sanitation measures** and **personal hygiene.** An effective **vaccine** is being sought.

(1) A **killed *S. typhi* vaccine** has been in use for many years but is not very effective.

(2) An **attenuated strain (Ty21a)** is also licensed. This strain is deficient in the gene coding for galactosidase, but other uncharacterized deficiencies seem to be responsible for its attenuated characteristics. The rates of protection obtained with Ty21a are rather variable.

(3) Two additional types of vaccines are currently under evaluation as potential replacements, both appearing to be more effective:

(a) A vaccine made of purified Vi polysaccharide

(b) Attenuated recombinant variants of Ty21a that lack one or several of the Aro genes

III. VIBRIONACEAE (Table 16-8)

A. *Vibrio cholerae*

1. Classification

a. O1 group

(1) Classic cholera, (a metabolic disturbance of the small bowel epithelium) is caused by a toxin-producing strain known as ***V. cholerae O1,*** which agglutinates with antiserum directed against the O1 antigen.

(a) This strain has **two biotypes: El Tor** and **classic.**

(b) The El Tor biotype, which is the major cause of the ongoing pandemic in the Western Hemisphere, seems to survive better in the environment and causes asymptomatic infection more often than the classic biotype. These factors are believed to account for the replacement of the classic biotype by the El Tor biotype as the major cause of human pandemic infection.

(2) The classification of *V. cholerae* is confused by the fact that some isolates reactive with the O1 antiserum do not release toxin and are known as **atypical (nontoxigenic) *V. cholerae) O1.***

b. Non-O1 group. Other toxigenic isolates, known as non-O1 *V. cholerae,* do not react with anti-O1 antiserum. These strains have been associated with isolated cases of cholera and small outbreaks of diarrhea.

TABLE 16-8. Defining Characteristics of Vibrionaceae

Gram-negative, comma-shaped rod
Oxidase-positive
Motile, with single polar flagellum

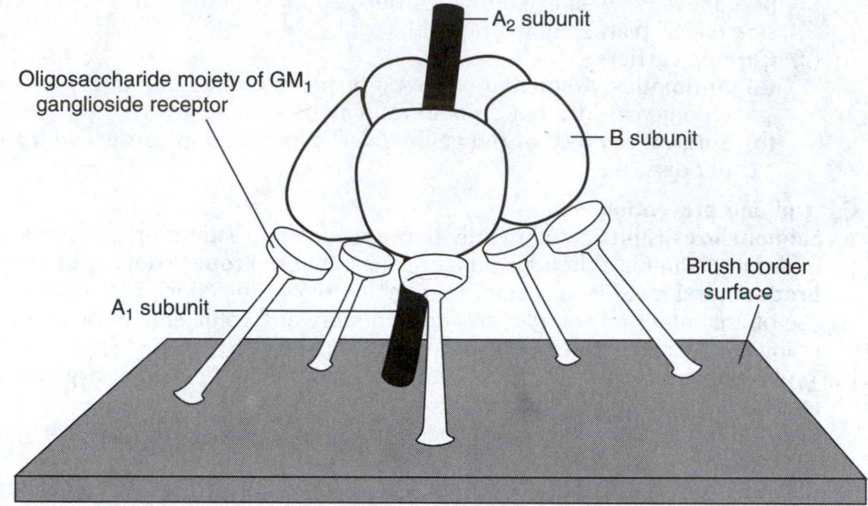

FIGURE 16-3. Subunit structure of cholera toxin (choleragen). After the B region binds to the GM_1 ganglioside receptor on the intestinal mucosal surface, the A region dissociates from the B region and penetrates the cell membrane. The disulfide bond that joins the A_1 and A_2 subunits is broken, and the A_1 subunit is activated. (Modified with permission from Rubino A, Guandalini S: Mechanisms of secretory diarrhea caused by bacterial enterotoxins. In *Chronic Diarrhea in Children,* edited by Lebenthal E. New York, Raven Press, 1984, pp 319–328.)

2. Determinants of pathogenicity

a. Enterotoxin. *V. cholerae* secretes the potent enterotoxin **choleragen.**

(1) Choleragen is a polymeric protein (molecular weight: 84,000 d) that consists of **two major non-covalently associated regions—** the A (active) region and the B (binding) region.

(a) The **A region** exhibits biologic activity.

(b) The **B region** facilitates the binding of choleragen to the intestinal cell.

(2) Both regions have **multiple subunits** (Figure 16-3).

b. Adhesion factors. Virulent *V. cholerae* adhere to the microvilli (brush border) of the small bowel mucosa and multiply. The mechanism of attachment is unclear; however, it is known that the *V. cholerae* O1 organism secretes the enzyme **mucinase,** which dissolves the glycoprotein coating of the intestinal cells.

3. Pathogenesis and clinical disease

a. Pathogenesis. A well-defined sequence of events occurs after *V. cholerae* ingestions, culminating in the onset of (copious, frequently life-threatening, secretory) diarrhea (Figure 16-4).

(1) Adherence and colonization. Virulent *V. cholerae* attach to the microvilli at the brush border and multiply.

(2) Secretion of cholera toxin. The toxin is released in close proximity to its specific cell membrane receptor **(GM_1 ganglioside).**

(3) Activation of the A_1 subunit. After the B subunit binds to the membrane receptor, the A subunit dissociates from the B subunit and penetrates the cell membrane. The disulfide bond that joins A_1 and A_2 is broken and the A_1 subunit is activated.

(a) Increased adenyl cyclase activity and accumulation of cyclic adenosine monophosphate (cAMP). Like pertussis toxin (see Chapter 15 II B 2 a), choleragen induces increased synthesis of cAMP, but through a slightly different mechanism. The activated A_1 subunit enzymatically transfers the adenosine diphosphate (ADP) ribose from a nicotinamide-adenine dinucleotide (NAD) to a guanosine triphosphate (GTP)-binding protein that regulates adenyl cyclase activity. Adenyl cyclase activity increases be-

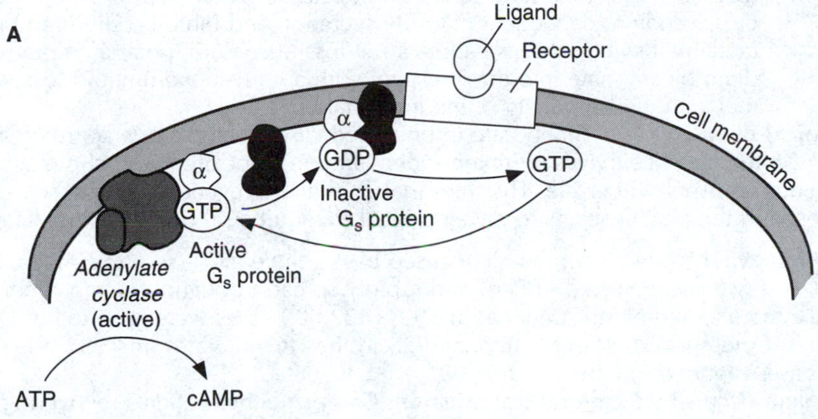

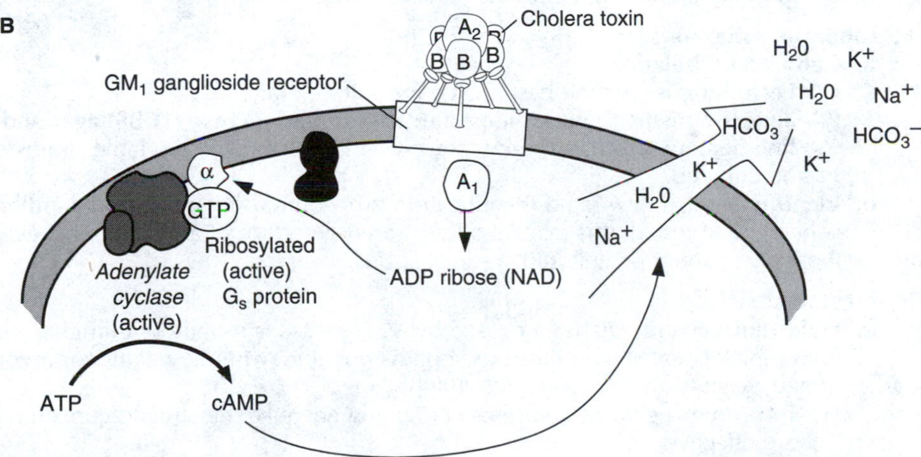

FIGURE 16-4. Cellular mechanism of action of cholera toxin. *(A)* Normal activation of adenylate cyclase by a G_s protein. In an inactive state, the G_s protein exists as a dimer with bound guanosine diphosphate *(GDP)*. The interaction of a receptor and ligand associated with the G_s protein causes a conformational change in the receptor, which, in turn, causes the GDP to dissociate from the G_s protein. The GDP is replaced by guanosine triphosphate *(GTP)*. GTP binding causes the G_s dimer to dissociate, and the α subunit, with bound GTP, activates the adenylate cyclase. Adenylate cyclase catalyzes the conversion of adenosine triphosphate *(ATP)* to cyclic adenosine monophosphate *(cAMP)*. Activation of adenylate cyclase is normally short-lived, because the α subunit has guanosine triphosphatase (GTPase) activity (i.e., it can break GTP into GDP). When GTP is converted to GDP, the G_s protein reassociates and becomes inactive. *(B)* Effect of cholera toxin. After binding to its receptor and penetrating the cell, the A_1 subunit of the toxin catalyzes the ribosylation of the α subunit of the G_s protein, activating the α subunit. The α subunit binds GTP and activates adenylate cyclase, but loses its GTPase activity, which renders the α subunit continuously active. The massive production of cAMP causes sodium-dependent chloride secretion and inhibits sodium *(Na^+)* and potassium *(K^+)* absorption. The resultant net flux of potassium, sodium, and bicarbonate *(HCO_3^-)* into the intestine is followed by hypersecretion of water *(H_2O)* and copious diarrhea. *ADP* = adenosine diphosphate; *NAD* = nicotinamide-adenine dinucleotide.

cause the normal GTP "turn-off" mechanism is inhibited, causing intracellular cAMP levels to mount.

(b) **Increased intestinal fluid loss.** The increased intracellular cAMP levels increase sodium-dependent chloride secretion and inhibit sodium and potassium absorption. This causes a net loss of sodium, potassium, and sodium bicarbonate into the intestine, with a corresponding fluid loss to maintain the isotonicity of the intestinal fluid.

b. **Clinical disease.** The mortality rate in untreated cases of cholera is approximately 60%. If the patient survives the intense dehydration associated with cholera, spontaneous recovery will ensue. The intestinal epithelium regenerates, diarrhea subsides, and the patient seems to develop local immunity, probably IgA-mediated.

4. **Epidemiology.** The ongoing epidemic (caused by *V. cholera* O1, serotype Inaba, biotype El Tor) was first detected in Peru and rapidly spread throughout South America, Central America, and North America. In 1991, 322,000 cases were reported in Peru, 46,000 in Colombia, 2690 in Mexico, and 25 in the United States. In 1992, the number of cases reported in Peru was 60,000.

a. Cholera occurs by **fecal-oral transmission.** Carriers (either patients recovering from the disease or chronic carriers) excrete the organisms, which contaminate water and food. Improperly cooked vegetables and seafood and nonpasteurized beverages present the greatest risk.

b. **Seasonal flooding** facilitates contamination of water supplies; flooding is often associated with cholera outbreaks in Asia.

c. Gastric fluid of normal acidity usually kills *V. cholerae;* **idiopathic tropical achlorydria** is relatively frequent in countries where cholera is epidemic, and it probably plays an important role in the spread of the disease.

5. **Laboratory diagnosis**

a. **Culture and isolation**

(1) **Fecal samples** are the best source for culture material.

(2) Selective media, such as **thiosulfate citrate bile sucrose (TCBS) agar** and **alkaline peptone broth,** are used to grow *V. cholerae.* Not all viable strains can be cultured.

b. **Identification.** A new rapid identification procedure using **monoclonal antibodies** is being field tested; this reagent allows rapid detection of all O1 strains, even those that cannot be cultured.

6. **Treatment.**

a. **Fluid replacement.** Diarrhea caused by *V. cholerae* is usually self-limiting, but fluid replacement should begin as soon as possible, without waiting for a confirmed diagnosis.

(1) **Intravenous glucose solutions** containing adequate electrolyte concentrations are effective.

(2) In underdeveloped countries, oral 2% glucose solution containing sodium chloride (3.5 g/L), potassium chloride (1.5 g/L), and sodium bicarbonate (2.5 g/L) has been an effective alternative measure.

b. **Antibiotic therapy** is reserved for serious cases. Drugs of choice are tetracycline, chloramphenicol, and cephalosporins.

7. **Prevention.** Classic killed vaccines have been extensively used, but the rate of protection is relatively low (i.e., they are effective in 60% of the vaccinated population) and the immunity is short-lived. Live attenuated vaccines have not fared better. Genetically engineered, nonpathogenic, living vaccines are being developed with the hope of achieving a better degree of protection.

B. *Vibrio parahaemolyticus* causes **food poisoning** characterized by **diarrhea.**

1. **General properties.** *V. parahaemolyticus* is a **halophilic marine organism;** it requires at least 2% sodium chloride to grow.

2. **Determinants of pathogenicity.** Pathogenic strains carry a **thermostable cytotoxin that causes hemolysis** and is cardiotoxic in certain animals. The existence of an en-

terotoxin, which would explain the diarrhea associated with *V. parahaemolyticus* infection, has not been proven.

3. **Epidemiology.** *V. parahaemolyticus* naturally inhabits brackish waters and infects estuarine and coastal water mollusks and crustaceans. Human disease is acquired by **ingestion of raw or improperly cooked seafood.**

4. **Treatment.**
The diarrhea caused by *V. parahaemolyticus* is usually self-limiting, requiring only supportive measures to compensate for fluid loss.

C. *Vibrio vulnificus* can cause **wound and systemic infections.**

1. **General properties**
   a. *V. vulnificus* is a **halophilic marine organism.**
   b. In contrast with other vibrios, it **ferments lactose.**

2. **Epidemiology and clinical disease**
   a. *V. vulnificus* grows in estuarine waters, where infections usually are contracted through **open wounds.** Swelling and erythema occur, and may evolve into gangrene within a few days.
   b. *V. vulnificus* can also contaminate shellfish. **Ingestion of raw oysters** may cause disease that is indistinguishable from other types of infectious gastroenteritis. The infection may become systemic, particularly in individuals with liver disease or other chronic conditions (e.g., chronic renal failure, congestive heart failure, diabetes, immunosuppression). The **septicemic form of infection** is associated with a **50% fatality rate.**

IV. *CAMPYLOBACTER* AND *HELICOBACTER*

A. *Campylobacter*

1. **General properties.** Campylobacter organisms are defined by the features listed in Table 16-9.

2. **Classification.** Main species include *C. jejuni* and *C. fetus.*

3. **Epidemiology**
   a. *Campylobacter* are **zoonotic bacteria** with a variety of animal reservoirs (e.g., cattle, poultry). Humans are infected via contaminated water or food.
   b. Once a human is infected, the bacteria can be transmitted from person to person by the **fecal-oral route.** Normal children can be carriers, and outbreaks in daycare centers have occurred.

4. **Clinical disease**
   a. ***C. jejuni*** causes **acute gastroenteritis,** which may be severe and ulcerative; systemic dissemination is rare. In children, the symptoms may mimic acute appendicitis. *C. jejuni* has also been reported to be associated with **Guillain-Barré syndrome,** an acute inflammatory demyelinating polyradiculoneuropathy associated with axonal motor neuropathy. An autoimmune response directed against neuron

TABLE 16-9. Defining Characteristics of *Campylobacter* species

Gram-negative, curved rods arranged in pairs (''gull wing'' appearance on Gram stain)*
Capnophilic (require 10% carbon dioxide for growth)
Thermophilic (grow best at 42°C)
Microaerophilic

* *Campylos* = ''curved'' in Greek

gangliosides is believed to be triggered by cross-reactivity between those gangliosides and *C. jejuni* LPS oligosaccharides.

b. ***C. fetus*** causes gastroenteritis less frequently, but is often involved in **systemic febrile infections in debilitated patients.**

5. **Laboratory diagnosis.** Diagnosis is confirmed by Gram stain and isolation in cultures of fecal material. The finding of blood or neutrophils in feces suggests invasion of the intestinal wall, which implies a more severe prognosis.

6. **Treatment.** Erythromycin and tetracyclines are effective against Campylobacter.

B. Helicobacter pylori (formerly *Campylobacter pylori*)

1. **General properties of** *H. pylori* are given in Table 16-10.

2. **Determinants of pathogenicity.** The main virulence factor is believed to be a **cytotoxin** that causes vacuolation in cultured gastric cells. The production of this toxin is a defining characteristic for type I strains of *H. pylori,* which predominate in specimens isolated from patients with gastric ulcers or gastric carcinoma.

3. **Clinical disease.** *H. pylori* is believed to be transmitted from **person-to-person** (cases tend to cluster in families). Infection is associated with chronic gastritis, gastric peptic ulcers, and gastric carcinoma.

4. **Diagnosis** requires a good degree of awareness by the physician and confirmation by adequate tests.

   a. **Clinical diagnosis** is complicated by the fact that symptoms are not typical of the classic dyspeptic syndromes and can easily be interpreted as nonspecific, psychogenic, or suggestive of some other type of intestinal pathology (e.g., irritable colon).

   b. The **"gold standard" approach** involves **gastric intubation, endoscopy,** and **biopsy.**

      (1) **Endoscopy** reveals inflammatory changes that would not be detected by an upper gastrointestinal series.

      (2) **Biopsy** supplies mucosa to be used for Gram stain analysis, histologic examination, and culture. In addition, a rapid test that detects *H. pylori* based on its production of urease can be performed on the biopsied tissue.

   c. **Tests of urease activity**

      (1) ***Campylobacter*-like organisms (CLO) test** is a direct test for urease production. A fragment of gastric mucosa is placed in urea-containing broth to which a pH indicator has been added. *H. pylori* will release urease, which breaks down urea and generates ammonia. The release of ammonia, a strong base, raises the pH and causes the broth to become dark pink. The greatest specificity for this test is obtained when the results are read within 20–60 minutes.

      (2) **Noninvasive tests of urease activity** have also been developed. The principle of these tests is simple: If an infected patient drinks a urea-containing solution, the urea will be broken down in the stomach and ammonia and carbon dioxide will be generated. Both compounds diffuse into the systemic circulation; carbon dioxide is eliminated by the lungs, and ammonia is eliminated in the urine.

         (a) **Breath test.** Breakdown of ^{14}C-labeled urea generates ^{14}C-labeled carbon dioxide, which can be traced in expired air.

TABLE 16-10. Defining Characteristics of *Helicobacter* species

Gram-negative, spiral-shaped (helical) rod
Capnophilic
Microaerophilic
Urease-producing

(b) **Urine test.** Breakdown of ^{15}N-labeled urea yields carbon dioxide and ^{15}N-labeled ammonia that can be traced by mass spectrometry.

(c) Both tests are noninvasive, and their positivity, usually measured at 20 minutes (breath test) and 2 hours (urine test), indicates infection.

5. **Treatment** is with a **combination of antacids** and one or two **broad-spectrum antibiotics.**
   a. **Antacids.** Omeprazole, a proton pump inhibitor, is preferred.
   b. **Antibiotics** are administered for 1–3 weeks. Options include **clarithromcin** (an acid-resistant macrolide, very effective for treatment of a gastric infection), **tetracyclines** (usually doxycycline), **amoxicillin,** and **metronidazole.**
   c. ***Bismuth subsalicylate*** is used in association with one or two of the antibiotics listed in (b) because *H. pylori* is susceptible to this compound.

Chapter 17

Gram-Negative Rods III: Opportunistic and Zoonotic Bacteria

Gabriel Virella

I. OPPORTUNISTIC BACTERIA

OPPORTUNISTIC BACTERIA are members of the normal flora that may cause severe systemic infection under certain circumstances (e.g., debilitation, immunocompromise).

A. Enterobacteriaceae

1. ***Klebsiella.*** Species include ***K. pneumoniae*** (***K. friedländeri***), ***K. oxytoca, K. ozaenae***, and ***K. rhinoscleromatis.*** *K. pneumoniae* is responsible for most infections.
   - a. **General properties** of *Klebsiella* are listed in Table 17-1.
   - b. **Determinants of pathogenicity**
     - (1) **Capsule.** A mucoid antiphagocytic capsule is *Klebsiella*'s major virulence factor.
     - (2) *Klebsiella* species participate in plasmid exchange with other enterobacteriaceae. Plasmid exchange is believed to be the basis for two inconstant characteristics of *Klebsiella* species:
       - (a) **Antibiotic resistance.** Many *Klebsiella* isolates are highly resistant to most antibiotics.
       - (b) **Toxins.** Some strains carry plasmids coding for toxins similar to the **heat-labile (LT)** and **heat-stable (ST) toxins** of *Escherichia coli.*
   - c. **Clinical disease**
     - (1) **Pneumonia.** *K. pneumoniae,* which is normally found in the respiratory tract of approximately 10% of the population, can cause pneumonia in immunocompromised individuals and diabetics. Lung abscesses may form.
       - (a) **Signs.** A significant clinical clue is the production of **thick, blood-tinged, viscous sputum.**
       - (b) **Prognosis.** Pneumonia as a result of *Klebsiella* infection carries a fatality rate of 50%. If bacteremia develops, the prognosis is even worse.
     - (2) **Urinary tract infections** are also commonly caused by *Klebsiella.*
     - (3) **Septicemia.** Newborns and alcoholics are susceptible.
     - (4) **Epidemic diarrhea** may be seen in newborns.
   - d. **Laboratory diagnosis.** *Klebsiella* species ferment lactose on MacConkey agar.
   - e. **Treatment.** Because these organisms are resistant to multiple antimicrobials, sensitivity testing is necessary to determine the drug of choice. Empiric therapy involves the use of an aminoglycoside and a cephalosporin.

2. ***Enterobacter*** species are often found in the normal intestinal flora, as well as in the environment. They are differentiated from other enterobacteriaceae on the basis of biochemical characteristics. The members of this genus are often involved in nosocomial infections, particularly of the **urinary tract,** in debilitated individuals. They are also associated with **bacteremia** and **septicemia.** Most commonly isolated species produce a potent β-lactamase that inactivates penicillins and first-generation cephalosporins.

3. ***Serratia***
   - a. **General properties.** Several species produce a **characteristic red pigment (prodigiosin).**
   - b. **Clinical disease.** In hospitalized patients, these organisms may be the cause of nosocomial surgical wound infection, urinary tract infection, respiratory tract infection, or severe systemic infection, including septicemia.
   - c. **Treatment.** Like many other Gram-negative bacteria, *Serratia* species are often resistant to multiple antibiotics.

TABLE 17-1. Defining Characteristics of *Klebsiella*

Gram-negative rod
Ferment lactose in MacConkey's
Mucoid capsule

4. ***Proteus.*** Species include ***P. mirabilis*** and ***P. vulgaris.***
   a. **General properties** of *Proteus* are listed in Table 17-2.
      (1) Numerous and long peritrichous flagella confer a **unique motility** on members of the *Proteus* genus. When growing in culture, the colonies have a **swarming** aspect.
      (2) The production of **phenylalanine deaminase** is common to *Proteus, Morganella,* and *Providencia* and allows differentiation of these species from other enterobacteriaceae.
   b. **Antigenic composition.** Like most Gram-negative enterobacteriaceae, *Proteus* species have **O, H,** and **K antigens.** The **Weil-Felix test,** which detects antibodies against certain rickettsiae in serum, uses specific *Proteus* strains that are agglutinated by cross-reactive antibodies directed against *Rickettsia* antigens.
   c. **Clinical disease**
      (1) **Urinary tract infections.** When urease-producing strains become involved in urinary tract infections, the production of urease results in the liberation of ammonia and raises the pH of the urine. The alkalization of the urine reduces the solubility of calcium, creating conditions favorable for the deposition of calcium and magnesium salts and the production of **kidney stones.**
      (2) **Wound infections.** *Proteus* is frequently isolated from infected wounds.
      (3) **Septicemia** may be caused by *Proteus.*

5. ***Morganella*** and ***Providencia*** are closely related to *Proteus.*
   a. **General properties.** All of these organisms are indole fermenters. *Morganella* species are urease producers, but most species of *Providencia* are not.
   b. **Clinical disease.** These organisms are most often involved in **nosocomial urinary tract infections, pneumonia,** and **bacteremia.** Clinical isolates are usually resistant to multiple antibiotics.

6 ***Citrobacter.*** The various species of *Citrobacter* are closely related to *Salmonella* and can be found in the environment or as part of the stool's normal flora. In debilitated patients, *Citrobacter* can cause urinary tract infections, diarrhea (especially in children), wound infections, septicemia, and neonatal meningitis.

7. ***E. coli*** can also be considered an opportunistic enterobacteriaceae (see Chapter 16 II B).

B. ***Pseudomonas. P. aeruginosa*** is the most important human pathogen; ***P. mallei*** and ***P. cepacia*** (recently segregated as a new species, *Burkholderia cepacia*) are the other species frequently isolated from humans. Soil and water are the natural habitat of *Pseudomonas* species, but they can behave opportunistically in debilitated or immunocompromised patients.

TABLE 17-2. Defining Characteristics of *Proteus*

Gram-negative rod
Extremely motile
Produce urease (several species)
Produce hydrogen sulfide from sodium thiosulfate
Ferment indole (*P. vulgaris*)
Produce phenylalanine deaminase

TABLE 17-3. Defining Characteristics of *Pseudomonas*

Gram-negative rod
Capsulated
Primarily aerobic, but can grow anaerobically
Oxidase-positive
Minimal growth requirements*
Does not ferment glucose or lactose
Motile
Pigment producers (many strains)

* *Pseudomonas* can grow at temperatures ranging from 25°C–42°C, in the presence of high concentrations of salt, and in spite of low concentrations of antiseptics and antibiotics.

1. **General properties** of *Pseudomonas* are listed in Table 17-3. *Pseudomonas* species can release three different pigments:
   a. **Pyocyanin** has the ability to catalyze the reduced nicotinamide-adenine dinucleotide (NADH)–dependent conversion of oxygen to superoxide and hydrogen peroxide.
      (1) The presence of superoxide and hydrogen peroxide inhibits the growth of other bacteria and causes cytotoxicity.
      (2) Pyocyanin causes the **blue discoloration** occasionally seen in the purulent exudates of infections caused by *Pseudomonas.*
   b. **Pyoverdin** is responsible for the **green discoloration** of the agar plates growing this organism.
   c. **Fluorescein** imparts a **green fluorescence** to bacterial colonies when they are examined under an ultraviolet light.
2. **Determinants of pathogenicity**
   a. **Alginate capsule.** Some strains of *Pseudomonas* produce an alginate capsule, which is formed by a polymer of mannuronic and glucuronic acids. Isolates producing this compound have a **mucoid (glistening) appearance.**
      (1) The alginate coat is important for survival in an aquatic environment, but it is also produced by bacteria infecting the lungs (probably in response to environmental changes, such as high osmolarity and low nitrogen).
      (2) It is believed that the alginate capsule functions both as an **adhesion factor** and as an **antiphagocytic factor.**
   b. **Pilin** and **non-pilus adhesins** are essential for initial colonization of epithelial tissue.
   c. **Hemolysins,** one of which is a phospholipase C, may destroy tissue surfactants and contribute to the development of pulmonary atelectasis.
   d. **Proteases** digest proteins, including elastase, and cause tissue destruction.
   e. **Toxins.** *Pseudomonas* produces several toxins, including **lipopolysaccharide (LPS, endotoxin),** an **enterotoxin,** and two exotoxins, **exotoxin S** (also known as **exoenzyme S**) and **exotoxin A.**
      (1) **Exotoxin A,** released by approximately 90% of the isolates, is the most important of the toxins released by *Pseudomonas.* Like diphtheria toxin (see Chapter 13 II B 3), exotoxin A has ADP-ribosyl transferase activity and inactivates elongation factor-2 (EF-2), inhibiting protein synthesis.
      (2) **Exotoxin S,** released by approximately 40% of the isolates, ADP-ribosylates host cell G proteins. Both exotoxins are believed to inhibit phagocytic activity.
   f. **Antibiotic resistance** results from the relative impermeability of the cell wall. Effective antibiotics are transported through porins or by diffusion after binding to LPS side-chains. Thus, mutations affecting porins and switches in LPS side-chain synthesis that result in charge changes are frequently responsible for the development of antibiotic resistance.

3. **Pathogenesis and clinical disease**
   a. **Pathogenesis.** *Pseudomonas* species are most often involved in opportunistic and nosocomial infections involving individuals with predisposing conditions (e.g., extensive burns, trauma to the skin or conjunctiva, urinary tract manipulations, cystic fibrosis).
      (1) Infection may remain localized at the site of the injury, but bacteremia develops frequently, leading to dissemination of the infection to distant foci and sepsis.
      (2) The unique association between *Pseudomonas* and cystic fibrosis has been the object of intensive investigation.
         (a) **Colonization.** The enhanced ability of *Pseudomonas* to colonize patients with cystic fibrosis seems to result from a combination of abnormalities.
            (i) The **high sialic acid content of the salivary mucin glycopeptides** in patients with cystic fibrosis enhances the adhesion of *Pseudomonas* to mucin-covered mucosal surfaces.
            (ii) Expression of **asialoganglioside$_1$ (aGM$_1$),** which serves as a receptor for *Pseudomonas,* is **increased** on the respiratory epithelium of cystic fibrosis patients.
            (iii) Damage of the mucosal epithelium by proteases, including a protease released by *Pseudomonas* and proteases released by inflammatory cells, leads to **exposure of cellular cytoskeleton components** with a strong binding affinity for *Pseudomonas.*
         (b) **Enhanced virulence.** The strains of *Pseudomonas* isolated from patients with cystic fibrosis produce **higher levels of exotoxin A.** The strains that establish chronic infection have a **well-developed alginate capsule** that increases resistance to phagocytosis.
   b. **Clinical disease**
      (1) **Ear infections.** *Pseudomonas* can cause outer and middle ear infections in healthy children.
      (2) **Bacteremia.** In debilitated patients, *Pseudomonas* accounts for 10% of all Gram-negative systemic infections and is associated with a 50% mortality rate.

4. **Epidemiology**
   a. **Transmission.** *Pseudomonas* are ubiquitous and resistant to disinfectants, a fact that accounts for the frequency with which they cause nosocomial infections. Hospitalized patients can be contaminated in a myriad of ways—via food, dirty hands, respiratory equipment, and intravenous fluids, for example.
   b. **Susceptibility. Burn victims, cystic fibrosis patients,** and **patients that have been catheterized for an extended period of time** are frequently affected.

5. **Diagnosis** of *Pseudomonas* infections requires **culture and isolation.**

6. **Treatment.** Antibiotic susceptibilities must be determined in all cases, because these organisms are resistant to a variety of antibiotics.

7. **Prevention.** General and often simple measures (e.g., hand washing) and the choice of adequate wound topical disinfectants can decrease the incidence of these infections in the hospital environment.

II. ZOONOTIC BACTERIA are bacteria, isolated from vertebrates other than humans, that sporadically are transmitted to and cause serious disease in humans.

A. *Brucella.* Species include *B. melitensis, B. abortus,* and *B. suis.*

1. **General properties** of *Brucella* species are summarized in Table 17-4.

2. **Determinants of pathogenicity**
   a. **Ability to resist phagocytosis.** It seems that low-molecular-weight substances on the bacterial surface inhibit fusion of lysosomal granules with the phagosomes.

TABLE 17-4. Defining Characteristics of *Brucella*

Gram-negative coccobacilli
Nonmotile
Facultative intracellular organisms
Fastidious; require enriched complex media and grow best in 5%–10% carbon dioxide*

* Colonies may take 2–5 days to develop

b. **Ability to survive intracellularly.** Once ingested by macrophages, the bacterium survives and multiplies intracellularly (e.g., in the lymph nodes, spleen, liver, and bone marrow). The ability to survive intracellularly complicates elimination by the immune system and treatment with antibacterial agents.

3. Pathogenesis and clinical disease

a. Pathogenesis

(1) Portal of entry

(a) **Gastrointestinal tract.** Ingestion of contaminated foods (e.g., goat and sheep milk and cheese) can lead to *B. melitensis* infection.

(b) **Dermal abrasions.** Direct contact with contaminated animal products presents a risk, especially to meat handlers, veterinarians, and abattoir employees.

(2) The bacteria localize in the reticuloendothelial system, eliciting a granulomatous host response. Focal abscesses and caseation may occur.

b. Clinical disease

(1) Clinical signs of brucellosis usually become apparent following an **incubation period of 3–16 days.**

(2) The acute disease, an **influenza-like syndrome with fever, headache, constipation,** and **severe limb, back, or abdominal pain,** may persist for several weeks. The fever and other symptoms tend to follow a protracted course with exacerbations and relapses.

(a) The **undulant fever** (Figure 17-1) may last for months.

(b) **Anemia, weakness,** and **easy fatigue** become prominent.

(3) **Sequelae.** The infection can disseminate to several organs and tissues, causing arthritis, spondylitis, meningitis, uveitis, and orchitis.

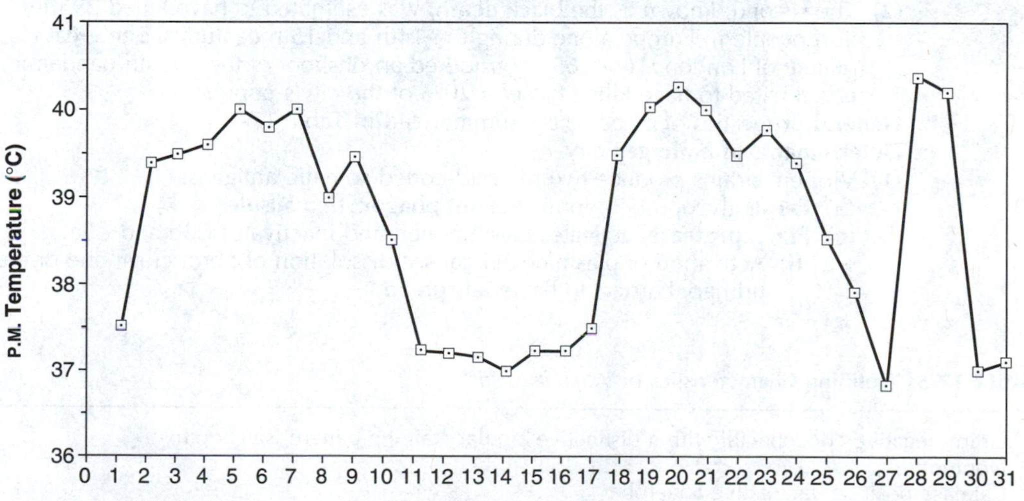

FIGURE 17-1. Plot of a typical undulating fever in an untreated case of brucellosis.

4. **Epidemiology**
   a. **Reservoirs.** Human infection by *Brucella* is a true zoonosis. In animals, *Brucella* multiplies in the uterus of gravid animals and in the mammary glands, particularly in goats and sheep. *Brucella* may be excreted in the milk for years.
   b. **Incidence.** Infection by contaminated milk products is prevalent in the Mediterranean basin, South America, Southeast Asia, and the Pacific region.
   c. **Mortality rate.** The mortality rate for untreated brucellosis is estimated to be 5%–10%.

5. **Laboratory diagnosis.** Diagnosis of brucellosis requires a high index of suspicion and is often based on the occupation, ethnic background, or travel history of the patient.
   a. **Culture and isolation** is necessary to confirm the diagnosis.
      (1) Because of the systemic nature of the infection, **blood cultures** are tried first.
      (2) If the disease has reached an advanced stage, **bone marrow aspirate** or **liver biopsy** may be required to obtain adequate samples for culture.
   b. **Serologic tests**
      (1) An **agglutination test** has been in use. This test requires verification of increasing antibody titers from acute to convalescent samples, or the finding of a titer greater than or equal to 160.
      (2) An **enzyme immunoassay (EIA) test** that detects specific IgM antibodies is now available and allows diagnosis of acute infection.

6. **Treatment**
   a. **Tetracycline** is the drug of choice.
   b. **Tetracycline and streptomycin.** Some epidemiological studies suggest that early treatment with tetracycline and streptomycin results in a lower rate of post-treatment relapse. Relapses result from the difficulty of eradicating intracellular bacteria.

7. **Control and prevention.** Herd vaccination, pasteurization of animal milk, and preparation of milk derivatives with pasteurized milk have contributed to the virtual eradication of this infection from most industrialized countries.

B. ***Yersinia*** belongs to the enterobacteriaceae family.

1. ***Y. pestis***
   a. **Historical significance.** *Y. pestis* is believed to have been responsible for at least two large pandemics of plague.
      (1) The first, during the reign of Justinian in 500 A.D., is estimated to have killed 100 million people.
      (2) The second, known as the **black death,** was estimated to have killed 25 million people in Europe alone during the 14th and 15th centuries. The great plague of London (1664–65), considered an offshoot of the second pandemic, is estimated to have killed close to 20% of the city's population.
   b. **General properties** of *Y. pestis* are summarized in Table 17-5.
   c. **Determinants of pathogenicity**
      (1) Virulent strains produce two plasmid-coded somatic antigens:
         (a) **F-1,** a glycoprotein, forms the **antiphagocytic capsule.**
         (b) **Pla,** a **protease,** activates plasminogen and inactivates C3b and C5a.
            (i) Activation of plasminogen causes dissolution of fibrin clots, one of the primary barriers to bacterial spread.

TABLE 17-5. Defining Characteristics of *Yersinia pestis**

Gram-negative coccobacilli with a distinctive bipolar staining pattern (safety pin)
Nonmotile
Catalase-positive, facultative anaerobe
Grows best at 28°C, colonies may take 2–5 days to develop

* Common to most other *Yersinia* species as well.

(ii) Inactivation of C3b and C5a leads to inhibition of C3b-mediated phagocytosis and C5a-mediated chemotaxis.

(2) In addition, virulent forms of *Y. pestis* carry the **W/V antigen,** which has antiphagocytic properties and seems to promote intracellular growth. (W is a protein, and V is a lipoprotein.)

d. Clinical disease. *Y. pestis* causes natural disease in rats and other rodents; when the host dies, if no other rodent is available for the flea to colonize, the fleas searching for a host will transmit the disease to humans. The plague has two distinct clinical forms.

(1) **Bubonic plague** is characterized by **large lymphadenopathies (buboes)** in the area draining the site of the flea bite and is usually associated with a **high fever.** If the disease progresses unchecked, **bacteremia** ensues following multiplication of the bacteria in the lymph nodes.

(2) **Pneumonic plague.** Bacteremia leads to secondary spread of the infection to many organs, including the lungs, and the plague becomes pneumonic.

(a) The **mortality rate** is **100%.**

(b) **Human-to-human transmission through infected droplets becomes possible.**

e. Epidemiology

(1) **Transmission.** Epidemiologically, two types of plague can be distinguished.

(a) **Urban plague,** which occurs mostly in cities, is the epidemic form transmitted by **rat fleas.**

(b) **Sylvatic plague** (from the Latin *silva,* wood) is acquired from infected **wild animals.** Sylvatic plague exists in the western United States, where the infection is endemic among pack rats, squirrels, and prairie dogs.

(i) Hunters and backpackers are susceptible, although transmission is accidental and infrequent.

(ii) Most cases of urban, and virtually all cases of sylvatic, plague are clinically bubonic, at least during the initial stages.

(2) **Incidence**

(a) The last pandemic, which started in Burma in 1894, caused an estimated 10 million fatalities over 20 years.

(b) The last outbreak recorded in this century took place in the North African city of Oran in the 1940s.

(c) Between 1958 and 1979, 47,000 cases of plague were reported worldwide.

f. Treatment. *Y. pestis* is susceptible to several antibiotics, including **streptomycin, chloramphenicol,** and **tetracycline.**

2. *Y. enterocolitica*

a. Determinants of pathogenicity. Virulence factors include:

(1) **Adhesins and invasins**

(2) **Antiphagocytic proteins**

(3) An **enterotoxin,** similar to the ST toxin of *E. coli*

b. Clinical disease

(1) **Gastroenteritis.** *Y. enterocolitica* causes food-borne gastroenteritis.

(2) **Reactive arthritis.** A cell wall component of *Y. enterocolitica* has been identified that induces T cell proliferation when it associates with a major histocompatibility complex (MHC) II molecule. This property is very similar to that exhibited by staphylococcal superantigen and it may be significant in the pathogenesis of reactive arthritis.

(3) **Ankylosing spondylitis.** The association of *Y. enterocolitica* with arthritis has been the cause of considerable speculation concerning the possible role of *Y. enterocolitica* in the development of ankylosing spondylitis.

c. Epidemiology

(1) **Reservoirs.** *Y. enterocolitica* infects a variety of domestic animals and rodents. It has also been isolated from lakes and well water.

(2) **Transmission**

(a) Humans may become infected by ingesting **contaminated food** and **water.**

(b) Transmission among humans by the **fecal-oral route** is also possible.

d. **Treatment.** The drugs of choice are **streptomycin, chloramphenicol,** and **tetracycline.**

C. *Francisella tularensis*

1. **General properties.** *F. tularensis* are small, pleomorphic, nonmotile Gram-negative rods.
2. **Determinants of pathogenicity.** This organism seems to evade humoral immunity by surviving as a facultative intracellular parasite; cell-mediated immunity (CMI) seems to be predominantly involved in protection.
3. **Transmission and clinical disease**
   a. **Transmission.** Rabbits, deer, and rodents can harbor *F. tularensis.* Transmission normally involves fleas or ticks, but humans can also contract the organism by handling the carcasses of infected animals or eating contaminated meat.
   b. **Clinical disease**
      (1) Tularemia is characterized by ulceration at the site of a bite or scratch, regional lymphadenopathy, fever, and malaise.
      (2) Ingestion of contaminated meat may cause a typhoid-like disease.
4. **Treatment. Streptomycin, chloramphenicol,** and **tetracycline** are the drugs of choice.

D. ***Pasteurella multocida*** infects a variety of animals and is usually transmitted to humans via **dog** and **cat bites.** Infection is usually mild, but can give rise to abscesses at the site of infection and regional lymphadenopathies. If untreated, the infection may become chronic. **Penicillins** are the drug of choice.

E. ***Campylobacter*** is discussed in Chapter 16 IV.

Chapter 18

Mycobacteria

John Manos
Gerald E. Wagner

I. INTRODUCTION

A. General properties

1. As a group, mycobacteria are slow-growing, aerobic bacteria with an unusual cell wall composition. They are slender, straight or slightly curved rods measuring 0.2–0.4 μm in diameter and 2–10 μm in length.
2. Some species are saprophytic. The most significant human pathogens are ***M. tuberculosis, M. avium-intracellulare***, and ***M. leprae.***

B. **Pathogenesis.** Mycobacteria characteristically survive after ingestion by macrophages and behave as **facultative intracellular organisms.**

1. The infected cells express major histocompatibility complex (MHC)-associated bacterial peptides that trigger T cell responses.
2. Activated $CD4^+$ and TH_1 cells release large amounts of interferon-γ-(IFN-γ), which activates the infected macrophages. The activated macrophages, in turn, destroy the intracellular mycobacteria. The activation of cell-mediated immunity (CMI) is responsible for the formation of the granulomatous lesions characteristic of most mycobacterial infections.

C. **Culture and isolation.** Mycobacterial isolation by culture should always be attempted, particularly when the patient is severely ill or when the diagnosis is unclear. At this time, culture and isolation is the **only practical method to determine antimicrobial agent susceptibilities.**

1. **Specimen selection and collection.** The choice of specimen is usually determined by the patient's clinical presentation and history.
   a. The **volume** of specimen submitted is important. Because body fluids may contain few organisms/ml, submission of larger volumes of fluid increases the likelihood of recovering the causative organism. Blood and feces from AIDS and other immunocompromised patients generally contain a high concentration of organisms.
   b. The **number** of specimens to be submitted is also important. One specimen per day of sputa, gastric aspirates, or urine should be submitted for 3–5 days.
   c. **Timing.** Early morning specimens are best because the organisms have accumulated overnight.
2. **Culture media.** Most laboratories use a combination of a broth and a solid medium to enhance recovery of organisms.
   a. **Broth.** Mycobacteria grow more quickly in broth media than on solid media.
      (1) Isolation of *M. tuberculosis* often occurs in 4–25 days in broth; on solid media, it averages 2–4 weeks, but may take as long as 8 weeks.
      (2) Special broth containing ^{14}C-labeled precursors can be used to detect growing mycobacteria, which metabolize the labeled nutrients and release $^{14}CO_2$.
   b. **Solid media**
      (1) **Egg-based media** (e.g., **Löwenstein-Jensen medium**) support good growth of most mycobacteria. Antimicrobial agents can be added to the media to inhibit undesirable bacteria present in specimens with numerous bacteria (e.g., sputum).
      (2) **Agar-based media** (e.g., **Middlebrook medium**) also support growth of myco-

bacteria. Middlebrook medium is transparent, allowing detection of minute mycobacterial colonies more quickly than with egg-based media.

D. Identification

1. **Staining.** Mycobacteria are **acid-fast** (i.e., they stain red) because of the N-glycolylmuramic (mycolic) acid in their cell walls. The **Ziehl-Neelsen stain** is the most commonly employed acid-fast staining technique.
   - **a.** The cell walls of mycobacteria are unique in that they contain N-glycolylmuramic acid rather than N-acetylmuramic acid.
   - **b.** The lipid content of the cell wall is very high (i.e., as much as 60% of the dry weight); therefore, mycobacteria are hydrophobic and impermeable to basic aniline bacteriologic stains.
2. **Biochemical characteristics**
   - **a. Growth rates** and **pigmentation** are the basis for categorizing mycobacteria.
     - **(1) "Rapid growers"** grow in less than 7 days.
     - **(2) "Slow growers"** require more than 7 days for growth.
       - **(a) Photochromogens** become pigmented after exposure to light.
       - **(b) Scotochromogens** are pigmented, regardless of exposure to light.
       - **(c) Nonphotochromogens** are nonpigmented under all conditions.
   - **b.** Each group has a set of key biochemical tests to help identify the members of that group. These tests can only be performed after the colonies have developed and may take 3–21 days to complete.
3. **Chromatographic analysis.** Gas–liquid or high-performance chromatography is used at the Centers for Disease Control (CDC) and at several state health department laboratories to identify the 27 most commonly isolated mycobacterial species.
   - **a.** Following chromatographic analysis of fatty acids extracted from the cell walls of an isolate, a computer program compares the resulting profile with profiles of known mycobacteria.
   - **b.** As with other identification methods, a sufficient amount of mycobacterial growth is required for chromatographic analysis. In addition, the technique is costly in terms of equipment, reagents, and specialized personnel.
4. **Nucleic acid hybridization** has had a strong impact on the identification of slow-growing mycobacteria.
   - **a.** Nucleic acid probes for *M. tuberculosis* complex, *M. avium-intracellulare* complex, *M. kansasii,* and *M. gordonae* (a common contaminant) are commercially available. The specificity and sensitivity of the probes is excellent, and results are available within 2–3 hours, once a sufficient amount of mycobacterial growth is available.
   - **b.** Limitations include costs related to equipment and reagents, the degree of technical expertise required, and the need to wait for significant mycobacterial growth.
5. **Polymerase chain reaction (PCR;** see Chapter 10 III B 2) does not require growth of organisms in order to detect mycobacteria, especially *M. tuberculosis,* in patient specimens. However, as of this writing, no method has been approved by the Food and Drug Administration (FDA) for commercial use.

II. *MYCOBACTERIUM TUBERCULOSIS*

A. General properties of *M. tuberculosis* are summarized in Table 18-1.

TABLE 18-1. Defining Characteristics of *Mycobacterium tuberculosis*

Acid-fast, slender rod
Slow-growing, fastidious bacterium
Microaerophic aerobe
Grows best at temperatures of 37°C

B. **Determinants of pathogenicity.** The virulence factors for *M. tuberculosis* have not been as well defined as those for many other bacteria.

1. **Cording factor** is a **glycolipid derivative of mycolic acid** that is present on the outer surface of *M. tuberculosis.*
   a. The glycolipid **inhibits migration of polymorphonuclear (PMN) leukocytes** and **elicits granuloma formation.** When released intracellularly, it **seems to damage mitochondrial membranes.**
   b. Cording factor causes bacilli to grow in culture in **serpentine "cords"** (i.e., parallel arrangements of bacilli form). Observation of this type of growth is usually indicative of pathogenicity.
   c. Cording factor is **immunogenic** and can induce protective immunity in animals.

2. **Sulfatides,** glycolipids located on the surface of mycobacteria, inhibit phagolysosome formation, permitting the bacterium to survive intracytoplasmically after being ingested by macrophages. Sulfatides may also prevent the pH inside the phagolysosome from dropping below 6.0 by preventing the insertion of proton adenosine triphosphatases (ATPases), which are responsible for intravesicular acidification.

3. **Antibacterial resistance.** The molecular mechanisms of resistance are being actively investigated. So far, they appear to involve mutations in the bacterial drug targets.
   a. **Isoniazid.** The antimycobacterial effect seems to involve blockade of mycolic acid synthesis, which is mediated by the binding of the drug to InhA protein, a receptor protein. Mutations in the InhA protein have been recently shown to correlate with resistance.
   b. **Rifampin.** Resistance is associated with a mutation of the gene coding for the B subunit of RNA polymerase.

C. **Pathogenesis and clinical disease**

1. **Primary infection.** Initially, infection with *M. tuberculosis* usually involves the mid- or lower lung field, and the focus is usually single. CMI will develop in most otherwise healthy individuals, controlling the infection and causing the patient to remain asymptomatic.
   a. The scar of the primary complex (i.e., the initial locus of infection and satellite lymphadenopathy) may calcify, making it visible on chest radiographs. Enlargement of the mediastinal lymph node may also be present.
   b. The bacilli in the lesions slowly die, although a few may remain viable for over 20 years. Several factors influence the outcome of infection with *M. tuberculosis,* particularly nutritional status and the competency of the immune system. Patients are at the most risk for developing active tuberculosis during the first year following the initial exposure.

2. **Active tuberculosis** may develop as a progression of primary infection or as a reactivation of a quiescent infection.
   a. **Progression of a primary infection.** If *M. tuberculosis* is not controlled at the site of the primary infection, phagocytosed bacilli will diffuse through the lymphatic vessels and the blood stream.
      (1) Any organ system can be infected. Lesions are most commonly seen in the apex of the lung; other body areas of high oxygen tension are frequently the sites of reactivation. The kidneys, bone and bone marrow, lymph nodes, brain, meninges, and intestines may be involved.
      (2) Microscopic granulomatous lesions develop, usually 2–6 weeks following infection. The lesions have a central area where epithelioid cells (modified macrophages) and giant cells predominate, surrounded by a lymphocytic infiltrate. In the lungs, the granulomatous lesions may become necrotic and form cavities by eroding bronchi and small blood vessels.
   b. **Reactivation of a latent infection** may occur 20 years or longer after the primary infection following deterioration of immune resistance to *M. tuberculosis.* This is the most commonly diagnosed form of the disease in western countries; men over the age of 50 are most commonly affected.

c. **Clinical signs** include coughing, hemoptysis, afternoon fever, night sweats, weight loss, and malaise. Symptoms may be more pronounced in reactivation tuberculosis.

3. **Disseminated (miliary) tuberculosis** is characterized by numerous small tubercles (granulomatous nodules).
   a. Very young or elderly individuals and immunocompromised patients are most frequently affected.
   b. Typically, a necrotic tubercle causes erosion of a blood vessel, leading to the hematogenous spread of the bacteria. Fulminant infection in every organ system results; therefore, this form of tuberculosis is associated with a high mortality rate.

D. Epidemiology

1. **Transmission.** Tuberculosis is not highly contagious but is acquired via inhalation of respiratory droplets.
2. **Incidence**
   a. The incidence of tuberculosis in western countries has declined dramatically during the last century; however, it is still a very prevalent disease in developing countries.
   b. In the United States, the introduction of tuberculostatic drugs substantially decreased the number of cases of active tuberculosis to approximately 20,000 cases per year. Unfortunately, the rate seems to be increasing.
3. **Susceptibility**
   a. **Socioeconomically disadvantaged people living in crowded urban areas** are at increased risk. The inner-city areas of Chicago and Washington, D.C. have the highest incidence of infection in the United States.
   b. **Native Americans** have a high incidence of tuberculosis.
   c. **AIDS patients** and **healthcare workers** are at increased risk.
   d. **Immigrants** from less developed countries show a higher prevalence of the disease.

E. Laboratory diagnosis.

The diagnosis may be strongly suspected when typical cavitary or calcified lesions are detected radiographically, but confirmation requires isolation of *M. tuberculosis.*

1. Finding acid-fast slender rods in sputum or any other adequate sample identifies *Mycobacteria* as the cause of disease.
2. Species identification requires culture for isolation and characterization of the isolate.
   a. Löwenstein-Jensen medium is the best medium for isolation of *M. tuberculosis.*
   b. Doubling times for isolates of *M. tuberculosis* are 6 hours or longer. Three to six weeks may be required before identifiable colonies appear.

F. Treatment.

Because of the increasing prevalence of resistant strains, antimicrobial sensitivity testing of isolates is essential.

1. **Regimen.** The treatment of tuberculosis involves simultaneous administration of at least two drugs (Table 18-2) to avoid the emergence of resistant strains of *M. tubercu-*

TABLE 18-2. Antituberculous Drugs

Primary	Secondary
Ethambutol	Capreomycin*
Pyrazinamide	Cycloserine
Isoniazid	Ethionamide
Streptomycin*	Fluoroquinolones
Rifampin	Kanamycin*
	Para-aminosalycilic acid (PAS)
	Rifabutin
	Viomycin*

* Injectables only

losis. The CDC recommends that four drugs should be used concurrently for the initial treatment in an effort to counteract the emergence and rapid spread of drug-resistant *Mycobacteria,* particularly among HIV-infected patients and their close contacts.

2. **Duration.** Treatment should be continued for several months, depending on the severity of the disease. Patient compliance is essential to minimize the emergence of resistant strains.

G. Control and prevention

1. **Immunoprophylaxis.** Administration of **bacille Calmette-Guérin (BCG),** an attenuated strain derived from *M. bovis,* has been used successfully as a vaccine in Europe and developing countries. Effectiveness trials in the United States showed minimal protection and results in other countries, although not as disappointing, have yielded variable results. At this time, this vaccine is not recommended for general use in the United States.

2. **Screening** for exposure is the preferred approach in the United States. The strong CMI elicited by this organism is used as the basis for a skin test.
   a. **Mantoux test.** Five units of *M. tuberculosis* antigen **(tuberculin** or its protein-purified derivative, **PPD)** are injected intradermally. The results are read 48–72 hours later. The appearance of an indurated erythematous reaction measuring at least 10 mm is considered a positive test result.
   b. **Interpretation**
      (1) **A positive Mantoux test does not necessarily mean the patient has tuberculosis.** It only means that the patient has been previously exposed to the bacterium (i.e., primary exposure has taken place). Vaccination can lead to a positive test result as well.
      (2) **False-positive reactions** may occur as a result of cross-reactions with other mycobacteria.
      (3) **False-negative reactions** occur in certain situations associated with **anergy** (e.g., overwhelming *M. tuberculosis* infection, immunosuppression).
   c. **Follow-up.** If a young tuberculosis-negative individual becomes tuberculosis-positive, he or she should be treated with isoniazid for 1 year in order to eradicate *M. tuberculosis.* In older individuals who test positive without evidence of recent conversion, treatment is not indicated because they may have been PPD-positive for many years.

III. MYCOBACTERIA OTHER THAN TUBERCULOSIS (MOTT).

Several species of mycobacteria other than *M. tuberculosis* can infect humans. With the exception of *M. leprae,* which is classified separately because of the unique characteristics of the disease it causes, these bacteria are generically designated MOTT, atypical mycobacteria, or nontuberculous mycobacteria (NTM).

A. Introduction

1. **Epidemiology**
   a. **Reservoirs and transmission.** The major reservoirs and modes of transmission for MOTT are summarized in Table 18-3. MOTT are usually acquired by inhalation or dermal inoculation.
   b. **Incidence.** MOTT are being detected more frequently, partly because of better identification techniques and partly because they are becoming more prevalent.
      (1) Nationwide, it is estimated that MOTT causes approximately 10% of all mycobacterial infections, but in some areas, the ratio is as high as 50%.
      (2) *M. avium-intracellulare* is the most commonly isolated MOTT.
2. **Clinical disease.** Presentation is variable. Some MOTT cause a disease similar to tuberculosis, whereas others tend to cause predominantly localized skin infections.

TABLE 18-3. Major Reservoirs and Sources of Transmission for MOTT

Organism	Reservoirs	Source of Transmission
M. kansasii	Unclear, possibly wild and domestic animals	Water, milk
M. avium-intracellulare	Birds, mammals	Aerosolized excreta or secretions
M. scrofulaceum	Moist soil	Unknown
M. marinum	Fish	Water, submerged objects

MOTT = mycobacteria other than tuberculosis.

3. **Diagnosis** requires identification of the organism. The acid-fast stain specific for *Mycobacterium* will not differentiate between *M. tuberculosis* and MOTT; differentiation requires biochemical tests.

B. ***M. kansasii*** can cause pulmonary disease as well as infections of the skin and subcutaneous lymph nodes. The disease tends to progress slowly and is susceptible to the usual antimycobacterial drugs.

C. ***M. avium-intracellulare* complex** includes several organisms that are not serologically distinct.

1. **Clinical disease.** These organisms cause opportunistic infections in immunosuppressed patients. The lungs are primarily affected, but infection can spread to other organs as well.
2. **Treatment.** Organisms in the *M. avium-intracellulare* complex are **highly resistant to antituberculous drugs.** Combinations of drugs, including some not usually used for tuberculosis (e.g., **clarithromycin)** may be required for effective therapy.

D. ***M. scrofulaceum***

1. **Clinical disease**
   a. *M. scrofulaceum* is the most common cause of **granulomatous cervical lymphadenitis** in children. The disease is characterized by enlarged lymph nodes, which may ulcerate or form draining sinus tracts.
   b. *M. scrofulaceum* may also cause lung disease, producing a **disease syndrome that resembles pulmonary tuberculosis.**
2. **Treatment** usually involves **surgical excision of the infected lymph node.** *M. scrofulaceum* is **generally resistant to antimycobacterial drugs.**

E. ***M. fortuitum* complex** is a group of free-living, rapid-growing mycobacteria that only rarely cause human disease. Injection-site abscesses among drug abusers are the most common form of disease. Infection also has been associated with implanted devices, such as heart valves and breast prostheses. Pulmonary infection occurs occasionally.

F. ***M. marinum*** grows at much lower temperatures than other mycobacteria (approximately 30°C) and is present in both fresh and salt water.

1. **Clinical disease.** *M. marinum* causes nodular ulcerative lesions of the skin at the site of trauma. The infection may spread to the liver through the lymphatic circulation.
2. **Treatment.** *M. marinum* is susceptible to tetracyclines, trimethoprim–sulfamethoxazole, and to the usual antituberculous drugs. When the infection is limited to the skin, surgical curettage is effective.

IV. *MYCOBACTERIUM LEPRAE*

A. Pathogenesis and clinical disease. *M. leprae* is the causative agent of **leprosy (Hansen's disease).** There are two major forms of leprosy. The type of helper T-cell population responding to the infection seems to dictate the form of the disease that develops— Patients with predominantly TH_1 responses develop tuberculoid leprosy with strong cell-mediated responses to *M. leprae* antigens, while patients with predominantly TH_2 responses have weak to absent CMI to *M. leprae* and develop lepromatous leprosy.

1. **Tuberculoid leprosy** is characterized by macules or extensive plaques on the trunk, face, and limbs.
   a. **Lesions.** The granulomatous lesions have a raised erythematous edge and a dry, hairless center that may be hypopigmented.
      (1) The lesions are **paucibacillary** (i.e., they contain few mycobacteria).
      (2) *M. leprae* invades sensory nerves, causing a **patchy anesthesia** in the lesions. Localized anesthesia often leads to injury and severe secondary bacterial infection.
      (3) Giant cells are abundant and lymphocytic infiltration is extensive in the lesions.
   b. Because CMI is intact in tuberculoid leprosy, patients show a **delayed-type hypersensitivity reaction to lepromin,** an *M. leprae* antigen derived from lepromatous tissue and analogous to tuberculin.
   c. Frequently, the disease is characterized by evidence of simultaneous slow progression and healing.

2. **Lepromatous leprosy.** The bacteria probably disseminate hematogenously, although the disease does not appear to be manifest in the deeper organs.
   a. **Lesions** are large, diffuse, and granulomatous.
      (1) The lesions are **multibacillary** (i.e., they contain large numbers of *M. leprae* organisms).
      (2) Sensory nerve involvement is diffuse and **patchy anesthesia** is common.
   b. **Facial disfigurement** is common. There is extensive skin involvement and mycobacteria accumulate in subcutaneous tissue, particularly in the loose folds of the skin and in the ear lobes. Extensive collagen destruction and scarring leads to thickening of the loose skin of the forehead, lips, and ears, resulting in the classic **leonine facies.**
   c. Patients with lepromatous leprosy are **anergic to lepromin.**

3. **Borderline cases** cannot be classified as tuberculoid or lepromatous.

B. Epidemiology

1. **Transmission.** Leprosy is not very contagious.
   a. Close contact with infected persons increases the risk of developing the disease, which is thought to be transmitted by **inhalation** of contaminated droplets.
   b. The **incubation period** is **extremely long,** lasting from several months to 20 years.

2. **Incidence.** It is estimated that there are between 15 and 20 million cases of leprosy worldwide. The disease occurs primarily in the tropics and subtropics, but a few cases are reported annually in the United States (most cases are imported). New York City has the largest population of people with leprosy in the United States, but there is no evidence of transmission of the disease.

C. Diagnosis is based primarily on clinical signs and symptoms.

1. **Scrapings** or biopsies from lesions reveal characteristic histopathology and, in lepromatous disease, large numbers of acid-fast bacilli.

2. **Culture and isolation.** *M. leprae* **cannot be cultured in bacteriologic media.** A cell culture system that supports the growth of *M. leprae* was recently developed; prior to its development, isolation required inoculation of seven-banded armadillos.

3. **Lepromin test.** In tuberculoid leprosy, a positive lepromin test has diagnostic value, but generalized anergy induced by a heavy antigenic load can lead to false-positive results.

D. **Treatment** is ongoing to prevent relapse. Combination treatment with three or more antileprotic drugs is showing promise in preventing relapses, which may be caused by drug-resistant strains of *M. leprae*.

1. **Dapsone (diaminodiphenylsulfone, DDS)** is the major drug employed in endemic areas. It is relatively inexpensive and usually effective; however, in some areas, mutational resistance has reached significant levels.

2. **Clofazimine, rifampin,** and **thalidomide** are also successfully used in the treatment of leprosy.

E. **Control and prophylaxis.** A vaccine has not been developed. Partial protection after administration of BCG has been reported, but the reports have been questioned.

Chapter 19

Spirochetes

John Manos
Victor Del Bene
Gerald E. Wagner

I. INTRODUCTION. The order Spirochaetales has two families: the **Spirochaetaceae,** which include two important genera of human pathogens (*Treponema* and *Borrelia*) and the **Leptospiraceae,** whose single genus, *Leptospira,* also includes human pathogens. The main common characteristics of the Spirochaetales are summarized in Table 19-1.

II. *TREPONEMA. T. Pallidum* is subdivided into four subspecies, three of which are pathogenic for humans. Only the subspecies *pallidum,* the etiologic agent of **syphilis,** the most important pathogen, and virtually the only one that causes disease in the United States, will be discussed in this chapter.

A. General properties are summarized in Table 19-2.

B. Determinants of pathogenicity. The virulence factors of *T. pallidum* are poorly characterized.

1. Virulence is related to the ability of the organism to attach to cells, which is potentiated by adsorption of fibronectin to the organism. In addition, binding to endothelial cells seems to be associated with upregulation of cell adhesion molecules, leading to enhanced binding of leukocytes, a necessary step for the induction of local inflammation.
2. The proteins in the outer coat of *Treponema* are poorly immunogenic.

C. Pathogenesis and clinical disease

1. **Pathogenesis**
   - **a.** *T. pallidum* travels from the site of infection (usually the skin) to the draining lymph nodes in approximately 30 minutes.
   - **b.** From the lymph nodes, the organism disseminates to the blood stream, where it adheres to the surface proteins of cells, especially endothelial cells. **Endarteritis,** the main lesion of syphilis, can lead to endothelial scarring and, over the long term, can cause an intense inflammatory reaction that may be followed by extensive tissue necrosis.
2. **Clinical disease**
   - **a. Adult syphilis** (Figure 19-1)
     - **(1) Primary syphilis.** Three to four weeks after initial penetration, a **chancre** (i.e., an ulcerated, indurated, well circumscribed, painless lesion) containing abundant spirochetes forms at the site of infection, heralding the onset of primary syphilis.
       - **(a)** The chancre usually heals spontaneously after approximately 14 days.
       - **(b)** In approximately 75% of patients, the disease will be cured. The remaining patients will develop secondary syphilis.
     - **(2) Secondary syphilis** usually starts to manifest itself 3–8 weeks after the disappearance of the primary chancre. This stage of the disease is characterized by systemic symptoms (evidence of dissemination of the infection).
       - **(a) Clinical signs** include **malaise,** a **low-grade fever, lymphadenopathy,** and

Table 19-1. General Characteristics of the Spirochaetales

Long, thin, corkscrew-shaped organisms; 0.1–0.3 μm wide
Contain axial fibrils responsible for the rotation and flexion movements associated with locomotion
Structurally Gram-negative (contain LPS), but some species are difficult to visualize using Gram's technique

LPS = lipopolysaccharide.

TABLE 19-2. Defining Characteristics of *Treponema pallidum*

Approximately 0.1–0.5 μm wide and 5–15 μm long, with 6–14 coils
Microaerophilic
Does not stain with Gram's technique
Can only be grown in tissue cultures

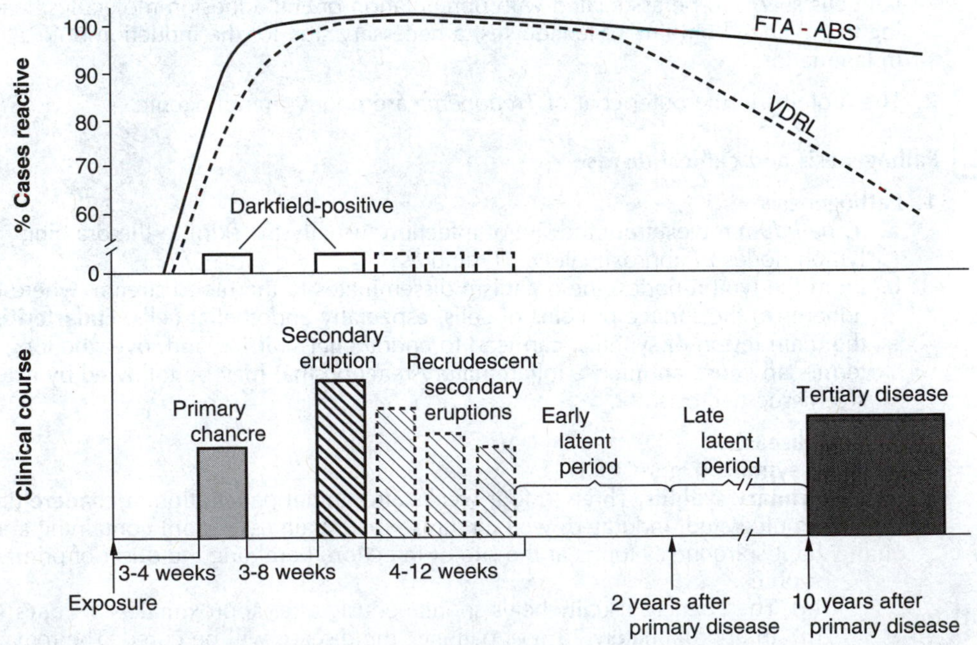

FIGURE 19-1. Correlation between clinical stages and diagnostic tests in untreated syphilis. *FTA-ABS* = fluorescent treponemal antibody absorption test; *VDRL* = Venereal Disease Research Laboratory test. (Modified with permission from Joklik WK, Willett HP, Amos DB, Wilfert CM: *Zinsser Microbiology,* 20th ed. Norwalk, CT, Appleton & Lange, 1992, p 662.)

alopecia areata (irregular hair loss). **Mucocutaneous eruptions** are also characteristic.

(i) On the **skin,** the rash is **maculopapular** and is found on the **palms** and **soles of the feet.**

(ii) The rash may also appear on **mucous membranes** in the form of **discolored patches.** On the anal mucosa, **condylomata latta** (i.e., raised, sessile lesions) are characteristic. Because the skin and mucosal lesions are infectious, gloves must be worn when examining patients.

(b) Most people with secondary syphilis will build a sufficient immune response and the disease will be cured spontaneously. Approximately 13%–15% of untreated secondary sufferers will progress to a latent stage and, finally, to the tertiary stage.

(3) Latent stage. Patients are arbitrarily classified as being in an **early latent** or **late latent stage,** depending on how much time has elapsed since the primary chancre (2 years is the usual benchmark). Patients test positive using serologic tests but are **asymptomatic.**

(4) Tertiary syphilis is characterized by degenerative and irreversible necrotic lesions that do not contain spirochetes.

(a) Clinical manifestations are varied and include severe aortitis (leading to aneurysm formation), blindness, mental incapacitation, and musculoskeletal problems secondary to neurologic involvement. Because of these diverse presentations and the diagnostic problems they cause, tertiary syphilis has been called the **"great imitator."**

(b) At this stage, therapy is rather ineffective.

b. Congenital syphilis. From about 16 weeks' gestation on, *T. pallidum* can cross the placental barrier.

(1) Twenty-five percent of infected fetuses die *in utero,* and another twenty-five percent die shortly after birth.

(2) Most surviving babies will have severe congenital and developmental anomalies.

(a) Evidence of intrauterine growth retardation, rhinorrhea, hepatosplenomegaly (often associated with **hyperbilirubinemia** and sometimes with obvious **jaundice),** and **lymphadenopathy** are commonly present at birth.

(b) Skeletal abnormalities may be evident at birth, either clinically or radiographically, but they tend to become more prominent later in untreated cases.

(c) Craniofacial alterations (e.g., a **prominent frontal region, short maxilla, saddle nose,** and **mulberry teeth**) are the most common manifestation. One or several of the elements of the so-called **Hutchinson's triad—notched teeth, interstitial keratitis,** and **eighth-nerve deafness**—are seen in approximately 75% of untreated children.

C. Epidemiology

1. Transmission. *T. pallidum* is transmitted by direct contact and transplacentally. Clinical laboratory workers, hospital personnel, and blood transfusion recipients may contract the disease accidentally.

2. Incidence. The incidence of syphilis, like that of most other sexually-transmitted diseases, is increasing. Recent figures indicate an average increase of 9000 cases per quarter.

D. Immunity.

The immune response to *T. pallidum* is easy to detect and useful for diagnosis, but there is considerable uncertainty about the protective role it plays.

1. The initial immune response to infection with *T. pallidum* is the formation of **antiphospholipid antibodies.** It is not clear whether *Treponema* has similar phospholipids, or whether the reaction is directed against host lipids absorbed by the parasite and rendered immunogenic by some modification associated with absorption.

2. There is a **specific temporary depression in cell-mediated immunity (CMI),** which may become persistent in some patients. Eventually, **IgG antitreponemal antibodies** able to immobilize and kill *T. pallidum* can be detected. Why *T. pallidum* causes persistent infection in individuals with strong humoral responses to this organism is not clear. The following may be contributing factors:
   a. It is believed that the delay in the synthesis of protective IgG antitreponemal antibodies may allow the organism to infect tissues that are fairly inaccessible to the immune response (e.g., the spinal column or the eye).
   b. CMI has not been characterized as protective.
   c. Once attached to endothelial cells, *T. pallidum* adsorbs several host proteins (particularly fibronectin) to its outer surface; these proteins may enhance attachment to the endothelium and represent an additional barrier to the immune system.

3. The immune response, even when unable to eliminate the infectious agent, **seems to play an important role in slowing down the evolution of the clinical disease.** This phenomenon is evidenced by the fact that an early, malignant form of meningovascular syphilis is often seen in immunocompromised patients.

E. Laboratory diagnosis. *T. pallidum* cannot be cultured in a clinical laboratory. Laboratory diagnosis is made by darkfield examination of material from the primary chancre or by serology.

1. **Adult syphilis.** Diagnosis is made on the basis of clinical signs and laboratory test results.
   a. **Darkfield examination** allows ready detection of the live, highly motile organisms. However, this method requires considerable skill, and is often unavailable in outpatient clinics.
   b. **Serologic tests**
      (1) **Types.** Serologic tests can be classified as **nonspecific (nontreponemal)** or **specific (treponemal).** In practice, most physicians obtain the nonspecific test result first and then confirm positive results with a specific test.
         (a) The **nonspecific tests** use **cardiolipin,** a phospholipid-rich lipid fraction obtained from bovine heart tissue, as antigen. The antiphospholipid antibodies produced by *T. pallidum* cross-react with cardiolipin. The nonspecific tests frequently give false-positive results in patients with viral influenza, infectious mononucleosis, or autoimmune or collagen disorders, in pregnant patients, and in elderly patients. The false-positive result is usually of a low titer.
            (i) The **Wassermann test,** which is based on complement fixation, detects IgG antibody.
            (ii) The **Venereal Disease Research Laboratory (VDRL) test** and the **rapid plasma reagin (RPR) test** are flocculation tests. The flocculation tests detect both IgG and IgM antibodies, and tend to be positive very early in the disease.
         (b) The **specific tests** use *T. pallidum* as antigen; therefore, they detect specific treponemal antibody.
            (i) Specific tests include the **fluorescent treponemal antibody absorption test (FTA-ABS),** the ***T. pallidum* immobilization (TPI) test,** and the **microhemagglutination *T. pallidum* (MHA-TP) test.**
            (ii) The specific tests can detect cross-reactive antibodies against other *T. pallidum* subspecies, but this is not a problem in the United States, where disease caused by those subspecies is virtually nonexistent.
      (2) **Positivity** (see Figure 19-1)
         (a) **Primary and secondary syphilis.** Both specific and nonspecific tests will give a positive result in almost 100% of those infected if the test is obtained after the appearance of the chancre.
            (i) The positivity rate during the primary phase varies from 85% for FTA-ABS to 50%–60% for MHA-TP; all tests have about a 100% positivity rate during secondary syphilis.
            (ii) If a patient with clinical signs and symptoms of primary syphilis has a

negative serologic test, he or she should be treated and the serologies repeated when the patient returns for follow-up.

(b) Tertiary syphilis. The specific tests tend to remain positive, while the nonspecific tests tend to become negative. Thus, if a patient presents with the signs and symptoms of late-stage syphilis, a specific test should be run in addition to a nonspecific test because the nonspecific tests may yield a false-negative result.

2. **Congenital syphilis.** Prenatal diagnosis is established by the diagnosis of maternal infection. Confirmation of the diagnosis in the infant requires visualization of *T. pallidum* in skin lesions or in cerebrospinal fluid (CSF), or detection of specific IgM antitreponemal antibodies using a serologic test.

F. Treatment

1. **Adult syphilis**

   a. **Penicillin** is the **drug of choice** for syphilis.

   (1) Principles underlying therapy

   (a) The cell wall of *T. pallidum* contains a peptidoglycan layer.

   (b) *T. pallidum* has never been observed to produce β-lactamase.

   (c) The rate of reproduction of *T. pallidum* is very slow. The doubling time has been estimated to be in the neighborhood of 20–30 hours.

   (2) Administration is timed so that the optimal killing concentrations are obtained and maintained over an extended period of time. Slow-release forms of penicillin, such as benzathine penicillins, are preferred.

   (a) A single large dose administered intramuscularly is sufficient for a patient who has had the disease less than 1 year.

   (b) Patients who have had syphilis for longer than 1 year should receive benzathine penicillin intramuscularly once weekly for 3 weeks.

   (c) Patients in the late stages of the disease are likely to have disseminated infection of endothelial cells and phagocytic cells. In addition, organs and tissues that antibiotics penetrate with difficulty [e.g., the eye, bones, and central nervous system (CNS)] may be infected. These patients are admitted to the hospital and administered penicillin intravenously around the clock for 10 days.

   b. **Proof of cure** depends on the results of serologic tests. Although the titers of specific tests remain positive virtually for life, the titers of nonspecific tests tend to decline with time if treatment is effective (Table 19-3).

   (1) The effectiveness of treatment is relative. In most clinically cured patients, viable organisms can be recovered from the lymph nodes for long periods of time (possibly for the rest of the patient's life). However, the remaining organisms seem to be controlled by the immune system and do not cause clinical disease.

   (2) If the patient is not treated until the tertiary stage, the nonspecific tests usually

Table 19-3. Percentage of Patients With Positive Titers Following Treatment for Syphilis

Test	Stage of Therapy	% Reactive 6 Months	% Reactive 1 Year	% Reactive >1 Year
Nonspecific				
RPR	Primary	30	20	5
RPR	Secondary	95	70	5
RPR	Late	95	95	50
Specific				
FTA-ABS	Primary	98	98	80

FTA-ABS = fluorescent treponemal antibody absorption test; RPR = rapid plasma reagin.

remain positive and it is impossible to know whether or not therapy has been successful.

c. **Complications associated with therapy.** Following administration of penicillin to a patient with active syphilis, a reaction known as the **Jarisch-Herxheimer reaction** may occur.

(1) The reaction is characterized by hypotension, cyanosis, high fever, and rigors. These symptoms are caused by the rapid destruction of large numbers of *Treponema* and the endotoxin-like effects of the cell wall products.

(2) It is important to recognize this entity, which is usually mild to moderate in severity and self-limited, and to distinguish it from a major (accelerated) penicillin allergic reaction. Fever, which is usually absent in anaphylactic reactions, is an important clue.

2. **Congenital syphilis.** Treatment is similar to that for adult syphilis and is instituted in all cases of confirmed or highly likely infection when the mother has not received adequate treatment prior to delivery.

III. *BORRELIA.* The major common characteristics of *Borrelia* are summarized in Table 19-4.

A. *B. recurrentis*

1. **Pathogenesis and clinical disease.** *B. recurrentis* causes **relapsing fever,** a febrile bacteremia that derives its name from the fact that three to ten recurrences are common.

a. **Pathogenesis**

(1) **Dissemination.** Judging from findings in severely ill patients and necropsy findings, *B. recurrentis* spreads to a variety of organs, including the spleen, liver, meninges, gastrointestinal tract, and kidneys.

(2) **Recurrence**

(a) *B. recurrentis* is capable of **antigenic variation** (see Chapter 8 V F) and **antigenic modulation** (i.e., selection of new strains), probably as a consequence of the immune response.

(i) High titers of lytic antibodies, agglutinins, and complement-fixing antibodies are induced during the course of a single infection.

(ii) Serotype specificity is determined by **variable membrane lipoproteins (VMPs),** which are expressed from genes located near the end of a linear plasmid. DNA rearrangements of the genes coding for VMPs result in sequential expression of new genes and are the basis for antigenic variation of this organism.

(b) Proliferation of a new mutant strain causes a recurrence, which is eventually controlled by a specific immune response, and the fever disappears. Successive recurrences are associated with the emergence of antigenically different strains.

b. **Clinical disease**

(1) The disease has a sudden onset with chills and a sharp rise in body tempera-

Table 19-4. Defining Characteristics of *Borrelia*

0.3–0.5 μm in diameter and 20–30 μm in length
Stainable with anyline dyes (Wright's or Giemsa stains); easily visualized with a light microscope after staining
Easy to culture in special cell-free media
Microaerophilic

ture after a 3- to 10-day incubation period. Numerous organisms are present in the blood at this stage, and the fever persists for 3–5 days.

(2) A second attack can occur in 4–10 days, and chills, fever, and severe headache are typical symptoms. Successive recurrences follow the same pattern.

2. **Epidemiology**

a. **Reservoirs and transmission.** *Borrelia* are zoonotic organisms transmitted by ticks and lice.

(1) Infected rats are the source of infection for ticks, which can pass the organism transovarially. Thus, infected populations of ticks tend to persist for long periods of time. Human sporadic disease is acquired either by a tick bite or by crushing a tick and inoculating minor skin lesions.

(2) Human lice become infected by a blood meal on an infected person. In 3–5 days, the infected louse can spread the disease to other humans. Louse-borne relapsing fever can be epidemic, and crowded living conditions can be a predisposing factor.

b. **Distribution.** Relapsing fever caused by *B. recurrentis* occurs worldwide.

(1) In the United States, infected ticks are most commonly found in the mountainous regions of the western states.

(2) Endemic areas tend to have large rat populations.

c. The **mortality rate** from relapsing fever is low in endemic areas. During epidemics, however, it frequently approaches 30%.

3. **Laboratory diagnosis**

a. **Examination of blood smears. Darkfield microscopy** or **staining with Wright's** or **Giemsa stains** may reveal spirochetes in the early stages of the disease.

b. **Blood cultures** will confirm the diagnosis as well.

c. **Serologic tests.** The **VDRL test** may be positive.

4. **Treatment.** A **single, large dose** of **erythromycin, tetracycline,** or **penicillin** is usually effective for eradicating *Borrelia.*

B. *B. burgdorferi*

1. **Determinants of pathogenicity.** The virulence factors of this spirochete are not well understood.

a. The cell wall of *B. burgdorferi* contains a toxic lipopolysaccharide, different from bacterial endotoxins, and the peptidoglycan has inflammatory properties.

b. Because *B. burgdorferi* is rarely isolated from tissues after the initial stages of disease, it is believed that the immune response plays a major pathogenic role. Antigenic modulation seems to take place in *B. burgdorferi,* although it seems not to be as well defined or as closely correlated with clinical evolution as it is in the case of *B. recurrentis.*

2. **Pathogenesis and clinical disease.** *B. burgdorferi* causes **Lyme disease** and is transmitted by ticks.

a. **Pathogenesis**

(1) After a variable incubation period (3–32 days), a skin lesion develops at the site of the tick bite. The spirochete migrates outward via lymph channels.

(2) Eventually, the spirochete may reach the blood stream and weeks to months after the apparent resolution of the initial episode, the patient develops symptoms suggestive of neurologic and cardiologic involvement. Marked increases of serum IgM and circulating immune complexes, including mixed cryoglobulins, are associated with or precede neurologic or cardiologic involvement.

(3) Even later, approximately 66% of patients develop arthritis. Serum IgM is usually normal, and immune complexes are only found in the synovial tissue.

b. **Clinical disease.** After the incubation period, the disease is characterized by remissions and exacerbations. Three stages of the disease have been identified; however, in any given patient, a single stage may be identified or stages may appear to overlap.

(1) **Stage 1** is characterized by **erythema migrans.**

(a) An annular lesion with a clear or necrotic center and a raised, red border develops at the site of the tick bite. The lesion is hot, but not painful. Multiple secondary (satellite) lesions with similar characteristics develop in approximately 50% of patients. Approximately 15% of patients do not develop skin lesions.

(b) Associated symptoms include malaise, fatigue, headache, fever and chills, generalized achiness, and regional adenopathy.

(2) Stage 2 is characterized by **neurologic symptoms** (e.g., meningitis, encephalitis, chorea, cranial neuritis) and **cardiologic symptoms** (e.g., atrioventricular block, cardiomegaly).

(3) Stage 3. Arthritis is the hallmark of stage 3 Lyme disease. Fatigue is the only common systemic symptom.

(a) Early symptoms include migratory musculoskeletal pain or swelling at one or two sites, lasting hours to days.

(b) Frank arthritis develops several months later. The large joints, especially the knees, are primarily affected, and joint swelling occurs.

(i) The joint manifestations may last weeks to months.

(ii) In 10% of patients, the arthritis becomes chronic, with erosion of cartilage and bone.

3. Epidemiology

a. Transmission. The spirochete is excreted in the saliva of *Ixodes dammini* or related ixodid ticks.

(1) Adult ticks acquire *B. burgdorferi* by feeding on infected deer.

(a) In the spring, the female ticks lay eggs in the soil.

(b) The eggs hatch larvae that feed on white-footed mice, the main animal reservoir.

(c) The following spring, the developed larvae parasitize mice and other mammals (including humans) to complete their maturation.

(d) When the ticks reach adulthood, they parasitize deer, mate, and complete their life cycle. *B. burgdorferi* is transmitted by the larvae during all the stages of maturation.

(2) In endemic areas, as many as 80% of the ticks are infected.

b. Distribution

(1) Initially recognized along the Atlantic seaboard of the United States, Lyme disease has now been reported in 35 states. Three major foci have been identified in the United States: the Northeast, which has a high deer population, the Midwest (especially Wisconsin and Minnesota), and the West (especially California and Oregon).

(2) Cases also have been reported in Australia and in many European and Asian countries.

c. Incidence. Most cases of Lyme disease are seen between May 1 and November 30, with 80% of clinical cases occurring in June and July. People younger than 40 years of age are most often affected; there are no gender predispositions.

4. Laboratory diagnosis. Because isolation or visualization of *B. burgdorferi* is only occasionally achieved, the diagnosis is often clinical. Erythema migrans is thought to be diagnostic, especially when followed by arthritis or neurologic symptoms.

a. Staining

(1) *B. burgdorferi* can be seen in **peripheral blood smears** or **CSF sediment** stained with **acridine orange, specific fluorescent antibody,** or **Giemsa stain.**

(2) Organisms can also be seen in **tissues** stained with a special **silver stain.**

b. Culture and isolation. *B. burgdorferi* can be cultured in broth from samples taken from the leading edge of the lesion, blood, or CSF.

c. Serologic tests. A number of serologic tests for diagnostic use are commercially available, but there are several problems associated with their use, ranging from the length of time required for antibody titers to develop (3–6 weeks for IgM, several months for IgG) to a general lack of specificity and poor sensitivity of most tests.

(1) Antibodies to *B. burgdorferi* cross-react with several other spirochetes, but the cardiolipin-based tests for syphilis remain negative in patients with Lyme disease.

(2) A **Western blot** method, based on the detection of antibodies to a 39 kDa protein that is believed to be unique to *B. burgdorferi* appears promising.

d. **Polymerase chain reaction (PCR).** There is considerable interest in developing a sensitive, PCR-based test for the detection of *Borrelia* antigen in tissues or body fluids.

5. **Treatment**
   a. **Early-stage Lyme disease**
      (1) **Doxycycline** is the drug of choice during the early stages of the disease. Other effective drugs include **amoxicillin** and **erythromycin.**
      (2) Treatment should be extended for **10–20 days.** A Jarisch-Herxheimer–like reaction may be observed when the treatment is started.
   b. **Late-stage Lyme disease.** In the second and third stages, the best treatment is **parenteral administration of ceftriaxone.** Approximately 50% of patients with arthritis improve with antibiotic therapy.

6. **Prevention.** A recombinant vaccine made with a surface-exposed lipoprotein (OspA) was found to induce protective immune responses in experimental animals and is in phase I of human trials.

IV. *LEPTOSPIRA*

A. **General properties** of *Leptospira* are summarized in Table 19-5.

B. **Pathogenesis and clinical disease.** ***L. interrogans*** includes several serotypes pathogenic for humans and causes a variety of clinical syndromes.

1. **Pathogenesis**
   a. **Transmission.** Infections are acquired through **contact with infected animals** or with products contaminated with **animal urine** (e.g., soil, food, water).
   b. **Portal of entry.** Spirochetes invade **intact mucous membranes or abraded skin,** but not intact skin.
   c. **Dissemination.** The organism enters the bloodstream (spirochetemia) and spreads **hematogenously** to a variety of organs and tissues.
      (1) **Hepatic involvement** is reflected by increased liver enzymes (transaminases), hyperbilirubinemia, and jaundice (icterus).
      (2) **Vascular involvement.** Diffuse vascular endothelial injury can lead to severe fluid loss and **hypovolemic shock.** In addition, the vasculitis precipitates **disseminated intravascular coagulation (DIC),** which is associated with thrombocytopenia and hemorrhagic diathesis.
      (3) **Kidney involvement** is reflected by acute tubular necrosis and **renal failure.**

2. **Clinical disease**
   a. **Subclinical (asymptomatic) leptospirosis** is detected in serological surveys of packing-house workers and veterinarians. The surveys show antibodies to the organism in individuals who do not recall having had clinical disease.
   b. **Anicteric leptospirosis** is difficult to diagnose.

Table 19-5. Defining Characteristics of *Leptospira*

Highly coiled and motile
0.1 μm in diameter and 6–20 μm in length with hooked end
Can be grown in enriched artificial medium
Microaerophilic, grow best at 30°C

(1) The early symptoms, which develop after an incubation period of 7–12 days, are influenza-like and nonspecific. The patient becomes afebrile and feels better, but then a secondary stage ensues.

(2) The secondary stage may last from a few days up to 1 month.

(a) The symptoms include severe headaches, myalgia, nausea, and vomiting. Physical examination may reveal splenomegaly in 15%–25% of patients, hepatomegaly (unusual), and signs of meningitis. The patient never becomes clinically jaundiced.

(b) During this stage, circulating antibody to *Leptospira* and immune complexes can be detected in the patient's serum.

(3) **Icteric leptospirosis (Weil's syndrome)** is the most severe form of disease associated with leptospirosis. Originally it was thought to be caused by the serotype *L. icterohaemorrhagiae,* but it was proven later that any serotype of *L. interrogans* can be associated with the syndrome.

(a) **Disseminated endothelial damage and vasculitis** may lead to impaired renal and hepatic function, internal hemorrhages, meningitis, cardiovascular collapse, and shock.

(b) **Hepatomegaly** is detected in 25% of cases and is usually associated with jaundice.

C. Laboratory diagnosis. Diagnosis of leptospirosis generally requires a high level of clinical awareness, but confirmation can be achieved through culture and isolation or serology.

1. **Culture and isolation.** *Leptospira* can be isolated from blood or CSF during the first week of illness or from urine later in the course of the disease. Significant growth may take up to 6 weeks. Material from the culture is examined weekly using dark-field microscopy.

2. **Serologic tests** are available, but antibody titers take approximately 4 weeks to peak, so this approach will not yield a quick diagnosis.

D. Epidemiology

1. **Reservoirs.** *L. interrogans* are animal parasites. Rats are the most significant vector worldwide, but dogs, cats, and livestock can also harbor the organism. Humans are dead-end hosts; that is, the organism cannot be transmitted among humans.

2. **Susceptibility.** Leptospirosis can be an occupational hazard for veterinarians and individuals involved in food processing (e.g., meat packers).

3. **Incidence.** Forty to fifty cases per year are reported in the United States. Cases are most frequently reported during the summer and fall months.

E. Treatment. Penicillin is the drug of choice; **tetracycline** is indicated in patients allergic to penicillin.

Chapter 20

Legionellaceae, Mycoplasmataceae, Actinomycetaceae, and Related Organisms

John Manos
Arthur Di Salvo

I. LEGIONELLACEAE. In 1976, following an American Legion convention in Philadelphia, many participants fell ill with a pneumonia that appeared to be caused by an unknown agent. The media coined the term **Legionnaires' disease** for this mysterious infection. The causative organism was eventually characterized as the first member of the Legionellaceae family, ***Legionella pneumophila.*** Previous outbreaks and epidemics of *Legionella* were identified by serological studies of stored sera. For example, *L. pneumophila* was identified as the cause of **Pontiac fever,** a disease of unknown etiology so named because of its initial occurrence in Pontiac, Michigan, a decade earlier.

A. *L. pneumophila*

1. **General properties** of *L. pneumophila* are summarized in Table 20-1. Eight serogroups of *L. pneumophila* have been described.
   a. The best culture medium is **charcoal yeast extract** buffered to a pH of 6.9 and supplemented with cysteine. *L. pneumophila* is unique in that it uses amino acids as a major source of carbon and energy.
   b. A **high carbon dioxide tension** (2.5%–5%) and **high humidity** favor growth, but even under optimal conditions, 2–6 days are required for growth.
2. **Determinants of pathogenicity**
   a. *L. pneumophila* is a **facultative intracellular organism;** the organism's best characterized virulence factors are related to its **ability to survive and multiply inside phagocytic cells.**
      (1) **Adhesion.** Outer membrane proteins mediate adhesion to and penetration of macrophages. After being ingested, the organism undergoes major changes in protein expression, reflecting adaptation to the intracellular environment.
      (2) **Ability to survive intracellularly.** Several factors seem to determine resistance to intracellular killing.
         (a) A **peptide toxin** inhibits the respiratory burst.
         (b) A **catalase** detoxifies residual hydrogen peroxide produced during the attenuated respiratory burst.
         (c) Undefined factors seem to prevent phagolysosome formation as well as the electron transport mechanisms responsible for acidification of the phagosome.
   b. **Inhibition of cell-mediated immunity (CMI).** As for most intracellular organisms, CMI immunity is essential for the elimination of *Legionella.* However, *Legionella* appears to depress CMI. One possible mechanism is the down-regulation of major histocompatibility complex (MHC)-I and MHC-II expression in the phagosomes of *Legionella*-infected macrophages, which may result in deficient antigen presentation to helper T cells.
   c. **Toxin production.** The precise pathogenic contribution of **several exotoxins** (e.g., hemolysins, cytotoxins) and of **endotoxin** has not been well defined, but may be important in determining tissue damage.
3. **Clinical disease.** The **incubation period** normally varies from 2–10 days. A short incubation is probably associated with a particularly high dose of bacteria or exposure to a virulent strain.
   a. **Legionnaires' disease.** The most typical pathologic consequence of infection with *L. pneumophila* is an **air space pneumonia** that may be patchy and diffuse or lo-

Table 20-1. General Characteristics of *Legionella pneumophila*

Thin, pleomorphic Gram-negative rod, 0.3–0.9 × 2.0–4.0 μm
Difficult to stain with conventional bacteriologic stains; best stained in tissues with silver stains
Flagellated, motile
Produces catalase and β-lactamase
Fastidious; best culture medium is charcoal yeast extract buffered to pH 6.9 and supplemented with cysteine

calized (lobar). Evidence of extrapulmonary spread (e.g., hepato- and splenomegaly) may also be seen.

(1) **Histopathology.** Alveolar inflammatory exudates containing neutrophils and macrophages (often with engulfed organisms) are the predominant feature.

(2) **Clinical signs** are nonspecific.

(a) **Fever** is seen in over 90% of patients and is associated with **chills, headache,** and a **cough** in over 75% of patients. The cough is usually nonproductive or productive of nonpurulent sputum.

(b) **Watery diarrhea** affects 30%–50% of patients.

(c) **Changes in mental status** (e.g., disorientation, confusion) may be seen.

b. **Pontiac fever** presents as a **flu-like syndrome** without lung involvement. It is a self-limiting disease, and usually carries a good prognosis. Pontiac fever is highly contagious, but the mechanism of transmission remains undefined. Treatment is supportive.

4. **Epidemiology**

a. **Distribution.** *L. pneumophila* and other *Legionella* species have worldwide distribution. They exist in a wide range of physical and chemical habitats, mostly aquatic, as parasites of many ameba species.

b. **Transmission.** *Legionella* is acquired through inhalation of airborne aerosolized microorganisms.

(1) Contaminated water cooling towers, air conditioning systems, shower heads, and faucets have been identified as sources of infection.

(2) There is no evidence of person to person transmission.

c. **Susceptibility.** Several predisposing factors seem to account for the development of clinical disease, including generalized immunosuppression and conditions that decrease the local defenses in the lungs (e.g., chronic lung diseases, smoking).

d. **Incidence.** Exposure and subclinical infection appear to be rather frequent (approximately 20% of the older population is serologically positive).

e. **Mortality rates** approach 15%–20%, despite adequate treatment.

5. **Laboratory diagnosis**

a. **Microscopic examination of specimens.** Rapid diagnosis may be provided by **silver staining** or **direct immunofluorescence** of biopsy tissues or sputum using fluorescein-labeled antibodies to *Legionella.*

b. **Culture and isolation.** Isolation of *L. pneumophila* is extremely difficult. *L. pneumophila* is virtually impossible to culture from sputum; a tissue sample is usually needed.

c. **DNA probes** may be used in the near future.

d. **Serologic tests.** Titration of anti-*Legionella* antibodies can be used for retrospective diagnosis; however, from the point of view of treating the acutely ill patient, serology is of limited value because it is impossible to wait 2–3 weeks (until the antibody titer has time to rise significantly) before starting therapy. An antibody titer of 256 or higher when the patient is acutely ill is presumptive evidence of infection with *Legionella.*

6. **Treatment.** Antibiotic therapy is essential for patients with Legionnaires' disease. Penicillins are ineffective, because most strains produce β-lactamase.

a. **Macrolide antibiotics** (e.g., **azithromycin, clarithromycin, erythromycin**) are the drugs of choice.
b. **Doxycycline** may be used if the patient cannot tolerate erythromycin.

7. **Prevention** involves identifying environmental sources that can constitute a source of human infection (e.g., the hospital water supply) and taking adequate measures once such sources are identified.

B. ***L. micdadei,*** the second most commonly isolated species of *Legionella*, is associated with a hospital-acquired pneumonia that is clinically very similar to Legionnaire's disease.

C. **Other species of *Legionella*** include ***L. bozemanii, L. gormanii, L. dumoffii, L. jordanis, L. longbeachae, L. wadsworthii,*** and ***L. oakridgensis.***

II. MYCOPLASMATACEAE.

The general characteristics of the family Mycoplasmataceae, which includes *Mycoplasma* and *Ureaplasma,* are summarized in Table 20-2. Members of the Mycoplasmataceae family are the smallest free-living bacteria. Many species infect a variety of animals and plants and a few infect humans.

A. **Historical information.** *Mycoplasma* was first isolated in 1898 from cattle with pleuropneumonia. In 1937, it was isolated from a human abscess and was designated **pleuropneumonia-like organism (PPLO).**

B. ***M. pneumoniae***

1. **Pathogenesis and clinical disease**
   a. **Pathogenesis**
      (1) *M. pneumoniae* is primarily a pathogen of the respiratory tract. Once it reaches the bronchi, a surface protein mediates adhesion to sialic acid-containing oligosaccharides found on the surface of ciliated mucosal epithelial cells. *M. pneumoniae* blocks the action of the respiratory cilia (i.e., it induces ciliostasis) and causes death of mucosal cells. Desquamation of the epithelium and an exudative bronchial and peribronchial inflammatory reaction that may extend to the alveoli follow.
      (2) The central nervous system (CNS), myocardium, skin, joints, and blood may also be affected.
         (a) Arthritis and cutaneous reactions are probably the result of deposition of immune complexes or of hypersensitivity reactions.
         (b) Hemolytic anemia may result from the production of cold agglutinins.
   b. **Clinical disease**
      (1) **Clinical signs and symptoms** develop insidiously after a relatively long incubation period (15–25 days).

Table 20-2. General Characteristics of Mycoplasmataceae

Pleomorphic, average diameter of 0.2 μm
Lack cell wall and do not stain with conventional bacteriologic stains
Requires sterols for growth in culture; lipopolysaccharide-rich molecules attach to the cholesterol-rich cell membrane
Fastidious; grow slowly on complex, enriched media
"Fried egg" colonies
M. pneumoniae grows aerobically; other species are facultative anaerobes
Species can be easily differentiated by metabolic characteristics

(a) At the onset, symptoms are vague (e.g., fever, malaise, headache).

(b) Most acute infections affect the respiratory tract.

(i) Patients may present with symptoms of pneumonia, tracheobronchitis, pharyngitis, or otitis media. The association of lower respiratory tract infection and otitis media in the same patient is highly suggestive of infection with *M. pneumoniae.*

(ii) Pneumonia caused by *M. pneumoniae* is not as serious as other bacterial pneumonias—the patient often remains ambulatory (atypical or walking pneumonia), the cough is not productive, and the systemic symptoms often disappear as the pulmonary symptomatology develops.

(2) **Chest radiographs** show a patchy lower lobe pneumonia, usually unilateral, but sometimes involving multiple lobes. Pleural effusions are seen in 25% of patients.

2. **Immunity**

a. The **humoral immune response** to *M. pneumonia* has been relatively well characterized, and includes:

(1) **Secretory IgA antibody** (short-lived; probably plays a limited role in recovery)

(2) **Complement-fixing IgG antibodies,** which can be detected for approximately 1 year after infection

(3) **Antibodies to *M. pneumoniae* surface glycolipids that cross-react with the I antigen of human erythrocytes.** These antibodies are of low affinity and the reaction is stabilized at low temperatures, therefore causing erythrocyte agglutination at 4°C (cold agglutinins).

b. Immunity to *M. pneumoniae* seems to be incomplete, because **reinfection is common.**

c. The increased severity of disease in older individuals suggests that **stronger secondary immune responses may actually play a pathogenic role.**

3. **Epidemiology**

a. **Transmission.** *M. pneumoniae* is spread by inhalation of aerosolized secretions from infected individuals. Infective organisms are shed for several weeks, starting days before the onset of symptoms and persisting for as long as 14 weeks.

b. **Susceptibility.** Crowding favors transmission and explains the high incidence among school children (5–15 years of age) and military recruits. In teenagers, 35% of pneumonia cases are caused by this organism.

c. **Distribution.** *M. pneumoniae* has a worldwide distribution, although it is more prevalent in temperate climates. Infection is seen most often during the late summer or early fall months.

d. **Incidence.** In the civilian population, the incidence is approximately 4%, but among military recruits, it is as high as 45%. Epidemics tend to recur every 4–8 years. The attack rate is approximately 60% in susceptible hosts, most of whom develop symptoms of respiratory infection.

4. **Diagnosis** is difficult to establish during the acute phase, because *Mycoplasma* cannot be stained in sputum, do not grow in conventional media, and the clinical symptoms are not sufficiently specific. Therefore, serological assays are used to confirm the diagnosis.

a. **Detection of cold agglutinins** is easy using O^+ erythrocytes, which express the I antigen but do not react with the anti-A and anti-B isohemagglutinins. However, detection of cold agglutinins can be indicative of several other infections (e.g., infectious mononucleosis and adenovirus infections).

b. **Specific antibody assays**

(1) **Antibody titers** are classically determined using **complement fixation tests.** Confirmation of the diagnosis requires verification of a significant increase in antibody titer when comparing specimens from the acute and convalescent stages.

(2) Assays for specific **IgM antibodies** to *M. pneumoniae* are also available. A high titer is indicative of an acute infection.

5. **Treatment. Tetracycline** and **erythromycin** are the drugs of choice, and can shorten the duration of clinical disease. Penicillin and cephalosporins are ineffective because these organisms lack a cell wall. The decision to start treatment is usually based on clinical grounds.

C. ***M. hominis*** **and** ***U. urealyticum*** are usually associated with infections of the urogenital tract. Both of these organisms have multiple serotypes.

1. **Clinical disease**
   a. ***M. hominis*** is most frequently involved in **puerperal fever,** but can also be associated with **nongonococcal urethritis, pyelonephritis,** and **pelvic inflammatory disease (PID)** in women. *M. hominis* can cause fever and other systemic symptoms in newborns.
   b. ***U. urealyticum*** is most commonly implicated in cases of **nongonococcal urethritis** and **puerperal fever.**
2. **Epidemiology.** Both *M. hominis* and *U. urealyticum* are found in the genitourinary tracts of asymptomatic individuals.
   a. Infants are often colonized at birth via the vaginal tract.
   b. Adults are infected via sexual transmission.
3. **Diagnosis.** *Ureaplasma* can be easily differentiated from other members of the Mycoplasmataceae family by its ability to produce urease. **Urease activity tests** are most commonly based on the release of ammonia as a result of urea degradation.
4. **Treatment**
   a. **Tetracyclines** (e.g., doxycycline) and **macrolides** (e.g., azithromycin) are preferred because they are also active against *Chlamydia,* the most common bacterial agent involved in cases of nongonococcal urethritis. Resistance to these antibiotics has been reported in approximately 10% of patients.
   b. **Fluoroquinolones** may be effective against resistant organisms.

III. ACTINOMYCETACEAE

ACTINOMYCETACEAE comprises three potentially pathogenic genera: ***Actinomyces, Nocardia,*** and ***Streptomyces.*** These organisms are closely related to the mycobacteria but were originally classified as fungi because they were thought to be transition forms between bacteria and fungi.

A. **General properties** of these three genera are summarized in Table 20-3. These organisms grow well at 35°C–37°C and assume the morphological appearance of delicate,

Table 20-3. Differentiating Characteristics of Actinomycetaceae

	Actinomyces	*Nocardia*	*Streptomyces*
Staining characteristics	Gram-positive	Gram-positive (stain poorly); weakly acid-fast	Gram-positive
Oxygen requirement	Strict or facultative anaerobes	Strict aerobes	Strict aerobes
Epidemiology	Part of normal flora (oropharynx, gastrointestinal tract)	Prevalent in soil; occasionally found in sputum of normal individuals	Prevalent in soil and water
Clinical disease	Produce abscesses with yellow granules	Cause subcutaneous and pulmonary infection	Cause subcutaneous infections with granules (mycetoma)
Reproduction	Non-spore former	Non-spore former	Spore former

branching filamentous forms, 0.5–0.8 μm in diameter. Some species form aerial mycelia in culture.

B. ***A. israelii***

1. **Pathogenesis and clinical disease. Actinomycosis** affects both humans and animals. In cattle, the disease often presents as an abscess located near the lower jaw ("lumpy jaw"). In humans, the organism also causes abscesses, frequently located around the jaw, but also in the thoracic area and abdomen.
   a. **Pathogenesis.** Injury of the oral mucosa (e.g., from a tooth abscess or extraction) provides the opportunity for *Actinomyces* to penetrate the deep tissues (where it finds anaerobic conditions). Eventually, a suppurative infection results.
   b. **Clinical disease.** The classic presentation is that of a draining abscess located around the lower jaw in a patient with a recent history of oral surgery or tooth extraction.

2. **Epidemiology.** *A. israelii* and other *Actinomyces* species are found throughout the world and can be isolated as part of the normal flora of the oral cavity of healthy people. Therefore, this organism is an endogenous opportunist.

3. **Diagnosis.** Macroscopic examination and culture of the purulent exudate draining from the abscess usually confirms the diagnosis.
   a. **Macroscopic examination.** Typical **yellow granules ("sulfur granules")** can be seen macroscopically in the exudate by rotating the vial containing the exudate or by running sterile water over the gauze used to cover the lesion.
   b. **Cultures** should be incubated anaerobically at 37°C. Colonies usually appear in 24–48 hours, but may take as long as 2 weeks to grow.

4. **Treatment** involves **draining the abscess** and administration of large doses (e.g., 20 million U/day) of **penicillin G.**

C. ***N. brasiliensis* and *N. asteroides***

1. **Clinical disease**
   a. **Pulmonary nocardiosis** is characterized by the formation of multiple abscesses in the lungs, often necrotic and confluent. The infection can spread hematogenously to other organs, particularly the brain, where it also causes abscess formation.
      (1) ***N. asteroides*** is usually the etiologic agent of pulmonary nocardiosis.
      (2) Pulmonary nocardiosis is the most common presentation in the **United States.**
   b. **Subcutaneous nocardiosis** presents as a subcutaneous draining abscess. The exudate may contain white granules, but this is an infrequent finding.
      (1) ***N. brasiliensis*** is frequently the cause of cutaneous lesions.
      (2) Subcutaneous nocardiosis is the most common presentation in **Latin America.**

2. **Epidemiology**
   a. **Distribution.** *Nocardia* are soil saprophytes distributed worldwide.
   b. **Transmission.** The infection is acquired either by wound contamination or by aspiration of contaminated particles.

3. **Diagnosis**
   a. **Macroscopic examination** of pus may reveal granules.
   b. **Isolation** of partially acid-fast branching filamentous organisms from sputum, pus, or biopsy material is diagnostic. Growth may require 1–2 weeks.

4. **Treatment** involves surgical **drainage of the abscesses** and the administration of sulfa drugs. **Trimethoprim–sulfamethoxazole** is particularly effective.

D. **Streptomycetes** are soil saprophytes acquired through wound contamination. Their distribution is worldwide.

1. **Clinical disease.** Streptomycetes can cause **mycetoma** ("fungus tumor"). True fungi may also cause this disorder. Mycetoma is characterized by subcutaneous abscesses in the lower extremities. The abscesses tend to drain and heal, but if left untreated, the infection may propagate to deeper tissues and invade the bone.

2. **Diagnosis** involves identification of the organism from cultures of exudates or biopsy material. Streptomyces grow on both bacterial and fungal (Sabouraud's dextrose agar) media. They produce a chalky aerial mycelium with extensive branching; spores eventually develop.

3. **Treatment.** The drugs of choice are **trimethoprim–sulfamethoxazole** and **amphotericin B.** If the disease is allowed to progress, **amputation** may be the only effective treatment.

Chapter 21

Intracellular Bacteria: Chlamydiae, Rickettsiaceae, and Bartonellaceae

John Manos
Victor Del Bene
John Sanders

I. INTRODUCTION.

As noted in previous chapters, many species of bacteria have acquired resistance mechanisms that allow them to survive intracellularly (Table 21-1). *Chlamydia* and *Rickettsia* are considered **obligate intracellular parasites** because they **can only survive and replicate inside mammalian cells.** *Bartonella* species also cause intracellular infections, but can be grown in artificial media.

II. CHLAMYDIAE

A. Introduction. The genus *Chlamydia* includes three species pathogenic for humans: *C. psittaci, C. trachomatis,* and *C. pneumoniae.*

1. **General properties** of these species are summarized in Table 21-2.
2. **Life cycle.** The life cycle of *Chlamydia* is fairly complex.
   a. The **elementary body** is the **infectious, extracellular form** of the organism.
      (1) It is the most differentiated form.
      (2) The elementary body is responsible for both spreading of the infection within a host and host-to-host transmission. The organism persists in this form in the extracellular milieu until it finds a proper target cell (usually columnar or transitional epithelial cells) to infect. It attaches to the surface of the target cell and is phagocytosed.
   b. The **reticulate (initial) body** is the **replicative, intracellular form.** The reticulate body evolves from the elementary body 5–6 hours after penetration of the target cell.
      (1) Once differentiated, the reticulate body begins to **divide by binary fission** and continues to divide for 18–24 hours.
      (2) **Inclusion bodies** are intracytoplasmic vacuoles that contain replicating organisms. They are usually located close to the infected cell nucleus, and can be visualized by conventional microscopy in infected cells.
         (a) Cells infected by *C. psittaci* and *C. pneumoniae* show multiple small inclusion bodies scattered around the nucleus.
         (b) Cells infected by *C. trachomatis* show a single large inclusion body.
   c. An **intermediate body** results from the condensation of the reticulate bodies and looks like a bull's eye when the infected cell is viewed under the microscope.
      (1) The intermediate bodies condense into elementary bodies that are again ready to leave the cell and infect other cells.
      (2) The cell dies in the process of releasing the elementary bodies.
3. **Determinants of pathogenicity.** All *Chlamydia* are highly infectious, but species differ in their degree of virulence. The pathogenic mechanisms are not fully understood, but the ability to replicate intracellularly and the production of both exotoxins and endotoxin are believed to play major roles. Intracellular survival seems to be associated with the ability of the reticulate body to inhibit the fusion of lysosomes with the phagocytic vesicle in which it is contained.
4. **Laboratory diagnosis.** *C. trachomatis, C. psittaci,* and *C. pneumoniae* are obligate in-

Table 21-1. Important Intracellular Human Pathogenic Bacteria

Obligate Intracellular	Facultative Intracellular
Chlamydia	*Bartonella*
Rickettsia	*Brucella*
	Legionella
	Listeria
	Mycobacteria
	Mycoplasma
	Salmonella

tracellular parasites, and as such, cannot be cultured on bacteriologic media. However, they can be grown on **cell culture monolayers.** Although there are a variety of antigen detection methods for *C. trachomatis,* **culture remains the most sensitive, specific method of detection of all** *Chlamydia* species.

a. After 48–72 hours of incubation, the monolayer is **stained with fluorescent antibodies** (which can be genus- or species-specific) **or** with **iodine,** which detects *C. trachomatis* only.

b. The identification of *Chlamydia* in culture is based on the presence of **inclusion bodies.**

(1) Inclusion bodies that stain with the anti-*Chlamydia* species antibody and the anti-*C. trachomatis* antibody are *C. trachomatis.*

(2) Inclusion bodies that stain with the anti-*Chlamydia* species antibody, but not with the anti-*C. trachomatis* antibody, are either *C. psittaci* or *C. pneumoniae.* There is currently no commercially available method of differentiating these organisms.

B. ***C. psittaci*** is the only zoonotic *Chlamydia* species pathogenic for humans. Birds, particularly parrots and parakeets, but also pigeons, are its normal host.

1. Clinical disease. *C. psittaci* causes **psittacosis** [also known as **ornithosis** (from *ornithos,* birds) or **parrot fever]** in humans.

a. The disease is systemic, but the lungs are primarily affected. The inflammatory response is lymphocytic, as is typical of many intracellular infections. Lymphadenopathy and hepatosplenomegaly are common.

b. Clinical presentation. After an incubation period of 1–2 weeks, the patient abruptly develops symptoms of pneumonia: **headache, malaise, anorexia, cough, chills,** and **fever.** Physical examination reveals a pulse rate slower than expected in a febrile patient, and occasionally a **maculopapular (morbilliform) rash** is seen.

2. Epidemiology

a. Transmission

(1) Inhalation of airborne particles (e.g., dried bird droppings) is the usual mode

Table 21-2. General Characteristics of *Chlamydia*

Cannot synthesize ATP; rely on cellular ATP for many of their metabolic reactions
Will not grow in artificial media
Possess ribosomes and synthesize their own proteins
Cell wall contains LPS but does not have a peptidoglycan layer
All three species share a common LPS antigen
Are not affected by β-lactam antibiotics

ATP = adenosine triphosphate; LPS = lipopolysaccharide.

of transmission. Infected birds appear normal or have diarrhea. The organism is present in the blood, tissues, feces, and feathers.

(2) **Human-to-human transmission** has been recorded but is rare.

b. **Distribution.** Psittacosis is distributed worldwide.

c. **Incidence.** In the United States, 50–150 cases of this disease are diagnosed every year.

d. **Susceptibility.** Psittacosis can be an occupational hazard.

3. **Diagnosis.** The clinical picture is similar to that of other types of pneumonia (particularly viral pneumonia and *Mycoplasma* pneumonia). A history of contact with birds helps in the diagnosis.
   a. **Isolation** is very difficult and is usually not attempted.
   b. **Serology** is the primary means of confirming the diagnosis. In a patient with a clinical presentation suggestive of psittacosis, the diagnosis is confirmed with a **complement fixation test,** showing either a fourfold rise in antibody titer (between acute and convalescent samples) or a significant single titer.

4. **Treatment**
   a. **Tetracyclines are the drugs of choice.** The mortality rate was approximately 40% before the introduction of tetracyclines; now it is less than 1%.
   b. **β-Lactam antibiotics are ineffective** because they penetrate mammalian cells poorly, and because *Chlamydia* lack a peptidoglycan layer.

C. **C. pneumoniae** is antigenically distinct from the other species and its inclusion bodies are pear-shaped.

1. **Clinical disease.** The disease has a 1- to 2-week incubation period. It may show a biphasic evolution, starting as an **upper respiratory infection** that later evolves into a mild **bronchopneumonia,** or it may present as a bronchopneumonia without the initial upper respiratory infection stage.

2. **Epidemiology**
   a. **Reservoirs and transmission.** *C. pneumoniae* is a strict human pathogen and is transmitted **person-to-person.**
   b. **Incidence.** Infection with *C. pneumoniae* seems to be rather common (seropositivity rates in adults are approximately 50%), but most infections are subclinical. Reinfection by different strains is possible.

3. **Diagnosis.** The diagnosis is usually made clinically, although differentiation from other types of bacterial and viral pneumonia is difficult. Diagnostic serological tests are not routinely available.

4. **Treatment. Tetracyclines** are the drugs of choice.

E. ***C. trachomatis*** is epidemiologically and medically the most important species of *Chlamydia.* Different strains are involved as etiologic agents of a number of clinical syndromes.

1. **Serotypes.** *C. trachomatis* can be classified into 15 different serotypes:
   a. **Types A, B, B_a,and C** are associated with endemic **trachoma,** the major cause of blindness in the world.
   b. **Types D through K** are associated with **nongonococcal urethritis** and **mucopurulent cervicitis** in adults, and **conjunctivitis** and **pneumonia** in neonates.
   c. **Types L_1, L_2,and L_3** are associated with **lymphogranuloma venereum (LGV).**

2. **Clinical disease.** Mucosal cells are the usual target cells of *C. trachomatis.*
   a. **Ocular disease. Trachoma (chronic follicular keratitis)** usually has an abrupt onset and is transmitted via close contact with an infected person. Poverty, crowding, and poor hygiene are associated with the condition. Trachoma is characterized by inflammation of the mucous membranes and conjunctiva that line the lid and sclera of the eye. If the disease is untreated, neovascularization of the cornea ensues and is followed by scar formation (pannus), which can lead to blindness.
   b. **Sexually transmitted diseases**

(1) **LGV,** a sexually transmitted disease with multisystem involvement, is not as common today as it was 30–40 years ago. After an incubation period of 3 days to 3 weeks, the disease evolves in three different phases.
   (a) The **primary stage** is characterized by a small, transient papulovesicular lesion in the genital area, which may ulcerate, be associated with urethritis symptoms, or go unnoticed.
   (b) The **secondary stage** begins 2–6 weeks later.
      (i) **Regional adenopathy** develops, usually in the groin. The enlarged, tender nodes are often present above and below the inguinal ligament. The indentation caused by the ligament is called the **groove sign.** Sometimes these nodes rupture and drain; when this occurs, they are referred to as **climatic buboes.**
      (ii) **Systemic symptoms,** including fever and anorexia, may be present. The white blood cell count and the sedimentation rate may be elevated.
   (c) The **tertiary stage** may develop in untreated patients. Fibrosis and scarring lead to urethral and rectal strictures. One to several years after the acute infection, blockage of lymphatic drainage leads to elephantiasis of the scrotum, penis, or labia (anogenital rectal syndrome).

(2) **Nongonococcal urethritis** is characterized by a scant urethral discharge that may be clear or milky, serous or mucoid. The discharge may or may not be accompanied by dysuria.
   (a) **Criteria commonly used to differentiate gonococcal from nongonococcal urethritis** are summarized in Table 21-3.
      (i) Gram-stain examination of urethral exudates and culture on Thayer-Martin agar should be performed to rule out gonococcal infection. The diagnosis of nongonococcal urethritis is corroborated by the finding of more than 5 polymorphonuclear cells on a urethral Gram stain in a patient in whom gonococcal urethritis has been ruled out.
      (ii) Because *C. trachomatis* is frequently cotransmitted with *Neisseria gonorrhoeae,* 20%–30% of men and 30%–60% of women who have gonococcal urethritis are concomitantly infected with *C. trachomatis.*
   (b) **Complications**
      (i) **Epididymitis** is a common complication of nongonococcal urethritis that can lead to sterility.
      (ii) **Reiter's syndrome** is characterized by a variable combination of **arthritis, conjunctivitis,** or **uveitis,** accompanied by **mucocutaneous lesions,** 1–4 weeks after the onset of **urethritis.** *C. trachomatis* is isolated in approximately 50% of the patients who present with this triad. It is believed that the ocular and joint manifestations of the syndrome result from a hypersensitivity reaction triggered by the infection.

(3) **Mucopurulent cervicitis** is the usual manifestation of chlamydial infection in women.
   (a) **Clinical signs.** Mucopurulent cervicitis is characterized by a mucopurulent discharge, inflammation of the cervix, and the finding of more than

Table 21-3. Clues for Differentiating Gonococcal Urethritis from Nongonoccal Urethritis

Gonococcal urethritis	Nongonococcal urethritis*
Gram-negative diplococci in Gram stain	No pathogenic bacteria in Gram stain
Symptoms <4 days	Symptoms appear within 4 days
Spontaneous, purulent discharge ("drip")	No discharge, or nonspontaneous mucoid discharge

* Etiologic agents include *Chlamydia trachomatis* (50% of cases), *Ureaplasma urealyticum* (20% of cases), *Trichomonas vaginalis* (5% of cases), herpes simplex virus type 2 (HSV-2), and other agents.

30 polymorphonuclear leukocytes per high-power field in a stained smear of the cervical exudate. The same clinical picture can be caused by other microorganisms, including *N. gonorrhoeae,* herpes simplex virus (HSV), and *Trichomonas vaginalis.*

(b) **Complications. Pelvic inflammatory disease (PID),** characterized by inflammation of the fallopian tubes (salpingitis) and adjacent structures, is the most common complication of chlamydial cervicitis in women.

c. **Neonatal infections** acquired during passage through an infected birth canal may remain asymptomatic, with colonization of the nasopharynx, or cause clinical disease.

(1) **Inclusion conjunctivitis** usually becomes evident soon after birth.

(2) **Pneumonia** may develop during the first 3 months of life, probably from organisms in the colonized nasopharynx. *C. trachomatis* is the most common cause of pneumonia in newborns.

3. **Epidemiology**

a. **Reservoirs.** *C. trachomatis* is a strictly human pathogen. Up to 5% of men and 10% of women are asymptomatic carriers. Asymptomatic carriers with active infection can act as reservoirs.

b. **Transmission** is **person-to-person** and may be **sexual, perinatal,** or via **direct contact with an infected person.**

c. **Distribution and incidence**

(1) **Trachoma,** while almost nonexistent in this country, is the leading cause of blindness in other parts of the world. It affects 400–500 million people each year; 10–20 million of the affected people are blind.

(2) **Sexually transmitted diseases.** *C. trachomatis* (serotypes D through L) is the most common bacterial cause of sexually transmitted disease in developed countries, accounting for approximately 50% of cases of nongonococcal urethritis in men and mucopurulent cervicitis and PID in women.

4. **Laboratory diagnosis.** A definitive diagnosis of *C. trachomatis* infection can be made via culture and isolation, antibody-based techniques, DNA hybridization, or polymerase chain reaction (PCR)-based assays.

a. **Culture and isolation** [see II A 4 b (1)] is the gold standard, but it is expensive, not readily available, and the results take several days to be reported. Except in the case of genital infections, isolation is seldom attempted because of the high cost of maintaining adequate cell cultures, and because some of the *Chlamydia* species are highly infectious.

b. **Antibody-based techniques**

(1) **Direct immunofluorescence.** Fluorescent monoclonal antibodies react with the elementary bodies and demonstrate *C. trachomatis* in clinical specimens. This technique requires a trained technician to carry it out and lends itself to subjective interpretation.

(2) **Enzyme immunoassays (EIAs)** have been developed to detect lipopolysaccharide (LPS) antigens in urethral and cervical specimens. These tests are up to 90% sensitive and more than 95% specific.

c. **DNA hybridization** with *C trachomatis*-specific gene probes is the basis for a rapid and simple test with good sensitivity and specificity. DNA hybridization has become the most widely used rapid diagnostic test for this bacteria.

d. **PCR**-based tests are entering clinical use.

5. **Treatment**

a. **Trachoma** is difficult to treat. Topical and systemic **sulfonamides** and **tetracyclines** are the drugs of choice. Reinfection is common.

b. **Nongonococcal urethritis** and **mucopurulent cervicitis**

(1) **Unconfirmed etiology.** If treatment is based on a clinical diagnosis with exclusion of gonorrhea but without confirmation of the etiology, an antibiotic regimen effective against *Chlamydia, Ureaplasma,* and *Mycoplasma* is preferred.

(a) A 7-day course of **doxycycline** is considered the first choice.

(b) **Erythromycin,** also given for a week, can be used in pregnant women or patients that are allergic to tetracyclines.

(2) **Confirmed etiology**
   (a) Treatment with **doxycycline** is usually adequate.
   (b) Because patient compliance is poor when relatively long administration schedules are involved, an alternative is to give a single dose (1 g) of **azithromycin** (a macrolide). This approach is 98% effective.
   (c) If the patient is **infected with *N. gonorrhoeae* as well,** treatment should include a **second- or third-generation cephalosporin.**

(3) **Treatment of complications.** PID and epididymitis are treated with the same antibiotics, administered for longer periods of time (10–14 days for PID, 21 days for epididymitis).

6. **Control and prevention**
   a. **Trachoma.** Sanitation and personal hygiene are the most effective means of preventing the spread of trachoma.
   b. **Sexually transmitted diseases**
      (1) The patient should abstain from sexual activity until he or she is symptom-free.
      (2) Sexual partners should be notified and asked to seek medical treatment, which includes cervical and rectal Gram stains, culture for *N. gonorrhoeae,* and diagnostic tests for *C. trachomatis.* Irrespective of the results of these tests, all sexual partners of nongonococcal urethritis or cervicitis patients should be treated for *C. trachomatis* infection.
      (3) The identification and treatment of asymptomatic carriers is believed to be very effective in reducing the rate of transmission.
   c. **Neonatal infections.** Neonatal inclusion conjunctivitis is best prevented by a 10–14 day course of oral erythromycin. Topical application of silver nitrate drops or antimicrobial ointments (e.g., erythromycin, tetracycline) have not been shown to be effective.

III. RICKETTSIACEAE.
The Rickettsiaceae family includes three genera: *Rickettsia, Coxiella,* and *Ehrlichia.*

A. **General properties** of the Rickettsiaceae family are summarized in Table 21-4.

B. **Pathogenesis.** Although the various rickettsioses vary, with the exception of Q fever, they share some similarities in the pathogenesis of disease.

1. After transmission (by insect bite or contamination of abraded skin with the fecal material from an infected insect), the rickettsiae multiply in the endothelial cells of microvessels close to the point of penetration. This stage of early multiplication (the **incubation period)** lasts approximately 1 week, during which time the patient has no symptoms or may present with a local eschar.
   a. During the first few days of the incubation period, a local reaction caused by hypersensitivity to tick or other vector products may be seen at the site of the bite and regional lymphadenopathy may be noted.

Table 21-4. General Characteristics of Rickettsiaceae

Small Gram-negative coccobacilli (0.3–0.5 μm in length) that stain poorly
Cell membrane is similar to that of Gram-negative bacteria; contains LPS and peptidoglycan
Obligate intracellular parasites, require growth cofactors (e.g., acetyl-CoA, NAD, ATP) provided by the cell
Will not grow on artificial media

Acetyl-CoA = acetylcoenzyme A; ATP = adenosine triphosphate; NAD = nicotinamide-adenine dinucleotide.

b. The rickettsiae multiply close to the penetration site, but after a few days, they disseminate via lymphatic drainage. Phagocytosis by macrophages, which takes place prior to the onset of the immune response, is the first barrier to rickettsial multiplication. Nonopsonized rickettsiae ingested by nonactivated macrophages tend to survive intracellularly and to proliferate. The enlargement of the lymph nodes reflects the inefficient inflammatory reaction induced by phagocytosis of nonopsonized rickettsiae.

2. After 7–10 days, the organisms begin to disseminate hematogenously. Replication of the rickettsiae in the nucleus or cytoplasm of endothelial cells causes a **vasculitis** that is characterized by perivascular mononuclear cell infiltrates. The infected cells show intracytoplasmic inclusions; intranuclear inclusions are also seen in cases of infection by *R. rickettsii.*
   a. As the infection disseminates, the endothelial damage and vasculitis become widespread, and the clinical manifestations become systemic. A generalized maculopapular skin rash develops as the vasculitis progresses, and perivascular tissue necrosis, thrombosis, and ischemia develop.
   b. The disseminated endothelial lesions lead to increased capillary permeability, edema, hemorrhage, and hypotensive shock. In addition, endothelial damage can lead to activation of the clotting system. As a consequence, disseminated intravascular coagulopathy (DIC) may develop. Death is usually caused by cardiac failure, secondary to circulatory disturbances or to direct cardiac damage.

C. Clinical disease

1. **Rocky Mountain spotted fever** is caused by ***R. rickettsiae.*** It is the most common rickettsial disease in the United States (0.2–0.5 cases/100,000 population); most cases are reported from the central and mid-Atlantic states.
   a. **Clinical presentation**
      (1) Rocky Mountain spotted fever is most prevalent in individuals **younger than 19 years of age,** with **males being affected twice as often as females.** The disease is seen most frequently during the **summer months.**
      (2) A **history of tick bite** is elicited from approximately 70% of patients. The risk of contracting Rocky Mountain spotted fever after being bitten by a tick is approximately 20%.
      (3) After a 7- to 10-day incubation period, the patient experiences **chills, fever (103°F–104°F), myalgia,** and **severe headache.** A **distinctive morbilliform rash** develops in 84%–100% of untreated patients 3–5 days after the onset of fever. The rash is papuloerythematous and begins peripherally (e.g., on the palms and soles), progressively spreading centripetally to the trunk.
   b. **Morbidity and mortality rates.** Rocky Mountain spotted fever is a serious disease; if untreated, permanent organ damage and death can result. The mortality rate is approximately 35% and the morbidity rate is even higher.

2. **Epidemic typhus,** caused by ***R. prowazekii***, is the most severe of the rickettsial diseases.
   a. **Clinical presentation**
      (1) The disease is most frequently seen in the **spring** and **summer months.**
      (2) The patient presents with **fever, headache, malaise, myalgia, prostration,** and a **rash** that is most pronounced on the trunk. As the disease progresses, **CNS** and **myocardial involvement** become clinically obvious and death may ensue.
   b. **Mortality rates** vary from 10%–60% in untreated patients.
   c. **Complications.** Patients who survive the initial infection may experience a relapse several years later **(Brill's disease).**

3. **Q fever** is caused by ***Coxiella burnetii.***
   a. The disease is characterized by **fever** and **influenza-like syndromes.** In some patients, a **bronchopneumonia** with patchy interstitial pulmonary infiltrates and occasionally with lobar consolidation, will develop. Rarely, the infection can become bacteremic and lead to hepatitis, endocarditis (in previously damaged valves), or meningoencephalitis.

Table 21-5. Major Pathogenic Species of Rickettsiae

Species	Disease	Vector	Reservoir	Geographic Distribution
Rickettsia rickettsii	Rocky Mountain spotted fever	*Dermacentor* ticks	Rodents, dogs	North and South America
Rickettsia conorii	Spotted (tick) fevers	Ticks	Rodents, dogs	Southern Europe, Africa, Middle East
Rickettsia prowazeckii	Epidemic typhus	Lice	Humans	Africa, Asia, South America
Rickettsia typhi	Murine typhus	Fleas	Rodents	Worldwide
Rickettsia tsutsugamushi	Scrub typhus	Mites	Rodents	Asia, South Pacific
Coxiella burnetii	Q fever	. . .	Sheep, goats, cattle	Worldwide
Ehrlichia chaffeensis	Ehrlichiosis	Ticks	. . .	Worldwide

b. Physical examination may reveal hepatosplenomegaly and a paradoxically low pulse rate. A skin rash is not seen in this disease.

4. Ehrlichiosis is caused by ***E. chaffeensis.*** *Ehrlichia* has special tropism for monocytes in tissues and peripheral blood. Clinically, the disease is characterized by fever with leukopenia, thrombocytopenia, and elevations in serum aminotransferase levels. Rash is an infrequent sign, and vasculitis is exceedingly rare.

D. Epidemiology.

Epidemiology. The basic epidemiologic facts for the major species of *Rickettsia* are summarized in Table 21-5.

1. Reservoirs and transmission

a. *Rickettsia.* All rickettsiae, with the exception of *C. burnetii,* are transmitted from infected to uninfected hosts via **ticks, fleas, lice,** and **other vectors.**

(1) The arthropods ingest the rickettsiae circulating in the blood of infected mammals, become infected, and transmit the disease to uninfected mammals.

(2) In addition, rickettsiae can be transmitted transovarially from tick to tick.

b. *Coxiella.* *C. burnetii* has a spore-like form that resists desiccation, allowing it to survive extracellularly and to spread without vector participation. *C. burnetii* is usually spread via inhalation of airborne organisms.

(1) Like all other rickettsioses, there are animal reservoirs for this disease. Cattle, sheep, and dogs are the main source of infectious material for humans. Q fever can be an occupational disease for those dealing with animals and animal products.

(2) Most human infections are acquired by inhalation of aerosolized particles containing the spore-like forms. Less frequently, the disease is acquired by ingestion of contaminated food.

c. *Ehrlichia.* Ticks are the likely vectors, and deer are the likely reservoirs.

2. Distribution. In the United States, some species are endemic (e.g., *R. rickettsiae* , *R. typhi* , *C. burnetii*) and others (e.g., *R. prowazeckii* , *R. akari*) are only sporadically isolated.

E. Laboratory diagnosis

1. Culture and isolation are difficult and dangerous because of the highly infectious nature of most rickettsiae.

2. **PCR** will confirm a clinical diagnosis of ehrlichiosis when the infection is active.

3. **Serologic tests** are widely used for the diagnosis of rickettsioses. Because even IgM antibody is seldom detected before the end of the first week of infection, serology is not useful as the basis for a decision concerning treatment, which must be started as early as possible. The main value of serological confirmation of a diagnosis is epidemiological.
   a. The **Weil-Felix test** is based on the cross-reactivity between some strains of *Proteus* and *Rickettsia.* Different strains of *Proteus* have surface antigens virtually identical to those found on several *Rickettsia* species. For example, patients infected with *R. rickettsii* have antibodies both to *Proteus* OX-19 and OX-2, whereas patients infected with *R. prowazeckii* have antibodies to *Proteus* OX-19 only.
   b. **Complement fixation** is not very sensitive and is somewhat time-consuming. Significant antibody titers take time to develop, and in order to be interpreted as positive, a significant rise in the antibody titer must be demonstrated.
   c. **Indirect fluorescence (EIA)** is more sensitive and specific. EIAs allow for discrimination between IgM and IgG antibodies, which helps in early diagnosis. However, false-negative results are possible, particularly early in the disease.
   d. **Direct immunofluorescence.** Identification of *R. rickettsii* in skin lesion biopsy samples by direct immunofluorescence or any other immunochemical technique is 100% specific and 70% sensitive, allowing a diagnosis as early as 3–4 days into the illness. It is the only serological test that is useful for confirming a clinical diagnosis, but it is not widely available.

F. Treatment.

Treatment. Antibacterial agents must be able to penetrate mammalian cells because the infection is mainly intracellular. The drugs of choice for most rickettsioses are **doxycycline** and **chloramphenicol,** the former being far less toxic.

1. It is essential to treat as early as possible (mortality rates of 3%–8% are reported if treatment is delayed or inappropriate) and to treat for 7–10 days.

2. It is important to remember that early treatment aborts the immune response and the majority of patients remain nonimmune after recovery. Therefore, there is a risk of relapse in approximately 15% of properly treated patients.
   a. The relapse is the result of residual persistence of intracellular rickettsiae in macrophages and occurs 2–3 weeks after the initial episode.
   b. To reduce the risk of relapse, antibiotics should be administered for 4–6 days after the fever has been resolved.

IV. BARTONELLACEAE.

BARTONELLACEAE. The Bartonellaceae family contains the genus *Bartonella.* The genus has been recently expanded by the addition of the *Rochalimaea* species, which used to be classified with the genus *Rickettsiae,* but has been reassigned on the basis of genetic homology.

A. Clinical disease

1. **Bartonellosis (Oroya fever, Carrión's disease).** Originally, the genus *Bartonella* contained a single human pathogenic species, ***B. bacilliformis.*** *B. bacilliformis* infects erythrocytes and causes a febrile disease associated with hemolytic anemia. Most cases are seen in South America.

2. **Cat-scratch disease** is usually a relatively benign infection characterized by lymphadenopathy and fever, sometimes with a protracted evolution and controversial etiology.
   a. **Etiology.** It was first believed to be caused by a Gram-negative rod, *Afipia felis,* but recent evidence (including DNA suggests that the true etiologic agent is ***B. (Rochalimaea) henselae***.
   b. **Clinical presentation**

Table 21-6. Major Pathogenic Species of Bartonella

Species	Disease	Vector	Reservoir	Geographic Distribution
Bartonella bacilliformis	Bartonellosis (Oroya fever, Carrión's disease)	*Phlebotomus* fly	Humans	South America
Bartonella (Rochalimaea) quintana	Trench fever; bacillary angiomatosis; peliosis hepatitis; endocarditis	Lice	Humans	Europe, Asia, Africa, North America
Bartonella (Rochalimaea) henselae	Cat-scratch fever; bacillary angiomatosis	Fleas (?), traumatic inoculation (?)	Cats, dogs	Worldwide

(1) The most common clinical presentation is that of an inflammatory adenopathy that may be associated with fever and other systemic symptoms (e.g., malaise, fatigue, anorexia). A scratch lesion distal to the adenopathy is often found, although in some cases the skin lesion has an appearance of a vesicle or pustule, more suggestive of an insect bite than of a scratch.

(2) The disease may become disseminated, with lymphadenopathy in multiple anatomical regions, exanthem, splenomegaly, arthralgias, and more pronounced and protracted systemic systems. Rarely, ocular or CNS involvement (e.g., seizures, coma, polyneuritis) may occur. Systemic involvement is more common in adults than in children.

3. **Bacillary angiomatosis** and **peliosis hepatis** are observed in immunocompromised patients. In these patients, ***B. henselae*** and ***B. quintana*** may disseminate, causing either **papular violaceus skin lesions** (bacillary angiomatosis) or a **persistent febrile bacteremia with hepatosplenomegaly** (peliosis hepatis).

B. Epidemiology. The general epidemiological characteristics of members of the genus *Bartonella* are summarized in Table 21-6.

C. Laboratory diagnosis. Bartonella grow in special artificial media and can be isolated from the peripheral blood of febrile patients. Most commonly, the diagnosis is based on **histologic demonstration using special silver stains** or by obtaining positive results with **serological tests.** An indirect immunofluorescence test is currently being evaluated and appears promising.

D. Treatment. There is no consensus about the best treatment. **Rifampin, doxycycline,** and **ciprofloxacin** have been reported to be effective. **Erythromycin** has been reported to be effective in cases of bacillary angiomatosis.

PART IV
BASIC VIROLOGY

Chapter 22

General Characteristics and Classification of Viruses

Gabriel Virella
John Manos

I. GENERAL CHARACTERISTICS. Viruses are not considered true living organisms because they lack the metabolic properties that enable the simpler forms of life to live and replicate autonomously. Rather, viruses are considered very simple **intracellular parasites,** essentially constituted by packs of genetic information enclosed in one or several protective layers. In addition, some viral particles may contain enzymes without which they could not initiate the replication cycle inside living cells.

A. Size. Viruses are very small, varying in size from 20 × 20 nm to 250 × 300 nm. Even the largest viruses are able to pass through filters able to retain bacteria, hence the designation "ultrafilterable agents."

1. Viral particles cannot be visualized by conventional microscopy, but are well within the limits of resolution of the electron microscope.
2. Parvoviruses (from the Latin *parvus,* small) and picornaviruses (from the Italian *piccolo,* small) are among the smallest viruses; poxviruses are the largest viruses (Figure 22-1).

B. Replication

1. **Viruses can only multiply in living cells.** Laboratory animals, embryonated eggs, and various cell lines (some primary, some immortalized) are commonly used to grow viruses. Cells that support full viral replication are known as **permissive.**
2. The **viral genome** coordinates the synthesis and assembly of viral components in the host cell. Replication strategies vary among viruses (see Chapter 23 II–III).

C. Host specificity

1. In most cases, the virus has a narrow range of host specificity, probably because access of the virus to the host cell is receptor-mediated. There are viruses that infect bacterial cells (bacteriophages), viruses that infect plants (e.g., tobacco mosaic virus), and viruses that infect specific species of animals.
2. Some viruses, however, have a wider range of host specificity:
   a. Some arthropod-borne viruses (arboviruses) are transmitted in a complex cycle involving birds, herbivores, mosquitoes, and, occasionally, humans.
   b. The rabies virus can infect several mammalian species, some of which act as vectors and transmit the disease to humans.
   c. It is believed that the influenza viruses can infect both humans and ducks, as a result of gene exchange between strains predominantly avian and strains predominantly human. This gene exchange results in the emergence of new human strains that can cause pandemics.

II. VIRAL STRUCTURE. The simplest naturally occurring infective viruses **(virions)** consist of **nucleocapsids** (i.e., a **nucleic acid core** surrounded by a protein coat, the **capsid**). Some viruses have an additional protective layer, the **envelope.** Viruses without an envelope are known as **naked.**

DNA viruses

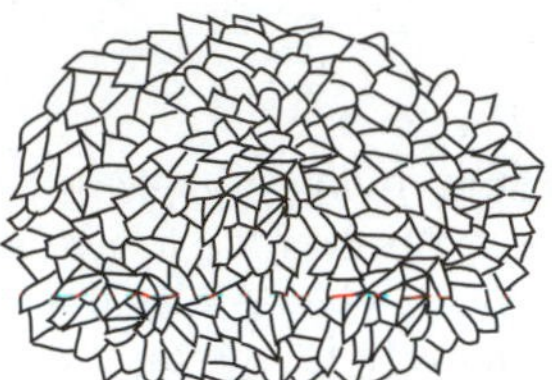

Poxviridae (300 nm)

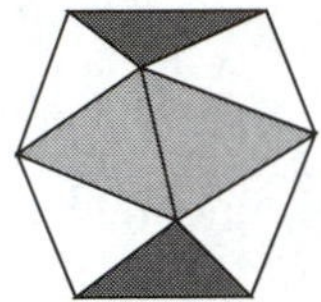

Iridoviridae (250 nm)

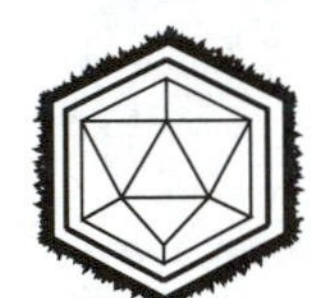

Herpesviridae (100–200 nm)

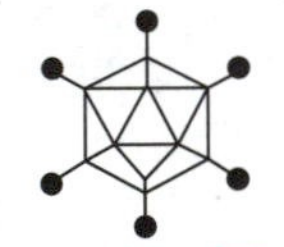

Adenoviridae (75 nm)

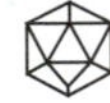

Papovaviridae (55 nm)

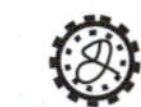

Hepadnaviridae (42 nm)

Parvoviridae (20 nm)

RNA viruses

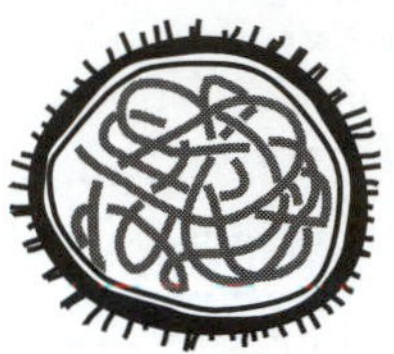

Paramyxoviridae (150–300 nm)

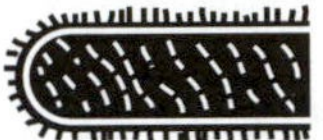

Rhabdoviridae (180 nm)

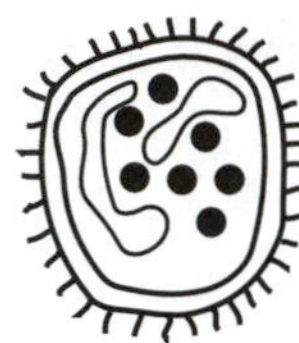

Arenaviridae (50–300 nm)

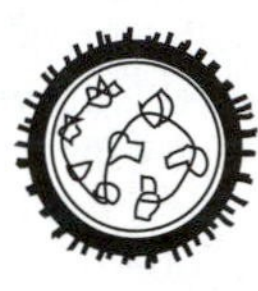

Orthomyxoviridae (80–120 nm)

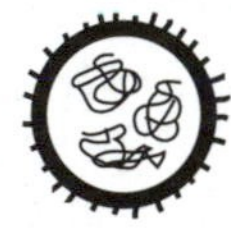

Bunyaviridae (100 nm)

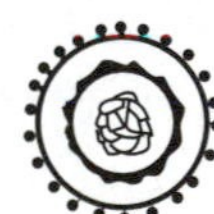

Retroviridae (80–110 nm)

Coronaviridae (60–220 nm)

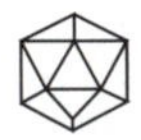

Reoviridae (60–80 nm)

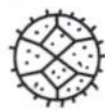

Togaviridae (60–70 nm)
Flaviridae (40–50)

Picornaviridae (25–30 nm)
Caliciviridae (35–40)

FIGURE 22-1. Size and morphology of the most important families of human viruses.

A. Nucleic acid core. The **viral genome** contains **either DNA** or **RNA.**

1. The nucleic acid can exist as a **single strand** (as is the case with most RNA viruses, except reoviruses) or as a **double strand** (the case with most DNA viruses, except parvoviruses).
2. The nucleic acid can exist as a **single segment** or as **several segments (polysegmented genome).**
3. Most viruses have **linear** genomes, with the exception of papovaviruses, which have a supercoiled **circular** genome.
4. The nucleic acid of viruses can be **infective** or **noninfective.** If an infective nucleic acid is introduced into a cell, viral progeny will be generated.
   - **a.** Infective DNA genomes are translated by cell polymerases into mRNA.
   - **b.** Infective RNA genomes are translated directly into protein by cellular ribosomes.

B. Viral capsid

1. **Functions.** The viral capsid:
   - **a.** Protects the nucleic acid core
   - **b.** Mediates viral adsorption to and penetration of cells through interactions with membrane receptors
2. **Composition.** Viral capsids are composed of varying numbers of **capsomeres (morphological units),** each of which is made up of one or more polypeptide chains, known as **protomers (structural units).** The structural units may be **monomeric** (constituted by a single repeating polypeptide chain) or **polymeric** (constituted by up to six different polypeptide chains).
3. **Nucleocapsid symmetry**
   - **a. Helical nucleocapsids.** The nucleic acid is surrounded by protein molecules arranged helically.
     - **(1)** All human viruses with helical symmetry are **enveloped** and include coronaviruses, rhabdoviruses, paramyxoviruses, orthomyxoviruses, bunyaviruses, and arenaviruses.
     - **(2)** Helical symmetry gives the virus a **rod-like appearance.**
   - **b. Icosahedral nucleocapsids.** The nucleic acid is surrounded by capsomeres arranged in icosahedrons (i.e., a solid with 12 vertices and 20 equilateral triangular faces).
     - **(1)** Viruses with icosahedral nucleocapsids include adenoviruses, reoviruses, iridoviruses, herpesviruses, and picornaviruses. Most viruses with icosahedral symmetry are **naked;** exceptions include togavirus, herpesvirus, retrovirus, and flavivirus.
     - **(2)** Icosahedral viruses have a **sphere-like appearance.**
4. **Resistance.** The protein capsid forms a tough protective layer; therefore, naked viruses are resistant to denaturation.

C. Viral envelope. In viruses that have an envelope, the envelope is derived from a cellular membrane and is acquired by the virus during the late stages of replication as the progeny virus undergoes budding (see Chapter 23 I E 2).

1. **Composition.** The envelope consists of a **lipid bilayer** derived from the cellular membrane and **viral-coded glycoproteins,** which are inserted in the bilayer and project to the outer surface. These glycoproteins replace the normal membrane proteins and serve two basic functions:
   - **a.** They promote interaction with nucleocapsid proteins, which is essential for the final stages of viral assembly.
   - **b.** They mediate attachment to cellular receptors, which is essential for infectivity.
2. **Denaturation.** Organic solvents and detergents dissolve the envelope, causing the particle to lose its infectiveness.

TABLE 22-1. Enzymes Contained in the Virion of Selected Human Viruses

Type of Virus	Enzyme
DNA viruses*	
Pox virus	DNA-dependent RNA polymerase
Hepatitis B virus (HBV)	DNA polymerase
+RNA viruses*	
Retroviruses	RNA-dependent DNA polymerase (reverse transcriptase); protease
−RNA viruses	RNA-dependent RNA polymerase; other enzymes

* Most do not pack enzymes.

D. **Viral proteins** can be classified by function into several groups:

1. **Structural proteins** are essential for the formation of infective viral particles.
   a. Some proteins are associated with the nucleic acid and are responsible for proper packing of viral genomes.
   b. Others form the protective layers of the virus (i.e., the capsid and envelope).
2. **Enzymes.** Table 22-1 summarizes the enzymes packed by some of the more important families of viruses.
   a. **Viral polymerases** are essential for nucleic acid replication. A viral particle carries only the components essential for replication. If the viral nucleic acid can be "read" by cellular polymerases, the viral polymerases will be expressed in infected cells but will not be packed in the virions. On the other hand, if the viral nucleic acid cannot be read by the cell polymerases, the virion will have to pack the necessary polymerase.
      (1) **DNA viruses.** Most DNA genomes can be read by the cellular polymerases. Those genomes are considered infective and the virions do not pack polymerases. Exceptions among DNA viruses include the poxviruses and hepatitis B virus (HBV), both of which carry their own polymerases and have replication strategies considerably different from those of other DNA viruses (see Chapter 23 II D,E).
      (2) **RNA viruses** are subclassified in two large families.
         (a) **Positive-stranded RNA (+RNA) viruses** pack RNA strands that can be read as protein messages by the host cell polyribosomes. These viruses do not carry polymerases, and their nucleic acid is infective. Retroviruses are an exception; the replication strategy of this family of viruses involves reverse transcription of +RNA into DNA. Because there is no enzyme in mammalian cells able to retrotranscribe RNA into DNA, retroviruses carry a **reverse transcriptase** in the viral particle.
         (b) **Negative-stranded RNA (−RNA) viruses** carry genomes of opposite symmetry to mRNA. Such strands are **noninfective.** These viruses need to carry a transcriptase to copy their negative RNA strands into positive strands, which can be translated into viral-coded proteins by the cellular ribosomes.
   b. **Proteases** are used by some viruses to process large transcripts into small, functional proteins. Others help release nucleic acids from the nucleocapsid.
   c. **Endonucleases** and **ligases** are specialized enzymes that some viruses require for replication.

III. NOMENCLATURE AND CLASSIFICATION

A. **Nomenclature.** Virus names are usually derived from the disease they cause (e.g., herpesvirus), the locality where the virus was first isolated (e.g., coxsackievirus, Norwalk

TABLE 22-2. Main Families of Human Viruses

	Nucleic Acid	Symmetry	Envelope
RNA Viruses			
Picornaviridae	SS+	Icosahedral	No
Togaviridae	SS+	Icosahedral	Yes
Caliciviridae	SS+	Icosahedral	No
Coronaviridae	SS+	Helical	Yes
Retroviridae	SS+	Helical/icosahedral*	Yes
Bunyaviridae	SS−	Helical	Yes
Arenaviridae	SS−	Helical	Yes
Orthomyxoviridae	SS−	Helical	Yes
Paramyxoviridae	SS−	Helical	Yes
Rhabdoviridae	SS−	Helical	Yes
Reoviridae	DS−	Icosahedral	No
DNA viruses			
Parvoviridae	SS	Icosahedral	No
Papovaviridae	DS	Icosahedral	No
Adenoviridae	DS	Icosahedral	No
Herpetoviridae	DS	Icosahedral	Yes
Poxviridae	DS	Complex	No
Hepadnaviridae	DS (partial)	Helical (?)	Yes
Unclassified viruses			
Hepatitis D virus†			

DS = double-stranded; SS = single stranded; + = positive-stranded RNA; − = negative-stranded DNA.
* Depending on the subfamily
† Circular, single-stranded, RNA-defective genome.

virus), the scientists responsible for isolating the virus (e.g., Epstein-Barr virus), or unique epidemiological characteristics of the virus (e.g., arboviruses).

B. **Taxonomic classification** of viruses is based on:

1. Homology of nucleic acids
2. Morphology, shape, and size
3. Presence or absence of an envelope
4. Nucleoplasmid symmetry
5. Nucleic acid characteristics, including:
   - **a.** Molecular weight
   - **b.** Type (DNA or RNA)
   - **c.** Polarity (positive or negative)
   - **d.** Number of nucleic acid strands and segments
   - **e.** Enzymes

C. The main families of human viruses and their general characteristics are summarized in Table 22-2.

Chapter 23

Viral Replication

Gabriel Virella
Salvatore Arrigo

I. RELATIONSHIP BETWEEN THE VIRUS AND THE HOST CELL.

RELATIONSHIP BETWEEN THE VIRUS AND THE HOST CELL. For many viruses, successful replication requires a delicate balance between the virus and the cell. The following factors affect the permissiveness of the cell with respect to the virus.

A. The cell must have receptors that allow the virus to attach and penetrate.

B. The cell has to be able to survive while infected until viral replication is completed and infectious progeny have been generated. Viral proteins may interfere with cell replication (in some infections, replication may cease entirely) but cell death only takes place after the virus has assembled full progeny particles in a permissive cell.

C. The cell has to provide an adequate environment for viral replication. For example, the virus may not be able to replicate unless the cell it infects is also replicating. In these cases, cellular transacting proteins that control the expression of cellular genes may also activate viral promoters and help activate the expression of viral genes. Thus, whether or not a cell synthesizes such transactivating factors will determine permissiveness.

II. STAGES OF VIRAL REPLICATION

A. **Adsorption** is the initial stage in the infectious cycle of any virus. The virus adheres to **specific receptors,** usually glycoproteins, on the plasma membrane.

1. Each cell can have **as many as 500,000** receptors. In most cases, the **infection is multiple** (i.e., hundreds of viral particles of the same type adsorb to the cell; however, once infected by a given virus, the cell usually becomes refractory to additional virus).
2. Some of the best characterized receptors are summarized in Table 23-1. Many viruses infect the **reticuloendothelial system** during the early stages of infection because in many cases, as soon as antibodies react with the viral particle, the resulting virus–antibody complexes are adsorbed and internalized through **Fc receptors.** Instead of being destroyed in the phagolysosomes, the viruses often start replicating inside the phagocytic cells.

B. **Penetration** is accomplished by two general mechanisms:

1. **Membrane fusion** is observed with enveloped viruses that have fusion-determining membrane glycoproteins (e.g., paramyxovirus, retrovirus). These proteins facilitate fusion of the viral envelope and the cell membrane soon after attachment of the virus to the host cell. The viral nucleocapsids are then released into the cytoplasm, and the viral envelope remains inserted in the plasma membrane.
2. **Receptor-mediated endocytosis (viropexis).** The receptor-bound virus is internalized through clathrin-coated vesicles, which become endosomal vesicles.

C. **Uncoating of the viral nucleic acid**

1. The nucleocapsids migrate into the cytoplasm.
   a. This migration is direct when the virus penetrates the envelope via membrane fusion.

TABLE 23-1. Viral Receptors

Virus	Receptor	Cell or Tissue
HIV	CD4 molecule	Helper T lymphocytes; monocytes and macrophages; antigen-presenting cells
Rhinovirus	Intracellular adhesion molecule-1 (ICAM-1)*	Nasal mucosa
Epstein-Barr virus	Complement receptor 2 (CR2)	B lymphocytes
Lactic dehydrogenase (LDH) virus†	Major histocompatibility complex molecules	Monocytes and macrophages; related cells
Reovirus‡	β-adrenergic receptors	Myocardial cells
Rabies virus	Acetylcholine receptors	Nervous tissue
B19 parvovirus	Erythrocyte P antigen	Erythroid precursor cells
Many viruses	Fc receptors	Monocytes and macrophages; related cells

* Over 90% of rhinovirus strains
† Infects mice
‡ Myocarditis-producing strains

b. When receptor-mediated endocytosis is the mechanism of entry, the acid pH in the endosomes promotes fusion of the viral envelope and the endosomal membrane, and the nucleocapsid is released into the cytoplasm.

2. Cytoplasmic proteases or viral proteases digest the protein layers, releasing the nucleic acid and some proteins that may have remained attached to the nucleic acid. Naked viruses either lose their capsids in the acid endosome, or they remain in the endosome until the phagolysosome is formed; in the latter case the proteases in the phagolysosome digest the capsid.

3. After uncoating is completed, infectious particles cannot be recovered from an infected culture. This inability to recover infective viruses marks the **beginning of the eclipse phase** of viral replication.

D. **Synthesis** involves replication of the nucleic acid and synthesis of viral proteins. Viral proteins are synthesized in the cytoplasm; the site of replication for the nucleic acid (viral genome) is variable. In general, enzymes necessary for replication of the nucleic acid and regulatory proteins are synthesized first, although some of these proteins may be carried into the cells by the virus. Later, the proteins necessary to construct progeny virions are produced, usually from messages derived from progeny nucleic acid.

1. DNA viruses (Figure 23-1)

a. Early period. The viral DNA diffuses to the nucleus and transcription by cellular DNA-dependent RNA polymerases is initiated. Only part of the viral genome is transcribed and translated, leading to the production of **early proteins** (i.e., regulatory proteins, viral-coded polymerases, and matrix proteins).

(1) Regulatory proteins have widely divergent functions.

(a) In classic lytic infections, the regulatory proteins inhibit host DNA, RNA, and protein synthesis, while at the same time promoting the expression of viral genomes. This is usually achieved by altering the specificity of the host polymerases and polyribosomes.

(b) Regulatory proteins induce cellular DNA replication following integration of the genomes of several DNA viruses and the genomes of retroviruses in the host genome. Induction of cellular DNA replication results in replication of the integrated viral genomes.

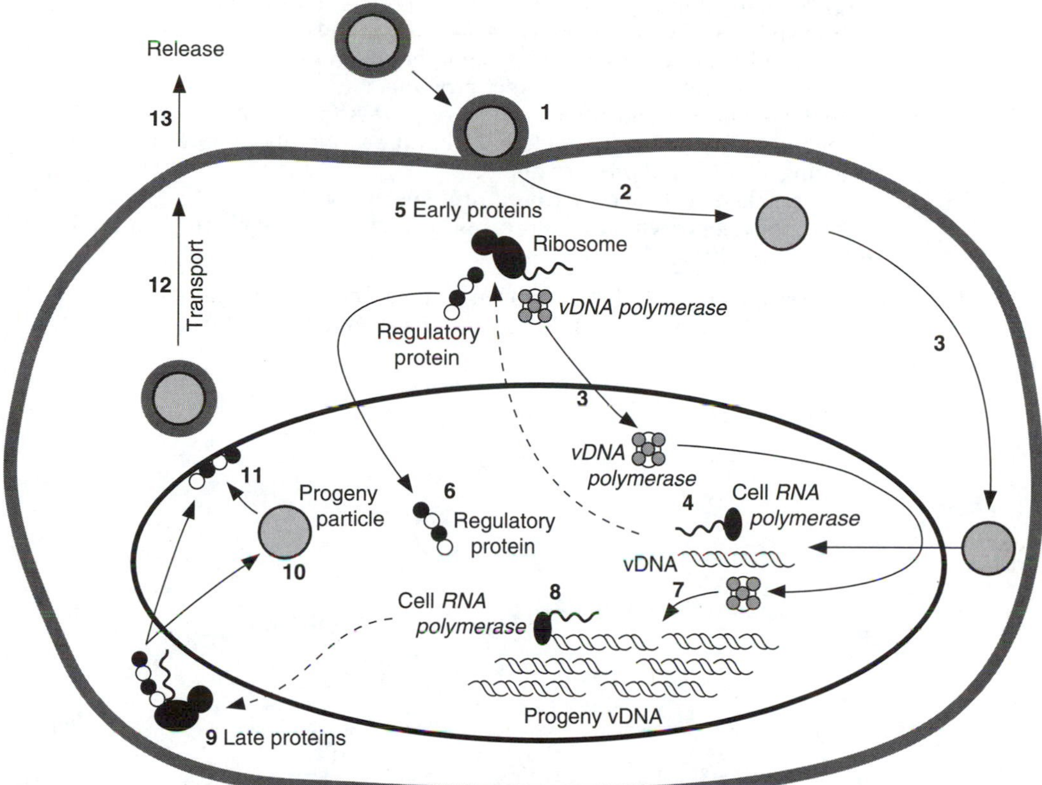

FIGURE 23-1. Replication cycle of a human DNA virus. Herpesvirus is represented here. Following adsorption to the host cell (*1*), the virus penetrates the cell via membrane fusion (*2*). The nucleocapsid is transported to the nuclear membrane (*3*) and the viral nucleic acid (*vDNA*) is released into the nucleus, where transcription takes place. Cellular DNA-dependent RNA polymerases begin transcribing the viral DNA (*4*). Translation of the early portion of the genome leads to the formation of the early proteins (*5*), which include regulatory proteins, viral-coded polymerases, and matrix proteins. The viral-coded polymerase diffuses to the host cell nucleus (*6*), where it allows replication of the viral genome so that progeny DNA strands can be generated (*7*). Some of the progeny DNA is transcribed by cell RNA polymerase (*8*) to induce the expression of the late proteins (*9*). The late proteins are used to assemble the progeny particle (*10*), which buds through the inner nuclear membrane (*11*), acquiring an envelope. After budding, the progeny viral particles are transported across the cytoplasm (*12*) and released by reverse phagocytosis or the Golgi apparatus (*13*).

(2) Viral-coded polymerases allow replication of the viral genome, generating progeny DNA strands.

(3) Matrix proteins are used to provide a scaffold for the replication of nucleic acid and assembly of viral progeny particles. Matrix proteins are found in electron-dense formations known as **inclusion bodies.**

b. Late period. Progeny nucleic acid is synthesized by viral-coded polymerases. However, not all "progeny" DNA is reserved to pack into new virions—some of it is transcribed by the viral polymerases or host-modified polymerases in its full length, so that the **late proteins,** structural proteins needed to assemble the progeny virions, can be expressed.

(1) The transcription of messenger RNA (mRNA) from the full length of the viral DNA strands during the late stages of replication depends on several mechanisms that are not mutually exclusive. As a result of any of these mechanisms, the polymerases will recognize different initiation and termination sites at different stages of the replication cycle, synthesizing different proteins. Mechanisms include:

(a) Sequential modification of DNA-dependent RNA polymerases
(b) Synthesis of viral-coded, DNA-dependent RNA polymerases
(c) Regulation by early proteins, some of which may act as transcription factors with affinities for different promoters
(d) Differences in the affinity of progeny DNA for host polymerases

(2) Regardless of the type of nucleic acid in the virion, the following rules pertaining to structural proteins apply:
(a) In **naked viruses,** only **capsid proteins** are produced.
(b) In **enveloped viruses,** both **capsid proteins** and **envelope glycoproteins** are synthesized.

2. **+RNA viruses** (Figure 23-2) have genomes that can be directly translated by cellular polyribosomes into large proteins, which are post-synthetically cleaved.

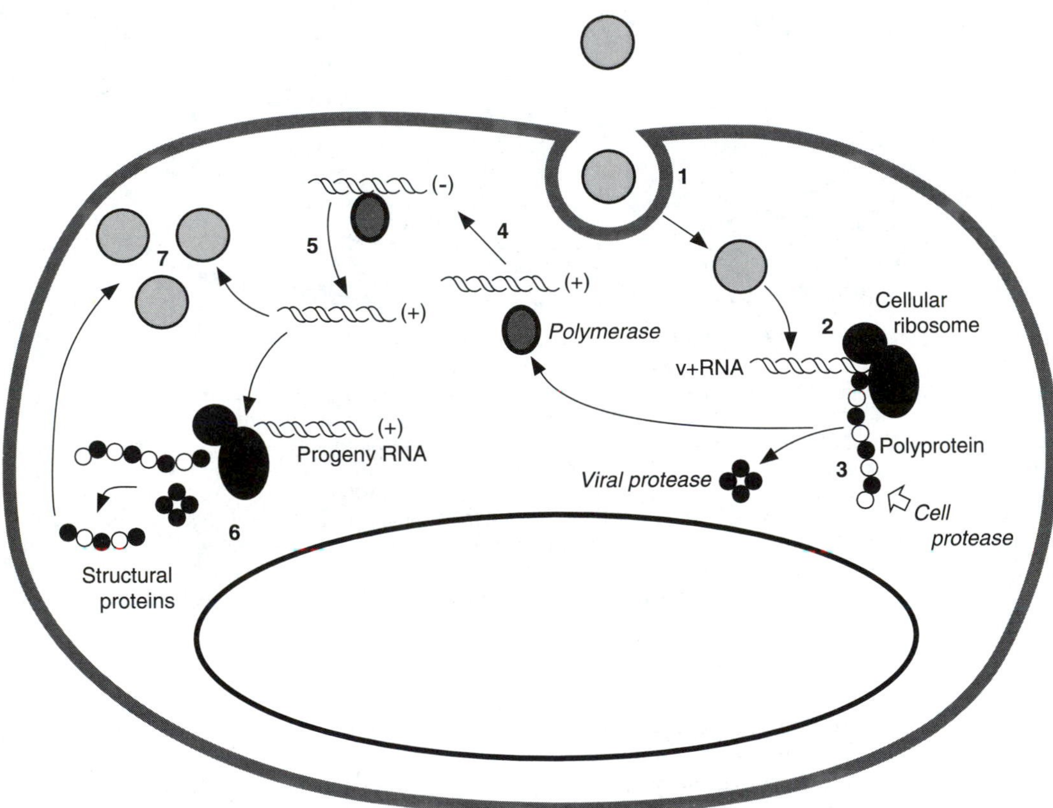

FIGURE 23-2. Replication cycle of a +RNA virus. Following adsorption to the host cell, the virus penetrates the cell via endocytosis (*1*). Replication begins as soon as the viral genome is released into the cytoplasm, because viral +RNA strands (*v+ RNA*) have the same molecular symmetry as messenger RNA (mRNA); therefore, they can be recognized and are directly translated by the cellular ribosomes (*2*). Cell proteases process the resultant viral polyprotein (*3*), forming a viral RNA-dependent RNA polymerase, a viral protease, and several structural proteins. The polymerase copies the +RNA strands into −RNA strands (*4*), which are used as templates to synthesize new +RNA strands (*5*). The newly synthesized +RNA is used in part to synthesize more structural proteins (6) and in part to be packed into the progeny virions (7).

a. **Early period.** In the early stages of replication, a **viral RNA-dependent RNA polymerase,** a **protease,** and several **structural proteins** are derived from the processing of polyproteins by cell and viral proteases.

b. **Late period.** The new polymerase copies the +RNA strands into −RNA strands that are used as templates to synthesize large numbers of new +RNA strands. The newly synthesized +RNA is packed in the progeny virions and used to produce more structural proteins.

3. **−RNA viruses** (Figure 23-3). The genomes of −RNA viruses need to be transcribed into +RNA strands (the equivalent of mRNA) before viral proteins can be synthesized. The cell has no RNA-dependent RNA polymerases, so **the virus has to pack its own polymerases.**

   a. **Early period.** The early stages of replication are concerned with the synthesis and transcription of +RNA strands. Both short and full-length transcripts are produced.

   b. **Later period.** The short +RNA strands are translated into the several viral proteins and enzymes necessary to form new viral particles, while the full-length +RNA strands serve as templates for progeny −RNA strands. As −RNA strands

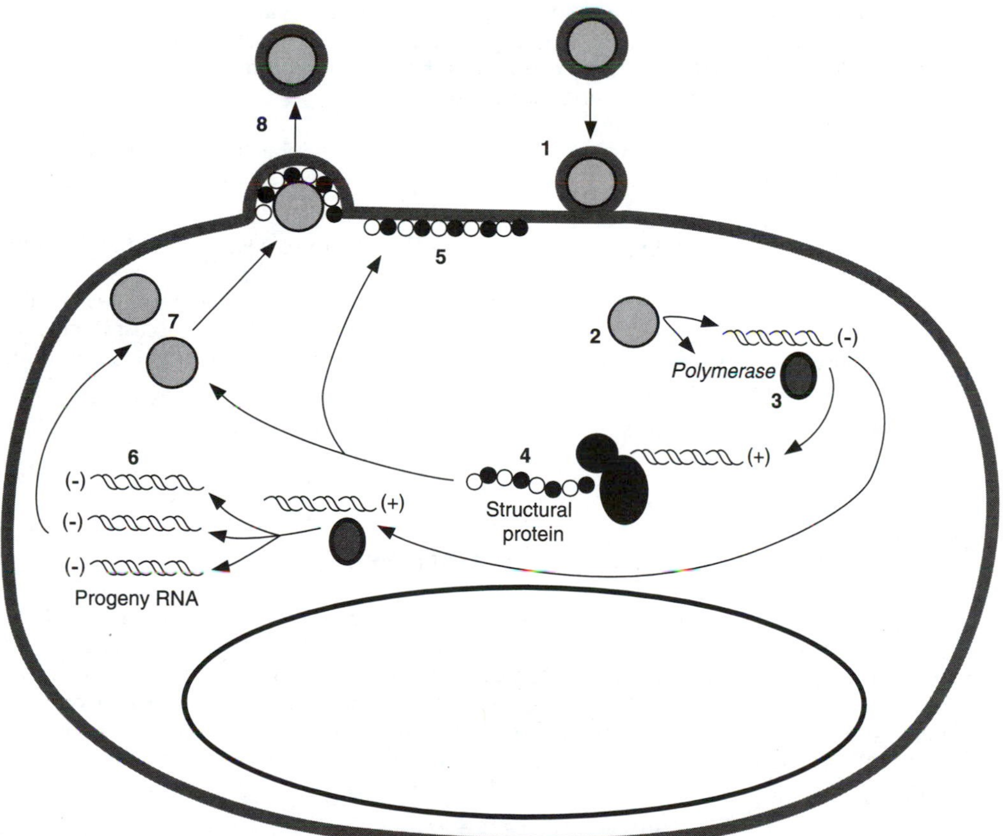

FIGURE 23-3. Replication cycle for a −RNA virus. Following adsorption to the host cell membrane (*1*), the virus penetrates the cell via membrane fusion. Following uncoating (*2*), viral −RNA is transcribed in +RNA by the RNA-dependent RNA polymerase packed by the virus (*3*). Both short and full-length transcripts are produced. The short +RNA strands are transcribed into viral proteins and enzymes for the progeny virions (*4*). One of these proteins is an envelope glycoprotein that is inserted into the cellular membrane (*5*) in preparation for budding. The full-length +RNA strands are used as templates for progeny −RNA strands (*6*). The progeny viral nucleocapsids, formed from structural proteins and progeny −RNA strands, are attracted to the modified patch of cell membrane (*7*). They pinch off pieces of the lipid bilayer membrane, completing the assembly process, and are released (*8*) by budding.

accumulate, they are also used as templates for additional short +RNA strands, which are needed to synthesize structural proteins and viral polymerase to be packed in the progeny particles.

E. **Assembly (morphogenesis).** Viral progeny are assembled, marking the **end of the eclipse phase.** In order to be infective, progeny particles must contain viral nucleic acid. The incorporation of nucleic acid into a nucleocapsid is facilitated by the production of protein and nucleic acid in close proximity and by **"packaging signals"** (i.e., specific sequences on the viral nucleic acid that determine interactions between core and internal capsid proteins).

1. **Naked viruses** can complete their maturation in the cytoplasm or in the nucleus. For a brief period of time, infective viruses are present in the cytoplasm; they are released when the cell bursts.
2. **Enveloped viruses** complete their maturation at the time of **budding.**
   a. After the **envelope proteins** are formed during the synthesis stage, they are glycosylated or myristylated, then transported and **inserted into a cellular membrane** (the nuclear membrane in the case of herpes virus, the membranes lining intracytoplasmic vacuoles in the case of some other viruses, or the plasma membrane for most enveloped viruses). The envelope glycoproteins are **arranged in patches** crosslinked to an inner viral-coded protein layer (equivalent to an outer capsid).
   b. The viral nucleocapsids, which are attracted to these modified patches of cell membrane, **pinch off pieces of the lipid bilayer membrane,** thus completing the assembly process by forming the envelope.

F. **Release.** The assembled virions are released to the extracellular fluid by one of two basic mechanisms:

1. **Budding** is the mechanism of release of enveloped viruses.
   a. Viral particles budding at the plasma membrane are released immediately to the outside.
   b. Viral particles budding at the nuclear membrane, ribosomal membranes, or at any other intracellular membrane are transported across the cytoplasm and eventually released. The transport systems used to secrete cellular proteins are usually involved in the transport of viral particles.
2. **Lysis** of the infected cell is the mechanism of release of naked viruses.

III. REPLICATION CYCLE OF MAJOR HUMAN DNA VIRUSES

A. **Papovaviruses.** This family of DNA viruses includes several oncogenic viruses such as **simian virus (SV) 40** and **polyomavirus,** which do not cause disease in humans, and two human pathogenic species: **BK** and **JC viruses** (named after the initials of the patients from whom they were initially isolated). The replication of papovaviruses follows the general process outlined for DNA viruses, but with some variations attributable to the fact that the virus genome exists as cyclic supercoiled, double-stranded DNA (Figure 23-4).

1. **Synthesis**
   a. **Early period.** Around the origin of replication, there are control regions (enhancers and promoters) that are activated by cellular factors. During the first 14–18 hours, genes A, H, I, and B (50% of the viral DNA) are transcribed into three precursor mRNAs of slightly different lengths. These precursor mRNAs are processed (spliced, capped at the 5′-termini, and polyadenylated at the 3′-termini) into the mRNAs coding for **three regulatory proteins [transforming (T) antigens],** which interfere with the control of cell division (see Chapter 27). In addition, the large T protein binds to the origin of replication and inhibits the synthesis of early genes, thus controlling the switch from the early to late phase of replication.

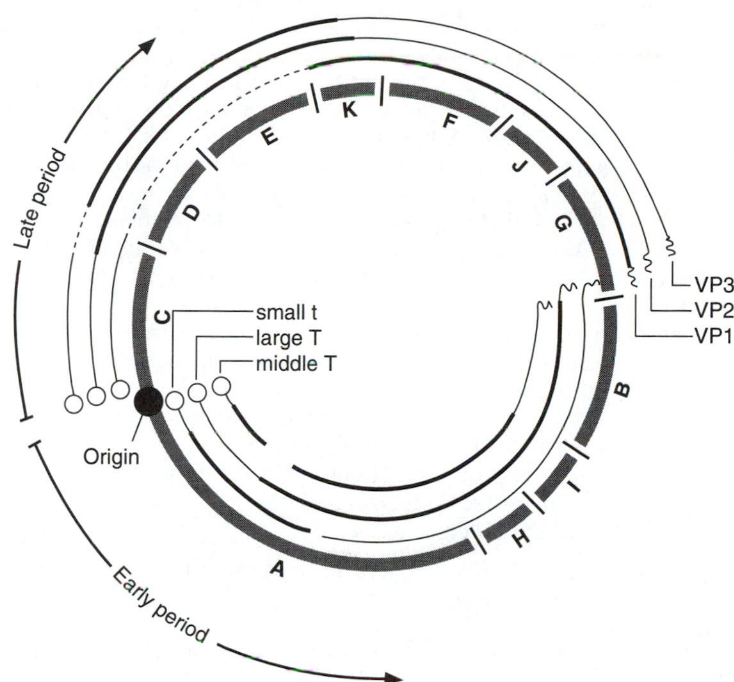

FIGURE 23-4. Replication of polyomavirus. The genome is cyclic supercoiled, double-stranded DNA. Early transcription starts at the origin and proceeds counterclockwise (in the direction of gene A), whereas late transcription proceeds clockwise (in the direction of gene C). Three messenger RNA (mRNA) strands are transcribed in each stage of replication. During the early stage of replication, the mRNAs coding for the transforming (T) antigens are produced: T (*large T,* 95 kDa), *middle T* (57 kDa), and t (*small t,* 17 kDa). During the late stage of replication, the mRNAs coding for capsid proteins (*VP1, VP2, VP3*) are produced. All resulting mRNAs are capped (*open circle*) and polyadenylated (*zig-zag line*). The *thick lines* represent translated mRNA segments. The *thin lines* represent untranslated segments. The *dashed lines* represent introns removed by splicing. The distal two-thirds of the mRNA coding for the middle T antigen and the mRNA coding for VP1 protein are read in a different frame than the mRNAs coding for other early or late proteins, respectively.

b. **Late period.** While transcription of the T antigens declines, genes C, D, E, K, F, J, and G are read in a clockwise direction. These genes are transcribed into at least three different mRNAs, coding for three different **capsid proteins (VP1, VP2,** and **VP3).** If the cell is fully permissive, the circular genomes remain unintegrated, replicating as autonomous elements.

2. **Assembly and release.** As many as 100,000 copies of viral DNA may accumulate in an infected cell; following assembly of the viral progeny in the host cell nucleus, the cell lyses, releasing the viruses.

B. **Adenoviruses.** The replication of adenoviruses closely follows the general procedure for DNA virus replication.

1. **Synthesis**
   a. **Early period.** During the first 8 hours, host cell DNA-dependent RNA polymerase II is responsible for viral replication. Only 30% of the genome is transcribed. The nuclear transcripts of this region are spliced, capped, and polyadenylated and code for a series of **regulatory proteins.**
      (1) The E1A and E1B genes code for proteins that activate the expression of viral genes and promote cell proliferation.

(2) The E2A gene codes for a DNA polymerase and a DNA-binding protein that serves as a primer for DNA replication.

(3) The E3 gene codes for a protein that binds to major histocompatibility complex-I (MHC-I) antigens, impairing their adsorption to the cell membrane and, consequently, reducing the antigenicity of the infected cell.

(4) The E4 gene codes for several proteins involved in the control of host and viral DNA replication.

b. **Late period.** The viral DNA polymerase begins to synthesize progeny DNA. The progeny DNA seems to have a different affinity for cellular RNA polymerases, which are able to transcribe the complete viral genome, generating messages for late proteins.

(1) During the late phase, the same DNA segments can be transcribed differently because promoters (initiation signals) and polyadenylation sites (termination signals) are staggered along the viral genome. The reading of the same nucleic acid segments in different reading frames has been described in other DNA viruses as well as in retroviruses.

(2) The repertoire of proteins that can be made from limited genetic information is expanded by processing common RNA nuclear transcripts in different ways, generating different mRNAs.

2. **Assembly and release.** Assembly takes place in the nucleus; progeny are released via lysis.

C. **Herpesvirus** (see Figure 23-1) is adsorbed after interaction with membrane receptors. The viral envelope and plasma membrane fuse, and the nucleocapsid is released into the cytoplasm. Uncoating takes place at nuclear pores, followed by migration of viral DNA into the nucleus.

1. **Synthesis**

a. **Early period.** The early proteins coded by the proximal third of the viral genome include phosphoproteins with regulatory functions, including transactivating proteins that initiate the transcription of the next set of viral genes. This set of genes, in turn, codes for a DNA polymerase and a DNA-binding protein necessary for viral DNA replication.

b. **Late period.** The viral-coded DNA polymerase replicates viral DNA, part to be packed in the progeny virions, and part to be read by cell polymerases, resulting in expression of the terminal genes that code for structural proteins (capsid proteins and envelope glycoprotein spikes).

2. **Assembly and release.** Assembly takes place in the nucleus, where progeny DNA strands are surrounded by capsid proteins to form the nucleocapsid. The final step of morphogenesis is the acquisition of a viral envelope at the level of the inner nuclear membrane. After budding, the progeny viral particles are transported across the cytoplasm and released either by reverse phagocytosis or via the Golgi apparatus.

D. **Poxviruses** are the most complex of all animal viruses, with more than 100 different proteins in their virions. Many of these proteins form a complex external protein coat.

1. The replication cycle of the poxviruses is unique in two main aspects:

a. **Replication takes place in the cytoplasm and is totally independent of cell polymerases** because, unlike other DNA viruses, poxviruses carry their own DNA-dependent RNA polymerase.

b. **DNA transcription is initiated before uncoating is completed** by the viral polymerase enclosed in the core.

2. **Synthesis**

a. **Early period.** One of the early proteins that is synthesized is a **protease (uncoating protein)** that completes the release of the nucleic acid into the cytoplasm, an essential step for the synthesis of progeny DNA. Other early proteins include **enzymes (thymidine kinase, DNA polymerase)** and **structural proteins.**

b. **Late period.** Synthesis patterns switch to late protein synthesis when DNA replication begins as a consequence of regulation at the translation level. That is, mRNA species coding for early enzymes cease to be translated, perhaps influenced by one of the first late proteins to be synthesized, while mRNA species coding for structural proteins continue to be translated.

3. **Assembly and release.** Morphogenesis takes place in the cytoplasm. The progeny is released when the cell lyses.

E. **Hepatitis B virus (HBV)** does not grow in culture, and information about its replication strategy is incomplete. The genome is constituted by double-stranded DNA, but the positive strand is shorter. The viral particle carries a viral polymerase that can transcribe both DNA and RNA. Two direct repeat segments exist near the ends of the double strand; these segments allow integration into the host genome.

1. **Synthesis**
   - **a.** After the virus is uncoated, the viral DNA and the polymerase migrate to the nucleus, where the **viral polymerase completes the positive strand,** using the negative strand as a template.
   - **b.** The complete double-stranded DNA is transcribed into several short mRNAs and into a complete +RNA strand (pregenomic RNA, the template for genome replication). The **viral genome can be read in three different open reading frames,** generating short mRNAs that code for different viral proteins and enzymes.
   - **c.** The replication of the viral nucleic acid is believed to follow a complex sequence.
     - **(1)** First, the pregenomic +RNA strand is encapsulated into cores that contain the viral polymerase. At this time, the polymerase acts as a reverse transcriptase, transcribing a −DNA strand using the +RNA strand as a template, while at the same time, the +RNA strand is degraded.
     - **(2)** The −DNA strand is then used as a template to transcribe a +DNA strand, but the transcription terminates before completion, resulting in a double DNA strand with a short positive strand.

2. **Assembly** of the virion involves the addition of an envelope containing the surface antigen (HBsAg).

3. **Integration.** During this complicated replication cycle, **viral DNA integrates into the host genome.** The viral DNA is usually fragmented and inserted in multiple sites. The only reading frame that remains open after integration is the one coding for HBsAg, which may be produced in large amounts in the absence of complete viral replication.

IV. REPLICATION CYCLE OF MAJOR HUMAN RNA VIRUSES.

The basic characteristics of RNA viruses and of their replication strategies are summarized in Figure 23-5.

A. **+RNA viruses.** Replication begins as soon as the viral genome is released into the cytoplasm, because +RNA strands have the same molecular symmetry as mRNA; therefore, they can be recognized and are directly translated by the cellular ribosomes.

1. **Picornaviruses** replicate like most other +RNA viruses (see I D 2). Replication of the genome involves transcribing −RNA from +RNA and using the −RNA strands as templates for progeny +RNA strands. All replication steps take place in the cytoplasm, where the progeny virions accumulate until they are released when the infected cells lyse.
   - **a.** The **translation of +RNA strands** may be complete or incomplete; the 5′ end of the coding region, which codes for structural proteins, is always translated, whereas the 3′ end, coding for the polymerase, is less frequently translated.
   - **b.** **Cleavage of the viral polyproteins** is carried out by cellular proteases.
     - **(1)** One of the products of this splicing is a **viral-coded protease** that continues the process in a more specific manner.

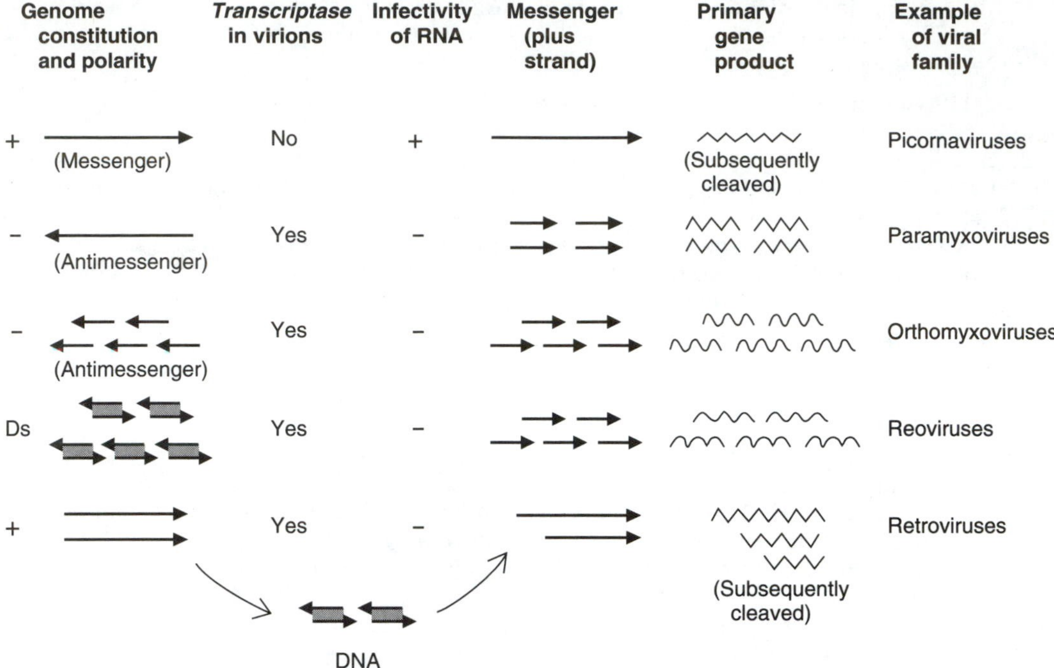

FIGURE 23-5. Diagram illustrating the general properties and replication strategies of RNA viruses. The **polarity** of the nucleic acid refers to its symmetry: +RNA is identical to messenger RNA (mRNA), whereas −RNA has a symmetry complementary to that of mRNA. **Infectivity** refers to the ability of the virion to initiate viral replication just by transfecting viral RNA to a suitable cell, a property shared by most DNA viruses and most +RNA viruses. Most −RNA genomes tend to be translated into short messages for individual proteins, whereas +RNA genomes are usually translated into large polyproteins that are post-synthetically cleaved. *DS* = double-stranded. (Modified with permission from Dulbecco R: Multiplication and genetics of animal viruses. In *Microbiology,* 4th ed. Edited by Davis BD, Dulbecco R, Eisen HN, Ginsberg HS. Philadelphia, JB Lippincott, 1990.)

(2) Another product of the polyprotein cleavage is a **viral RNA-dependent RNA polymerase** that is necessary for the replication of the genome.

2. **Togaviruses.** The replication cycle is similar to that of picornavirus. The main difference is that because togaviruses are enveloped, they mature by budding from the cell membrane of the infected cell.

3. **Retrovirus.** The replication strategy of retrovirus is summarized in Figure 23-6.
   a. The replication of retroviruses is unique because it involves a **DNA intermediate.** Because reverse transcription and integration must precede viral replication, the +RNA strands carried by retroviral particles are **not infective.**
      (1) **Reverse transcription.** A **reverse transcriptase,** packed in the virion, synthesizes DNA using RNA as a template. By reading the +RNA strand in the 3′-5′ direction, −DNA strands are generated.
         (a) +DNA strands are copied from the newly synthesized −DNA strands, generating double-stranded DNA. The double-stranded DNA is transported into the host cell nucleus.
         (b) The terminal sequences of the +RNA strand are duplicated, resulting in the synthesis of identical sets of repeating sequences at each end of the viral DNA. These repeating sequences are essential for integration of the viral DNA into the host DNA.
      (2) **Integration.** A second enzyme with both **endonuclease** and **ligase** (**integrase**) activities splices the host DNA, allowing end-to-end recombination of viral

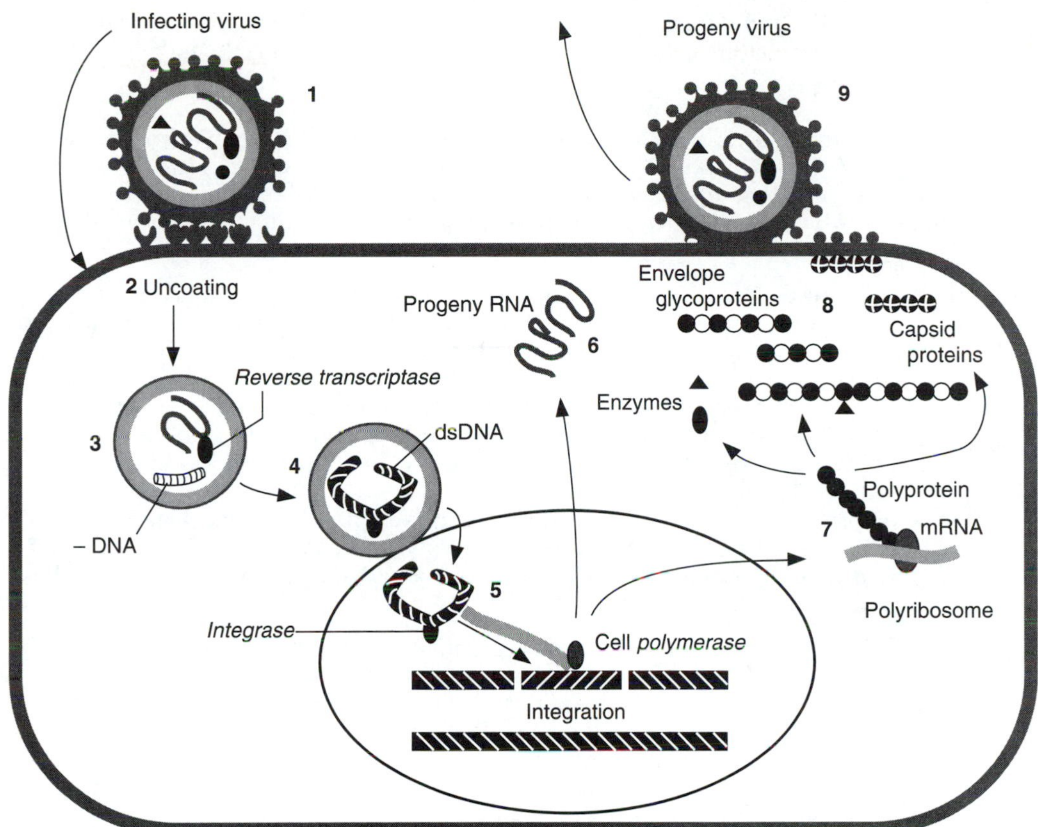

FIGURE 23-6. Replication cycle of retroviruses. Following adsorption to the host cell wall (*1*), the infecting virus enters the cytoplasm via membrane fusion. Following uncoating (*2*), a reverse transcriptase (packed in the virion) synthesizes −DNA using RNA as a template (*3*). +DNA strands are copied from the newly synthesized −DNA strands, generating double-stranded DNA (*dsDNA, 4*). The double-stranded DNA is transported into the host cell nucleus, where integrase splices the host DNA, allowing end-to-end recombination of viral DNA with the spliced host DNA (*5*). The integrated DNA is transcribed by host DNA-dependent RNA polymerase into +RNA strands. Intact +RNA is used for progeny genomes (*6*). Some of the +RNA is translated as mRNA into polyproteins that are cleaved to produce structural proteins and enzymes for the virion (*7*), and some of the +RNA is spliced into short mRNAs that encode for envelope proteins, regulatory proteins, and other accessory proteins (*8*). The progeny virus is then released by budding (*9*).

DNA with the spliced host DNA. Then, the same enzyme ligates the fragments into a single double strand of DNA.

(3) Transcription. The integrated DNA is transcribed by host DNA-dependent RNA polymerases into +RNA strands. The primary RNA full-length transcripts can:

- **(a)** Remain intact to be used as progeny genomes
- **(b)** Be translated as mRNA into large polyproteins, which are post-synthetically cleaved to generate the structural proteins and enzymes needed to assemble the virion
- **(c)** Be spliced into short mRNAs encoding envelope proteins, regulatory proteins, and other accessory proteins

b. Assembly and release. Viral assembly takes place in the cytoplasm; maturation takes place at the cell membrane when the progeny particles exit the cell by budding.

B. **−RNA viruses.** The virion must contain an **RNA-dependent RNA polymerase** because −RNA is noninfective, and replication cannot begin until the genome is transcribed into a +RNA strand. Mammalian cells lack transcriptases able to perform this task, so the infecting virus has to carry its own preformed polymerase. As a rule, replication takes place in the cytoplasm.

1. **Rhabdoviruses.** Replication involves transcription of the −RNA strand either as a complete +RNA strand, which is used as a template for progeny −RNA strands, or as five short +RNA strands that are translated into nucleocapsid proteins, envelope glycoproteins, and a viral polymerase.
   a. The transcription of −RNA into short mRNAs involves a polycistronic polymerase of viral origin that begins transcribing at the initiation site close to the 3′ end. The polymerase stops at intercalated polyadenylation "signals" to yield five short mRNAs (Figure 23-7).
   b. As protein N accumulates, it forms a complex with the polyadenylation regions, which became obliterated. Transcription then proceeds in an uninterrupted fashion, yielding complete +RNA strands that are used as templates for the synthesis of progeny −RNA strands.
2. **Orthomyxoviruses** are unique because the initial transcription of orthomyxovirus −RNA to +RNA takes place in the nucleus (Figure 23-8).
   a. Viral mRNAs need transcription primer. In the case of the orthomixovirus, the primer is a cap from cellular nuclear RNA.
   b. The infective virus contains a transcriptase, an endonuclease, and several proteins. The endonuclease is used to break nascent host RNA strands, and the fragments are then bound by a protein (P2).

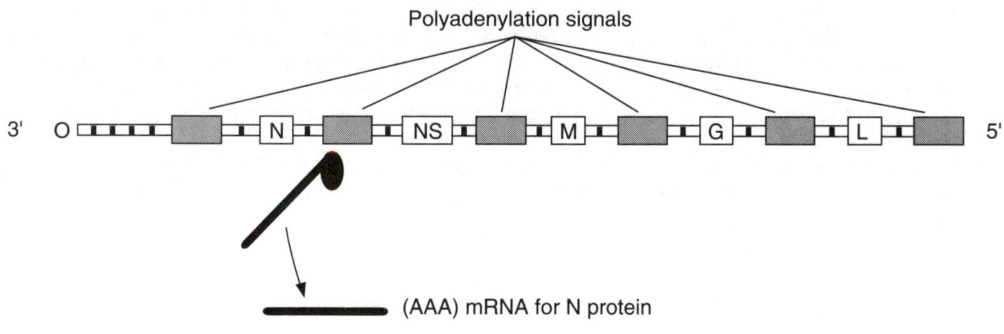

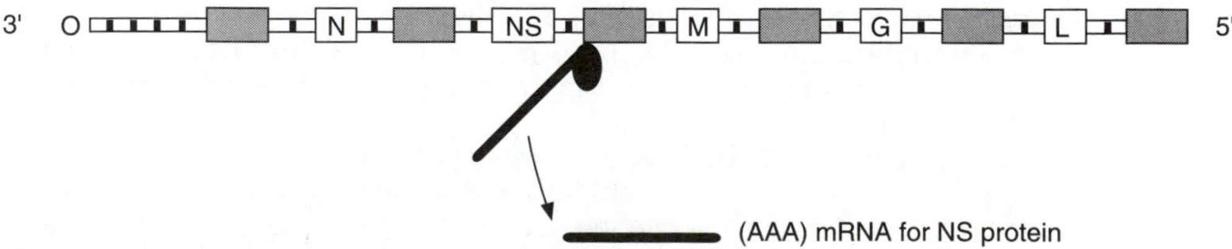

FIGURE 23-7. The mechanism responsible for the synthesis of short messenger RNA (*mRNA*) strands from the rhabdovirus genome. Genes N, NS, and L code for nucleocapsid proteins and genes M and G code for envelope glycoproteins. The gene products from genes N, NS, and L form a complex in the nucleocapsid that functions as an RNA-dependent RNA polymerase.

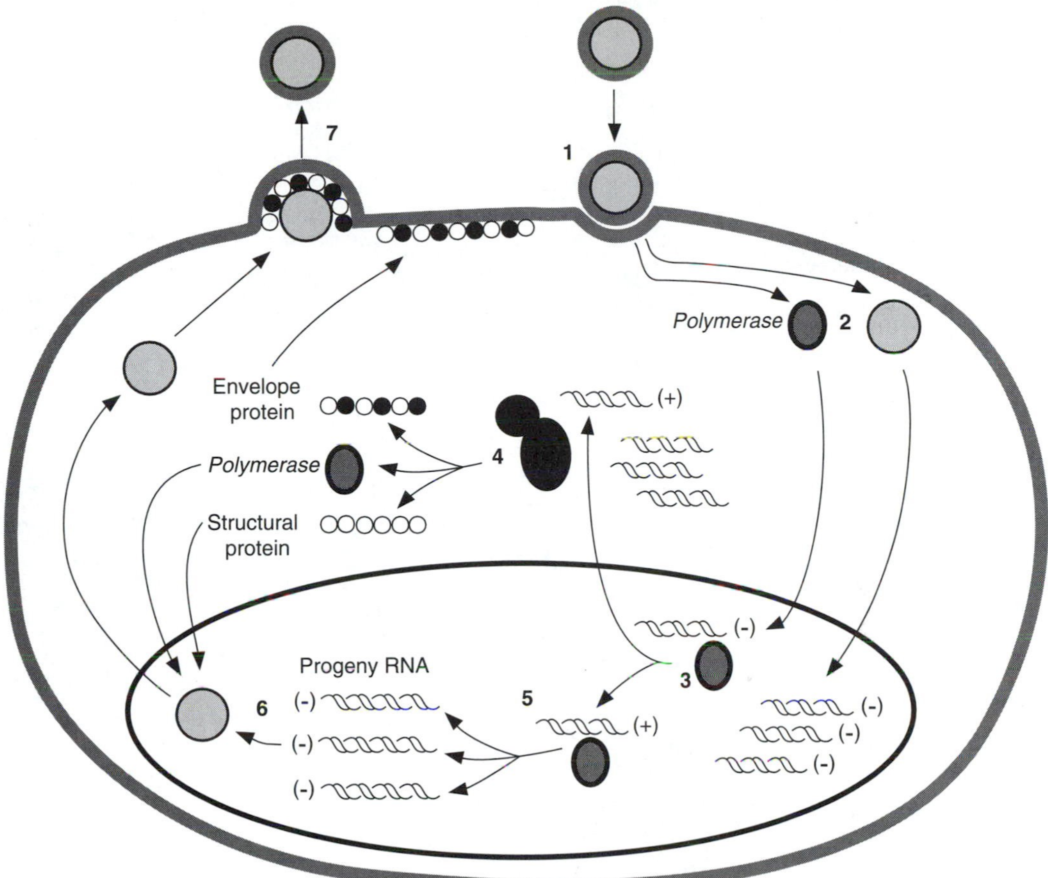

FIGURE 23-8. Orthomyxovirus replication cycle. The virus binds to a clathrin-coated vesicle on the host cell membrane and enters the cytoplasm via membrane fusion in endosomic vesicles (*1*). After uncoating (*2*), transcription of viral −RNA to +RNA by virion-packed polymerase takes place in the nucleus (*3*). Cellular nuclear RNA acts as a transcription primer for the translation of short viral mRNAs into viral proteins and enzymes (*4*). Transcription of complete +RNA strands, which serve as templates for genomic replication, does not require the host primer (*5*). The viral nucleocapsids are assembled in the nucleus (*6*). Maturation takes place at the cell membrane, when the virus exits by budding (*7*).

c. The complex P2-capped mRNA 5′ end is then bound at the 3′ end of the different segments of viral −RNA and serves as a primer for the viral transcriptase, which begins transcribing short viral mRNAs that will be translated into viral proteins and enzymes.

d. Transcription of complete +RNA strands, which serve as templates for genomic replication, does not require the host primer. A specific capsid protein (NP) seems to determine the transcription of complete strands, which are not used as messages for protein synthesis.

e. The viral nucleocapsids are assembled in the nucleus and maturation takes place at the cell membrane when the virus exits by budding.

Chapter 24

Viral Genetics

Gabriel Virella
Salvatore Arrigo

I. VIRAL GENOMES. Viral particles may contain DNA or RNA, but never both. Several characteristics of the nucleic acid (e.g., the number of strands, polarity, infectivity) determine the biological properties and mechanisms of genetic variation exhibited by different viral families (Table 24-1).

A. DNA viruses. The genomes of most DNA viruses are **double-stranded, monosegmented,** and **infective.**

B. RNA viruses. The genomes of most RNA viruses (except reovirus) are **single-stranded** and can be **mono-** or **polysegmented.** Retroviruses have two partially linked identical RNA strands.

1. **Positive-stranded RNA (+RNA)** is **infective** (with the exception of retrovirus).
2. **Negative-stranded RNA (−RNA)** is **not infective** (i.e., it needs to be transcribed into +RNA to be translated).

II. VIRAL MUTATION. Like all nucleic acids, the nucleic acids of viruses are susceptible to mutations. Biologically important implications of viral mutations include the loss or acquisition of pathogenicity and the development of mechanisms that may allow viruses to escape the host immune system. In addition, the study of viral mutants provides insight into the constitution of the viral genome and definition of viral gene function.

A. General characteristics of viral mutations

1. **Rate of occurrence.** Viral mutations occur spontaneously, usually at an average rate of 10^{-8} particles. The rate of mutation of retroviruses is considerably higher, as a consequence of errors that occur during reverse transcription that are not corrected because the reverse transcriptase lacks the ability to "copyedit."
2. **Experimental induction** of mutations is possible using **chemical agents** or **ultraviolet irradiation** (in the case of DNA viruses).

B. Types of viral mutations

1. **Point mutations** occur when a single nucleotide base is changed. Point mutants with specific characteristics are often selected in the laboratory:
   a. **Conditioned lethal mutants** can multiply under some conditions but not under the conditions that allow the multiplication of wild viruses.
      (1) **Temperature-sensitive mutants** do not replicate well at temperatures between 36°C and 41°C; therefore, they are attenuated strains in humans. Their antigenic make-up is virtually identical to that of the wild strain, and, consequently, these mutants are often used for immunization purposes.
      (2) **Host-dependent mutants.** The mutation results in the replacement of an amino acid codon by a termination codon. Bacteriophages with these mutations will replicate on bacteria that have mutated transfer RNA (tRNA) that can recognize the termination codons as coding for a given amino acid. Although the new amino acid may be different from the original one, in some cases, transcription results in a functional protein.

TABLE 24-1. General Characteristics of Viral Genomes

Virus	Nucleic Acid	Number of Strands	Number of Segments	Polarity	Infectivity of Naked Nucleic Acid
Poxvirus	DNA	2	1	N/A	−
Herpesvirus	DNA	2	1	N/A	+
Adenovirus	DNA	2	1	N/A	+
Papovavirus	DNA	2	1	N/A	+
Hepadnavirus	DNA	2*	1	N/A	−
Parvovirus	DNA	1	1	+ and −	+
Picornavirus	RNA	1	1	+	+
Calicivirus	RNA	1	1	+	+
Togavirus	RNA	1	1	+	+
Flavivirus	RNA	1	1	+	+
Coronavirus	RNA	1	1	+	+
Retrovirus	RNA	1†	2†	+	−
Rhabdovirus	RNA	1	1	−	−
Paramyxovirus	RNA	1	1	−	−
Orthomyxovirus	RNA	1	8	−	−
Arenavirus	RNA	1	2	−	−
Reovirus	RNA	2	10 or 11	N/A	−

* Of unequal length.
† Two identical + RNA strands; thus the genome is considered single-stranded but contains two identical segments.

b. **Plaque-size mutants** induce changes in the diameter of the zone of viral lysis seen in infected monolayers. The mutation usually affects the capsid protein, allowing easier adsorption to and penetration of permissive cells. Mutants inducing larger plaques grow faster in cell culture and are usually more virulent *in vivo.*

c. **Host-range mutants** infect cell types or species not infected by the wild strain. The basic mutation affects either proteins that mediate adsorption to host cells or genes that modulate the interplay between cellular replication and viral expression.

d. **Drug-resistant mutants** are not susceptible to antiviral agents successfully used to treat infections caused by the wild strain. The mutation usually affects an enzyme that is inhibited by the antiviral drug; for example, the enzyme may lose affinity for the antiviral drug, allowing the virus to replicate in the presence of the drug.

e. **Enzyme-deficient mutants** are strains that lack an enzyme or have a mutant enzyme. The mutation may or may not be lethal, depending on whether or not it affects an enzyme essential for replication.

f. **Hot mutants** grow well at 41°C and are extremely virulent.

2. **Deletion mutants** occur when a whole segment of the viral genome is lost. **Defective virus particles** (see III B) are examples of deletion mutants.

III. INTERACTIONS BETWEEN VIRUSES

A. Interactions between viral genomes. Viral infection is multiple; that is, many virions gain access to the cell more or less simultaneously. The co-infecting viruses are usually identical or very closely related. Because of this multiplicity of infection, the genomes of the infecting particles may interact in a variety of ways.

1. **Recombination**

a. **DNA viruses.** Recombination classically involves double-stranded DNA viruses. Recombination is inconsequential when the recombination involves two normal

A

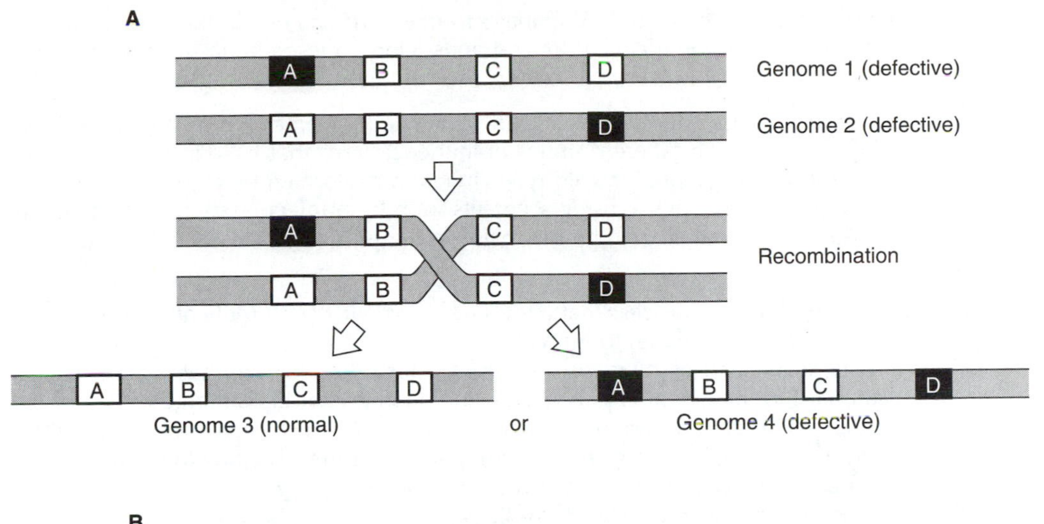

B

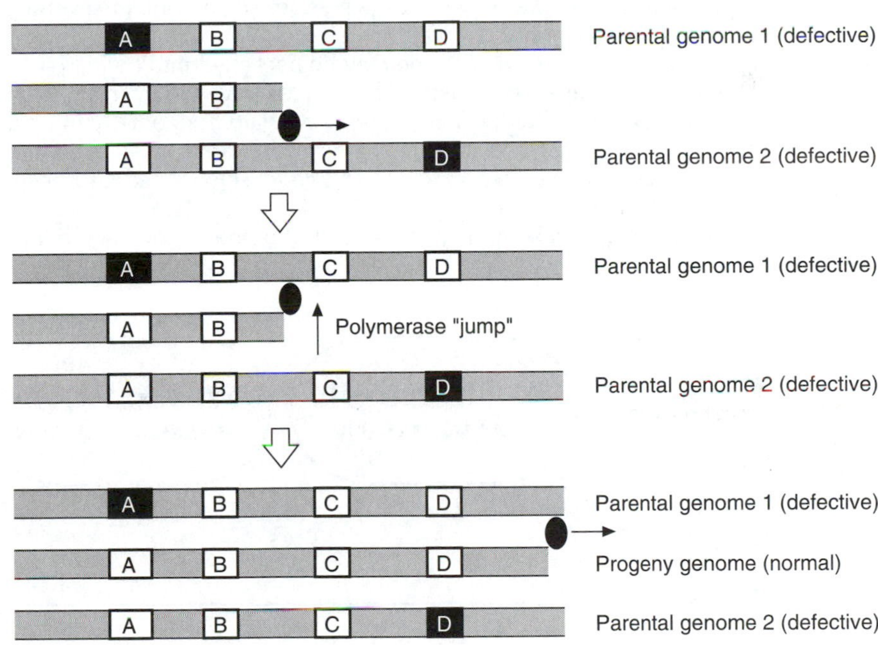

FIGURE 24-1. (*A*) Recombination between DNA viruses. (*B*) Recombination between RNA viruses.

genomes and the resultant genome is also normal, but recombination may result in the creation of a complete wild-type genome from two mutant genomes (Figure 24-1A).

b. RNA viruses. When copying positive strands into negative strands to be used as templates for replication, the polymerase may "jump" from one positive strand to another, producing a hybrid −RNA template (Figure 24-1B). A similar mechanism may contribute to the generation of genetic diversity of HIV. The genome of HIV is constituted by two strains of +RNA. In the process of transcribing DNA from RNA, the reverse transcriptase often "jumps" from one RNA strand to the other. Such jumps are inconsequential if the strands are identical; however, if two different mutant strains of HIV manage to infect the same cell, the progeny virions will contain non-identical RNA strands. Under these circumstances, the polymerase "jumps" may cause the emergence of recombinant genomes.

2. **Reassortment** occurs only in viruses with segmented genomes. For example, if a cell is co-infected with two different strains of influenza virus that have mutated in different segments of the genome, a wild-type virus may be formed by reconstituting a normal set of genome segments, using segments from **both** infecting mutants (Figure 24-2). Reassortment is believed to be the **major cause of antigenic shift** in influenza virus.

3. **Complementation** is a process that allows defective viruses to replicate and spread horizontally (from individual to individual).
   - **a.** If a cell is infected by two defective viruses (for example, one that lacks the gene that codes for an essential polymerase and another that lacks the gene that codes for the glycoprotein envelope spikes), the defective viruses may assist each other in producing infective progeny by coding for all of the structures necessary to assemble nondefective particles between the two of them. However, the packed genomes remain defective (Figure 24-3).
   - **b.** Alternatively, if a defective virus (e.g., one lacking one or several genes essential for its full replication) co-infects a cell with a nondefective virus of very similar structure, the defective genome may be packaged into a viral particle whose structural components are coded by the nondefective virus. This is the way in which defective tumor-causing retroviruses propagate horizontally in nature.
   - **c.** Phenotypic mixing and pseudotype formation are special examples of complementation that may take place when two closely related viruses (e.g., poliovirus I and II) co-infect a cell.
     - **(1) Phenotypic mixing** (Figure 24-4). In the process of assembling progeny viri-

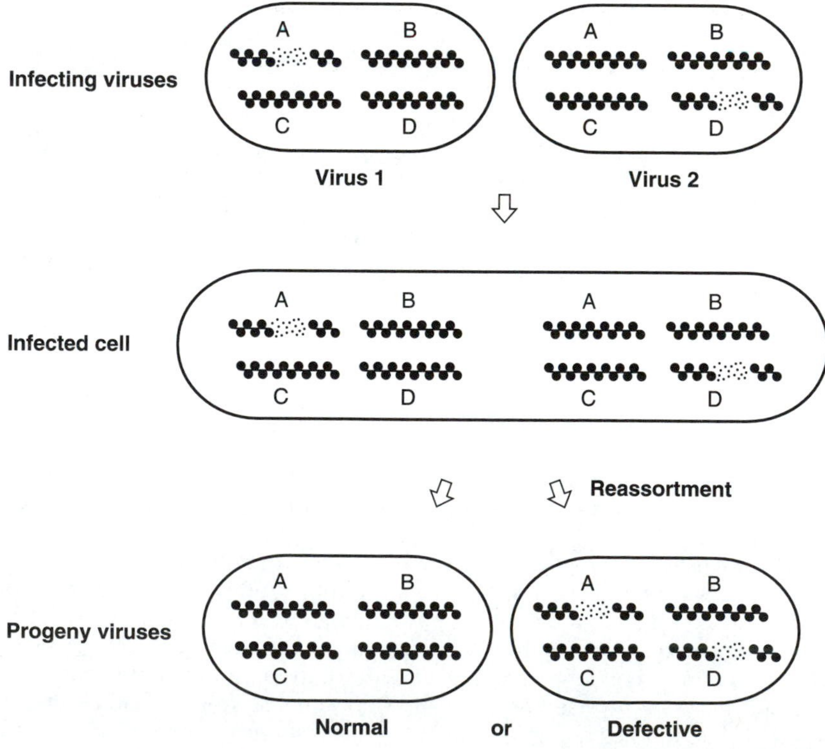

FIGURE 24-2. Reassortment between RNA viruses.

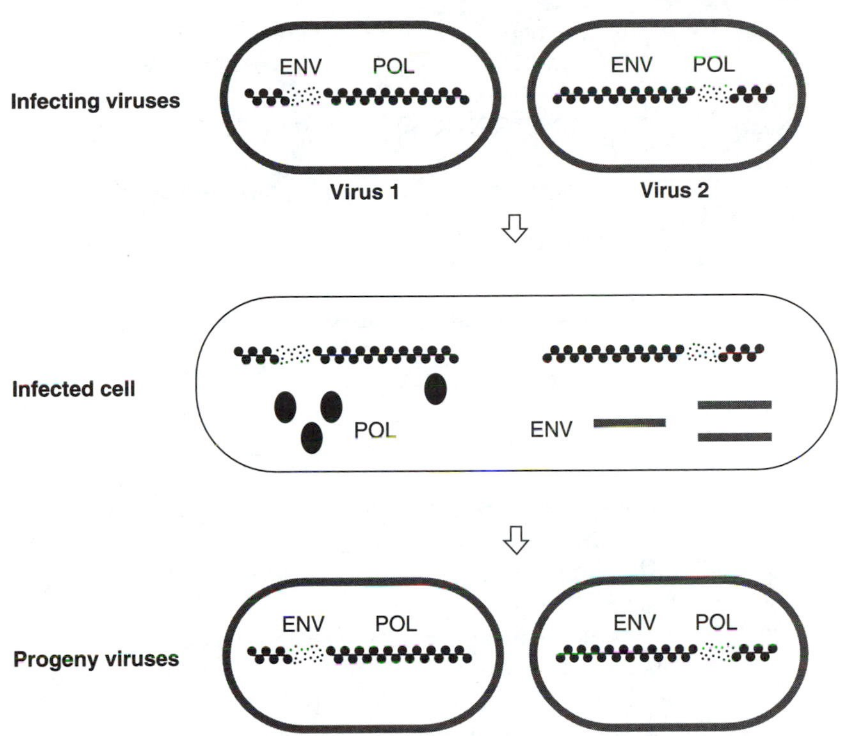

FIGURE 24-3. Complementation between defective viruses. In complementation, two defective viruses work together to assemble a virus that is capable of being transmitted. For example, if virus 1 lacks the gene that codes for the glycoprotein envelope spikes (*ENV*) and virus 2 lacks the gene that codes for the polymerase (*POL*) essential for viral replication, each virus can supply the part the other lacks. However, the progeny viruses will still have a defective genome.

ons, hybrid capsids constituted by subunits coded by the two different viruses may be generated.

(2) **Pseudotype formation.** At the time of encapsulating progeny nucleic acid, viral genomes of one virus may be encapsulated in the capsids of the second virus, or vice versa. The genetic process resulting in pseudotype formation is known as **phenotypic masking.** Phenotypic masking is reversed when a single pseudotype infects a cell. If the particle carries a type II genome inside a type I capsid, the progeny will necessarily carry type II capsids and genomes, because all progeny components will be coded by a type II genome.

B. Defective interfering (DI) particles. Viral particles that contain defective genomes usually cannot multiply on their own. Their successful replication (defined as the transfer of defective genomes to other cells) depends on simultaneous infection with an infectious **"helper" virus.** However, the defective particle often interferes with the replication of the "helper" virus, hence the designation **defective interfering particle.** High multiplicity of infection at the single-cell level favors the creation of DI particles.

1. The adsorption and penetration of DI particles is determined by their normal capsids. Once released, the defective nucleic acid is expressed, causing a variety of effects (e.g., inhibition of host biosynthesis, synthesis of viral proteins, transformation) while simultaneously interfering with the replication of complete homologous viruses.
2. Interference with normal virus replication is believed to result from the fact that the RNA of the DI particle is smaller than the complete genomic RNA. As a result, the RNA of the DI particle has a higher affinity for RNA polymerase and is preferentially expressed and replicated.
3. DI particles cause persistent infection when co-infecting with a complete, "helper" virus for the following reasons:

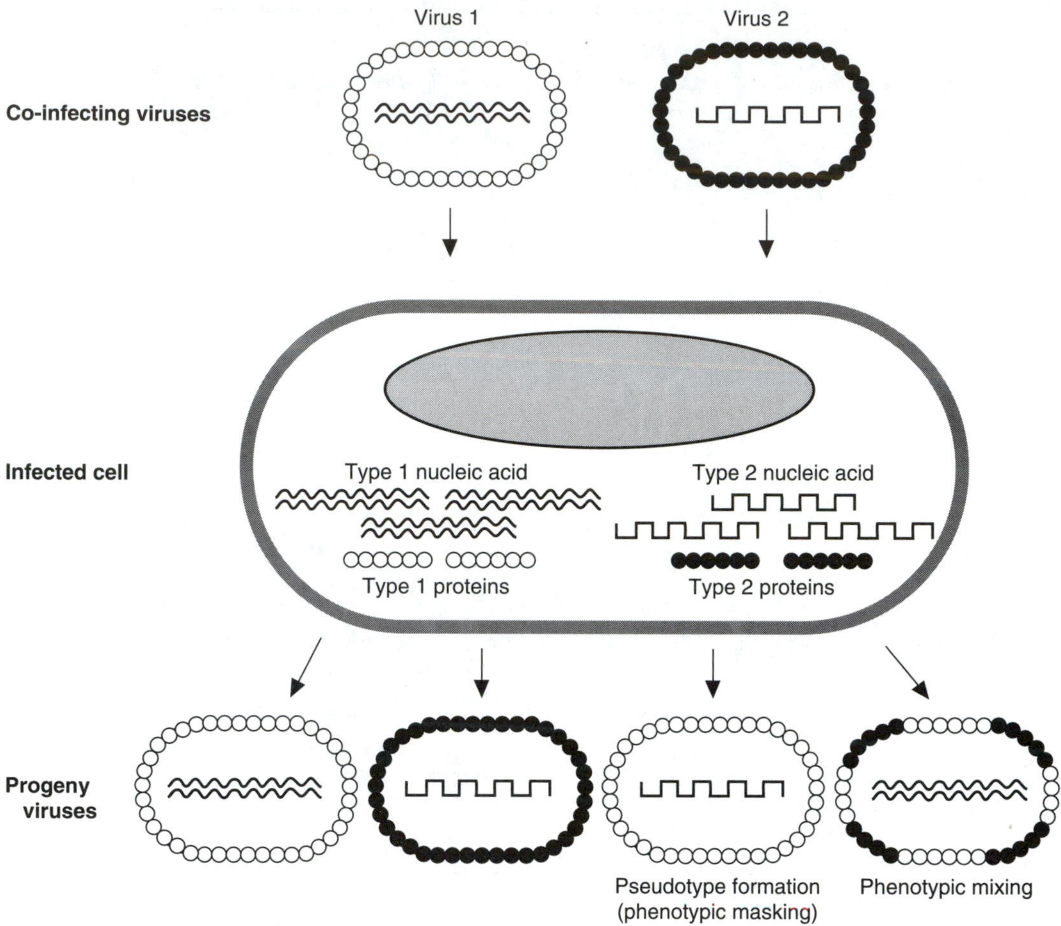

FIGURE 24-4. Pseudotype formation (phenotypic masking) and phenotypic mixing.

a. The genome of the DI particle is preferentially expressed and replicated. Because of the defective nature of the genome, DI particle replication tends to cause less cytopathology than replication of complete virions.
b. The progeny DI particle RNA has recognition structures that allow it to be encapsulated; therefore, it tends to be more effectively propagated than the complete genome of the helper virus.

C. Effects of viral infection of a cell on the behavior of other viruses. When one type of virus infects a cell, two possible outcomes concerning infection by another virus are possible.

1. **Infection may prohibit a second virus from infecting the cell** (i.e., the cell may become refractory). Several non-mutually exclusive factors may account for this phenomena:
   a. Synthesis of interferon, preventing the propagation of a second virus in an infected culture
   b. Blocking the transport of proteins, used as receptors by other viruses, to the plasma membrane
   c. Inhibition of the translation of the mRNA of a second virus, possibly as a result of alterations in the cap-binding protein (induced by the first virus or by the formation of inactive complexes between the second viral genome and the polymerase carried by the first virus)

d. Down regulation of the expression of cellular genes that are required by the second virus for the early stages of replication, leading to inhibition of the transcription of the nucleic acid of the second virus

2. **Infection may enable a second virus to replicate on a cell that is usually not permissive to it** if the first virus enhances the translation of the second virus' messenger (mRNA).
   a. A well known example of this "helper" effect is the enhancement of adenovirus replication in kidney cells by simian virus (SV)-40.
   b. The same helper function can be carried out by nonreplicative defective particles that remain silent except for facilitating the infectiveness of an unrelated virus. Thus, the virulence of some viruses may depend on a co-infecting defective particle that performs a "helper" function.

IV. THE ROLE OF GENETIC VARIATION IN THE EVOLUTION OF VIRUSES.

Viral mutations and genetic interchange between related viruses are responsible for viral genetic diversity. The success of the mutants depends on several factors:

A. The ability of the virus to replicate effectively cannot be compromised.

B. The mutant must have a survival advantage over the original strain.

The ability to evade the host immune system is a common benefit derived from mutations. Mutations may affect:

1. **Viral surface proteins.** These proteins, which interact with the host cell through plasma membrane receptors, are usually the targets of the immune system. Mutations that alter these surface proteins are therefore often advantageous. In addition, it must be noted that changes in surface proteins may not affect viral assembly and replication as drastically as changes in capsid proteins, matrix proteins, or replication enzymes.
2. **Viral hemagglutinin.** Mutations of the viral hemagglutinin of the influenza virus reduce the virus' reactivity with pre-existing neutralizing antibodies, allowing the virus to spread rapidly among the population. This type of mutation is an example of natural selection of mutants.
3. **Immunodominant domain of gp120.** HIV is extremely prone to mutations. The mutations affecting the immunodominant domain of gp120, the major envelope protein of HIV and a major target of the immune system, are very effectively selected by their ability to allow viral escape from the immune system. The emergence of this type of mutant is believed to be one of the major determinants of progression from asymptomatic HIV infection to clinical AIDS.

Chapter 25

Interferons and Antiviral Agents

Victor Del Bene

I. INTRODUCTION.

In order for a virus to infect a mammalian cell, it must attach, penetrate, uncoat, reproduce its genome, take over the host's synthetic machinery, assemble progeny particles, and complete the viral replication cycle before killing the host cell. The development of antiviral compounds has depended on progress in the understanding of viral replication.

II. CLASSES OF ANTIVIRAL AGENTS

A. Natural antiviral compounds. Interferons are natural substances that have antiviral properties in adjacent, noninfected cells (as opposed to in infected cells).

1. **Types of interferons.** Three interferon molecules have been characterized:
   - a. **Type I interferons**
     - (1) **Interferon-α (IFN-α)** has maximal antiviral activity.
     - (2) **Interferon-β (IFN-β)** has intermediate antiviral activity.
   - b. **Type II interferons. Interferon-γ (IFN-γ)** is more active as a lymphokine than as an antiviral agent.

2. **Regulation of interferon expression.** The interferon genes are not expressed in a normal, resting cell. Expression of the IFN-α and IFN-β genes seems to be regulated by labile repressors that bind to promoter (enhancer) elements and block transcription. Many viruses produce regulatory proteins or special forms of messenger (mRNA) that diffuse to the nucleus and shut down cell protein synthesis. If the termination of host protein synthesis is gradual, the drop in synthesis of the short-lived interferon repressors will remove the block to interferon synthesis while the cell is still able to synthesize some proteins, including interferons.

3. **Mechanism of action.** Once synthesized, interferons are secreted, diffuse, bind to specific cellular receptors, and are taken up by uninfected neighboring cells where they inhibit viral replication. Inhibition of viral replication by interferons is mediated by cellular enzymes whose expression is regulated by interferons.
   - a. **Type I interferons**
     - (1) Type I interferons **inhibit viral protein synthesis.** The antiviral effect is very specific, and cellular protein synthesis is not affected. Type I interferons inhibit viral protein synthesis by activating the following enzymes:
       - (a) Two oligo-A synthetases, which, in the presence of double-stranded RNA, synthesize an adenine nucleotide with unique 2′-5′ phosphodiester linkages that digests viral mRNA
       - (b) A 68-kilodalton protein kinase that autophosphorylates in the presence of double-stranded RNA and then phosphorylates and inactivates elongation factor-2 (EF-2), blocking protein synthesis
     - (2) Type I interferons **may block other stages of viral replication, including budding.**
   - b. **Type II interferons.** IFN-γ also has antiviral effects, mediated by:
     - (1) **Induction of nitric oxide synthetase,** which inhibits viral replication by increasing intracellular nitric oxide levels
     - (2) **Upregulation of major histocompatibility complex-I and -II (MHC-I and MHC-II) expression,** which facilitates the activation and effector function of cytotoxic T cells capable of destroying virus-infected cells

(3) **Activation of monocytes, macrophages,** and **natural killer (NK) cells,** which are able to kill virus-infected cells by nonimmune mechanisms

4. **Clinical uses**
   a. **IFN-α** is used:
      (1) In the treatment of viral infections, especially condylomata acuminata and chronic hepatitis B and C
      (2) As a prophylactic or therapeutic agent in immunocompromised patients predisposed to varicella-zoster infections (e.g., chickenpox, shingles) or to infections caused by herpes simplex virus, types 1 and 2 (HSV-1, HSV-2)
      (3) As a prophylactic against cytomegalovirus (CMV) infection in patients who have undergone renal transplantation
      (4) In the treatment of AIDS-associated Kaposi's sarcoma and hairy cell leukemia (the mechanisms responsible for the therapeutic effects of IFN-α in these patients are not well understood)
   b. **IFN-γ** has been used primarily as an immunostimulant in the treatment of oncologic disorders and some immunodeficiency diseases.

B. Synthetic antiviral agents. Antiviral compounds can be grouped according to their point of action in the viral replication cycle (Figure 25-1).

1. **Agents that block attachment, uncoating, or both**
   a. **Anti-gp120** and **recombinant (hybrid) CD4** inhibit HIV in permissive cells *in vitro.*
      (1) Recombinant genetic hybrid molecules in which the binding site of CD4 substitutes the V regions of human immunoglobulin have been developed and tested clinically, but the results so far have been disappointing. Hybrid molecules have the advantage of a longer half-life relative to soluble CD4.
      (2) **Mechanism of action.** Both anti-gp120 and CD4 bind to gp120, a viral envelope glycoprotein that interacts with the CD4 molecule in target cells to mediate adsorption of the virus. The mechanism of action of anti-gp120 and CD4 was thought to be the blocking of viral attachment; however, it has been shown that viral neutralization *in vivo* requires binding to a single gp120 molecule on the viral envelope, and it is believed that the mechanism of action of anti-gp120 (and probably of soluble and hybrid CD4) is to prevent viral uncoating in the cell.
   b. **Recombinant intercellular cell adhesion molecule-1 (ICAM-1).** ICAM-1 has been identified as the cellular receptor for 80%–90% of the 130 different rhinovirus strains that cause 50%–60% of all "common colds." Recombinant ICAM-1 blocks infectivity *in vitro* and *in vivo,* minimizing symptoms of the "common cold," but this type of therapy is too costly to be used routinely for a disease with such low mortality, and the wide variety of viruses and viral strains involved makes vaccination impractical.
   c. **Amantadine** and **rimantadine** can be used prophylactically and therapeutically in influenza A infections. These drugs bind to M2, a viral protein that forms ion channels in the lipid bilayer of the viral envelope. It is believed that these ion channels are involved in transporting protons into the virion interior and facilitating virus uncoating. Either by interfering with the function of the M2 protein or by some unknown mechanism, amantadine and rimantadine inhibit the fusion of the viral envelope with the endosome membrane, preventing release of the nucleocapsid into the cytoplasm.

2. **Agents that inhibit DNA polymerase.** The discovery that certain nucleoside-like molecules could be recognized as substrate by DNA polymerases was an important breakthrough in antiviral therapy. These nucleoside-like molecules lack the proper radicals for crosslinking to other nucleotides, so when added to a normal DNA chain, termination of DNA synthesis results. In addition, these nucleoside-like molecules have a greater affinity for the binding site of the polymerase than the natural nucleosides. Although these compounds affect primarily viral DNA synthesis, they also affect cellular DNA synthesis; as a result, these agents can have severe side effects.
   a. **Vidarabine [adenine arabinoside (ara-A)]** has a tertiary structure similar to that of

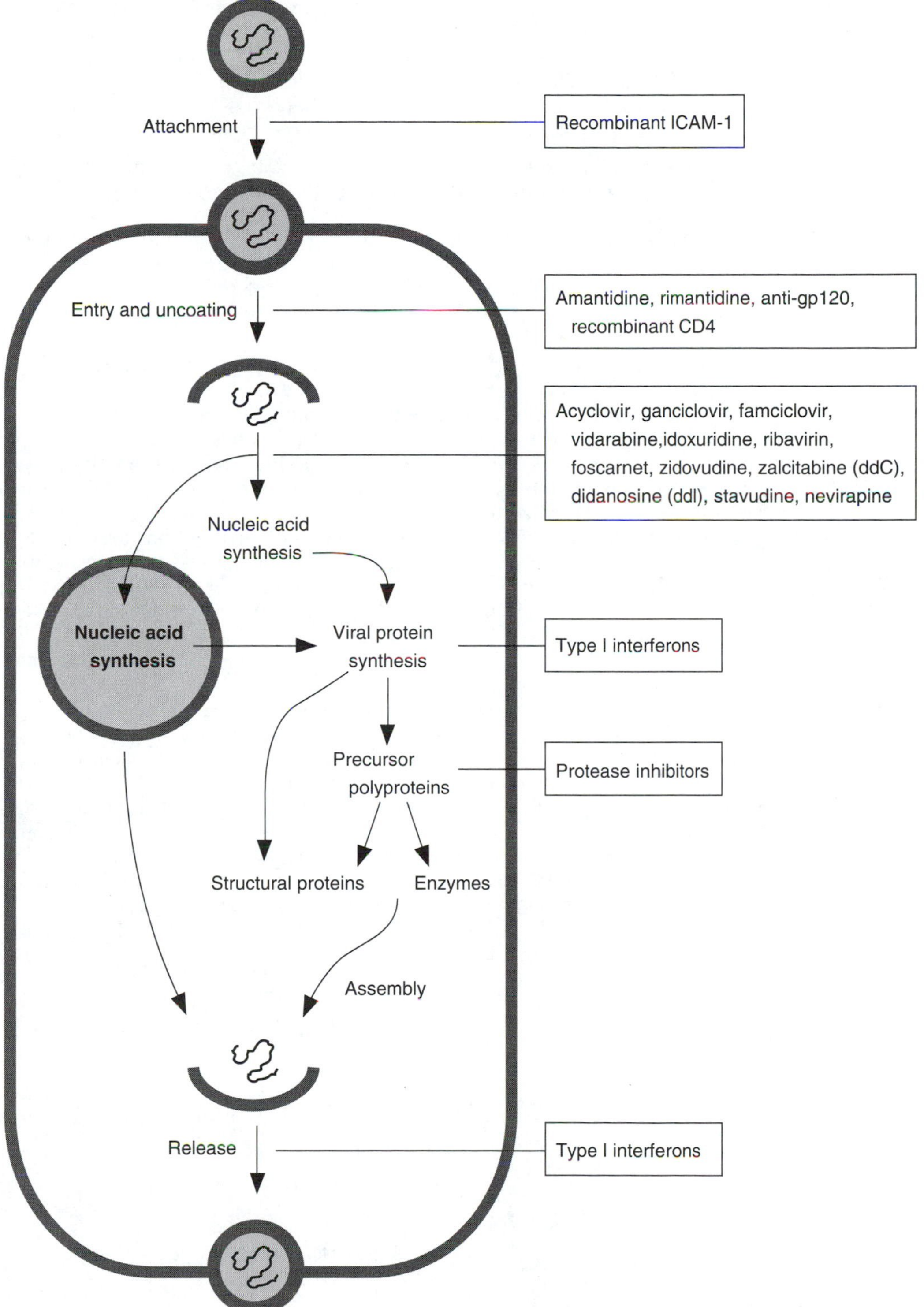

FIGURE 25-1. Sites of action of major antiviral compounds. *ICAM-1* = intercellular cell adhesion molecule-1.

deoxyadenosine, except for an extra hydroxyl group that prevents attachment of the next nucleoside. Therefore, once vidarabine is incorporated into a nascent DNA chain, synthesis is terminated. Vidarabine was the first compound shown to greatly improve the outcome of herpes simplex encephalitis.

b. **Idoxuridine (IDU)** is a uridine analog with a mechanism of action similar to that of vidarabine. IDU is used as a topical agent for herpes infection of the cornea.

3. **Target-activated nucleoside analogues** were developed with the hope that they would be active in infected cells, without affecting DNA synthesis in cells not infected by the virus.

a. **Acyclovir** was the first agent that successfully interfered specifically with the synthesis of viral genetic material. The molecule resembles guanosine (Figure 25-2) except that it is acyclic (i.e., the sugar moiety is incomplete).

(1) **Mechanism of action.** Acyclovir, as it is administered to the patient, is inactive. Incorporation of acyclovir into a nascent DNA molecule requires conversion of the drug into a high-energy form, which requires triple phosphorylation. The first phosphate group is added almost exclusively by a **viral thymidine kinase,** which is expressed in infected cells soon after infection. After the first phosphate is added, mammalian cell kinases complete the phosphorylation steps. Thus, **the inactive nucleoside-look alike is promptly phosphorylated only in cells actively infected by the virus and DNA synthesis in uninfected cells is not affected.**

(a) **Prevention of crosslinking.** The viral DNA polymerase adds acyclovir to the DNA chain. The next nucleoside is not able to crosslink with acyclovir because it lacks the necessary hydroxyl group.

(b) **Binding to DNA transcriptase.** Acyclovir is irreversibly bound to DNA transcriptase, rendering the enzyme unavailable for natural substrates.

(2) **Administration.** Acyclovir can be administered orally and intravenously, and it crosses the blood–brain barrier.

(3) **Clinical uses.** Acyclovir is effective against certain viruses of the herpes group. Other viruses of the herpes group, such as Epstein-Barr virus and CMV, do not have a viral-specified thymidine kinase; therefore, acyclovir is not activated or effective in diseases caused by those viruses.

(a) **Herpes encephalitis.** As a result of its ability to cross the blood–brain barrier, acyclovir is efficient in the treatment of herpes encephalitis. The survival rate of patients with herpes encephalitis has increased from 25% (untreated) to 48% (treated with vidarabine) to 75% (treated with acyclovir). Treatment also improves the quality of life of survivors.

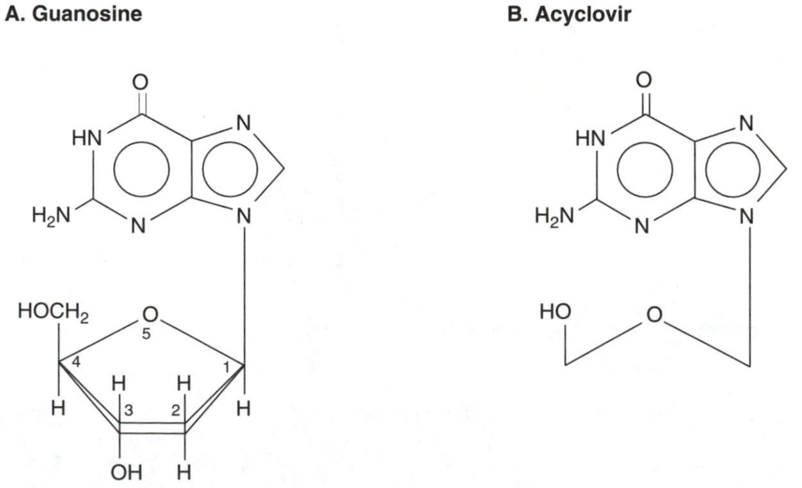

A. Guanosine **B. Acyclovir**

FIGURE 25-2. Comparison of the molecular structures of (*A*) guanosine and (*B*) acyclovir.

(b) **Recurrent labial or genital herpes.** Acyclovir has been successfully used as prophylaxis against recurrent labial or genital herpes.

b. **Famciclovir.** The mechanism of action and clinical uses of famciclovir are identical to those of acyclovir. Famciclovir can be given orally with less frequency than acyclovir and seems to be better tolerated.

c. **Ganciclovir,** a derivative of acyclovir, also becomes active after phosphorylation, which appears to depend on mammalian kinases and a viral phosphotransferase. Ganciclovir is more toxic than acyclovir.

(1) **Administration.** Previously, ganciclovir was administered exclusively by the intravenous route, but a formulation suitable for oral administration is now available.

(2) **Clinical uses.** The viral DNA polymerase of CMV has a high affinity for the active form of ganciclovir. Therefore, this drug is effective in infections caused by this virus (i.e., retinitis, encephalitis).

4. **Agents that inhibit reverse transcriptase.** A specialized group of polymerase inhibitors are those that interfere with the reverse transcriptase of the retroviruses.

a. **Zidovudine [azidothymidine (AZT)]** structurally resembles thymidine except for the substitution of a hydroxyl group by a nitrogen in the 3′ position of the pentose ring (Figure 25-3).

(1) **Mechanisms of action.** Zidovudine has at least two mechanisms of action:

(a) **Competitive inhibition.** Zidovudine has greater affinity for reverse transcriptase than the natural substrate; therefore, the binding of natural nucleosides by the reverse transcriptase is blocked.

(b) **Chain termination.** Cellular kinases phosphorylate zidovudine, which is preferentially bound to the reverse transcriptase during transcription of viral DNA. If instead of thymidine zidovudine is added to the nascent DNA chain, elongation will be terminated because zidovudine lacks the 3′ hydroxyl group essential for the formation of 5′–3′ diester linkages between nucleic acid molecules. Thus, the synthesis of DNA is interrupted as soon as a zidovudine molecule is incorporated.

(2) **Clinical uses** of zidovudine in AIDS patients and HIV-positive patients are discussed in detail in Chapter 57 VII A 1 a. In general, zidovudine has proven to be most useful in reducing transplacental and perinatal transmission of the virus to neonates.

(3) **Toxicity.** Major side effects include anemia and neutropenia. Obviously, neutropenia is undesirable in a patient who may be already immunocompromised.

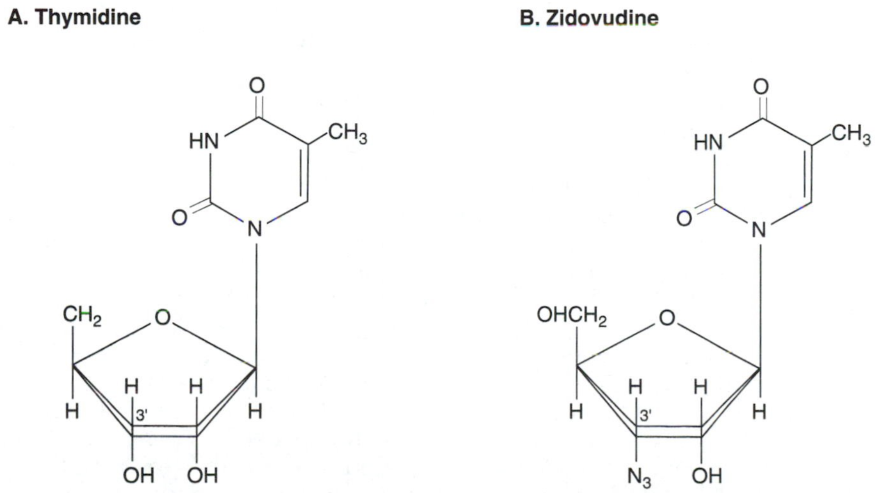

A. Thymidine **B. Zidovudine**

FIGURE 25-3. Comparison of the molecular structure of (*A*) thymidine and (*B*) zidovudine.

b. **Zalcitabine [dideoxycytidine (ddC)]** is another chain terminator that has been used successfully. It is particularly useful in cases of HIV that show resistance or fail to improve with zidovudine. However, zalcitabine has serious side effects, including painful sensorimotor peripheral axonal neuropathy (reported in 22%–35% of patients receiving the drug) and pancreatitis (reported in 1.1% of patients).

c. **Didanosine [dideoxyinosine (ddI)]** is related to zalcitabine and is associated with the same type of side effects, although toxicity is less common.

d. **Stavudine [didehydrodeoxythymidine (d4T)]** is a thymidine analog that inhibits reverse transcriptase much the same way as zidovudine does. It is hepatotoxic and neurotoxic, but seems to be better tolerated than zidovudine.

e. **Lamivudine [2′-deoxy-3′-thiacytidine (3TC)],** a zidovudine analogue, has been heralded as beneficial when used in conjunction with zidovudine in the treatment of HIV-positive patients and patients with AIDS.

f. **Nevirapine (dipyridodiazepinone)** is a non-nucleoside reverse transcriptase inhibitor that is currently under evaluation. The drug binds to a hydrophobic pocket of the reverse transcriptase at a site different from the sites to which other reverse transcriptase inhibitors bind. Therefore, strains of HIV resistant to several of the other reverse transcriptase inhibitors are not cross-resistant to nevirapine.

5. **Protease inhibitors. Saquinavir, ritonavir,** and **indinavir** are synthetic, nonhydrolyzable synthetic peptides.

a. **Mechanism of action.** These agents are competitive inhibitors of the HIV protease, thereby inhibiting the processing of polyproteins. HIV-infected cells exposed to these compounds accumulate uncleaved *gag* polyprotein precursors, which are cytotoxic.

b. **Clinical uses.** HIV appears to develop resistance to these agents, which may limit their use as single-agent anti-HIV agents. However, the use of protease inhibitors with reverse transcriptase inhibitors may represent an important breakthrough in the treatment of AIDS.

6. **"Broad-spectrum" nucleoside analogues** have multiple points of action.

a. **Ribavirin** is a nucleoside analogue of guanosine.

(1) **Mechanisms of action.** Ribavirin affects viral replication by blocking viral protein synthesis in two different ways:

(a) It competes with guanosine for the enzymes producing guanosine triphosphate (GTP), the initial compound necessary for capping of mRNA synthesis.

(b) It binds to RNA polymerase and blocks its activity.

(2) **Clinical uses**

(a) **Respiratory syncytial virus infections in neonates and infants.** However, there is some controversy regarding ribavirin's efficacy and clinical value in treating these infections.

(b) **Hantavirus infections.** Early administration of ribavirin seems to be associated with clinical improvement.

b. **Foscarnet**

(1) **Mechanisms of action**

(a) It inhibits DNA chain elongation by binding to the pyrophosphate receptor on the DNA polymerase, preventing pyrophosphate exchange from deoxyribonucleoside triphosphate.

(b) It inhibits HIV reverse transcriptase by a similar mechanism, although it binds to a site different from the pyrophosphate binding site of the reverse transcriptase.

(2) **Clinical uses.** Foscarnet is effective predominantly against viruses of the herpes group, particularly CMV and HSV. Because of its dual effects on CMV DNA polymerase and HIV reverse transcriptase, foscarnet is effective in the treatment of CMV infections in HIV-positive patients. However, the cost of the drug and the need to administer it through an infusion pump reserve its use to patients not responding to ganciclovir.

III. RESISTANCE TO ANTIVIRAL AGENTS

A. Acyclovir. HSV and varicella-zoster virus strains that lack or express a modified thymidine kinase are resistant. These strains are usually not pathogenic for immunocompetent hosts but can cause severe disseminated disease [including infection of the central nervous system (CNS)] in immunocompromised individuals. More rarely, resistance has been associated with mutations in the viral DNA polymerase, which concomitantly confer resistance to other DNA polymerase inhibitors.

B. Ganciclovir. Resistance of CMV to ganciclovir can result from decreased phosphorylation of the drug in infected cells. Decreased phosphorylation seems to be caused either by alterations in the viral phosphotransferase, or by alterations of the DNA polymerase.

C. Zidovudine. Resistance is common in HIV isolates obtained from patients treated with zidovudine for more than 6 months, which could explain the decline of long-term survival in AIDS or AIDS-related complex (ARC) patients treated for longer than 15 months. The resistance is associated with mutations in the reverse transcriptase, which decrease the transcriptase's binding affinity for zidovudine without impairing its ability to transcribe the HIV RNA.

D. Nevirapine. Resistance develops rather quickly, sometimes after only a few weeks of therapy. Resistance is caused by point mutations that affect the configuration of the binding pouch for this compound in the reverse transcriptase, decreasing the affinity for the drug.

Chapter 26

Viral Infections: Epidemiology, Pathogenesis, and Pathology

John Manos
Gabriel Virella

I. EPIDEMIOLOGY

A. Transmission of viral diseases

1. **Horizontal transmission** is the transmission of disease from **person to person.** Common routes include the:
   a. **Respiratory route.** The respiratory tract is probably the most common way by which viruses are spread from person to person. Viruses that cause localized respiratory infections are excreted when the infected person sneezes and coughs, even if the infected person is asymptomatic.
      (1) Most viruses are fairly rapidly inactivated by desiccation; therefore, **close contact** is necessary for the transmission of virus-containing droplets. This is one reason why many upper respiratory viral infections predominate during the winter months, when more people stay crowded indoors for long periods of time.
      (2) In some cases, the initial infection of the respiratory tract may not be apparent. For example, the measles virus infects the upper respiratory tract mucosa first; however, clinical disease is only manifested when the virus spreads to the skin following the second viremia.
   b. **Fecal-oral route.** Fecal-oral transmission is the second most common way of spreading viral infections, particularly among the enterovirus group of the *Picornaviridae,* the *Reoviridae,* and the *Calciviridae.*
      (1) The resistance of viruses to inactivation in the gastrointestinal tract is related to their structure. For example, the enteroviruses are naked viruses and are not affected by compounds with detergent effects (e.g., bile), which destroy the lipid bilayers of viral envelopes. Their protein capsids are also resistant to stomach acidity and intestinal proteases.
      (2) The viruses that colonize the gastrointestinal tract may be excreted in the feces for many days or even weeks. The patient will remain infective for as long as he excretes the virus, and the virus excreted from an infected carrier can be spread to other individuals, usually by fecal contamination of food or water.
   c. **Venereal route.** Venereal transmission is involved in the spread of the viruses that cause AIDS, herpes, hepatitis, molluscum contagiosum, and genital warts. Disruption or inflammation of the mucosa (such as could occur with trauma or bacterial infection) may facilitate the transmission of some of these viruses during intercourse.
   d. **Cutaneous route.** Mechanical abrasions (possibly microscopic) and animal or insect bites can facilitate penetration of a virus.
   e. **Inoculation.** Theoretically, any viral infection can be transmitted if virus-containing blood is collected from an infected donor and transfused into a noninfected recipient. Modes of transmission include sharing of needles among drug abusers and transfusion of blood or blood components.
2. **Vertical transmission** is the transmission of disease from **mother to infant.**
   a. **Transplacental transmission** causes **congenital infections** [e.g., HIV, rubella, herpes, cytomegalovirus (CMV) infection, hepatitis B].
   b. **Perinatal transmission** occurs as the fetus passes through an infected birth canal.
   c. **Transmission during lactation.** Some human viruses (e.g., HIV) can be transmitted via breast milk.

3. **Zoonotic transmission.** Viral zoonoses are diseases that normally occur in **animals** (the natural hosts) but may be sporadically transmitted to humans. In most zoonoses, man is the terminal host (i.e., because infection is usually via bite wounds, propagation of the disease stops with the human host).
   a. Rabies virus can be transmitted through the bite of an infected animal or through contact with infected animal excreta or secretions.
   b. Some viruses can be transmitted to humans by vector arthropods (most frequently mosquitoes), which pick up the virus when feeding on an infected animal host and transmit it to humans.
   c. Hantaviruses, which cause acute respiratory distress and hemorrhagic fever, can be acquired by contact with materials contaminated by the urine of infected rodents.

B. Viral infections from the community perspective

1. **Public health concerns**
   a. **Inapparent infections** are subclinical (i.e., the infected person is asymptomatic). Because an infected but asymptomatic person is still infectious to other people, inapparent infections are a major source of viral dissemination.
   b. **Latent infections.** Many viruses (e.g., herpesviruses) cause latent infections. Once individuals are infected, they harbor the virus for the rest of their lives. Infected individuals excrete these viruses and pass them onto contacts under a variety of conditions, some of which may not involve clinical evidence of disease.
2. **Role of resistance.** The degree of resistance (innate or acquired) of a population influences the severity and propagation of viral disease.
   a. **Ways of acquiring resistance**
      (1) **Previous infection.** Viruses are excellent antigens and induce strong humoral immune responses.
         (a) Antibodies play a very significant role in terms of preventing reinfection. For example, in the case of measles, residual antibodies and memory cells ready to be activated persist in the circulation after the first incidence of disease. If the virus infects an immunized individual, the infection will be stopped during the first viremic stage, before it has time to multiply and reach target tissues.
         (b) Mucosal infections can be prevented if secretory IgA antibodies are present, either as a result of a previous infection or vaccination.
      (2) **Mass immunization** has resulted in the eradication of smallpox and in significant reductions in the number of cases of measles, rubeola, poliomyelitis, and yellow fever.
   b. **Herd immunity.** The degree of immunization necessary to prevent spread of a disease is not 100%. When 60%–70% of the population is immune, the chain of transmission will be broken. The principle of herd immunity explains the self-limiting nature of an epidemic. After some time, the individuals who have survived the epidemic will have protective antibodies, the infectious agent will be unable to spread, and the incidence of cases will progressively decline until the epidemic is over.
3. **Periodicity of epidemics.** Several factors may contribute to the periodic recurrence of viral epidemics.
   a. Herd immunity may disappear with time.
   b. Nonimmune babies continue to be born, and if prophylactic immunization is not practiced, a population of susceptible individuals will emerge, eventually reaching the numbers necessary for effective transmission of the disease.
   c. Some viruses undergo continual antigenic variation. New strains are able to cause epidemics in previously immune populations.

C. Seasonal fluctuation

1. **Summer.** Many viral diseases are more common in the summer months. This is particularly true in the United States for **diseases transmitted by mosquitos.**

2. **Fall.** Diseases caused by **enteroviruses** (**coxsackievirus, echoviruses,** and **poliovirus)** are more prone to occur in the late summer and early fall. The reason is not clear.

3. **Winter. Rhinoviruses,** which cause the common cold, are more prevalent during the winter months, when indoor crowding facilitates the transmission of infections by the respiratory route.

II. PATHOGENESIS

A. Determinants of pathogenicity

1. **Virus factors that influence the outcome of infection.** For the most part, the factors that determine virulence are poorly understood. The following are some of the best understood factors.
   a. **Cell tropism.** While some viruses infect a wide range of cells, others infect only specific cell types.
      (1) Specificity is related to factors such as:
         (a) Specific interaction with a cell receptor of very limited expression
         (b) Control of viral replication by cellular promoters unique to one or few cell types
      (2) The nature of the infected cells, a direct consequence of cell tropism, can be a major virulence determinant. The rabies virus is a good example—G protein, a major envelope glycoprotein, has special affinity for acetylcholine (ACh) receptors in the nervous tissue, enabling the virus to infect neural cells. In general, viruses able to infect the nervous tissue cause very severe disease because of the inability of neural cells to regenerate. Furthermore, the immune response to these infections may contribute to the degeneration of irreplaceable tissue.
   b. **Mutations** may significantly increase the virulence of a virus. For example, the virulence of influenza virus seems critically dependent on the primary structure of the virus' hemagglutinin. Avirulent strains can become virulent as the result of critical point mutations affecting this protein. It is believed that the mutations result in increased susceptibility of the hemagglutinin for proteolytic enzymes; proteolysis, in turn, exposes a latent hydrophobic N terminal that allows the influenza envelope to fuse with the cell membrane of endothelial cells, resulting in the liberation of free nucleocapsids into the cytoplasm.

2. **Host factors that influence the outcome of viral infection**
   a. **Age.** The age of the host plays a significant role in the virulence of a virus. Several viruses, including respiratory syncytial virus, hepatitis B virus (HBV), coxsackievirus B, and enterovirus, cause more serious or chronic disease in infants than in older children and adults. On the other hand, diseases of childhood, such as measles and chickenpox, have a relatively benign course in young patients but are more severe in older patients.
   b. **Nutrition.** Viruses cause more serious disease in malnourished individuals, probably because malnutrition is associated with depressed cell mediated immunity (CMI).
   c. **Genetic factors** have been shown to influence the outcome of infectious diseases. In the case of viral diseases, the most interesting associations are emerging in HIV-infected individuals.
      (1) HLA-B35–positive individuals seem at greater risk for developing AIDS, while HLA-B8– and HLA-DR3–positive individuals are underrepresented among those that develop clinical disease.
      (2) HLA-DR2 is associated with greater risk to contract opportunistic infections.
      (3) HLA-DR5 is associated with greater risk of developing Kaposi's sarcoma.

B. Sequence of events in viral infection

1. **Entry.** The portal of entry is most commonly the respiratory tract, intestinal tract, or skin. In some cases, the infection remains localized to the site of entry, but in most cases, the infection at the portal of entry is asymptomatic or only mildly symptomatic and the virus eventually spreads to secondary target tissues.
2. **Spread** may be contiguous or systemic.
   a. **Contiguous spread** is characteristic of those infections that remain limited to the portal of entry. Most viral upper respiratory infections and some viral skin infections (e.g., warts) follow this pattern of spread.
      (1) The **incubation period** is short in this type of infection (2–3 days).
      (2) **Viremia** does occur, but only after the disease has already been clinically manifested. Under these circumstances, viremia does not lead to additional clinical manifestations.
      (3) **Reinfection** is common with these viruses because circulating antibodies are not protective. Secretory IgA responses may offer some protection against reinfection of mucosa, but the protection is short-lived.
   b. **Systemic spread.** After gaining access to the body, the virus enters the blood stream, viremia ensues, and the virus disseminates to other tissues before the disease is clinically detectable.
      (1) Because the viremia precedes the onset of disease, the **incubation period** is longer (2–3 weeks).
      (2) The **viremia** associated with systemic spread usually has two stages. The first stage ends when the virus is taken up by the reticuloendothelial system. Activation of the reticuloendothelial system may lead to:
         (a) Elimination of the virus (abortive infection)
         (b) Viral multiplication in the reticuloendothelial system, leading to a second viremia of greater magnitude that immediately precedes the onset of clinical symptoms
      (3) **Reinfection.** Systemic antibodies play a significant role in protection against reinfection.
3. **Target organs.** Most viruses have a predilection for certain organs (Figure 26-1). These predilections are not absolute; some viruses have a predilection for certain organs but may infect other tissues as well (e.g., herpesvirus can cause meningoencephalitis; poliovirus can infect and replicate in the gastrointestinal tract).

C. Types of viral infection

1. **Productive infection** is only possible if the infected cells are permissive (i.e., they allow the viral particle to replicate and produce infectious progeny).
2. **Abortive infection** occurs when a virus gains access to a cell, but the cell dies before the virus completes its replicative cycle. Infection of a nonpermissive or marginally permissive cell can lead to abortive infection. Abortive infection can also occur when a virus infects a permissive cell that has been pretreated with interferon (see Chapter 25 II A).
3. **Persistent infection** results from a stable relationship between cell growth and viral multiplication. Viruses that cause persistent infections (Table 26-1) do not disturb essential cell functions (i.e., DNA, RNA and protein synthesis) significantly enough to cause cell death. Therefore, infected cells multiply and the offspring cells are infected; soon all cells are infective, producing large amounts of virus. Although cell death does not occur, infection may alter some functions of the cell, leading to clinical disease. Persistent infections are caused by the following types of viruses:
   a. **Viruses released by budding** are most likely to be involved in persistent infections because cell lysis is not required for viral release.
   b. **Viruses that infect cells that do not express major histocompatibility complex-I (MHC-I) molecules.** MHC-I molecules are involved in the presentation of viral-derived peptides to the immune system. Lack of MHC-I molecules is probably one of the factors contributing to the persistence of viruses in neuronal cells, which do not express MHC-I molecules.

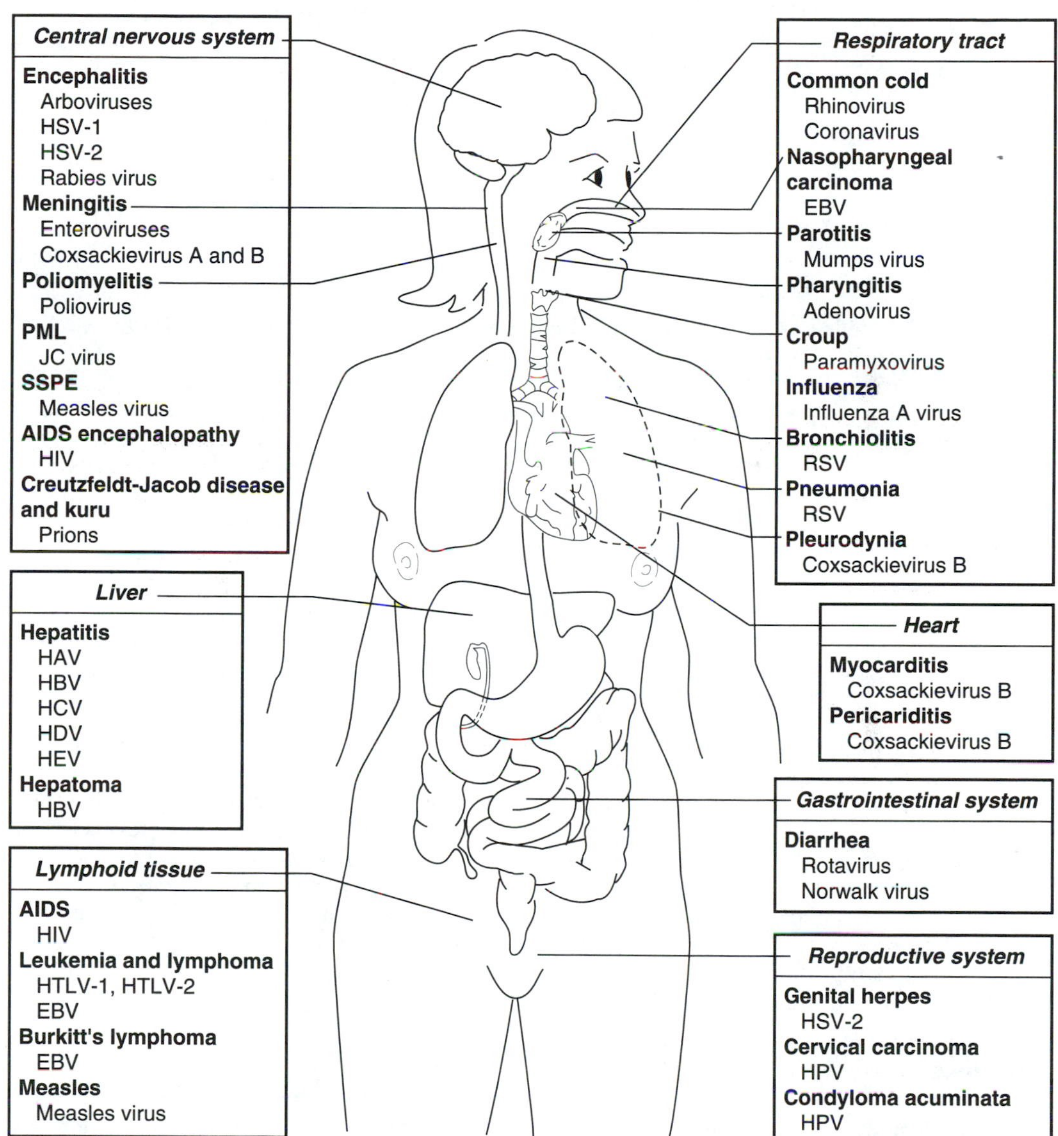

FIGURE 26-1. Target organs and tissues for the most important human pathogenic viruses. *EBV* = Epstein-Barr virus; *HAV* = hepatitis A virus; *HBV* = hepatitis B virus; *HCV* = hepatitis C virus; *HDV* = hepatitis D virus; *HEV* = hepatitis E virus; *HPV* = human papillomavirus; *HSV* = herpes simplex virus; *HTLV* = human T-lymphotropic virus; *PML* = progressive multifocal leukoencephalopathy; *RSV* = respiratory syncytial virus; *SSPE* = subacute sclerosing panencephalitis.

TABLE 26-1. Viruses That Cause Persistent Infection in Humans

RNA Viruses	DNA Viruses
Measles virus	Herpesviruses
Rubella virus	Cytomegalovirus
Retroviruses	Epstein-Barr virus
HTLV-1	Herpes simplex virus, types 1 and 2
HTLV-2	Herpes zoster
HIV	Papovaviruses
	Papillomaviruses
	Poliomaviruses
	Adenoviruses
	Hepatitis B virus

HTLV = human T lymphotropic virus.

c. **Lytic viruses that are prevented from disseminating by antiviral antibody or interferon**

d. **Viruses of reduced virulence,** which grow better at 31°C–33°C than at 37°C. Such strains are often isolated from persistently infected cell cultures and animals.

e. **Defective interfering (DI) particles,** which lack a portion of the genome, do not multiply by themselves, but interfere with the multiplication of infective viruses (see Chapter 24 III B).

4. **Latent infection.** Whereas persistent viral infections are associated with the release of significant amounts of virus from the infected cells, latent viral infections are associated with sporadic release of progeny virus (Table 26-2). Viral multiplication begins, but is arrested at a later stage. Latent infections are uniquely associated with DNA viruses, particularly those of the herpes group. By mechanisms that are not fully understood, the latent infection can be reactivated, causing cyclic disease that is not progressive.

5. **Inapparent infection.** Special assays are required to reveal the presence of a virus causing an inapparent infection. For example:

   a. The BK virus infects most individuals by adolescence and sets up inapparent infectious foci in the kidneys, where it is believed to replicate at such low levels that it is undetectable using conventional assays. If the individual becomes immunocompromised, the virus proliferates, and its presence becomes detectable.

   b. The JC virus, a papovavirus related to the BK virus, causes an inapparent but persistent infection of the brain associated with progressive multifocal leukoencephalopathy.

TABLE 26-2. Latent versus Persistent Asymptomatic Viral Infections

Characteristics	Latent Infection	Persistent Infection
Production of infectious virus	No	Yes*
Viral nucleic acids detected by *in situ* hybridization	Yes	Yes
Viral antigen detectable by antibodies	No	Yes
Potential for viral replication in response to external stimuli	Yes†	Yes‡

* Usually at very low levels (enough to elicit a sustained antibody response but usually not enough for the virus to be seen by light or electron microscopy).

† The individual then becomes symptomatic.

‡ These individuals are "latent carriers."

III. PATHOLOGY

A. Cellular level. The effects of viral infection on infected host cells vary considerably. The infection may be **inapparent,** induce **cytopathology** (which often results in cell death), or induce **cellular transformation** (which is associated with immortalization of the infected cell; see Chapter 27).

1. **Cytopathic effects** (Table 26-3) are always associated with the presence of live viral particles in the material studied.
   a. **Morphologic changes.** For example, cell rounding is caused by disruption of the cytoskeleton.
   b. **Nuclear changes.** Examples include pyknosis, changes in nuclear structure, and margination of chromatin.
   c. **Cell membrane changes** are caused by replacement of the normal membrane glycoproteins by virus-coded proteins.
      (1) Changes in the cell membrane are a **prominent phenomenon in infections caused by enveloped viruses,** but viral proteins can also be detected at the cell membrane of cells infected with naked viruses.
      (2) **Effects.** Cell membrane changes can have the following effects on host cells.
         (a) The permeability of the host cell membrane may increase.
         (b) Cells may show a tendency to agglutinate with glycoprotein-binding lectins, such as concanavalin A.
         (c) Cells may express new antigens that are not detected in uninfected cells (e.g., tumor-specific antigens).
         (d) Cells may exhibit a tendency to fuse with uninfected cells. Fusion results from the interaction of cell membranes of uninfected cells with certain viral glycoproteins, also called **fusion proteins,** expressed on the membranes of infected cells.
            (i) Fusion may affect a relatively low number of cells, leading to the formation of **giant multinucleated cells** [e.g., the **Tzanck cell** seen in fever blister lesions caused by herpes simplex virus (HSV)].
            (ii) It may result in **syncytia,** large masses of cytoplasm containing hundreds or even thousands of nuclei.

TABLE 26-3. Cytopathic Effects of Various Viruses

Virus	Nucleic Acid	Envelope	Genome Replication	Maturation	Inclusion Body	Cytopathic Response
Poxvirus	DNA	No	Cytoplasm	Cytoplasm	Cytoplasm	Foci, pocks*
Herpesvirus	DNA	Yes	Nucleus	Nuclear membrane	Nucleus	Giant cells†
Adenovirus	DNA	No	Nucleus	Nucleus	Nucleus	Transformation
Papovavirus	DNA	No	Nucleus	Nucleus	None	Transformation
Hepadnavirus	DNA	Yes	Nucleus	Cytoplasm	None	None
Picornavirus	+RNA	No	Cytoplasm	Cytoplasm	None	Cell lysis
Togavirus	+RNA	Yes	Cytoplasm	Membranes	None	None‡; cell lysis§
Retrovirus	+RNA	Yes	Nucleus	Membranes	None	Cell lysis; syncytia
Rhabdovirus	−RNA	Yes	Cytoplasm	Membranes	Cytoplasm	None
Paramyxovirus	−RNA	Yes	Cytoplasm	Membranes	Nucleus and cytoplasm	Syncytia
Orthomyxovirus	−RNA	Yes	Nucleus	Membranes	Nucleus	Cell rounding

* On embryonated eggs.
† Some members of the family.
‡ Rubella virus.
§ Eastern equine encephalitis virus.

(e) Cells may show an inability to adhere, leading to disruption of cell monolayers (foci).

d. **Inclusion bodies,** visible using a conventional microscope, are characteristic (but not exclusive) of some viral infections.

(1) In some cases, these intracellular bodies function as "virus factories," while in others, they represent the accumulation of debris and byproducts.

(2) The **location** of inclusion bodies is reflective of the site where viral assembly takes place. Therefore:

(a) Inclusion bodies tend to be located in the **nucleus of cells infected with DNA viruses.** The inclusion bodies (**Guarnieri bodies**) of poxviruses, DNA viruses that replicate in the cytoplasm, are an exception.

(b) Inclusion bodies tend to be located in the **cytoplasm of cells infected with RNA viruses.** Examples include **Negri bodies,** seen in the cytoplasm of brain cells infected by rabies virus.

e. **Necrotic** and **degradative changes** may be visible during the late stages of viral infection, preceding cell lysis.

2. **Causes of cell death in viral-infected cells.** The functional alterations that result in cell death can be grouped as follows:

a. **Inhibition of host macromolecular biosynthesis.** The translation of host messenger RNA (mRNA) may be adversely affected by various factors, including:

(1) Changes in the cytoplasm's electrolyte balance that preferentially impair the translation of cell mRNA

(2) Inactivation of cap-binding proteins

(3) Preferential translation of viral mRNA

(4) Overwhelming production of viral mRNA

(5) Increased degradation of cellular mRNA

b. **Abnormal membrane permeability**

(1) Abnormal permeability of the plasma membrane disrupts normal metabolic processes.

(2) Increased permeability of lysosomal membranes allows spillage of hydrolytic enzymes into the cytoplasm.

c. **Inhibition of host DNA and RNA synthesis** is usually secondary to interference with transacting proteins that control gene expression and cell proliferation. More rarely, inhibition of host DNA and RNA synthesis is caused by the synthesis of specific viral proteins that inhibit cellular nucleic acid synthesis.

3. **Histopathic effects.** The reactions to viral infection seen in infected tissues result from a combination of **cell damage** and **inflammatory changes.** The inflammatory cells in viral infections are predominantly mononuclear (lymphocytes and monocytes), in contrast to those seen in bacterial infections [which typically show a polymorphonuclear (PMN) infiltration].

a. **Lungs. Interstitial pneumonia,** characterized by mononuclear cell infiltrates in the alveolar wall, is a consequence of viral infection. **Alveolar pneumonia** is usually associated with secondary bacterial infections; in this case a PMN infiltrate within the alveoli may be seen.

b. **Viscera**

(1) **Hepatic tissue.** Viral hepatitis is usually associated with cell necrosis and fatty infiltration. Clinically, the infection may be asymptomatic or fatal, with all possible gradations in between.

(2) **Renal tissue.** Although viruses, particularly cytomegalovirus (CMV), can be isolated from the urine, there is some controversy about whether viruses other than CMV can actually infect the kidney. Desquamated cells with typical inclusion bodies can be detected in the urine of patients with rubella, mumps, measles, and CMV infection (especially in patients who have undergone renal transplantation).

c. CNS

(1) **Viral encephalitis** can be primary or secondary.

(a) **Primary viral encephalitis.** The virus actually invades the brain, causing neuronal damage. Herpes simplex virus, the arboviruses, and less frequently, the mumps virus and rabies viruses, cause encephalitis. Viruses may lyse infected neurons, cause intense inflammation, or induce demyelination (believed to be secondary to a hypersensitivity response triggered by the virus).

(b) **Secondary viral encephalitis** can be **postinfectious** or **postvaccinal.** The pathogenesis of secondary encephalitis may involve **spread of the virus to the brain,** such as it happens in some cases of measles, or what appears to be a **hypersensitivity reaction** causing demyelination rather than neuronal death, as seen in chickenpox.

(2) **Viral meningitis.** Typically, the cerebrospinal fluid is clear, with slightly elevated proteins, normal glucose, and few leukocytes (predominantly lymphocytes). Enteroviruses are most often involved in viral meningitis.

Chapter 27

DNA Tumor Viruses and Retroviruses

Gabriel Virella
Salvatore Arrigo

I. INTRODUCTION

A. Viruses associated with malignancies in humans

1. **Human DNA tumor viruses,** including papillomaviruses, the Epstein-Barr virus, and hepatitis B virus (HBV)

2. **Human tumor-associated retroviruses,** including the human T lymphotropic viruses, types I and II (HTLV-I and -II).

B. Definitions

1. **Immortalization** refers to the ability of virus-infected cells to grow indefinitely provided that adequate nutrients are available.

2. **Transformation** refers to the ability of virus-infected cells to cause malignant growth in immunosuppressed or immunodeficient animals. While transformed cells are always immortalized, the reverse is not true. Transformation is induced by **tumor viruses,** viruses that are able to cause (by themselves or in association with other factors) malignant cell growth.

C. Characteristics of transformed cells.

Virus-transformed cells differ from their normal counterparts in several ways.

1. **Possession of a viral genome.** Transformed cells contain all or part of a viral genome.
   a. Most commonly, the viral genome and the cell DNA are integrated. Integrated genomes are often poorly expressed or not expressed at all; therefore, rescue techniques are often employed in an attempt to reveal the integrated genome.
      (1) Cells may be treated with mutagens, in an attempt to activate the transcription of viral genomes.
      (2) Cocultivation or fusion of the infected cells with a cell line that may be more permissive to the virus can lead to viral replication. Rescue by coculture with permissive cells will only yield an infective virus if complete genomes are present in the infected cells.
      (3) Integrated defective viruses can be rescued by coinfecting the cells carrying the defective virus with a second, complete, and related virus through the process of complementation (see Chapter 24 III A 3).
   b. Rarely, the viral genome exists as a plasmid-like entity (episome).

2. **Morphologic changes.** Transformed cells in culture often grow with random orientation and assume a rounded shape and increased refractivity.

3. **Loss of contact inhibition.** Normal cells in culture tend to grow in monolayers and their growth is inhibited by neighboring cells—a phenomenon known as contact inhibition. Transformed cells do not exhibit this property, causing them to multiply randomly and in overlapping layers. As a consequence, conventional microscopic examination of a cell culture infected by a transforming virus often shows cell growth in large clumps known as foci.

4. **Reduced growth factor requirements.** Normal cells usually require the addition of fetal serum to the culture fluid to provide essential growth factors. The need for serum supplementation is considerably reduced in transformed cells.

5. **Changes in membrane transport properties.** Simple sugars and other nutrients are transported at a considerably higher rate through membranes of transformed cells, reflecting a state of metabolic activation that is consistent with the proliferative activity of the cell.

6. **Expression of tumor-associated surface antigens.** Virus-transformed cells express tumor-associated antigens. Most are virus-specific; others are products of de-repressed host genes that are not normally expressed.

7. **Changes in the composition of the plasma membrane** occur in transformed cells. Major changes include:
   a. **Reduced density and size of cellular glycolipids,** molecules that seem to play a significant role in contact inhibition of the growth of normal cells
   b. **Increased content of glycoprotein oligosaccharides,** which contributes to the increased agglutinability by lectins
   c. **Reduced fibronectin content,** which increases the fluidity of the membrane and may contribute to the morphologic changes associated with malignant transformation

8. **Chromosomal changes,** such as partial deletions, translocations, and partial or complete duplications, occur in transformed cells.

D. Identifying viral oncogenic behavior

1. The best evidence supporting the oncogenic role of viruses is obtained when an isolated virus causes a tumor in an experimental animal, and reisolation or cloning of the same virus causes a second tumor in another animal host.

2. Less strict criteria can be used to define a virus as the causative agent of a given type of malignancy:
   a. Visualization of viral structures (antigens or genomes) on tumor cells
   b. Establishment of an epidemiologic link between a given malignancy and a given virus
   c. Isolation of a suspect virus from tumor tissue and determination of the ability of the suspect virus to transform cells *in vitro*

II. DNA TUMOR VIRUSES.

As a rule, DNA tumor viruses have limited oncogenic potential in humans. Among several of the DNA tumor viruses, the mechanism of transformation is remarkably similar: the viral genome codes for proteins that **inactivate proteins coded by tumor suppressor genes.**

A. **Polyoma viruses** and **simian virus 40 (SV40)** have been extensively studied for their transforming properties.

1. **Oncogenic potential.** The oncogenic potential of these viruses in humans is limited.
   a. Polyoma viruses can cause a variety of histologically distinct tumors in newborn mice and hamsters. **BK virus** and **JC virus** are human polyoma viruses named after the two patients in whom they were first isolated. Both viruses, which are structurally homologous to SV40, can transform cultured cells and cause tumors in a variety of animals, but have never been shown to be associated with malignancies in humans.
   b. SV40, isolated from cultures of monkey kidney cells, causes leukemias and sarcomas in baby hamsters.

2. **Conditions that may contribute to transformation.** Polyoma viruses and SV40 cause a lytic type of infection in fully permissive cells, but under certain conditions, the viral genome may integrate and cause transformation *in vitro.* Conditions that may lead to transformation include:
   a. **Infection of cells that are not fully permissive.** Cells that are not fully permissive may not support full replication.

b. **Inactivation of the viral genome.** For example, the photodynamic induction of point mutations may prevent full replication of the viral genome.
c. **Exposure of the cultured cells to chemical carcinogens.** Chemical carcinogens may provide additional transforming signals.

3. **Mechanism of transformation.** The transforming polyoma virus–host cell interaction is characterized by the integration of viral DNA into the host cell DNA (usually 1 to 3 viral genomes per cell, but sometimes up to 50 viral genomes can be integrated in a single cell). Only part of the integrated viral DNA is expressed in the transformed cell, particularly the portion that codes for early antigens (large T, middle t, and small t for polyoma; large T and small t for SV40).
   a. The **large T antigen,** which is expressed on the membrane of cells infected with the polyoma virus, triggers antitumor immune responses. Large T antigen performs several key functions in transformation, most of which are related to interactions with the products of tumor-suppressor genes.
      (1) Large T antigen **binds and inactivates p53,** a cellular phosphoprotein whose expression is increased in the presence of damaged DNA.
         (a) Normally, p53 enhances the synthesis of a protein that binds and inactivates two important cyclines that promote cell division. As a result of the arrest in cell division, DNA repair can take place, after which the levels of p53 decrease and the cell divides.
         (b) Large T antigen inactivates p53, thus causing it to lose its regulatory capacity in a cell expressing large amounts of abnormal DNA.
      (2) Large T antigen **binds and inactivates the retinoblastoma (Rb) gene product,** the first tumor suppressor gene identified.
         (a) Normally, the Rb gene codes for a protein that binds and inactivates several transcription factors, preventing progression into the S phase of cell division.
         (b) Interaction with the T antigen inactivates the Rb gene product, thus removing a second means of controlling cell proliferation.
   b. The **middle T antigen,** expressed only in cells infected by a polyoma virus, is considered an acute transforming gene because it can cause transformation by itself (if it is strongly expressed) and the transformed cells have highly tumorigenic properties. In SV40, the functions of the middle T antigen are carried out by the large T antigen.
      (1) Middle T antigen is located in cytoplasmic membranes, including the plasma membrane, in close association with pp60, the product of the cellular proto-oncogene *c-rc*. pp60 is a cell membrane–associated protein kinase that phosphorylates tyrosine residues in phosphoproteins. (Normal cells usually phosphorylate serine and threonine residues.)
      (2) After association with the middle T antigen, the kinase activity of pp60 is enhanced and the aberrant phosphorylation of phosphoproteins involved in cell activation is believed to result in uncontrolled proliferation.
   c. The **small t antigen** has accessory functions related to transformation. Its expression is usually associated with the loss of contact inhibition, probably secondary to the dissolution of the intracellular cytoskeleton.

B. **Papillomaviruses,** such as the **human papillomaviruses,** cause both spontaneous benign and malignant tumors in animals, and probably in humans as well. Most human papillomaviruses cause benign warts, but a variety of carcinoma-associated genotypes have been defined.

1. **Oncogenic potential**
   a. Almost 100% of **cervical, vulvar,** and **penile cancers,** as well as **precancerous lesions of the cervix** (including cervical dysplasia), contain human papillomavirus genomes. Cervical carcinoma is close to being defined as a sexually transmitted disease as a result of the epidemiologic associations among cervical carcinoma, penile carcinoma, and the recovery of human papillomavirus from the semen of partners of infected women.

(1) Human papillomavirus types 6 and 11 are predominantly recovered from differentiated cervical carcinomas, laryngeal papillomas, and condylomas.
(2) Human papillomavirus types 6, 11, 16, and 18 are predominantly recovered from vulvar carcinoma.
(3) Human papillomavirus types 16 and 33 are predominantly recovered from papillomavirus-associated penile intraepithelial neoplasm, which develops in partners of women with cervical intraepithelial neoplasm.

b. Papillomaviruses appear to behave as **cocarcinogens:** their genomes are often found in benign lesions that become malignant after long periods of quiescence. During latency, the expression of the viral genome is tightly controlled; smoking, other infections (e.g., genital herpes), and chronic inflammatory lesions appear to be associated with a loss of the cellular control and the emergence of malignant lesions. For example, human papillomavirus types 6 and 11 cause **anogenital warts (condylomata acuminata)** and **respiratory papillomatosis;** both types of lesions can become malignant. **Flat warts (epidermodysplasia verruciformis),** also caused by some types of human papillomavirus, become malignant in 25% of patients.

2. **Mechanism of transformation.** Only 10% of the papillomavirus genome is usually transcribed in cells that carry it, probably because it is hypermethylated. The expressed 10% includes the regions that code for the transforming antigens E7 and E6. The proteins coded by these two genes **bind and inactivate the Rb gene product and p53.**

C. Adenoviruses

1. **Oncogenic potential.** Adenoviruses are not associated with human malignancies, but several strains can immortalize cells in culture and several others (including strains infecting humans) can cause tumors in rodents.

2. **Mechanism of transformation.** Usually only part of the viral DNA is integrated. Even when most of the genome is integrated, it is done in fragmented form. Transformation depends on the expression of the region coding for the "early" genes, E1A and E1B.
   a. **E1A** codes for two transactivating proteins that promote transcription of both viral and cellular genes. In addition, E1A codes for proteins that modify the activity of the Rb gene product and of a cyclin-binding cellular protein (p107).
   b. **E1B** codes for a protein that inactivates p53.

3. The **degree of tumorigenicity of adenovirus-transformed cells** is inversely related to the intensity of expression of major histocompatibility complex-I (MHC-I) antigens. Those with minimal expression of MHC-I antigens are most capable of evading the immune system. Two mechanisms have been proposed to explain the poor expression of MHC-I in adenovirus-infected cells:
   a. A down-regulating effect of E1A proteins on the transcription of MHC-I genes
   b. Interference with the transport of MHC-I antigens to the cell membrane as a consequence of the binding of gp19, a viral glycoprotein, to newly synthesized MHC-I polypeptides

D. Herpesviruses

1. **Oncologic potential.** Herpesviruses have been shown to be tumorigenic in animals (e.g., the Marek's disease virus in chickens) and have been epidemiologically linked with human malignancies.
   a. **Epstein-Barr virus** has been associated with spontaneously occurring tumors in humans, namely **Burkitt's lymphoma** and **nasopharyngeal carcinoma.** A solid epidemiologic link between Epstein-Barr virus and both African Burkitt's lymphoma and nasopharyngeal carcinoma has been established, suggesting that this virus at least acts as a cocarcinogen in these two malignancies. Epstein-Barr virus may be one of several cofactors that lead to malignant transformation.
   b. Recently, a novel herpesvirus has been reported to be associated with **Kaposi's sarcoma** in AIDS patients.

2. **Mechanism of transformation in Epstein-Barr virus–related malignancies.** The Epstein-Barr virus infects B lymphocytes, causing them to become immortalized lymphoblastoid cells that do not release progeny. A small part of the viral genome is expressed in infected cells.

   a. **Burkitt's lymphoma**

      (1) **Epstein-Barr nuclear antigen-1 (EBNA-1)** is overexpressed in Burkitt's lymphoma. This nuclear protein is responsible for latent infection, which is associated with persistence of Epstein-Barr virus episomes in the host cell.

      (2) **Chromosomal translocations in Burkitt's lymphoma** have been extensively studied. A common denominator is that they affect **chromosome 8** and result in the exaggerated expression of an **abnormal c-*myc*** product.

         (a) The c-Myc protein, a nuclear-binding phosphoprotein, has a positive effect on normal cell proliferation, and is also involved in the control of apoptosis. In Burkitt's lymphoma, the c-Myc protein is more active than its normal counterpart, due to mutations that make the transactivating domain resistant to inhibition by p107, a protein that normally modulates its transactivating activity.

         (b) The translocations affecting chromosome 8 result in increased expression of the c-*myc* gene through several mechanisms:

            (i) Most commonly, the c-*myc* coding sequence is translocated to the unrearranged chromosome 14. That chromosome has active transcription enhancers that induce the expression of c-*myc*.

            (ii) In addition, as a consequence of the 8:14 translocation, regulatory sequences that control c-*myc* expression remain in chromosome 8 and the expression of the translocated c-*myc* gene becomes unregulated.

            (iii) In other translocations (8:2, 8:22), c-*myc* is translocated near enhancer sequences that activate cryptic promoters.

         (c) The consequences of the increased synthesis of an abnormally active product include increases in the rate of cell proliferation and in apoptosis.

         (d) Chronic Epstein-Barr virus and *Plasmodium* infections can induce chronic B cell proliferation and create conditions favoring the emergence of chromosomal translocations. The overexpression of c-*myc,* EBNA-1, and other unregulated proto-oncogenes will result in malignant growth.

   b. **Non-Burkitt B cell lymphoma.** The nuclear antigens EBNA-5 and EBNA-2, latent membrane protein-1 (LMP-1), and LMP-2 are overexpressed in non-Burkitt B cell lymphoma.

      (1) **EBNA-5** binds and inactivates p53 and the Rb suppressor protein.

      (2) **EBNA-2** interacts with a nuclear-binding protein; the complex then transactivates both viral and host cell promoters.

      (3) A complex of EBNA-5 and EBNA-2 activates a G1 cyclin and promotes cell proliferation, playing an essential role in B cell immortalization.

      (4) **LMP-1 and LMP-2.** LMP-2 is associated with a tyrosine kinase of the *src* family and is probably responsible for the phosphorylation of the epidermal growth factor (EGF) receptor, which becomes hyperresponsive to EGF. Other effects of LMP-1 and LMP-2 include activation of a calcium/calmodulin–dependent protein kinase, increased synthesis of interleukin-10 (IL-10), activation of receptors involved in growth signaling, and transactivation of the *bcl-2* proto-oncogene. These activities appear to be the basis of the essential role that LMP-1 and LMP-2 play in Epstein-Barr virus–induced B lymphocyte transformation.

   c. **Nasopharyngeal carcinoma. EBNA-1, LMP-1,** and **LMP-2** are overexpressed in nasopharyngeal carcinoma cells.

E. HBV

1. **Oncogenic potential. Primary hepatoma** can develop in chronic HBV carriers (particularly neonatally-infected children). HBV may be only one cofactor leading to malig-

nancy; other possible cocarcinogens include aflatoxin B1, a mutagenic mycotoxin that is a common food contaminant in austral Africa and China, the regions with the highest prevalence of hepatocellular carcinoma.

2. **Mechanism of transformation.** The integration of viral DNA is most often associated with fragmentation of the viral genome, loss of genetic material, and complex rearrangements with multimeric inserts and translocations involving chromosomes 17 and 18.
   a. Several mechanisms have been proposed to explain malignant transformation, including inactivation of cellular tumor suppressor genes (e.g., p53), gene amplification, genome destabilization, and recessive mutations in the chromosomes most often affected by HBV genome insertions.
   b. One region is always retained in the integrated virus, and it is believed to contain a super promoter such as the one contained on the long terminal repeat (LTR) sequences of retroviruses, which may be responsible for activation of cellular proto-oncogenes.

III. RETROVIRUSES

A. Structure and classification

1. **Structure.** Most retroviral particles are constituted by a **core,** which contains the genome and enzymes and is surrounded by an inner **nucleocapsid shell** with icosahedral or spherical symmetry. The core is protected by an outer **envelope,** constituted by a lipid bilayer membrane with inserted glycoprotein spikes.

2. **Classification**
   a. **Subfamilies** of retroviruses have been defined, all of them sharing the same general characteristics:
      (1) **Oncovirus** (tumor-causing viruses)
      (2) **Lentivirus** (includes the HIV viruses)
      (3) **Spumaviruses** (animal viruses)
   b. **Morphotypes.** Under the electron microscope, retroviruses can be subclassified according to their core morphology and location:
      (1) **Oncoviruses**
         (a) **Type C oncoviruses** have centrally located spherical cores.
         (b) **Type B oncoviruses** have an eccentrically located spherical core.
      (2) **Lentiviruses** have elongated cores.

3. **Genome.** The unintegrated viral genome (Figure 27-1) is constituted by two identical +RNA strains linked together close to the 5′ end.
   a. **Genes.** All complete retroviruses contain the *env, gag,* and *pol* genes. The *onc* gene is unique to the oncoviruses.
      (1) The ***env*** gene codes for **envelope glycoproteins.**
      (2) The ***gag*** gene codes for **group antigens,** proteins that constitute the nucleocapsid shell.

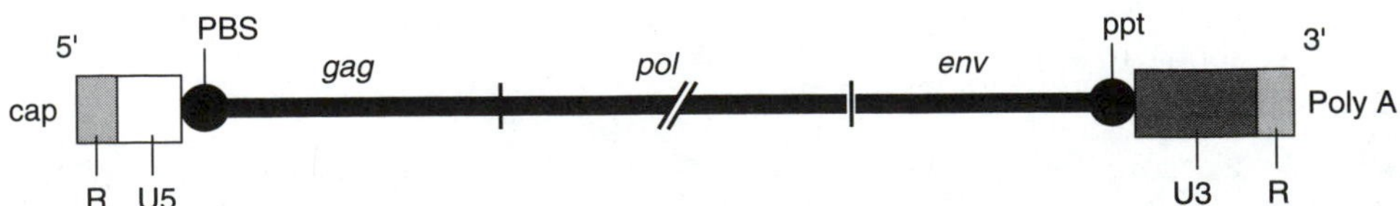

FIGURE 27-1. Typical retroviral genome. *PBS* = polymerase-binding site.

(3) The ***pol*** gene codes for the **reverse transcriptase** (RNA-dependent DNA polymerase).
(4) The ***onc*** gene codes for **products responsible for transformation.**

b. Regulatory sequences flank the coding regions and include:
(1) Identical terminal **redundancy regions** (**R regions**) near the 5′ and 3′ ends
(2) Two unique sequences, one at the 5′ end and one at the 3′ end (the **U5** and **U3 regions,** respectively)
(3) A **primer-binding site (PBS)** near the 5′ end
(4) A **purine-rich tract (ppt region)** located just inside the U3 region
(5) A strong **transcription promoter** located in the U3 region, near the 3′ terminus

c. Long terminal repeats (LTRs). During reverse transcription, the regulatory sequences are duplicated. As a result, the **integrated viral DNA** is flanked by two identical LTRs.
(1) Each LTR contains (in the 5′ to 3′ direction) a transcript of the U5, R, and U3 regions of the retrovirus RNA.
(a) The U3 region contains a **transcription enhancer** that can be activated by transactivating factors of both viral and cellular origin. In addition, it contains "TATA" and "CAT" boxes, which serve as binding sites for the cellular polymerases.
(b) A "cap" site, situated between the U3 and R regions, marks the beginning of messenger RNA (mRNA) transcription.
(c) The R region contains a site for the addition of poly A, marking the end of mRNA transcription.
(2) Both ends of each LTR are flanked by direct repeat sequences, recognition units for integration. Many copies (as many as 100 or more) of retroviral genomes can be integrated in a given cellular genome.

B. Oncogenic potential. Oncoviruses cause leukemias and solid tumors in a variety of animals, including humans. Depending on their genomes, oncoviruses can be classified as **nondefective (complete)** or **defective.**

1. **Nondefective oncoviruses** carry all the structural and regulatory genes (*gag, pol*, and *env*) needed for replication. With the exception of the Rous sarcoma virus, these genomes do not include oncogenes (transforming genes). Nondefective oncoviruses are infective but in most cases are nontransforming and **cause malignancies only sporadically.**
   a. When nondefective oncoviruses cause malignancy, it is due to the insertion of the viral genome near a cellular oncogene that is subsequently overexpressed as a result of the influence of viral transcription enhancers contained in the LTR regions. The c-*onc* product is often abnormally active, probably as a result of **insertional mutagenesis** (i.e., mutations in the host genome induced by the insertion of the retrovirus).
   b. The **Rous sarcoma virus** is a unique retrovirus that has a complete genome and also **carries an oncogene** (*src*). This virus is highly infective, has transforming properties, and causes malignant growth with high frequency. It infects chickens, quails, and some mammals, including marmoset monkeys. Most knowledge about oncoviruses has been acquired through studies of this virus.

2. **Defective oncoviruses.** The genome contains an oncogene but is missing one or several of the genes essential for viral replication. Defective oncoviruses are believed to result from the incorporation of a transforming gene into an integrated retrovirus.
   a. Defective oncoviruses cause tumors with high frequency because their LTRs enhance the transcription of the oncogene they carry. Defective oncoviruses frequently cause tumors of the hematopoietic system (e.g., acute leukemia), sarcomas, endotheliomas, and neural tumors in a variety of animal species.
   b. The transforming gene usually replaces one of the genes essential for replication so that even when the defective genome is expressed, infective progeny are not generated. Thus, defective viruses tend to remain integrated, and their transmis-

sion is usually vertical (i.e., through the genomes of germ cells). Defective viruses may be transmitted horizontally if complementation with a co-infecting helper virus takes place (see Chapter 24 III A 3).

C. **Oncogenes** are transforming genes that have homologous counterparts (proto-oncogenes) in normal cells. While the cellular proto-oncogenes have introns and are under the influence of cellular regulatory genes, the viral oncogenes lack introns and are controlled by viral regulatory genes.

1. **Nomenclature.** Viral oncogenes are designated by placing the letter *v* before the specific designation of the gene; cellular oncogenes are designated by the letter *c*. For example, the viral copy of the oncogene *src* is designated as v-*src,* while the homologous cellular proto-oncogene is designated as c-*src*.

2. **Origin.** Oncogenes are believed to be cellular genes with regulatory properties that became integrated in the viral genome as a consequence of recombinational events taking place during viral replication. Most proto-oncogenes are involved in the regulation of cell growth and differentiation. Their tumorigenic potential may result from:
   a. Loss of transcription control mechanisms and exaggerated expression under the influence of viral enhancer regions
   b. Structural and functional differences between the proto-oncogene products and the viral oncogene products, probably a result of mutations that occur as a consequence of the integration of the proto-oncogene into the viral genome

3. **Role in cell transformation.** Oncogenes code for a variety of proteins that can be directly implicated in the process of malignant transformation. These proteins influence cell growth by a variety of mechanisms:
   a. **Growth factor activity.** The *sis* gene product is identical to the β chain of platelet-derived growth factor (PDGF). Cells expressing a receptor for that growth factor are susceptible to transformation.
   b. **Protein kinases.** Several oncogenes code for amino acid-specific kinases. For example, v-*src* codes for a tyrosine kinase that phosphorylates cytoskeleton constituents, causing abnormalities in the cellular adhesive plaques and leading to a loss of contact inhibition.
   c. **Autoactivation of protein kinases.** The v-*erb* A and B gene products are truncated versions of receptors mediating cell activation. These truncated receptors lack the extracellular domain but contain the transmembrane and intracellular domains. The intracytoplasmic portions of these receptors are protein kinases with tyrosine specificity and appear to be in a state of autoactivation.
   d. **Transactivating proteins.** Some oncogenes code for transactivating proteins that diffuse to the nucleus and activate transcription enhancers for both viral and cellular genes. The enhanced transcription of DNA is of special significance if a protein controlling cell replication or differentiation is overexpressed. Examples of these mechanisms include the proteins coded by v-*fos* and v-*jun,* which regulate the transcription of genes controlling cell growth and multiplication, and two phosphorylated proteins, coded by the v-*myc* gene, that act on regulatory genes involved in the control of cellular proliferation and differentiation.

4. **Identification of oncogenes.** Neoplastic cell populations can be shown to contain activated proto-oncogenes by transfecting tumoral DNA into immortalized cell lines, such as the 3T3 cell line. If the transfected cells develop the ability to induce malignancies in immunoincompetent animals, it is considered proof that there was an active oncogene in the DNA isolated from the tumor. Identification of the oncogene in question is attempted using DNA probes for known oncogenes.
   a. It must be noted that proving that tumoral DNA carries sequences homologous to known viral oncogenes does not prove that that particular sequence is actively expressed. Even if it can be established that a given oncogene has been activated in a given tumor, that fact does not prove the viral etiology for that tumor; some

TABLE 27-1. Proto-oncogenes Demonstrated in Human Tumors

Tumor	Genes	Chromosomes
Bladder carcinoma	c-*Ha-ras*	6, 11, 12, X
Lung cancer	c-*Ki-ras*	6, 11, 12, X
Small-cell lung carcinoma	c-*myc*	8
Colon adenocarcinoma	c-*myc*, c-*Ki-ras*	8, 12
Neuroblastoma	c-*sis*	22
Mammary carcinoma	c-*erb-A*, c-*erb-B*	3, 17
Chronic and acute myelogenous leukemia	c-*abl*	4, 9
Burkitt's lymphoma	c-*myc*, c-*bcl-2*	8, 18
B cell leukemias and lymphomas	c-*bcl*	8, 18

other type of mutagenic event (e.g., chemical mutagens) may have caused the activation.

b. Table 27-1 contains a list of proto-oncogenes identified in human malignancies.

D. Mechanisms of transformation. Retroviruses can induce malignancy by a variety of mechanisms. These mechanisms are not exclusive.

1. **Insertion of a viral transforming gene in the host genome**
2. **Activation of a pre-existing oncogene.** The viral genome may integrate near a proto-oncogene and activate its expression through its transcription enhancers. This mechanism has been demonstrated in nondefective leukemia viruses that do not carry oncogenes.
3. **Gene amplification.** For unknown reasons, some malignant tissues show extensive replication of proto-oncogene-containing DNA segments, which may or may not be associated with chromosome duplication. The amplified expression of the corresponding gene products (probably altered by coexisting mutations) leads to transformation.
4. **Mutation.** The integration of a retrovirus may cause mutations in cellular proto-oncogenes that result in the synthesis of a gene product of increased activity with transforming capacity.
5. **Translocation.** Coincidentally or as a consequence of viral genome insertion, chromosomal translocations can occur and affect DNA segments containing proto-oncogenes or oncogenes. Translocations may expose the genes in question to enhancer sequences that activate cryptic promoters, or repressors may be left behind during the translocation.

E. HTLV-I and HTLV-II are human exogenous retroviruses (i.e., they have complete genomes and can be transmitted horizontally).

1. **Oncogenic potential.** HTLV-I and HTLV-II are associated with:
   - **a. Acute T cell leukemia,** relatively rare in the United States, but common in southern Japan
   - **b. Spastic tropical paraparesis,** a degenerative disease of the central nervous system (CNS) seen predominantly in South America
2. **Mechanism of transformation.** The HTLV-I and -II genomes contain genes that code for proteins that modify nuclear transactivating proteins and appear responsible for malignant transformation. However, there are no homologous cellular genes for the viral transforming genes; therefore, these genes are not technically oncogenes.
   - **a.** Both viruses are replication-competent and infect many different types of cells, but only $CD4^+$ T cells have been shown to be immortalized as a consequence of infection by HTLV-I.

(1) In patients with leukemia, the proliferating $CD4^+$ T cells display membrane interleukin-2 (IL-2) receptors, and in some cases, produce IL-2, suggesting that a deregulated autocrine growth stimulatory circuit may cause immortalization.

(2) The infected T cells are not destroyed; there is a state of polyclonal activation of T cells and a mild immunodeficiency.

b. The genomes of the two HTLV viruses contain a region (*X*) with two open reading frames located between the *env* gene and the 3′ LTR. This region codes for several transregulatory proteins that are probably responsible for the immortalization of infected cells. The best studied of these proteins is the *tax* (p40, x-lor, x-tat) protein, which diffuses to the nucleus, where it seems to modify nucleoproteins involved in transcription control [e.g., nuclear factor kB (NFkB)], increasing their activity.

(1) Binding sites for NFkB have been located upstream of the IL-2 receptor gene, explaining why this gene is overexpressed by infected cells.

(2) NFkB is believed to interact with the LTR region of HTLV, and, as a consequence, the transcription of the integrated provirus may increase by as much as 100-fold.

(3) NFkB and other *tax*-modified nucleoproteins are believed to interact with promoter/enhancer sequences for a variety of other genes, including those that code for IL-2 and IL-4.

(4) NFkB activates HIV replication; thus, simultaneous infection with HTLV-I and HIV is particularly dangerous because HIV will tend to be overexpressed under the influence of the *tax* gene product.

F. Retroviruses and medicine

1. Applications

a. Research. Retroviruses, naturally occurring genetic vectors, are extensively used in research.

b. Therapy. Retroviruses have been successfully used as vectors for gene therapy in children with congenital adenosine deaminase deficiency. Other applications involving retroviral vectors include experimental attempts at tumor therapy.

2. Problems include difficulty in obtaining large amounts of vectors, problems controlling vector stability and insertion points, inadequate expression of the transfected genes, and the transient nature of gene therapy when the target cells have a limited rate of replication and a short life span. Considerable efforts are underway to develop techniques for the infection of stem cells, which should solve the problems related to the short life span of transfected cells.

IV. TWO-HIT THEORY OF MALIGNANT TRANSFORMATION.

While retroviruses containing one single oncogene can transform cells, and single transforming oncogenes, when expressed vigorously, can achieve the same result, in most cases it appears that malignant transformation requires the synergistic effects of at least two transforming signals. Several observations support this theory:

A. Several oncogenes (e.g., v-*ras*) can induce transformation of immortalized 3T3 cells but do not transform cultures of primary cells. Thus, the oncogene would represent a second hit to a cell that had already been hit once by an immortalizing agent.

B. Many malignant cells express products of several activated proto-oncogenes. In Burkitt's lymphoma, c-*myc* is actively expressed, but this gene is also expressed in Epstein-Barr virus–immortalized, nontransforming lymphocytes. Malignant growth appears to be always associated with the activation of a second proto-oncogene (e.g., c-*bcl-2*).

C. Most DNA tumor viruses carry more than one oncogene—for example, the large T, middle T and small t genes of the polyoma virus, the T and t genes of SV40, the E1A and E1B genes of adenovirus, the E6 and E7 genes of papillomaviruses. Some of the proteins coded by those genes activate cell proliferation while others block the antiproliferative effects of tumor suppressor gene products, synergistically contributing to malignant transformation.

Chapter 28

Viruses and the Immune System

Gabriel Virella

I. INTRODUCTION.

I. INTRODUCTION. Most viruses are acquired either through mucosal infection or via direct inoculation into the blood stream. The **skin** and **secretions of the mucous membranes** represent **natural barriers to viral infection.** When those mechanisms are overwhelmed or bypassed, the virus multiplies at the portal of entry and disseminates throughout the body. The final outcome of the infection depends on the efficiency of the immune system, which acts to limit dissemination or promote elimination of the virus after it has reached its target organ.

A. Acute infection. Recovery depends primarily on nonimmunologic defense mechanisms, such as fever and the production of interferons. The role of humoral immunity in acute viral infections is limited on account of the typically short incubation periods—the virus proliferates at the portal of entry, spreads hematogenously, and infects the target tissue before neutralizing antibodies are synthesized in sufficient concentrations.

B. Chronic infection. Recovery is more likely to depend on the activation of cytotoxic T cells, which are able to recognize and destroy viral-infected cells. Antibodies are not effective for preventing cell-to-cell spread through syncytia or destroying infected cells.

II. ANTIBODY-MEDIATED (HUMORAL) IMMUNITY.

II. ANTIBODY-MEDIATED (HUMORAL) IMMUNITY. The capsid protein(s) in naked viruses and the envelope glycoproteins in enveloped viruses are immunogenic.

A. Types of antiviral antibodies

1. **Neutralizing antibodies** prevent viral replication and play an important protective role.
   - **a.** Neutralizing antibodies usually react with surface antigens (e.g., the capsid proteins of naked viruses or the glycoprotein spikes of enveloped viruses).
   - **b.** Originally, it was theorized that neutralizing antibodies directly blocked interaction between viral proteins and their cellular receptors. However, it has been proven that very few antibody molecules are required to neutralize a single viral particle (in some cases, a single antibody molecule is sufficient) and that phenotypically mixed particles (whose capsid is constituted by proteins of two different serotypes) can be neutralized by a single antibody as well. Mechanisms involving **steric hindrance** appear most likely involved:
     - **(1)** A single neutralizing antibody molecule crosslinking two epitopes of contiguous capsomers is likely to trigger a generalized configurational alteration of the viral capsid that impairs interaction with cellular receptors or the release of the viral genome once the nucleocapsid has gained access to the cytoplasm.
     - **(2)** The binding of antibody to envelope glycoproteins may prevent the fusion of the envelope with either the cell membrane or the membrane of acidified endosomes, preventing release of nucleocapsids into the cytoplasm.
2. **Mucosal antibodies** are believed to prevent infection at the portal of entry by blocking attachment to mucosal cell receptors.
3. **Complement-fixing antibodies** are important from a diagnostic point of view. In addition, they may play a protective role, either by promoting complement-mediated lysis of virus-infected cells or by causing complement-mediated disruption of the viral envelope.

B. The role of viral antibodies in long-term immunity. Lasting immunity to most viral infections depends on the rapid synthesis of neutralizing antibodies, or the activation of preexisting neutralizing antibodies.

1. Immunologic memory is triggered either by natural exposure to the virus or by immunization.
2. Diseases caused by antigenically stable viruses with very few serotypes and no animal reservoirs (e.g., measles, mumps, smallpox, chickenpox, rubella, hepatitis B, polio) are most effectively prevented by vaccination.

III. CELL-MEDIATED IMMUNITY (CMI).

The major mechanism of defense against an established viral infection is elimination of the infected cells. Viruses that cause self-limited diseases in the normal host cause severe, difficult to treat infections in individuals with CMI deficiencies.

A. Immunocompetent cells

1. **Cytotoxic T lymphocytes** are believed to play a key role in the destruction of infected cells. The effector cells are $CD8^+$ T lymphocytes, which recognize and kill cells with self major histocompatibility complex (MHC) molecules modified by a viral peptide.
2. **Helper T lymphocytes** play an essential role in promoting the activation, proliferation, and differentiation of cytotoxic T lymphocytes. A predominance of the TH_1 subpopulation seems essential for proper activation of cytotoxic effector mechanisms.
3. **Natural killer (NK) cells.** NK cell-mediated cytotoxicity and **antibody-dependent CMI** are thought to play a role in the elimination of virus-infected cells. For example, HIV-infected cells can be killed by normal K lymphocytes after pre-incubation with serum containing anti-HIV antibodies—a clear demonstration of **antibody-dependent cell-mediated cytotoxicity (ADCC).**

B. Viral interaction with immunocompetent cells.

The protection offered by CMI is complicated by the fact that the cells themselves can become infected. Furthermore, the activity of lymphocytes engaged in the destruction of virus-infected cells may be more deleterious than the infection itself.

1. **Reticuloendothelial system.** The infection of macrophages and related cells is common during a viral infection. In most cases, the initial infection at the portal of entry is followed by replication in the reticuloendothelial system, then by a second viremia, immediately followed by infection of the target tissue. In most cases, the infection of the reticuloendothelial system is transient, but certain viruses (e.g., HIV) cause persistent infection of phagocytic cells, which then become a continual source of virus. Macrophages and related cells can be infected as a consequence of two types of interactions:
   a. **Virus receptors on macrophage membranes** permit direct infection by viruses. A well-defined example is the expression of a slightly modified CD4 molecule that allows infection by HIV. A variety of receptors would have to be available to account for the almost universal infection of these cells.
   b. **Ingestion of antibody–virus complexes** occurs through FcRγ-mediated phagocytosis. The complexes may dissociate in the acidic endosomic compartment, and the virus, "freed" from the neutralizing antibody, may be able to penetrate the cytoplasm and initiate its replicative cycle. This pathway would allow many different viruses to infect macrophages but requires IgG antibody synthesis; therefore, it is not likely to be involved in the early infection of macrophages that precedes the second wave of viremia.
2. **Lymphocytes.** The infection of T lymphocytes is significant because it can lead to a state of functional depression.

a. **Depletion of helper T cells.** In some cases, the functional depression is a consequence of the depletion of helper T cells. For example:
   (1) HIV-infected patients develop a severe depletion of the $CD4^+$ cell population, which, along with several other factors discussed in detail in Chapter 57, leads to a progressive and eventually profound state of immunodeficiency.
   (2) A recently isolated strain of lymphocytic choriomeningitis virus (LCMV), an RNA virus of the arenavirus family, may cause non-lethal infections in normal mice. The infections are associated with a state of immunodepression that is believed to be caused by the elimination of infected $CD4^+$ T cells and accessory cells by LCMV-specific $CD8^+$ cytotoxic lymphocytes, a mechanism of immunosuppression that may also be involved in AIDS.

b. **Infection of immunocompetent cells.** A variety of viruses are able to infect immunocompetent cells and cause functional alterations without inducing numerical depletion.
   (1) Human T-lymphotropic virus-I (HTLV-I) infects $CD4^+$ cells.
   (2) Measles virus depresses ADCC, NK activity, and T and B cell function in measles-infected lymphocytes. By causing arrest of the cell cycle in the G1 stage, the measles virus inhibits the T cell proliferative response. This functional depression of infected lymphocytes is probably the mechanism explaining the **anergy** often seen during the acute phase of measles.

c. **Other mechanisms**
   (1) Infected cells may release soluble viral proteins that then act as blocking factors by binding to antibodies before they can bind to the infected cell membrane. The release of soluble HIV gp120 by infected lymphocytes is an example of this mechanism.
   (2) Infected cells may release soluble factors that suppress noninfected cells. One such factor is released during the lytic cycle of Epstein-Barr infection in approximately 50% of Epstein-Barr virus–transformed cell lines and has been recognized as an analogue of interleukin-10 (IL-10), an interleukin with down-regulating effects on T helper cells.

IV. PATHOLOGIC CONSEQUENCES OF THE ANTIVIRAL IMMUNE RESPONSE

A. Virus–antibody complex deposition.

Virus–antibody complex deposition. Formation of virus–antibody complexes takes place whenever antibody synthesis coincides with active viral replication or with the expression of viral proteins in infected cells. If the virus or viral antigens gain access to the circulation, soluble immune complexes are formed and deposited in tissues, where they may cause inflammatory changes.

1. In infants with **congenital cytomegalovirus (CMV) infection,** circulating complexes are deposited in the kidney, causing kidney damage.
2. In patients with **hepatitis B virus (HBV) infection** and **chronic HBV carriers,** immune complexes containing the HBV surface antigen (HBsAg) can be found in circulation. These immune complexes can be deposited in the joints, kidneys, or small cutaneous blood vessels, leading to arthritis, glomerulonephritis, or vasculitis, respectively.

B. Virus–antibody complex facilitation of infection.

Virus–antibody complex facilitation of infection. Virus–antibody complexes may promote infection of cells by a virus that otherwise would not infect them. For example:

1. Virus–IgG antibody complexes promote the infection of phagocytic cells.
2. Epstein-Barr virus–dimeric IgA complexes formed in the submucosa are believed to facilitate the infection of mucosal cells by the Epstein-Barr virus through the interaction of virus-associated dimeric IgA with the polyIg receptors on the mucosal cell. This mechanism of infection has been proposed to explain how Epstein-Barr virus induces nasopharyngeal carcinoma in spite of the fact that the natural tropism of this virus is for B lymphocytes.

C. Tissue damage as a consequence of the antiviral response

1. The original strains of LCMV cause an acute form of choriomeningitis that is rapidly fatal in adult, immunocompetent mice. However, when neonatal (or adult immunosuppressed) mice are infected with heavy inoculums of this virus, they develop a state of tolerance and suffer from a chronic infection that is not fatal in the short run. The obvious conclusion is that a normal, energetic immune response is directly linked to inflammation in the central nervous system (CNS) and death.

2. Chronic hepatitis is believed to result from the cytotoxic cell-mediated immune response directed against hepatocytes chronically infected by HBV, which, by itself, might not cause significant cell damage. Experimental evidence in support of this theory has been obtained with transgenic mice that express HBV-coded antigens on their hepatocyte cell membranes. These mice develop $CD8^+$-mediated anti-HBV cytotoxic responses, that lead to hepatocyte destruction *in vivo.*

V. EVASION OF THE IMMUNE RESPONSE.

Viruses have acquired a variety of mechanisms that allow them to escape the immune response that otherwise would eliminate them. Some strategies rely on interference with the immune response, as discussed in III B. Other strategies rely on avoidance mechanisms:

A. Genomic integration is seen exclusively with DNA viruses and retroviruses. Once the genome is integrated, the virus can multiply and spread horizontally to other cells, and be transmitted vertically to the progeny of the infected cell. The latter mode of transmission will happen even in cells in which the virus is minimally expressed, and allows effective persistence of the infection with minimal involvement of the immune system.

B. Direct cell-to-cell propagation has been observed with a variety of viruses (e.g.,herpesviruses, paramyxoviruses, HIV). These viruses are able to induce the formation of giant multinucleated cells and syncytia.

C. Infection of cells lacking MHC-I antigens (e.g., neurons) allows the virus to evade the immune response. Cells lacking MHC-I antigens are not easily recognized by the immune system because they do not express MHC–viral peptide complexes on their membranes.

D. Inhibition of MHC–viral peptide complex expression has been observed in some viral infections. The transport of MHC-I viral–peptide complexes to the cell membrane requires association with transport proteins. Some viruses (e.g., adenoviruses) disturb this process, reducing the expression of MHC-I viral–peptide complexes on the infected cell membrane, thus preventing effective recognition by cytotoxic T lymphocytes.

E. Antigenic variation has been well characterized for HIV and is believed to result from errors introduced by the reverse transcriptase during synthesis of viral DNA from the RNA template. The mutations modify the antigenicity of gp120 to the point that previously synthesized antibodies are not able to recognize the mutant, allowing its escape and proliferation.

F. Antigenic modulation (i.e., the loss of antigens involved in the recognition of infected cells by the immune system) seems to play an important pathogenic role in subacute sclerosing panencephalitis (SSPE), a progressive degenerative neurological disease caused by the measles virus. SSPE patients have high titers of antibodies to several viral antigens, but measles virus cannot be directly recovered from the brains of infected patients. It has been shown that the infected brain cells do not express viral antigens on the membrane, although large amounts of viral polypeptides and glycoproteins are found in the cytoplasm.

1. The lack of expression of viral antigens by infected cells could be a consequence of antigenic modulation induced by suboptimal concentrations of antiviral antibody. *In vitro,* suboptimal concentrations of anti-measles hemagglutinin antibody induce shedding of hemagglutinin from the membrane of infected cells.
2. The amount of antibody needed to induce antigenic modulation (10 molecules/cell) is approximately 1/50 of the amount needed to cause complement-mediated lysis and 1/5 of the amount needed to induce ADCC.

G. Inhibition of immune effector mechanisms

1. Several poxviruses release soluble molecules homologous to the interferon and tumor necrosis factor-α (TNF-α) receptors, known as **viroceptors.** These proteins block the antiviral effects of the cytokines.
2. A major secretory protein encoded by vaccinia virus has been found to be homologous to a C4 inhibitory protein; therefore, it is capable of preventing the progression of the classical pathway of complement activation.
3. HBV induces the synthesis of large quantities of soluble surface antigen (HbsAg) by the infected host cells. The circulating HBsAg blocks antiviral antibodies before they reach the infective particles, acting as a "deflector shield" to protect the virus from neutralizing antibodies.

PART V

CLINICAL VIROLOGY

Chapter 29

Diagnosis of Viral Infections

John Manos

I. CULTURE AND ISOLATION is the gold standard in viral diagnosis, but it has some major drawbacks, such as the time that it takes for many viruses to replicate (several days to weeks for some viruses) and the risk of infection of laboratory personnel.

A. Culture. Because viruses do not grow on artificial media, viruses must be cultured on cell cultures or some other type of **living system.**

1. **Embryonated eggs.** Inoculation of embryonated eggs is used for growing some viruses, such as mumps and influenza viruses. (The influenza vaccine is obtained from virus grown in the allantoic cavity of embryonated eggs, which is why individuals who are allergic to eggs may not be candidates for vaccination.)
2. **Laboratory animals.** In the past, mice and chimpanzees were inoculated with viruses, but inoculation of laboratory animals has been largely replaced by the use of cell cultures.
3. **Cell cultures.** Growing viruses on cell cultures is the most widely used isolation technique. Cultures of monkey kidney cells were the first to be developed, and poliovirus was one of the first viruses to be grown on kidney cell cultures. With time, cell culture systems were developed that allowed isolation and growth of a variety of viruses, making studies of viral replication, the development of attenuated mutant strains, and the development of vaccines possible.
   - **a. Types**
     - **(1) Primary cultures** are prepared with freshly isolated cells, cannot be subcultured, and need to be used within 2–3 weeks.
     - **(2) Diploid cultures** are prepared with cells that can be subcultured twenty to thirty times.
     - **(3) Heteroploid cultures** are prepared from immortalized cell lines that can be subcultured indefinitely.
   - **b. Permissiveness.** Not all viruses will grow in all cell lines; a virus will only infect and replicate in a cell that carries the proper receptor for the virus. Thus, when trying to isolate an unknown virus, the specimen is inoculated on three or four cell lines with the hope that at least one of them will be permissive for the unknown virus.
   - **c. Detecting viral growth in cell cultures**
     - **(1) Observation of cytopathogenic effects.** Cytopathogenic effects are seen in cell monolayers as a consequence of viral replication. The changes can be suggestive of infection by a family or group of families, but in general do not allow determination of the species of virus involved with certainty. For example:
       - **(a)** Herpesviruses will induce **loss of architecture** and **rounding of cells** in the cell monolayer in 24–48 hours.
       - **(b)** Paramyxoviruses (measles virus, respiratory syncytial virus) cause the cells of the monolayer to coalesce into large multinucleated **syncytia** in 3–5 days. Syncytia are formed by membrane fusion of neighboring infected and noninfected cells.
       - **(c)** Cytomegalovirus (CMV) causes the appearance of characteristic **foci of cell lysis** in 2–3 weeks.
       - **(d)** Viruses may cause the appearance of **inclusion bodies** in infected cells. Inclusion bodies are visible by conventional microscopy after adequate staining; the location and appearance of the inclusion bodies can provide information about the infecting virus.
     - **(2) Hemadsorption.** Enveloped viruses may replicate and exit infected cells with-

out causing visible morphologic changes in infected cells; however, in some cases, the virus inserts hemagglutinins in the cell membrane. The presence of hemagglutinins allows the virus to be detected indirectly through the technique of hemadsorption, which consists of adding a suspension of red blood cells to a cell culture 3–5 days after inoculation with suspected material. If a hemadsorbing virus infects the monolayer, the red blood cells will be adsorbed to the cell surface through the viral hemagglutinins, giving the cells a grape-like, clustered appearance.

(3) **Hemagglutination** can be used to detect a virus carrying hemagglutinins in its envelope after the virus is shed into the culture medium. If the virus is present in the medium and the medium is mixed with red blood cells, the virus will cross-link the red cells and cause agglutination.

(4) **Cytopathogenic effect interference** can be used to detect the growth of viruses that do not cause morphologic changes in the infected cells, but that will prevent infection of the cell line with a second virus that produces characteristic cytopathogenic effects. A classic example is the interference of rubella virus with echovirus. A cell line inoculated with rubella virus will look normal 10–12 days after inoculation. If an echovirus, which normally produces cytopathogenic effects, is inoculated in a cell line that has previously been inoculated with rubella virus, no cytopathogenic effects will be observed.

B. Isolation. The precise identification of a virus growing in culture requires additional testing.

1. **Morphologic examination** is only possible by electron microscopy, which is technically difficult and expensive, and may not lead to successful identification of the virus.

2. **Serologic techniques.** In most cases, serologic techniques are used to precisely identify the virus.

   a. **Neutralization** is performed by mixing a known antibody with the unknown virus recovered from the cell culture medium. After incubating the antibody–virus mixture, it is inoculated into a fresh cell culture. A lack of cytopathogenic effects indicates that the unknown virus was neutralized by the known antibody, allowing identification of the virus.

   b. **Hemadsorption inhibition** can be used to identify a virus that causes hemadsorption to infected cells. Medium from the culture is mixed with antibody to a specific virus and the mixture is added to a fresh cell culture. After appropriate incubation, the second culture is tested for hemadsorption. A negative result means that the antibody reacted with the virus, allowing identification of the virus.

   c. **Cytopathogenic effects interference inhibition** can be used to confirm the identity of a virus that has interfered with the infection of a cell line by a virus that normally causes cytopathogenic effects. Specific antibody to the interfering virus (e.g., rubella virus, if this is the suspected identity of the interfering virus) is added to medium obtained from the cell culture and the mixture is used to inoculate a second culture; after 1–2 days, the cytopathic virus (e.g., the echovirus) is added to the second culture. If cytopathogenic effects are observed, it can be concluded that the first culture was infected with the interfering virus against which the antiserum was directed.

   d. **Direct immunofluorescence** is the preferred technique because of its speed, specificity, and relative simplicity. For example, while identification of CMV by cytopathogenic effects inhibition takes 2–3 weeks, CMV can be detected with fluorescent monoclonal antibodies in an infected cell culture as soon as 24 hours after inoculation. If a cell culture has been inoculated with a given specimen and there is evidence of viral multiplication in the culture, the virus can be identified by adding a fluorescent monoclonal antibody to the suspected virus to a scraping obtained from the infected culture. After a relatively short incubation period, followed by washing to eliminate unreacted antiserum, the scraping is observed under the fluorescent microscope. If the cells fluoresce, the virus in question has infected the monolayer.

e. **Immuno-electron microscopy** can be used for the precise identification of a virus visualized by electron microscopy. For example, herpesviruses can be easily visualized by electron microscopy, but precise identification of the virus (e.g., as herpes simplex, varicella-zoster, CMV, or Epstein-Barr) is not possible on a morphologic basis alone. Immuno-electron microscopy uses a specific antibody labeled with an electrodense tag to specifically identify the virus. Unfortunately, this technique is expensive and slower than the conventional immunofluorescence technique.

II. SEROLOGY.

In many cases, it is simpler to establish the identity of a virus indirectly, by testing the presence of specific antibodies in the patient's blood.

A. General considerations

1. **Total antibody assays versus solid-phase immunoassays**
   a. **Total antibody assays** do not allow distinction between antibodies produced in response to an acute infection and residual antibodies from a previous infection from which the patient has recovered. Because diagnosis usually requires verification of a significant rise in the titer of specific antibodies to a suspected virus on two samples, the first one collected when the patient is ill with a suspected viral disease and the second collected when the patient is convalescent (in 2–3 weeks), the diagnosis is usually retrospective and has mainly epidemiologic value.
   b. **Solid-phase immunoassays (enzymoimmunoassays, radioimmunoassays)** allow distinction of IgG antibodies from IgM antibodies. The finding of increased concentrations of specific IgM antiviral antibodies is considered evidence of a recent infection, and the results can be valuable for the management of the patient.
2. **Practical guidelines**
   a. Blood samples should be obtained as soon after the onset of illness as possible, and then 2–3 weeks later.
      (1) It is of paramount importance to **submit two samples.** The test is unlikely to be run until the convalescent sample is submitted, because, in most cases, a single antibody titer does not discriminate recent exposure from past exposure.
      (2) A fourfold or greater increase in antibody titer between the two samples strongly suggests that the patient was infected at the time the first sample was drawn.
   b. **The virus that is suspected of causing the disease must be indicated** on samples sent to the laboratory for analysis.

B. Techniques

1. **Hemagglutination inhibition** is a technique specially suited for the measurement of antibodies directed against hemagglutinating viruses, such as influenza viruses. An infected patient will produce antibodies to the viral hemagglutinins, which can be detected by their ability to inhibit viral hemagglutination.
2. **Complement fixation** is the mainstay for serologic diagnosis of viral diseases and for some viruses, this is the only technique available to confirm a diagnosis. Complement fixation is a time-consuming test that requires trained personnel for its proper execution, and it can only detect complement-fixing antibodies (i.e., IgG and IgM). Complement fixation cannot differentiate between IgG and IgM antibodies.

3. **Direct immunofluorescence** can be used to confirm the diagnosis of a viral infection if a sample of infected tissue and a fluorescein-conjugated antiviral antibody are available. The labeled antiserum is incubated with the tissue sample, and then unbound antibody is washed away. Examination under a fluorescent microscope permits identification of the virus.

4. **Enzyme immunoassay (EIA)** has largely replaced most other immunoassays because of its relative simplicity, specificity, and versatility.

   a. **EIA can be adapted to allow detection of either antigen or antibody.** Although total antibody assays by EIA suffer from the same pitfalls as other serologic assays, particularly the need for repeated assays, EIA can be easily adapted to the assay of specific IgM antibodies, which are indicative of recent exposure. Antigen assays, although not as widely available, have the advantage of allowing the rapid diagnosis of a viral infection. Some antigen-detection assays have been adapted into rapid and easy-to-perform diagnostic procedures that take 5–10 minutes to run with minimal equipment.

      (1) **To measure antibody,** a known antigen is adsorbed to a solid phase (e.g., a test tube, microtiter plate well, disc, magnetic sphere) and then proper dilutions of the patient's sera are incubated with the antigen-coated solid phase. If there are antibodies in the patient's sera, they will attach to the antigen. After washing unreacted immunoglobulins off of the solid phase, an enzyme-labeled anti-human antibody is added to the solid phase. The unreacted antibody is washed off and a substrate is added to the solid phase. The enzyme-labeled antibody binds to the patient's antibody that has reacted with the immobilized antigen. After washing off unreacted labeled antibody, a chromogenic substrate is added and the intensity of color (proportional to the quantity of antibody present in the patient's serum) is measured using a spectrophotometer.

      (2) **To measure antigen,** a specific antibody is adsorbed to the solid phase. The patient's serum is added, and if viral particles or viral antigens are in the circulation, they will be bound by the immobilized antibody. After washing the solid phase, enzyme-labeled antibody of the same specificity as that adsorbed to the solid phase is added. After incubating and washing off unbound reactants, a chromogenic substrate is added. A positive reaction is reflected by the development of color.

   b. **Western blot (immunoblot)** is the most widely used confirmatory technique for a positive HIV antibody enzyme immunoassay. The technique has three main steps:

      (1) Electrophoresis is used to separate HIV antigens on polyacrylamide gel, which, due to its sieving properties, separates viral antigens by size. Electrophoresis is followed by blotting onto a nitrocellulose membrane.

      (2) The blotted nitrocellulose membrane is then overlaid with the patient's serum.

      (3) After washing off unbound proteins, an enzyme-labeled anti-human immunoglobulin antiserum is placed over the membrane. The labeled antibody binds to any antibody captured by the viral antigens, and when a chromogenic substrate is finally added, the antigen–antibody complexes are revealed as stained bands.

III. DNA HYBRIDIZATION is based on the detection of viral genomes through hybridization with a complementary strand.

A. In its simplest form, the ability of viral DNA to hybridize with a labeled complementary strand of DNA is tested. (The specificity of the test is directly proportional to the length of the complementary strand.) A variety of tags (e.g., enzymes, radioactive material) can be coupled to the complementary strand, but detection of hybridization usually requires electrophoretic separation on a sieving gel. Electrophoretic separation allows comparison of the mobility of the complementary DNA by itself versus that of the complementary DNA–viral DNA complex.

B. **Polymerase chain reaction (PCR)** increases the sensitivity of DNA hybridization by increasing the amount of viral DNA obtained from the patient. This approach is useful when a rapid response is necessary and the amount of viral DNA likely to be present in the patient's sample is small.

Chapter 30

DNA Viruses I: Herpesviruses

John Manos

I. INTRODUCTION

A. Human pathogenic viruses of the herpes group are listed in Table 30-1. As a group, these viruses are the most common causes of human viral infection.

B. The general characteristics of the herpesviruses are summarized in Table 30-2.

II. HERPES SIMPLEX VIRUS (HSV). There are two types of HSV: **HSV-1** and **HSV-2.**

A. Pathogenesis and clinical disease

1. **Pathogenesis.** The virus invades the cutaneous vascular endothelium, causing epithelial cell necrosis and inflammation and leading to the formation of vesicles. The incubation period is usually 5–6 days.
   a. **Primary infection.** The virus replicates actively in skin or mucosal vesicular lesions but is not eliminated.
   b. **Latent infection.** Following primary infection with HSV, the virus becomes localized in the **sensory ganglia,** either the **trigeminal ganglion** (HSV-1) or the **sacral ganglion** (HSV-2), where it remains latent. Individuals with latent infection remain seropositive for the rest of their lives.
   c. **Recurrences** may occur frequently or not at all, depending on the individual. Trigger mechanisms may include **fever, colds, sunlight, menses, certain foods,** and **stress.** Two theories have been proposed to explain latency and the emergence of recurrences.
      (1) **Static theory.** This theory postulates that the virus exists in the ganglia, possibly integrated in the host cell's DNA. Different stimuli induce viral replication, and the viral progeny propagate centrifugally through the neuraxon to the skin nerve endings. From these nerve endings, the virus propagates to the epidermal cells, replicates actively, and causes the appearance of vesicular lesions.
      (2) **Dynamic theory.** This theory postulates that the virus is constantly replicating at low rates and constantly traveling down the neuraxon to the skin. However, the number of viral particles normally reaching the skin is too low for a vesicular lesion to develop. Exposure to trigger mechanisms enhances viral replication, causing larger numbers of viruses to travel down the neuraxons, and leading to the development of vesicular lesions.

2. **Clinical disease.** Generally, HSV-1 causes perioral lesions, whereas HSV-2 causes genital lesions. Both viruses cause vesicular lesions and can usually be recovered from the vesicles.
   a. **Herpetic gingivostomatitis**
      (1) **Primary herpetic gingivostomatitis** (see also Chapter 56 III E). The vesiculoulcerative lesions typical of primary herpetic gingivostomatitis tend to be localized at the level of the mucocutaneous junctions in the perioral region and are associated with a high fever and dysphagia. Recovery is usually complete and uneventful after 7–10 days.
      (2) **Recurrent herpetic gingivostomatitis.** After primary infection, the virus will re-

TABLE 30-1. Herpesviruses Pathogenic to Humans

Herpes simplex virus (HSV), types 1 and 2
Varicella-zoster virus
Epstein-Barr virus
Cytomegalovirus (CMV)
Human herpesvirus-6 (HHV-6)

main latent for life but episodically will cause recurrent eruptions in some individuals, often coinciding with fever **(fever blisters).** In a given individual, fever blisters tend to recur in the same general location.

b. Genital herpes. Recovery from primary infection is usually complete, but recurrent episodes of vesicular lesions with the same general distribution are frequent.

c. Complications

(1) Encephalitis is a demyelinating disease of rapid progression. Patients first show personality aberrations and then develop localized neurologic signs. Early diagnosis and treatment with intravenous acyclovir is essential for survival. Once the patient has become semicomatose, therapy is usually ineffective and the patient dies.

(2) Meningitis is usually mild and most patients recover without sequelae.

(3) Keratitis is the most common cause of **corneal blindness** in the United States. The lesion takes the appearance of a dendritic ulcer. It eventually heals, but may leave scars that can impair vision if they are located over the pupil. Herpes keratitis tends to be recurrent and as a result of repeated scarring, the cornea becomes clouded.

(4) Eczema herpeticum (Kaposi's varicelliform eruption) is the appearance of herpetic lesions at the sites of preexisting eczematous lesions.

B. Transmission in the absence of active fever blisters or genital lesions is considered possible, but exceptional.

1. Direct contact with vesicular discharge

a. Transmission of mucocutaneous herpes usually occurs via person-to-person contact when active lesions are present. (Fever blisters are fairly contagious.) Transmission can also occur through contact with contaminated objects.

b. Genital herpes is also usually transmitted by direct contact between an uninfected individual and one with active lesions. Venereal transmission is facilitated by the fact that women may have asymptomatic intravaginal lesions.

2. Sexual transmission via semen is believed to be possible.

3. Perinatal transmission can occur when the mother has an outbreak of vaginal herpes at the time of delivery. Passage through an infected birth canal is the most common mechanism of transmission, but the virus may spread to the fetus *in utero,* perhaps through a small hole in the amniotic membrane or if the membranes rupture prematurely. Lesions develop in the newborn 5–10 days later. Perinatal transmission can often be avoided by delivering the baby via caesarian section.

4. Congenital transmission. HSV is very rarely transmitted across the placenta. In order

TABLE 30-2. General Characteristics of the Herpesviruses

Double-stranded DNA
Nucleocapsid with icosahedral or cubic symmetry
Surrounded by an envelope derived from the nuclear membrane
Latency

for congenital transmission to occur, the mother must be viremic, which only occurs if she is primarily infected during pregnancy. Infection early in the course of the pregnancy places the infant at risk for microcephaly and organomegaly.

C. Diagnosis

1. **Clinical diagnosis.** In most cases of mucocutaneous herpes, the diagnosis is established clinically based on the typical vesicular lesions. However, in some cases, the lesions may not be obvious and diagnosis may be critical. This is particularly true in the case of a pregnant woman with a history of genital herpes who is approaching term.

2. **Laboratory diagnosis**
   a. **Microscopic examination** of a scraping from the base of a vesicle may reveal **Tzanck cells,** giant multinucleated cells with intranuclear inclusions that push the chromatin to the margins. These cells are relatively easy to detect in Pap smears or smears of vaginal exudates from women with genital HSV infections.
   b. **Culture and isolation.** Culture of material from suspicious lesions is indicated in women who have had a history of genital herpes, or who develop a suspicious genital lesion at any time during gestation. HSV grows rapidly in a variety of cell lines. It should be noted, however, that culture may not help to decide whether to proceed with natural birth or to perform a caesarian section because the result of isolation may be negative one day and positive the next.
   c. **Serology**
      (1) In cases of suspected **herpes encephalitis,** confirmation of the diagnosis requires examination of biopsied brain tissue by **direct immunofluorescence** using specific monoclonal antibodies to detect viral particles in the biopsied tissue.
      (2) Serologic tests for IgM antibody are available.

D. **Treatment** depends on the clinical situation. Uncomplicated fever blisters and genital lesions are self-limiting; their evolution does not seem to be changed by antiviral therapy.

1. **Acyclovir** is indicated for all serious HSV infections (e.g., generalized infection, herpes encephalitis, and infections in immunocompromised patients). Acyclovir can be administered orally or parenterally, and therapy should be initiated within 72 hours. An ointment for topical therapy of common herpetic lesions is available as well.

2. **Famciclovir** can be given orally with less frequency than acyclovir and seems to be better tolerated.

III. VARICELLA-ZOSTER VIRUS

A. **Pathogenesis and clinical disease.** Varicella-zoster virus is the etiologic agent of **chickenpox (varicella)** and of **shingles (herpes zoster).**

1. **Pathogenesis.** The mechanism of vesicle formation is the same as that for HSV.
   a. **Chickenpox** is always seen as a consequence of a **primary infection.** The incubation period is usually 13 days, but varies from 10–21 days.
   b. **Shingles** is believed to result from the **reactivation of the virus,** which remains latent for life in the sensory ganglia of patients who had chickenpox. The trigger mechanisms that provoke the development of shingles are not well understood, but reactivations are often seen in cancer patients, patients taking immunosuppressive drugs, and trauma patients.

2. **Clinical disease**
   a. **Chickenpox** is a highly contagious childhood disease.
      (1) The **vesicular rash** of chickenpox (see also Chapter 56 II A) typically shows le-

sions at different stages of development. The lesions begin as small red spots (papular lesions), then vesiculate and finally crust over and heal without scarring. The number of lesions in a chickenpox rash can be minimal, in which case the diagnosis may be difficult.

(2) **Complications.** In children, the disease usually follows a benign course, but in adults, the disease is more severe and may be life-threatening to immunocompromised individuals.

(a) **Reye's syndrome** may occur in children following varicella-zoster virus infection.

(b) **Large-cell pneumonia** may be seen in immunocompromised individuals.

(c) **Postinfectious encephalitis** or **meningitis** can occur in immunocompromised as well as immunocompetent patients.

b. **Shingles** (see also Chapter 56 III B)

(1) The **vesicular rash** occurs in a dermatomal distribution and is most often seen on the chest, but it may be located anywhere. The vesicles have a sharply demarcated border that is not seen in other types of herpes lesions. The rash is very painful; in some cases, the pain precedes the rash, making diagnosis difficult.

(2) **Recurrences** of shingles have been reported, but are unusual.

(3) **Complications** include **keratouveitis** if the ophthalmic branch of cranial nerve V is involved.

B. **Transmission.** Varicella-zoster virus usually spreads by the **respiratory route,** although the vesicles are infectious and **transmission through vesicular fluid** can occur. Susceptible children who have close contact with a patient with herpes zoster may develop chickenpox.

C. **Diagnosis** is usually established clinically. When confirmation is deemed necessary, two options are available:

1. **Microscopic examination** of material obtained from lesions (including bronchoalveolar lavage from patients with pneumonia) may show **Tzanck cells.**

2. **Culture and isolation** is easy and may be the only way to establish a diagnosis, particularly when the infection is generalized.

D. **Treatment** is usually supportive. **Acyclovir** is used in severe cases, such as when the infection becomes disseminated.

E. **Immunoprophylaxis.** A live, attenuated vaccine for chickenpox is available and is recommended for all children, starting at 1 year of age.

IV. EPSTEIN-BARR VIRUS

A. Pathogenesis and clinical disease

1. **Pathogenesis.** Epstein-Barr virus targets the B lymphocytes, which carry the CR2 molecule, a specific receptor for the virus. The virus remains latent for years (possibly for life) in the B lymphocytes of infected individuals.

2. **Clinical disease**

a. **Infectious mononucleosis** is the most common manifestation of acute Epstein-Barr virus infection in the United States and most other industrialized countries. The infection is frequently subclinical in children, whereas college students and young adults tend to be symptomatic.

(1) **Acute mononucleosis.** Patients present with an acute exudative pharyngitis, disseminated lymphadenopathy (typically in the submandibular region), fever, and, occasionally, a faint maculopapular (morbilliform) rash. Some patients

only complain of lethargy and moderate fever in the afternoon. Recovery may be slow and relapses can occur; however, recurrences are rare.

(2) **Chronic Epstein-Barr virus infection** is diagnosed in cases with an evolution period that exceeds 6 months. Epstein-Barr virus has been suggested to be the cause of the **chronic fatigue syndrome,** characterized by unexplained fatigue and depression.

b. **Burkitt's lymphoma** is a peculiar type of lymphoma, localized to the soft tissues surrounding the jaw. In Africa, Burkitt's lymphoma is strongly associated with Epstein-Barr virus infection, although there is no evidence for the presence of this virus in the tissues of similar lymphomas that affect American patients.

c. **Nasopharyngeal carcinoma,** prevalent among Asian men, is also strongly associated with the Epstein-Barr virus.

B. Transmission.

Epstein-Barr virus is spread predominantly via respiratory secretions, mainly through oral contact. The virus can also be transmitted through blood transfusions and venereally.

C. Diagnosis

1. **Blood work.** In patients with infectious mononucleosis, the **complete blood count and differential** often show atypical lymphocytes (e.g., T lymphoblasts, precursors of cytotoxic T cells involved in a reaction against infected B cells). However, other viral infections, including hepatitis B virus (HBV) infection, may cause similar changes.

2. **Serology** is most often used to confirm the diagnosis.

a. The **monospot test** is based on the detection of cross-reactive heterophile antibodies that agglutinate horse erythrocytes. The test is cheap and fast, but is not entirely specific for infectious mononucleosis. In addition, positivity does not distinguish between recent mononucleosis and mononucleosis acquired in the past.

b. **Epstein-Barr virus–specific antibody tests** detect specific antibodies to **viral capsid antigen (VCA), early antigens (EA),** and **Epstein-Barr nuclear antigen (EBNA).**

(1) **VCA antibody test.** This test can discriminate among IgG, IgA, and IgM antibodies.

(a) A positive VCA-IgM antibody test indicates recent infection with the Epstein-Barr virus.

(b) A positive VCA-IgA antibody test is associated with nasopharyngeal carcinoma.

(2) **EA antibody test.** Early antigens are found in Burkitt's lymphoma and nasopharyngeal carcinoma.

(3) **EBNA antibody test.** A positive test is indicative of past infection.

D. Treatment

Treatment is supportive.

V. CYTOMEGALOVIRUS (CMV)

A. Pathogenesis and clinical disease

1. **Pathogenesis.** CMV is a prevalent virus that causes minimal symptoms or asymptomatic infection in otherwise healthy adults, but may cause severe disease when the immune system is not well developed or compromised. Polymorphs, monocytes, B lymphocytes, and epithelial cells may all be latently infected.

2. **Clinical disease.** Primary infection is usually subclinical; therefore, epidemiologic studies are difficult. Clinical disease is most often seen under the following conditions:

a. **Following transfusion or transplantation.** Some patients develop a **mononucleosis-like syndrome** caused by CMV after receiving multiple transfusions or an organ transplant. The infection may become disseminated and life-threatening if the patient is immunocompromised. Patients who are seronegative for CMV should receive blood and organs from seronegative donors.

b. In the setting of immunosuppression. CMV can be recovered from more than 90% of immunosuppressed patients (particularly those that are taking immunosuppressive drugs following organ transplantation).

(1) CMV infection can present as fever, pneumonia, esophagitis, enteritis, hepatitis, retinitis, uveitis—virtually any type of infection. The development of CMV hepatitis in a patient with a liver transplant is difficult to differentiate from rejection because there are no reliable laboratory tests on which this differentiation can be based.

(2) CMV can exist in a latent form in the transplanted organ and the infection may be reactivated after the patient is immunosuppressed. Because of the tropism the virus exhibits for the kidneys, kidney infections are common. Reactivation of the virus may impair the survival of the transplanted kidney.

c. In neonates. CMV infection is estimated to occur in 1% of all neonates. Given the immaturity of the immune system at birth, neonates are particularly susceptible to CMV infection.

(1) Transfusion of CMV-positive blood to a neonate may be followed by **disseminated infection,** including hepatitis, pneumonia, eye infections, and central nervous system (CNS) involvement.

(2) Some evidence suggests that children infected during the neonatal period, even if apparently asymptomatic, may be later diagnosed as **autistic** or may develop **personality problems,** a variety of **mild mental abnormalities,** or both.

B. Transmission

1. **Respiratory route.** Although this virus is usually excreted in large amounts in the urine, it is believed that it is transmitted by the respiratory route.

2. **Venereal transmission** has also been suggested.

3. **Perinatal transmission.** CMV can be acquired following passage through the birth canal of an infected mother.

4. **Congenital transmission** is rare but when it occurs, is rather severe (particularly when the mother is infected during the first trimester). The newborn may show chorioretinitis or hydrocephalus with periventricular calcification (the latter is also a feature of congenital toxoplasmosis). Infection may be associated with a rash and hepatosplenomegaly.

C. Diagnosis

1. **Optical microscopic examination** of stained smears of urinary sediment and stained kidney biopsy tissue may show cells with a dark intranuclear inclusion surrounded by a clear halo **(owl-eye inclusion).** These cells are fairly typical of CMV infection.

2. **Culture and isolation** is the gold standard of diagnosis. Urine is the most widely used source of CMV in most patients, given the tropism that the virus has for the kidneys.

3. **Serology** is widely used for the diagnosis of congenital infections. In cases of suspected congenital infection, it is usual to order a panel of tests known as **TORCH** [**T**oxoplasmosis, **O**ther (e.g., syphilis), **R**ubella, **C**ytomegalovirus, **H**SV]. TORCH titers are obtained in the mother and the child; an infected child will have titers to one of these agents that is considerably higher than that of the mother. The tests currently included in the TORCH panel are often able to distinguish between IgM and IgG antibodies, the former indicating fetal infection (IgM is not transported across the placenta).

D. Treatment. Ganciclovir and foscarnet are the drugs of choice. These drugs are mostly indicated for the treatment of CMV infections in immunocompromised patients.

VI. HUMAN HERPESVIRUS-6 (HHV-6, HBLV).

HUMAN HERPESVIRUS-6 (HHV-6, HBLV). Because HHV-6 was first isolated from the peripheral blood of patients with B-cell lymphoma, it was designated human B cell lymphotropic virus, or HBLV. However, this designation is not accurate because the virus can infect a variety of other cells.

A. Clinical disease

1. **B-cell lymphoma.** Integrated DNA sequences with homology to the HHV-6 genome are detected in many B cell lymphomas, although a precise etiologic role has not been elucidated.
2. **Roseola infantum (exanthema subitum),** a benign exanthematous disease of childhood, is caused by HHV-6 (see Chapter 56 II C).
3. **Chronic fatigue syndrome.** HHV-6 has been implicated as a possible etiologic agent for chronic fatigue syndrome. Antibodies to HHV-6 have been detected in these patients. However, up to 90% of healthy individuals have positive HHV-6 serologies.

B. Epidemiology

1. **Prevalence.** Serologic studies have revealed that this virus is ubiquitous. Infection seems to take place during the first few months of life. By adulthood, the rate of positivity is 80%–90%.
2. **Transmission.** The mechanism of transmission is unknown.

Chapter 31

DNA Viruses II: Papovaviruses

John Manos

I. INTRODUCTION. There are two serologically distinct genera of human pathogenic papovaviruses: **papillomaviruses** and **polyomaviruses.** Both are naked DNA viruses, with the capability of transforming cells *in vitro.*

II. PAPILLOMAVIRUSES. There are many species of papillomaviruses. Some infect animals and others infect humans, but all of them have special tropism for the skin and mucosae. Diversity among human papillomaviruses can be recognized serologically as well as at the DNA level. More than 60 distinct genotypes have been identified by DNA hybridization techniques.

A. Epidemiology

1. **Prevalence.** Infection with papillomaviruses is common and often asymptomatic. It is estimated that 20%–60% of adults in the United States are infected, and according to some statistics, genital infection may be the most common viral venereal disease.
2. **Transmission.** Papillomaviruses are transmitted by direct contact, through minor abrasions, sexually, and perinatally.

B. Clinical disease depends on the interplay between the type of papillomavirus (Table 31-1), the location of the infection, and the effectiveness of the host's antiviral defense mechanisms.

1. **Skin warts** can occur anywhere, but the most common site is on the hands. Children and young adults tend to be affected most often. In immunocompromised individuals, warts may become widespread.
2. **Genital warts** are also common. After venereal transmission of the virus, the incubation period is long and variable (ranging from several weeks to several months). In some cases, the virus will cause minimal lesions that may go undetected but are still infectious. In other cases, the lesions become vegetative and very obvious **(condyloma acuminatum).**
3. **Cervical carcinoma** can evolve in patients with genital warts. Papillomavirus genomes can be demonstrated by *in situ* hybridization techniques in the vast majority of cervical carcinomas, irrespective of the stage.
4. **Laryngeal warts** are rare. Children younger than 5 years of age are most commonly affected following perinatal transmission of the virus. After a few months or years, the child develops vocal cord papillomas that can eventually hinder speaking and breathing. Treatment usually involves surgical excision, but the lesions recur and with repeated surgery, permanent damage of the vocal cords may result.
5. **Epidermodysplasia verruciformis** is a very rare, lifelong disease, with onset during infancy or early childhood. The disease is characterized by multiple, polymorphic, wart-like lesions widely distributed throughout the body. The lesions tend to become confluent. One-third of patients develop multiple foci of malignant transformation in the plaques (particularly on areas exposed to sunlight). Eventually the lesions evolve into squamous cell carcinomas, which are slow-growing and do not tend to metasta-

TABLE 31-1. Clinical Diseases Caused by Papillomaviruses and Associated Genotypes

Disease	Associated Genotypes
Skin warts	1, 2, 4, 10
Genital warts (including condyloma acuminatum)	6, 11, 16, 18, 31
Epidermodysplasia verruciformis	5, 8
Cervical carcinoma	16, 18, 31, 33, 35
Laryngeal warts	6, 11

size. Genetic, and possibly immunologic, host factors seem to determine the abnormal pathogenicity of the papillomavirus genotypes associated with this disease, which are seldom recovered from normal individuals.

C. Diagnosis is usually clinical because the virus does not grow in conventional tissue cultures and serology tests are not useful—the viruses are immunogenic, but the levels of antibodies are low, making antibody measurement impractical. In the case of genital warts, confirmation by *in situ* hybridization using a probe for the viral DNA may be indicated.

D. Treatment depends on the type of lesion.

1. **Skin warts.** Most benign warts regress spontaneously, but removal using chemicals (e.g., salicylic acid, tincture of iodine, formaldehyde, acetone), freezing, or cauterization may be indicated for cosmetic reasons. Recurrences are frequent. Surgery should be avoided because a satellite wart may occur at the incision site at a later time.

2. **Venereal warts** can also be treated with a variety of agents, including laser therapy, freezing, interferon-α (IFN-α), podophyllin, and surgery. Refractory warts may respond to administration of an autogenous vaccine prepared from an extract of the patient's own wart tissue.

3. **Premalignant and malignant lesions** are usually treated surgically.

III. POLYOMAVIRUSES include several animal viruses, including simian virus 40 (SV40), and two human viruses, the BK virus and the JC virus (see Chapter 27 II A).

A. BK virus

1. **Epidemiology.** The BK virus infects children early in life. By the age of 3 or 4 years, 50% of children have antibodies to BK virus and by the age of 10 years, 100% of the children have seroconverted.

2. **Pathogenesis and clinical disease.** Primary infection is not associated with recognizable clinical symptoms, although some clinicians think BK virus may be associated with mild upper respiratory tract infections. The virus tends to infect renal epithelial cells, where it remains latent. Reactivation can occur in immunocompromised patients (e.g., renal transplant patients receiving immunosuppressive drugs).

B. JC virus

1. **Epidemiology**
   a. **Prevalence.** The JC virus is also prevalent, but seropositivity in the adult population usually does not exceed 75%.
   b. **Transmission.** The route of transmission is unclear, but is most likely respiratory or fecal-oral.

2. Pathogenesis and clinical disease

a. Pathogenesis. Primary infection is not associated with illness. After the primary infection, the virus remains latent, but may become reactivated in immunocompromised patients.

b. Clinical disease. Progressive multifocal leukoencephalopathy (PML) is a rare, slowly degenerative neurologic disease that is usually fatal (see Chapter 50 III).

Chapter 32

DNA Viruses III: Adenoviruses, Poxviruses, and Parvoviruses

John Manos

I. ADENOVIRUSES were first isolated in 1953 from adenoidal and tonsillar tissue.

A. General characteristics

1. **Structure.** Adenoviruses are naked, icosahedral, and contain a double-stranded DNA genome.

2. **Serotypes.** There are over 40 antigenically distinct serotypes. Approximately half of the serotypes are not known to cause disease in humans. Some serotypes have transforming properties, but an association with human malignancy has not been established.

B. Epidemiology

1. **Prevalence.** Adenoviruses are ubiquitous, widely distributed viruses. The first infection usually takes place early in life. By the age of 10 years, virtually everybody has been infected with one or another adenovirus.

2. **Transmission.** The viruses are spread person-to-person by aerosol droplets; crowding facilitates transmission. Adenoviruses can also infect the eyes by direct contact.

C. Pathogenesis and clinical disease

1. **Pathogenesis**
   a. **Portal of entry.** Symptoms are caused by the local spread of infection on the upper respiratory mucosa, which is the portal of entry for the virus. Viremia occurs after the onset of symptoms, but it is inconsequential.
   b. The **incubation period** is 4–5 days.
   c. **Types of infection.** Adenoviruses can cause three kinds of infections at the cellular level:
      (1) **Lytic infection.** Following infection of a permissive cell, the virus actively replicates; rupture of the host cell membrane releases the progeny particles and causes the cell to die. For every infected cell, between 10,000 to 1 million virus particles are released, but only 1%–5% are infectious.
      (2) **Persistent infection** occurs when viral replication is relatively slow and normal cell replication can compensate for the cells lost as a result of the infection. Persistent adenovirus infections are generally asymptomatic and chronic; eventually the infections resolve.
      (3) **Transforming infection** seems to be favored by conditions adverse to complete replication (e.g., marginally permissive host cells). The viral DNA is integrated into the host DNA; in adequate experimental systems, integration is associated with transformation.

2. **Clinical disease** is generally mild. In some individuals, the infection may be subclinical.
   a. **"Common cold."** One of the classic presentations is an acute upper respiratory infection that is indistinguishable from the common cold caused by rhinoviruses.
   b. **Lower respiratory tract infections (bronchiolitis, pneumonia)**
      (1) In infants, adenoviruses can cause lower respiratory tract infections that are indistinguishable from infections caused by parainfluenza type 3 virus and respiratory syncytial virus. The infection is particularly severe when adenoviruses of serotypes 1, 2, or 5 are involved.

(2) In young adults (particularly military recruits), adenoviruses may cause acute upper and lower respiratory disease, including pneumonia.

(3) In immunocompromised patients, adenoviruses may cause a severe form of pneumonia as well as encephalitis.

c. **Conjunctivitis.** Adenoviruses are a common cause of conjunctivitis. In older children, the conjunctivitis can be associated with pharyngitis **(pharyngoconjunctival fever).** The conjunctivitis usually starts unilaterally and then spreads to the other eye. Secondary bacterial infection is possible, and is usually evidenced by the formation of purulent secretions in the inflamed eye or eyes.

d. **Hemorrhagic cystitis** may be seen in older children infected with an adenovirus.

e. **Diarrhea** sometimes occurs in older children as a result of adenovirus infection.

f. **Meningoencephalitis** is a rare consequence of adenovirus infection in older children.

g. **Intussusception,** probably secondary to infection of the abdominal lymph nodes, is another rare manifestation of adenovirus infection in children. Intussusception may cause acute intestinal obstruction requiring emergency surgery and may be difficult to differentiate clinically from acute appendicitis.

h. **Epidemic keratoconjunctivitis** is an acute infection of the cornea and conjunctiva that tends to occur in individuals whose jobs predispose them to trauma (e.g, welders). It is usually a self-limited disease.

D. **Diagnosis** is usually clinical, and is strongly suggested by the finding of a preauricular adenopathy in a patient with upper respiratory infection. If indicated, confirmation can be achieved via culture and isolation (adenoviruses grow in conventional cell culture systems) or serology.

E. **Treatment** is usually supportive. In patients with conjunctivitis that becomes purulent, topical antibiotic treatment might be indicated.

F. **Prevention.** An oral live vaccine that contains the two most common serotypes responsible for acute respiratory disease is being used successfully by the military services.

II. POXVIRUSES

POXVIRUSES are a complex group of viruses that cause primarily vesicular lesions in the host.

A. **Structure.** Poxviruses, the largest animal viruses, are brick-shaped and nonenveloped. They have a protein-rich multilayered coat that makes them relatively resistant to disinfectants and antiseptics. The nucleic acid is double-stranded DNA, but, unlike the other DNA viruses, the entire replicative cycle takes place in the cytoplasm (see Chapter 23 III D).

B. **Diseases caused by orthopoxviruses.** Orthopoxviruses that cause disease in humans include **variola virus** (the etiologic agent of **smallpox),** the **vaccinia virus** (used for vaccination against smallpox), the **cowpox virus,** and the **monkeypox virus.**

1. Smallpox

a. **Epidemiology.** Smallpox was the first human disease for which effective immunoprophylaxis was developed (see Chapter 9 II A). The last case of recognized smallpox in the United States was reported in 1949, and the last known case of smallpox in the world was reported in 1977, in Somalia, Africa. A few years later, the World Health Organization (WHO) declared the world "smallpox-free" and vaccination of children was discontinued. Laboratory accidents pose the main problem now, but only a few designated laboratories are permitted to maintain virus stocks.

b. **Clinical disease.** Smallpox was a moderately contagious exanthematic disease that carried a high mortality rate. Evidence suggested the existence of two strains of the virus—one that caused **variola major,** the most serious form of the disease (with a mortality rate as high as 50%), and one that caused **variola minor (alastrim),** a milder disease with a mortality rate of less than 1%.

(1) After an average incubation period of 12 days, the patient developed prodromal symptoms (fever, myalgia, malaise).

(2) The rash of smallpox was vesicular, with lesions that were characteristically all at the same stage of development and centripetally distributed (i.e., they were more numerous on the extremities and face). The vesicular lesions eventually developed a scab, and often left a scar.

(3) Patients with variola major developed severe complications, including encephalitis and hemorrhagic forms of the disease associated with disseminated intravascular coagulation (DIC), mucosal bleeding, and general toxemia. Once these complications developed, the prognosis was very poor.

c. Diagnosis, which was usually clinical, was supported by the microscopic observation of cytoplasmic inclusion bodies known as **Guarnieri bodies** in infected epithelial cells. The virus can be grown in embryonated eggs and tissue culture.

2. Cowpox is characterized by vesicular lesions on the teats and udders of cattle. Humans can acquire cowpox through direct contact with lesions; clinical disease in humans most often entails vesicular lesions on the hands.

3. Monkeypox resembles smallpox clinically. There are a few known cases of humans contracting monkeypox from monkeys, but no transmission of monkeypox among humans has been documented.

C. Diseases caused by parapoxviruses. Parapoxviruses cause primarily zoonoses that can be transmitted to humans.

1. Pseudocowpox (milkers' nodule), which can be transmitted from cattle to humans, represents an occupational hazard for dairy workers. The disease is usually self-limiting and reinfection can occur.

2. Contagious pustular dermatitis (orf) is a disease of sheep and goats that can be transmitted to humans following close contact with infected animals.

D. Diseases caused by unclassified poxviruses. Molluscum contagiosum is a venereally transmitted disease caused by a poxvirus of the *Leporipox* genus, which includes viruses that usually infect rabbits. The virus is distributed worldwide and the infection is characterized by the appearance of papules that resolve spontaneously.

III. PARVOVIRUSES include the genus *Parvovirus* and the genus *Dependovirus.* Dependoviruses require a helper virus to replicate in a susceptible cell and are not known to be pathogenic for humans.

A. Structure. Parvoviruses, the smallest DNA viruses, are naked virions with a single-stranded negative DNA genome.

B. Epidemiology. Parvovirus-like agent (PVLA) strain B19 is a fairly ubiquitous human virus, first isolated from peripheral blood. By the age of 16 years, one-third of the population is seropositive.

C. Clinical disease. PVLA strain B19 has received considerable attention because of its clinical associations:

1. Aplastic crisis. Infection of precursor cells of the erythroid lineage in the bone marrow by PVLA strain B19 is the trigger for aplastic crisis in children who have homozygous sickle cell disease. In a study of children with sickle cell anemia and aplastic crisis, 37 out of 40 showed evidence of PVLA strain B19 infection.

a. The susceptibility of these cells is believed to be the result of at least two factors:

(1) Expression of the erythrocyte P antigen, the receptor for the virus

(2) The existence of transcription factors in erythroid precursors that promote viral replication

b. As a consequence of infection with PVLA strain B19, the infected erythrocyte precursors are destroyed and the patient develops a profound anemia characterized by marked depletion of erythroblastoid elements in the bone marrow.

2. **Erythema infectiosum ("fifth disease")** is a very mild, febrile, self-limiting disease that affects infants (see Chapter 56 II E). It is associated with a faint rash that has a reticular appearance on the limbs. The face has a "slapped cheeks" appearance.

3. **Hydrops fetalis.** There is some evidence to suggest that the B19 strain may play a significant role in miscarriages due to the development of nonimmune hydrops fetalis.

Chapter 33

RNA Viruses I: Picornaviruses

John Manos

I. OVERVIEW.

OVERVIEW. Picornaviruses are small, naked viruses, with a +RNA genome. There are two major groups of picornaviruses that infect humans:

A. **Enteroviruses** are acid-stable and infect the gastrointestinal tract. They replicate best at 37°C and are stable at a low pH; therefore, they can withstand the acidity of the stomach. Because they lack an envelope, they resist the detergent effects of bile acids as well. The main mode of transmission for enteroviruses is the fecal-oral route. The following viruses are included in this group:

1. **Poliovirus** (types 1, 2, and 3)
2. **Coxsackievirus A** (24 serotypes) and **coxsackievirus B** (6 serotypes)
3. **Echovirus** (34 serotypes)
4. **New enteroviruses** (strains 68 through 72)

B. **Rhinoviruses** are acid-labile and infect the upper airway mucosae. Transmission is by inhalation of aerosolized particles that contain the virus. The optimal temperature for replication is 33°C. Temperatures below 37°C are prevalent in the upper airways, particularly during cold weather, which may explain why rhinovirus infections are prevalent during the colder months.

II. ENTEROVIRUSES

A. Polioviruses

1. **Epidemiology**
   a. **Incidence and distribution.** Poliomyelitis was a sporadic disease before the 1800s, but became epidemic thereafter. Poliomyelitis outbreaks were reported in all continents, with maximal incidence in the temperate climates of the northern hemisphere. Most cases occurred during the late summer or early fall months. As a result of successful mass vaccination, polio is now an almost extinct disease, except in underdeveloped countries (Figure 33-1).
   b. **Transmission** is by the fecal-oral route.

2. **Pathogenesis**
   a. **Multiplication.** The **portal of entry** is the intestinal epithelium, where the virus multiplies. The **incubation period** is 9–12 days.
   b. **Initial viremia.** From the intestinal epithelium, the virus spreads to the adjacent lymph nodes and enters the circulation. The patient may form antibody at this stage, preventing the infection from spreading **(abortive infection).**
   c. **Second viremia.** In patients who are unable to control the initial viremia, there is a second, major viremia, and the virus spreads throughout the body. Many types of cells have receptors for polioviruses, including the neurons of the anterior horn of the spinal cord, as well as nerve cells in the medulla oblongata and in the bulbar pons.

3. **Clinical disease**
   a. **Inapparent infection.** Most polio infections are inapparent.
   b. **Abortive infections** are associated with nonspecific symptoms.

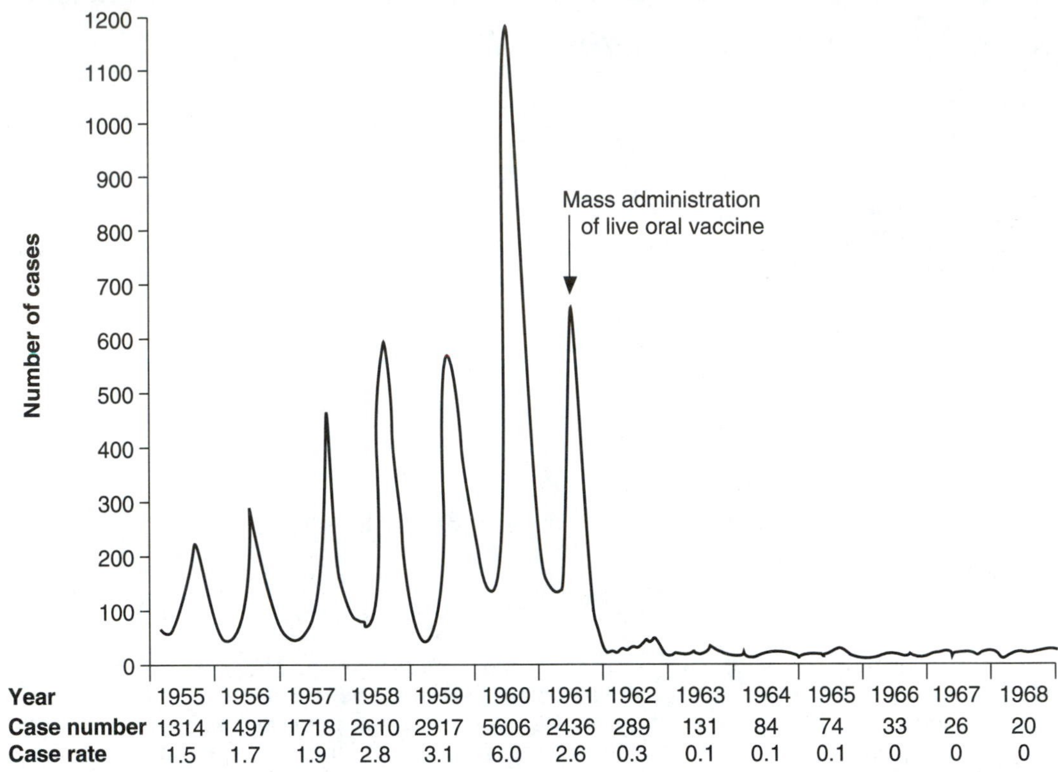

FIGURE 33-1. Effect of mass vaccination with the oral polio vaccine on the incidence of poliomyelitis in Japan from 1955–1968. Case rates are calculated per 100,000 population. (Redrawn with permission from Sabin AB: Oral poliovirus vaccine: history of its development and use and current challenge to eliminate poliomyelitis in the world. *J Infect Dis* 151:420, 1985.)

c. Aseptic meningitis. Approximately 1% of patients present with a self-limiting meningitis that usually leaves no sequelae.

d. Paralytic poliomyelitis. Approximately 0.1% of patients develop paralytic poliomyelitis.

(1) Spinal poliomyelitis is characterized by flaccid paralysis because the disease process involves motor neurons.

(a) The **paralysis** is usually **asymmetrical.** The proximal muscles are more likely to be involved than the distal muscles, and the lower extremities are involved more often than the upper extremities. The paralyzed muscles eventually become atrophic as a result of a lack of motor innervation.

(b) Sensory loss is **unusual;** if the patient presents with both sensory and motor loss, the diagnosis of poliomyelitis is considered highly unlikely.

(2) Bulbar poliomyelitis involves the base of the brain and is a much more serious condition than spinal poliomyelitis. The involvement of cranial nerves and the respiratory and circulatory centers in the medulla compromises vital functions, particularly the control of respiratory muscles. Bulbar poliomyelitis is more common in adults.

(3) Bulbospinal poliomyelitis. In some patients, there is bulbospinal involvement; the prognosis for these patients is very poor.

e. Encephalitis as a result of poliovirus infection is rare, but carries a grave prognosis.

f. Postpolio syndrome. Twenty to thirty percent of individuals who experienced a paralytic episode of polio in their youth experience fatigue, muscle pain, weakness, and atrophy 25–35 years later. The recurrence seems to be associated with

TABLE 33-1. Comparison of Polio Vaccines

Characteristic	Sabin's Vaccine	Salk's Vaccine
Immunizing agent	Live, attenuated virus	Killed virus
Administration route	Oral	Parenteral
Immunity	Mucosal (IgA) and systemic	Systemic
Induction of herd immunity	Yes	No
Reversion to virulent form	Possible, but very rare	No

further denervation of previously affected groups. The cause for this denervation is unknown.

(1) Usually, the affected muscles are those involved in the original episode, although weakness may affect muscle groups originally not involved.

(2) The progression of symptoms is slow and usually does not cause significant disability.

4. **Laboratory diagnosis.** Because of the low prevalence of polio in the United States and in most industrial countries, any suspected case needs to be confirmed and the virus should be isolated and characterized.

   a. **Serology.** The quantitation of IgM antibodies in serum or cerebrospinal fluid (CSF) can be considered evidence of recent or ongoing infection.

   b. **Culture and isolation.** Isolation in tissue culture is essential for proper characterization of the virus as a wild-type poliovirus or as a vaccine revertant.

5. **Prevention**

   a. **Two vaccines** for polio are available (Table 33-1).

      (1) **Killed vaccine (Salk).** The inactivated polio vaccine is administered parenterally, does not colonize the intestine, and causes only a systemic immune response.

      (2) **Attenuated vaccine (Sabin).** The attenuated vaccine is administered orally. Oral administration has several advantages.

         (a) Oral immunization is **simpler** and **more suitable for mass immunizations,** particularly in underdeveloped countries where the disease is still relatively common.

         (b) **Both local and systemic immunity** are induced by the oral vaccine—local immunity is stimulated by proliferation of the virus in the intestine, and systemic immunity is triggered by the spread of the attenuated virus from the intestinal tract to the systemic circulation.

         (c) The attenuated vaccine is **transmitted by the fecal-oral route to nonimmunized children,** because viable attenuated viruses are excreted in the feces during the stage of intestinal proliferation. Thus, the oral vaccine has been heralded as biologically superior based on the fact that it favors the transmission of attenuated viruses among nonimmunized individuals. Theoretically, the widespread use of the oral polio vaccine will result in the replacement of the pathogenic strains of polioviruses in the environment by their attenuated counterparts.

   b. The **oral vaccine is preferred in most countries,** including the United States. Some advocate a return to the killed vaccine, at least for the initial immunization, because the few cases of paralytic poliomyelitis currently seen in the United States (9 cases per year) are caused by the attenuated vaccine, which seems to have the capacity to mutate to virulent forms upon replication in the intestine. However, the recommended policy still calls for use of the oral vaccine because postvaccination polio is a rather rare event, occurring once for every 2.6 million doses of oral vaccine.

TABLE 33-2. Associations between Coxsackieviruses and Clinical Disease

Disease	Coxsackie Virus A	Coxsackie Virus B
Herpangina	Serotypes 2–6, 8, 10	. . .
Infantile diarrhea	Serotypes 18, 20–22, 24	. . .
Hand-foot-and-mouth disease	Many serotypes	. . .
Multisystemic disease in neonates	. . .	Serotypes 2–5
Pleurodynia	. . .	All serotypes
Pericarditis, myocarditis	. . .	All serotypes

B. Coxsackieviruses

1. **General characteristics**
   a. **Structure.** The coxsackieviruses are morphologically similar, and **morphologically indistinguishable from poliovirus.**
   b. Antisera to polioviruses do not neutralize coxsackieviruses, which are **totally non–cross-reactive with polioviruses.**

2. **Classification.** Two major types of coxsackieviruses (types A and B) have been defined on the basis of their effects in laboratory animals. Multiple strains in each type (24 strains of type A, 6 strains of type B) have been defined serologically.

3. **Clinical disease.** Young children are most commonly affected.
   a. **Inapparent** or **subclinical** infections comprise over 90% of coxsackievirus infections.
   b. **Upper respiratory infections** (the **"common cold"**) and **undifferentiated febrile illness** are common, totally nonspecific presentations.
   c. **Aseptic meningitis** and **meningoencephalitis** are seen in association with all enteroviruses, including coxsackievirus A and B.
   d. **Strain-specific manifestations.** The different strains show prevalent associations with certain clinical presentations (Table 33-2). However, there is considerable overlap.
      (1) **Coxsackie A viruses** are most frequently associated with:
         (a) **Infantile diarrhea**
         (b) **Herpangina,** clinically characterized by the occurrence of herpes-like ulcerations on the posterior pharynx
         (c) **Hand-foot-and-mouth disease,** a self-limiting disease clinically characterized by ulcerations in the mouth and buccal mucosa, and similar vesicular ulcerations on the palms and soles of the feet
      (2) **Coxsackie B viruses** are most frequently associated with:
         (a) **Myocarditis** and **pericarditis.** In older children, the myocarditis or pericarditis is essentially benign. In young adults, the symptoms may mimic a myocardial infarction. Chronic evolution as a result of cross-reactive autoimmunity has been well documented following an episode of viral myocarditis caused by coxsackieviruses.
         (b) **Multisystemic disease of the newborn.** The neonate presents with variable combinations of myocarditis, encephalitis (encephalomyocarditis syndrome), hepatitis, and adrenal cortex involvement. Multisystemic disease of the newborn is associated with high morbidity and mortality rates.
         (c) **Pleurodynia** is painful inflammation of the intercostal muscles, and, to a lesser degree, the pleura, usually accompanied by fever.

4. **Treatment** is supportive.

5. **Prevention.** Vaccines against coxsackieviruses are not available.

C. Echoviruses. In the search for enteroviruses that followed the successful culture of poliovirus in nonneural cells, unidentified viruses were isolated from the stools of healthy children. These viruses were designated ECHO viruses (E for enteric, C for the cytopathogenic effect they caused, H for human, and O for orphan because they were viruses that had not yet been associated with a disease).

1. **Clinical disease**
   a. **"Common cold."** Like most other enteroviruses, echoviruses can cause upper respiratory tract infections and undifferentiated febrile illness.
   b. **Aseptic meningitis.** Echoviruses are the most common cause of viral meningitis in the United States (see Chapter 49 III A). The symptoms (e.g., nausea, vomiting, headache) are of moderate intensity and the mental status of the patient remains clear.
   c. **Ascending paralysis or encephalitis.** Rarely, some echoviruses cause a polio-like ascending paralysis or encephalitis.
   d. **Morbilliform rash.** Clinical infection with enteroviruses (except for poliovirus) is often associated with a measles-like rash.

2. **Treatment.** Viral meningitis is basically a self-limiting disease. Treatment is essentially supportive, but exclusion of other types of meningitis is imperative.

D. Newer enteroviruses. Additional enteroviruses have been reported and designated sequentially by order of discovery (enteroviruses 68 through 72). Most of these viruses are medically unimportant, except for types 70 and 72. The others may cause a rash and occasionally, meningitis.

1. **Enterovirus type 70**
   a. **Epidemiology**
      (1) **Distribution.** Disease caused by enterovirus type 70 is most prevalent in the Near Eastern, Middle Eastern, and other third-world countries where crowded living conditions are common.
      (2) **Transmission.** The virus is transmitted via close personal contact, rather than by the fecal-oral route, and is more contagious than influenza virus.
   b. **Clinical disease.** Enterovirus type 70 is associated with an acute, hemorrhagic conjunctivitis. The disease is usually self-limiting and leaves no permanent damage, but occasionally, keratitis may develop and lead to blindness. Secondary bacterial infections can also worsen the situation.

2. **Enterovirus type 72** is **hepatitis A virus (HAV),** which, in the last few years, has been classified as an enterovirus (see Chapter 38 II).

III. RHINOVIRUSES.

Over 100 antigenically distinct rhinoviruses have been identified so far, and all of them appear to be able to cause the **"common cold."**

A. Epidemiology. Rhinovirus infections occur worldwide and year-round, with higher prevalence in the winter. Crowding and close contact favors transmission, which is by the respiratory route.

B. Pathogenesis and clinical disease

1. The **incubation period** is **2–5 days.** The patient is infective from right before the onset of symptoms until approximately 2–3 days into the disease.

2. **Symptoms.** Coryza is the most common symptom. Fever is common in children but relatively rare in adults. Systemic symptoms are mild, and the clinical disease seldom lasts more than 7 days.

3. **Complications** include:
   a. **Chronic bronchitis,** which tends to develop in children with preexisting lung disease
   b. **Sinusitis,** commonly associated with rhinovirus infections and sometimes involving superinfecting bacteria
   c. **Otitis media**

C. **Diagnosis** is usually clinical. To make a specific diagnosis, culture and isolation is required; nasal secretions are the best specimens for culture.

D. **Treatment** is supportive, except when the rhinovirus infection is associated with or followed by a bacterial infection.

E. **Immunity** depends on the production of secretory IgA antibodies. Because IgA memory fades relatively quickly, a person may be reinfected with the same serotype. In addition, the rhinoviruses show antigenic drifting, which results in the emergence of new strains. **Prophylaxis** by vaccination is virtually impossible.

Chapter 34

RNA Viruses II: Arboviruses and Rubella Virus

John Manos

I. OVERVIEW

A. **Arboviruses** are transmitted by blood-sucking arthropod vectors.

1. The arbovirus group is **defined epidemiologically** and **includes members of several virus families** (Table 34-1). Over 200 arboviruses have been identified, most having been isolated from arthropod vectors. Approximately 80 of these arboviruses have been shown to cause disease in humans.
   a. **Alphaviruses** are members of the ***Togaviridae*** **family.**
   b. **Flaviviruses** are members of the ***Flaviviridae*** **family,** which is closely related to the *Togaviridae* family. One major characteristic common to members of both families is the possession of an envelope with inserted glycoproteins that have the ability to cause hemagglutination.
   c. **Bunyaviruses** are members of the ***Bunyaviridae*** **family.**
   d. **Reoviruses** are members of the ***Reoviridae*** **family.**
2. Most of the arboviruses have been named according to where they were discovered (e.g., California encephalitis virus).

B. **Rubella virus** is the only member of the genus ***Rubiviridae,*** which is also a member of the *Togaviridae* family. However, because rubella virus is transmitted from person to person, it is not an arbovirus. The characteristics of the rubivirus group are summarized and contrasted with the characteristics of the alphavirus and flavivirus groups in Table 34-2.

II. ARBOVIRUSES

A. Pathogenesis

1. When the infected vector bites a suitable host, the virus is **injected into the capillary circulation.** The first round of viral replication takes place in the vascular endothelium.
2. Viral replication is followed by a **viremia** that precedes the onset of clinical symptoms.
   a. Because these viruses are introduced directly into the bloodstream, the **incubation periods** are short (approximately 1 week).
   b. Patients often present with a morbilliform **rash,** secondary to **endothelial cell damage** and an associated **increase in vascular permeability.** If the endothelial damage is severe and disseminated, the rash may become hemorrhagic and involve the mucous membranes and the gastrointestinal mucosa as well as the skin. **Disseminated intravascular coagulation (DIC)** and **thrombocytopenia** may evolve, aggravating the hemorrhagic diathesis.
3. The circulating virus reaches the organ for which it has special **tropism;** for example, the liver in the case of yellow fever virus or the brain in the case of the encephalitis viruses.

B. **Clinical disease.** Arboviruses cause three clinical syndromes:

1. **Arthralgia syndrome,** exemplified by **Dengue fever.** Dengue fever is clinically characterized by:

TABLE 34-1. Major Families and Genera of Arboviruses

Family	Structural Characteristics	Genus	Examples
Togaviridae	+ RNA, enveloped	Alphaviruses	Eastern equine encephalitis virus, Western equine encephalitis virus, California equine encephalitis virus, Venezuelan equine encephalitis virus
Flaviviridae	+ RNA, enveloped	Flaviviruses	Yellow fever virus, dengue virus, St. Louis encephalitis virus, Japanese B encephalitis virus, Central European encephalitis virus
Bunyaviridae	− RNA, enveloped	Bunyaviruses	California encephalitis virus, LaCross encephalitis virus
		Phleboviruses	Sandfly fever virus
		Nairoviruses	Crimean-Congo hemorrhagic fever virus
Reoviridae	Segmented double-stranded RNA, naked	Orbiviruses	Colorado tick fever virus

a. A **flu-like syndrome** with chills, a "saddle back" fever (i.e., one in which the temperature drops and then rises again), headache, retroocular pain, and conjunctivitis

b. **Severe muscular and joint pain** (hence the nickname **"breakbone fever"**)

c. A **measles-like (morbilliform) rash** lasting 2–3 days

2. **Hemorrhagic syndrome,** exemplified by **yellow fever.** The infection with yellow fever virus can be subclinical or associated with disease of variable severity. The overall mortality rate is approximately 10%. Survivors recover completely and have permanent immunity.

   a. In **mild cases,** yellow fever may present as a **flu-like syndrome** with fever, chills, headache, backache, nausea, and vomiting, and is difficult to distinguish from many other viral infections.

   b. More **severe cases** are associated with **extensive hemorrhaging** in the mucous membranes of the nose, gastrointestinal tract, and bladder.

      (1) **Melanemesis** (i.e., vomiting of digested blood) is a typical symptom.

      (2) A **decrease in blood pressure** is accompanied by a **paradoxical decrease in pulse rate** (usually when blood pressure decreases, the pulse rate increases).

TABLE 34-2. Comparison of the General Characteristics of Rubivirus, Alphavirus, and Flavivirus

Characteristic	Rubivirus	Alphavirus and Flavivirus
Nucleic acid	+ RNA	+ RNA
Hemagglutinin-containing envelope	Yes	Yes
Serotypes	One	Variable
Transmission	Human-to-human	Arthropod vectors
Capable of causing congenital infection	Yes	No

(3) The development of **jaundice** or **proteinuria,** indicative of hepatic or renal involvement, respectively, is ominous.

3. **Encephalitis syndrome** can be caused by alphaviruses, flaviviruses, and bunyaviruses. The clinical presentation mimics a **severe flu-like syndrome** (e.g., headache, fever, musculoskeletal aches). If the disease progresses, new symptoms develop, such as **drowsiness** (in viral encephalitis there is involvement of the sensorium, whereas in viral meningitis the sensorium remains clear), **nuchal rigidity,** and **focal neurologic symptoms** (e.g., tingling, weakness, paraesthesias, confusion, paralysis, convulsions, coma, and death). However, full recovery is the rule and is associated with life-long immunity to the causative virus.

C. **Epidemiology.** Most arboviruses cause disease in nonhuman vertebrates, which serve as reservoirs for the virus, and are transmitted by blood-sucking arthropods (e.g., mosquitoes, ticks). The vertebrate host often recovers from the infection, but the vector will carry the virus for life. As a rule, humans are not necessary for the propagation of arboviruses; they serve as dead-end hosts.

1. **Dengue fever** is epidemic in the **Caribbean** and is one of the exceptions to the rule of arboviruses having nonhuman vertebrates as hosts. Humans are the natural reservoir for the dengue virus, which is transmitted by a **mosquito-man-mosquito cycle.**

2. **Yellow fever** is still prevalent in **South** and **Central America**—the importance of mosquito abatement programs is well exemplified by the disease-free status of the Panama Canal Zone, in contrast with the relatively high incidence in neighboring Panama.
   a. **Urban yellow fever** involves a **mosquito-man-mosquito transmission cycle.** The urban type can be controlled by immunization and mosquito extermination programs.
   b. **Sylvatic yellow fever** refers to the jungle or wild type of yellow fever; the transmission cycle is **mosquito-monkey-mosquito.** Sylvatic yellow fever is considerably more difficult to eradicate than urban yellow fever, and there is always the possibility that a human may be bitten by an infected mosquito from the sylvatic cycle and become the source of an urban yellow fever outbreak in an area that had been previously disease-free.

3. **Encephalitis**
   a. **Transmission.** Birds are the natural reservoirs for the arboviruses that cause encephalitis, but mosquitoes can transmit the disease to horses and humans.
   b. **Distribution.** Eastern equine encephalitis virus, Western equine encephalitis virus, California equine encephalitis virus, St. Louis encephalitis virus, and Venezuelan equine encephalitis are common in the United States.
      (1) Eastern equine encephalitis virus is the cause of epidemics, large and small, which occur throughout the United States with Texas, New Jersey, Florida, and the western states being the most common locations.
      (2) Venezuelan encephalitis virus is restricted to Texas and Florida.
   c. **Incidence.** In 1994, 674 cases of encephalitis were reported to the Centers for Disease Control (CDC). Of these, the vast majority were caused by Eastern equine encephalitis virus, Western equine encephalitis virus, or St. Louis encephalitis virus. Some cases were probably caused by herpesviruses. In 75% of cases, the etiology is undetermined.
   d. **Mortality rates.** Eastern equine encephalitis virus causes the most serious form of clinical disease, with a mortality rate of approximately 20%. The other encephalitis viruses have epidemic mortality rates of 5%–10%.

D. **Diagnosis**

1. **Culture and isolation** is usually the cornerstone of viral identification, but in the case of arboviruses, it is difficult as well as dangerous. If isolation is to be attempted, pe-

ripheral blood samples must be obtained from the patient very early in the disease, during the viremic stage. By the time symptoms are evident, the patient is past the viremic stage. It is then difficult to isolate the organism unless liver or brain biopsy or autopsy are performed.

2. **Serology** is most often the basis for the confirmation of a diagnosis of arbovirus encephalitis. Antiviral antibodies are detected by **hemagglutination-inhibition** or by **complement fixation.** A fourfold or greater increase in specific antibody titer between the acute and convalescent sera is necessary to establish the diagnosis.

E. Control and prevention

1. **Control**
   a. **Mosquito abatement programs** are very effective in reducing the incidence of yellow fever and the viral encephalitides.
   b. **Exposure avoidance** (e.g., by using mosquito nets) is also effective.
2. **Prevention.** Immunoprophylaxis is available for yellow fever and Japanese B encephalitis. Several equine vaccines have also been developed and are effective in preventing infection in horses.

III. RUBELLA VIRUS

A. Clinical disease

1. **Rubella (German measles)**
   a. **Typical course.** Patients are typically young. Following an incubation period of 12–23 days (18 days on average), a mild maculopapular rash develops (primarily on the face and thorax), accompanied by retroauricular lymphadenopathy (usually bilateral), a mild fever, and joint pain (especially in girls).
   b. **Complications.** Usually the disease follows a benign course, but occasionally it may be followed by evidence of systemic infection, including:
      (1) **Migratory arthritis,** seen mostly in women
      (2) **Thrombocytopenia** and **hemorrhagic diathesis**
      (3) **Postinfectious encephalitis,** which is rare, but tends to occur predominantly in adults and is associated with a high mortality rate (20%–50%)
2. **Congenital rubella**
   a. **Fetal defects** can be transient or permanent (the latter are usually the result of developmental abnormalities).
      (1) **Transient abnormalities** include **low birth weight, thrombocytopenic purpura ("blueberry muffin" baby), hepatosplenomegaly, metaphyseal radiolucencies,** and **pneumonitis.**
      (2) **Permanent abnormalities** include **cataracts, cardiac lesions** (e.g., patent ductus arteriosus, pulmonic stenosis), **microcephaly** (associated with mental retardation), and **deafness.**
   b. **Risk and severity.** Infection during the **first trimester** is associated with the greatest risk for the fetus.
      (1) Maternal infection during the first 2 months of pregnancy is associated with a 40%–60% chance of fetal defects. The defects are likely to be multiple. Spontaneous abortions may also occur.
      (2) Maternal infection during the third month is associated with a 30%–50% chance of fetal defects; defects are more likely to be singular.

B. Epidemiology

1. **Incidence.** Before the vaccine was introduced, over 50,000 cases of rubella per year were reported, but this incidence is much lower than the true frequency of the disease, which is mild, often subclinical, and difficult to diagnose. The last epidemic

outbreak occurred in 1964. Most infections occur during the late winter and early spring months.

2. **Transmission** is from person-to-person through inhalation of infected aerosolized respiratory secretions. Viral shedding is highest while the rash is present, but patients can be infectious for several days before and several days after the appearance of the rash (a total period of approximately 15–20 days).

C. Diagnosis. Clinical diagnosis may be difficult, particularly in an infant. Once suspected, the diagnosis is established by isolation of the virus, or, more commonly, by serology.

1. **Diagnosis in infants. TORCH titers** (see Chapter 30 V C 3) are usually obtained because of the difficulty of differentiating congenital infections from one another. A negative result in a serologic test is not necessarily conclusive.

2. **Diagnosis in pregnant women.** If a pregnant woman is thought to be exposed to the rubella virus, she should be tested immediately.
   a. If her serum is positive for rubella virus antibodies, then she has been infected previously. To determine if the infection is recent, specific antirubella IgM should be assayed.
   b. If the result of the serologic test is negative (i.e., there are no detectable antirubella antibodies), then the woman should be tested again in 28 days (18 days' incubation time plus 10 days to develop antibody). If the patient tests positive on the second test, then she has been recently infected. The rise in IgM antibodies may require less time for detection, allowing a faster diagnosis.

D. Treatment is supportive; no specific antiviral treatment is available. γ-Globulin can be administered to a pregnant woman who has been exposed to rubella virus in an attempt to prevent infection. However, if the infection has occurred, γ-globulin will not prevent viremia or fetal infection, and the results of future serologic assays on the newborn will be confused by the persistence of transplacentally transferred antibodies from the γ-globulin.

E. Prevention

1. **Vaccination.** An effective live, attenuated vaccine is available. Although the attenuated virus has not been shown to cause clinical infection or fetal abnormalities, vaccination should be withheld from pregnant women and vaccinated women should avoid pregnancy for 3 months following vaccination.

2. **Booster shots.** Lifelong immunity follows natural infection. Reinfection was believed to act as a natural booster, but the protective effect of natural infection was lost following the implementation of widespread vaccination programs; therefore, periodic boosters are necessary to maintain an adequate level of protection.

Chapter 35

RNA Viruses III: Orthomyxoviruses

John Manos

I. GENERAL CHARACTERISTICS.

The **influenza viruses (types A, B, and C),** a group of highly contagious human pathogenic viruses, are orthomyxoviruses.

A. Structure

1. **Genome.** The nucleic acid consists of eight attached segments of **-RNA.**
2. **Envelope.** The envelope is a lipid bilayer with inserted **hemagglutinin (H)** and **neuraminidase (N) glycoprotein spikes** that project to the outside. Hemagglutinin is the component on the viral membrane that attaches to a specific receptor on a susceptible cell.
   a. The H and N spikes are **coded by the viral genome.** During viral replication, these spikes are synthesized early in the replication cycle, and become attached to the plasma membrane at specialized patches where budding takes place. Cellular membrane proteins are displaced out of those patches.
   b. Both H and N molecules are **immunogenic.** The antibodies reacting with the hemagglutinin molecule inhibit hemagglutination and neutralize viral infectiveness. The serotype of a given influenza virus isolate is determined by the reactivity of a viral isolate with antisera directed against different types of hemagglutinins.

B. Classification.

All strains of influenza virus are designated and differentiated by the combination of H and N antigens that is unique to them. Three major hemagglutinin components (H1, H2, and H3) and two neuraminidase components (N1 and N2) have been identified for influenza A virus.

II. EPIDEMIOLOGY

A. Incidence.

Of the three types of influenza virus, types A and B tend to cause epidemics that recur every 1–3 years, while type C usually does not cause epidemics. Worldwide epidemics (pandemics) occurred in the past. The worst pandemic occurred in 1918—21 million people died, mostly as a result of secondary bacterial pneumonia.

1. **Antigenic shift and drift** are responsible for the unique epidemiologic features of influenza virus.
   a. **Antigenic drift** refers to minor antigenic changes resulting from point mutations in the viral hemagglutinins and neuraminidase glycoproteins.
   b. **Antigenic shift** refers to major antigenic changes that result from the reassortment of the eight nucleic acid segments that constitute the viral genome.
      (1) When a major antigenic shift takes place, the new viral strain infects a primarily susceptible population, one that has never been exposed to that particular strain before. The result is a pandemic. As most of the survivors develop antibody, the pandemic subsides.
      (2) Every 2–3 years, there is another epidemic caused by the new strain, but the subsequent epidemics are weaker than the original pandemic as a result of the increasing level of immunity in the population. Eventually, the virus strain in question disappears.
      (3) After many years, the population is no longer protected against that strain, which may reemerge and start a new cycle of infection.
2. **Major strains responsible for pandemics.** Three strains have emerged as causes of

pandemics in the last 30 years: 1957—the Asian influenza strain (H2N2), 1967—the Hong Kong influenza strain (H3N2), and in 1977—the Russian influenza strain (H1N1).

   a. H3N2 and H1N1 substrains derived by antigenic drifting from the original strain are involved in current influenza outbreaks, which have not reached pandemic proportions.

   b. Because resistance to the H2N2 strain is waning (as the population gets older), this strain is the most likely candidate to cause the next pandemic outbreak.

3. **Seasonal variation.** In the northern hemisphere, in countries with temperate climates, the incidence of viral influenza peaks in **late December** or **January.**

B. **Prevalence** of influenza is usually lower in the older population, which has developed immunity to the prevalent strains over the years.

C. **Transmission** is person-to-person via respiratory secretions. Patients are contagious from approximately 24 hours before the onset of clinical symptoms until approximately 48 hours after the onset of symptoms.

III. PATHOGENESIS AND CLINICAL DISEASE

A. The **portal of entry** is the **upper respiratory tract,** where the virus attaches to and infects the mucosal epithelial cells.

B. **Symptoms** develop following an **incubation period** of **1–3 days.** Influenza types A and B cause a virtually identical disease (although type B tends to cause milder disease than type A) and can only be differentiated by isolation or through serologic studies.

1. Classic influenza is characterized by the **sudden onset** of **fever, chills,** and **myalgia.** There may be nasal discharge or redness of the mucous membranes and adenopathy. A dry cough is prominent.

2. **Duration.** The fever may be high and lasts approximately 3 days. The other symptoms may persist for up to 1 month after the acute disease has subsided.

C. **Convalescence.** The convalescent period lasts 1–2 weeks. It takes approximately 10 days to 2 weeks for antibodies to the viral hemagglutinin to peak. The antibodies persist, but their concentration decreases with time, and their effectiveness declines as new antigenic strains emerge.

IV. DIAGNOSIS.

The diagnosis of sporadic influenza cases is usually clinical. However, clinical diagnosis of influenza is uncertain because many viral and other types of infections cause "flu-like" symptoms. The identification of the type of influenza virus responsible for an outbreak requires either isolation and typing of the virus from infected individuals, or the performance of serologic studies.

A. **Isolation** can be achieved by culture in a variety of cell lines. Throat swabs are the preferred sample for culture.

B. **Serologic diagnosis** is based on the detection and quantitation of antibodies directed against the viral hemagglutinin (hemagglutination-inhibiting antibodies).

1. The concentration of hemagglutination-inhibiting antibodies is estimated by incubating a standardized viral suspension with serial dilutions of a patient's serum and determining the highest dilution able to inhibit hemagglutination.

2. The confirmation of a recent infection is based on the verification of a significant rise in the antibody titer (fourfold as a minimum) between a sample collected during the acute phase of the disease and a sample collected 2–3 weeks later, during convalescence.

V. TREATMENT

A. **Amantadine** prevents viral penetration of the target cell or uncoating and must be administered prophylactically or early in the infection. When administered early after the onset of symptoms, amantadine will diminish the symptoms and accelerate convalescence. Side effects include insomnia, dizziness, and difficulty concentrating.

B. **Rimantadine** is a newer drug with fewer side effects than amantadine.

VI. COMPLICATIONS.

Influenza is a more serious disease (with more frequent complications) in older individuals and the mortality rate increases with age. A variety of complications can occur in patients with (or recovering from) viral influenza.

A. **Complications related to the spread of viral infection. Croup, myositis, myocarditis,** and **pericarditis** are the result of the spread of the viral infection.

B. **Complications related to secondary infection. Secondary bacterial pneumonia** and **exacerbation of chronic obstructive pulmonary disease** can occur secondary to virally induced compromise of the immune response, especially in older patients.

C. **Complications related to hypersensitivity reactions**

1. **Reye's syndrome** affects younger patients following a variety of **acute febrile infections,** particularly viral influenza (type B) and chicken pox.
   a. There is an unequivocal link with the **administration of aspirin,** which seems to precipitate the onset of the syndrome in genetically predisposed individuals. At least in some patients, there seems to be an underlying defect in the ability to oxidize fatty acids, which is aggravated by the inhibition of the deficient enzyme by salicylates.
   b. Clinically, Reye's syndrome is described as an **acute metabolic encephalopathy associated with fatty degeneration of the liver and other viscera.** Symptoms that reflect central nervous system (CNS) and liver involvement predominate, including lethargy and drowsiness that may progress to irreversible coma. Liver enzyme levels and ketone bodies become grossly elevated.
   c. The **mortality rate** is **10%–40%.**
2. **Guillain-Barré syndrome (ascending paralysis)** is a rare complication of influenza and other acute infections believed to result from an autoimmune response directed against neuron gangliosides as a result of a cross-reactive immune response triggered by the infection. Pathologically, it is an acute inflammatory demyelininating polyradiculoneuropathy associated with an axonal motor neuropathy.

VII. PREVENTION

A. **Prophylactic administration of amantadine** is indicated during high-risk periods for elderly patients (particularly institutionalized patients) and for patients with chronic obstructive pulmonary disease or heart disease.

B. **Vaccination** is recommended for patients with underlying diseases known to be associated with more severe infection, elderly patients with chronic diseases, and healthcare workers. The vaccine is produced in the allantoic cavity of embryonated eggs and may cause reactions in individuals allergic to egg proteins.

1. The vaccine is a killed vaccine, and includes the three prevalent strains, the two most recent type As (H2N3 and H1N1) and the most recent type B. Because it is a killed vaccine, maintenance of the immunized state requires annual boosting. Antigenic drifting necessitates revaccination with the most updated vaccine.
2. The effectiveness ranges from 0%–60%, depending on the study and the conditions of administration.
3. Efforts to design a universally efficient polyvalent vaccine containing the three H components and the two N components of influenza A are under way.

Chapter 36

RNA Viruses IV: Paramyxoviruses

John Manos

I. INTRODUCTION

A. General characteristics. Paramyxoviruses are enveloped viruses with helical symmetry and a −RNA genome. Some have envelope glycoproteins with neuraminidase and hemagglutinating properties, others have only hemagglutinins; others do not express either type of glycoprotein.

B. Classification. There are three genera in the *Paramyxoviridae* family:

1. **Paramyxovirus.** These viruses have both hemagglutinins and neuraminidase on their envelopes. The **parainfluenza viruses** and the **mumps virus** are paramyxoviruses.
2. **Morbillivirus.** These viruses express hemagglutinins only. The **measles (rubeola) virus** is a morbillivirus.
3. **Pneumovirus.** These viruses do not express neuraminidase or hemagglutinins. **Respiratory syncytial virus** is a pneumovirus.

II. PARAINFLUENZA VIRUSES

A. Classification. There are **four major serotypes** of parainfluenza virus.

1. **Parainfluenza virus types 1** and **2** usually infect infants and children, and tend to cause biennial epidemics, usually in the fall.
2. **Parainfluenza virus type 3** infects infants younger than 2 years of age year-round and tends to cause more severe disease than that caused by parainfluenza viruses types 1 or 2.
3. **Parainfluenza virus type 4** causes mild disease.

B. Clinical disease. The primary infection is most serious; subsequent infections tend to produce milder symptoms.

1. **"Common cold."** All of the parainfluenza viruses can cause colds, which are usually mild.
2. **Laryngotracheobronchitis (croup)** is commonly associated with parainfluenza viruses types 1 and 2.
3. **Bronchiolitis** and **pneumonia** are usually caused by parainfluenza virus type 3.

C. Epidemiology. Transmission is via the inhalation of infectious aerosolized secretions.

D. Diagnosis. The precise viral etiology of a case of upper respiratory infection cannot be established clinically. Isolation or serologic tests are required. In many cases, however, physicians establish a clinical diagnosis of viral upper respiratory tract infection and treat supportively without confirming which virus is causing the symptoms.

E. Treatment. There is no specific therapy, but adequate supportive therapy is very important.

III. MUMPS VIRUS

A. Clinical disease. Mumps is an acute, generalized viral infection that primarily affects the parotid glands. It is usually a mild disease that follows a benign course. Immunity is lifelong after a case of mumps.

1. **Subclinical disease.** Approximately one-third of infections are subclinical.
2. **Clinical disease.** Following an incubation period of 2–3 weeks, a nonsuppurative swelling of the salivary glands, predominantly the parotid gland, occurs. The disease evolves in several defined stages:
   a. **Prodromal symptoms** are nonspecific, and include aches, mild fever, and swelling of Stenson's duct. Prodromal symptoms usually occur 1 or 2 days before the classic parotid swelling begins.
   b. **Parotitis** can be unilateral or bilateral, and may cause discomfort while chewing or speaking.
3. **Complications**
   a. **Central nervous system (CNS)**
      (1) **Encephalitis** is usually postinfectious, mild, and without sequelae. Occasionally, the encephalitis occurs in the absence of parotid swelling or may precede the swelling (in which case, it is preinfectious). The encephalitis is believed to be caused by an autoimmune process triggered by cross-reactivity between a virus-coded peptide and a brain tissue–derived peptide.
      (2) **Meningitis.** One in ten cases of viral meningitis is caused by the mumps virus.
      (3) **Deafness** occurs in approximately 4% of patients and is usually transient.
   b. **Glandular**
      (1) **Epididymoorchitis** is most likely to occur in adolescents. It is rarely bilateral, and infertility is a very rare consequence.
      (2) **Oophoritis** may occur but usually does not cause sequelae.
      (3) **Pancreatitis** is extremely rare. The possibility that subclinical pancreatic involvement may be involved as a cause of juvenile diabetes has been investigated but not proven.
      (4) **Hepatitis** is also rare.

B. Epidemiology

1. **Susceptibility.** Mumps tends to affect school-aged children. It is unusual to see mumps in infants because the mother's antibody remains protective for the first year. Most cases occur during the late winter or early spring months.
2. **Incidence.** Before the mumps vaccine was introduced, the incidence of mumps was high (more than 200,000 cases per year). After 1975, the year the vaccine was introduced, the number of cases dropped to 60,000 per year and in 1985, only 3000 cases were reported. In 1987, there was an increase in the number of cases to 13,000, apparently as a result of less aggressive immunization programs. The number of cases per year has declined over the last few years, down to 1322 in 1994.
3. **Transmission** is by inhalation of contaminated aerosol droplets and is favored by close contact.

C. Diagnosis is usually clinical, but can be confirmed by isolation in tissue culture or by serology. Detection of antibodies to an envelope antigen (V antigen) by complement fixation is indicative of past infection; detection of soluble (S) antigen is indicative of a recent or current infection.

D. Treatment is supportive.

E. Prevention

1. A safe and efficient **live attenuated vaccine** is available.
2. **Mumps immune globulin** can be used to prevent the disease in nonimmunized individuals exposed to the virus.

IV. MEASLES (RUBEOLA) VIRUS

A. Clinical disease

1. **Measles (rubeola).** Subclinical cases of measles are rare.
   a. The **incubation period** lasts 10–20 days.
   b. The **prodromal phase** lasts several days and is characterized by:
      (1) **Coryza** (i.e., runny nose)
      (2) **Conjunctivitis,** which results from hematogenous spread, not from a direct infection of the eye, and is usually associated with **photophobia**
      (3) **Cough**
   c. **Koplik spots,** a tiny, punctuate, whitish rash with an erythematous base that appears on the buccal mucosa just above the lower molars, is pathognomonic for measles. It occurs bilaterally at the end of the prodromal period, 24–36 hours before the rash appears.
   d. The **exanthematic stage** is characterized by the typical **morbilliform rash,** which begins on the face and thorax and spreads peripherally. The rash lasts approximately 5 days.

2. **Modified measles** is a mild form of measles that occurs in infants who are still protected by maternal antibodies, and in individuals who have been administered hyperimmune measles γ-globulin or regular γ-globulin (which also contains anti-measles antibodies) close to the time of infection.

3. **Atypical measles** occurs in people who have received either the early killed vaccine or the killed vaccine followed by live vaccine and are later exposed to a wild strain. It is a serious, prolonged illness that lasts for several days. Virus is not recovered from the patient, who is not contagious.
   a. **Pathogenesis.** Atypical measles is believed to result from a hypersensitivity reaction to measles, elicited by the killed vaccine. These patients are believed to be partially immune as a result of vaccination. Consequently, full viral replication does not take place but the virus still infects permissive cells, where it undergoes limited replication. Very little or no progeny are detected, but the infected cells, modified by the virus, are likely to stimulate an immune response. The clinical picture is thus believed to be mainly determined by the immune response to infected cells.
   b. **Signs and symptoms**
      (1) In contrast to the classic measles rash, the rash starts peripherally (on the arms and hands) and spreads centrally. In addition, the rash, rather than being maculopapular, may be urticarial, maculopapular, hemorrhagic, or vesicular (the latter type can lead to a misdiagnosis of chickenpox).
      (2) Other signs and symptoms include edema of the extremities, high fever, interstitial pulmonary infiltrates, and pleural effusions.

4. **Complications of measles virus infection** can be life-threatening.
   a. **Respiratory tract**
      (1) **Measles pneumonia,** often referred to as **giant cell pneumonia** because of the detection of giant, multinucleated cells in infected tissues, is a rare but devastating complication of measles virus infection, especially in immunocompromised patients. No effective antiviral therapy is available.

(2) **Reactivation of tuberculosis** is seen in purified protein derivative–positive patients who contract measles. Diagnosis can be difficult because measles, like many other viral infections, causes temporary anergy, causing purified protein derivative–positive patients to become purified protein derivative–negative for approximately 1 month.

b. CNS

(1) **Postinfectious encephalitis** is a rare complication that occurs as the rash fades and fever wanes. Prior to measles immunization, the measles virus was the second most common cause of postinfectious viral encephalitis (second to mumps virus).

(a) The clinical course may be mild or severe (particularly in patients under the age of 2 years). Surviving patients may be left with permanent sequelae (e.g., mental retardation).

(b) Measles virus is not recovered from the brain; the encephalitis is believed to result from an autoimmune-type reaction (as is the case with postinfectious encephalitis following mumps or the chickenpox).

(2) **Subacute sclerosing panencephalitis (SSPE)** is a chronic degenerative neurologic disease with a high mortality rate that occurs several years after infection with the measles virus (see Chapter 50 II).

B. Epidemiology

1. **Transmission.** Measles is spread via respiratory droplets and indirectly by fomites; it is highly contagious (particularly during the late prodromal stages). Crowding facilitates spread of the disease.

2. **Prevalence.** The prevalence of measles declined significantly after the introduction of the vaccine in 1963, and with this decline the natural boosting provided by the spread of the wild virus has been lost. As a consequence, the disease is now more often seen in the college student population, where a combination of lack of immunization and loss of vaccination-related immunity creates ideal conditions for epidemic outbreaks.

C. Diagnosis. The diagnosis of measles usually can be made during the prodromal phase on the basis of the patient's symptoms, particularly if the patient is seen during the coldest months of the year, when measles is prevalent. The diagnosis may be more difficult in older children and young adults, or during the warmer months. Under these circumstances, measles may not be suspected.

1. **Differential diagnoses** include the many other infectious and hypersensitivity diseases in which maculopapular rashes are also seen—enteroviral infections, rubella, infectious mononucleosis, AIDS, rickettsial infections (e.g., Rocky Mountain spotted fever), and drug reactions.

2. **Confirmation of the diagnosis** requires isolation of the virus, usually from throat swabs or respiratory secretions, or detection of a significant increase in specific antibody titers.

D. Prevention. The measles virus is serologically monotypic and antigenically stable—qualities that facilitated the development of a vaccine. A killed vaccine was introduced in 1963, but was later replaced by a live, attenuated vaccine.

1. The vaccine is given after the first year of life (so as not to react with maternal antibodies) and is 95%–98% efficacious.

2. Vaccination is contraindicated in immunocompromised individuals.

3. To prevent atypical measles, it is recommended that persons who received the killed vaccine, or the killed vaccine followed by the live vaccine, receive a booster of live vaccine.

V. RESPIRATORY SYNCYTIAL VIRUS

A. Pathogenesis and clinical disease

1. **Pathogenesis.** Respiratory syncytial virus infects the respiratory tract, where it replicates. The incubation period is approximately 5 days.
2. **Clinical disease.** Respiratory syncytial virus is a major cause of respiratory illness in young children, and causes devastating disease in children younger than 24 months of age. Infection of infants younger than 4 months of age is possible because systemic maternal antibodies are not protective
   a. **Lower respiratory tract infections** (e.g., pneumonia, bronchiolitis, and tracheobronchitis) are the more common manifestations of primary infection with respiratory syncytial virus.
   b. **Upper respiratory tract infections** present as a common cold. Coughing is a major symptom; the cough does not resemble that of whooping cough.
   c. **Complications** of respiratory syncytial virus infection tend to occur in infants and include **otitis media,** which is common, and **myocarditis,** which is rare.

B. Epidemiology

1. **Seasonal occurrence.** Infections occur in December and January. Respiratory syncytial virus infection should be suspected when an unusually high number of bronchiolitis or pneumonia cases are seen in the pediatric population during the winter months.
2. **Transmission.** Respiratory syncytial virus is highly contagious and spreads by the respiratory route. Outbreaks reaching epidemic proportions are common. Reinfection with respiratory syncytial virus is common; the first infection is more severe than subsequent infections.

C. Diagnosis. Quick diagnosis is critical and is usually made on a clinical and epidemiologic basis. Definitive diagnosis is based on viral isolation or serology. The importance of confirming a diagnosis depends on the emphasis placed on treatment with ribavirin (see IV D).

1. **Viral isolation** is attempted from nasal swabs.
2. **Serology.** A quick diagnostic technique of satisfactory sensitivity and specificity based on **enzyme immunoassay (EIA)** detection of viral antigen in a nasal swab is available. Specificity and sensitivity values ranging from 75%–95% have been reported for this technique. Negative results in this test do not rule out a possible infection with respiratory syncytial virus, but positive results confirm the diagnosis.

D. Treatment. Ribavirin is considered the drug of choice by some groups, and ineffective by others. It is usually administered as an aerosol.

E. Prevention. Live attenuated vaccines have been tried but none has been approved.

Chapter 37

RNA Viruses V: Other RNA Viruses

John Manos
David T. Kingsbury
Gabriel Virella

I. RHABDOVIRUSES.

RHABDOVIRUSES. Among the many different species of rhabdoviruses, the **rabies virus** is particularly important as a human and animal pathogen.

A. General properties. Rhabdoviruses are −RNA enveloped viruses with helical symmetry.

B. Epidemiology

1. **Sylvatic rabies** is rabies occurring in wild animals (e.g., skunks, raccoons, foxes, wolves, coyotes, mongoose, weasels, bats).
   - **a.** Overall, in the United States, skunks are the most common carriers. On the east coast, raccoons are most often involved.
   - **b.** Twenty species of bats, including fruit and herbivorous bats, are known to transmit rabies in North America. Bat rabies has been reported in almost every state in the United States.
2. **Urban rabies** is rabies in domestic animals (e.g., dogs, cats, horses, cattle). Vampire bats in South America are an important source of rabies in cattle.
3. **Transmission.** Rabies virus primarily affects wild mammals. Humans and domestic animals are accidentally infected and their role in perpetuation of the virus is negligible. In a majority of cases, the disease is transmitted by an animal bite. Occasionally, transmission may occur via a scratch or, even more rarely, inhalation of contaminated aerosolized animal materials.
   - **a.** The virus is found in the saliva of infected animals for a few days before clinical signs become recognizable. If the virus is present in the animal's saliva at the time of the bite, the risk of transmitting the infection is 30%–40%. If the virus is only found in the brain, the risk of transmission is lower (10%–15%).
   - **b.** Bat infection may be latent because bats excrete virus in saliva for months. Humans can acquire the infection by inhalation of contaminated particles in bat-populated caves.

C. Pathogenesis and clinical disease

1. **Pathogenesis**
   - **a. Replication and dissemination.** After multiplying in muscle cells at the site of a bite, the virus invades peripheral nerve fibers at the neuromuscular junction and spreads to the spinal cord and brain via nerve pathways. In the brain, the virus replicates in the gray matter and propagates via autonomic nerve fibers to peripheral tissues (including the salivary glands), from which it is excreted.
   - **b.** The **incubation period depends on the portal of entry** (the farther away from the brain, the longer the incubation period) and **virus dose.**
     - **(1)** On average, the incubation period is 1–3 months; it can be as short as 1 week or as long as 1 year.
     - **(2)** The incubation period of bat-transmitted human rabies is relatively short (3–4 weeks).
   - **c. Pathologic effects.** Histologically, rabies is characterized by degenerative changes in the nerve cells and diffuse perivascular mononuclear cell infiltration. Characteristic eosinophilic intracytoplasmic inclusion bodies (Negri bodies) are

found in the central nervous system (CNS) tissue, particularly in the area of the hippocampus.

2. **Clinical disease**
   a. **Subclinical disease** is not known to occur in humans.
   b. **Clinical disease**
      (1) The onset of clinical disease is marked by discomfort at the site of the animal bite (e.g., paraesthesias), headaches, insomnia, and apprehension.
      (2) As the disease progresses, the patient develops dysphagia (for fluids at first, and then solids), generalized convulsions, delirium, and coma. In the delirium stage, the patient may show manic behavior and require isolation. Rarely, the patient develops flaccid paralysis. Death occurs in more than 90% of cases.

D. Treatment. The treatment of an animal bite wound inflicted by an animal suspected of carrying rabies includes general measures and specific anti-rabies prophylaxis.

1. **General measures** include the following:
   a. **Aggressive cleansing** of the wound
   b. **Administration of a tetanus toxoid booster,** if needed
   c. **Administration of a broad-spectrum antibiotic** effective against *Pasteurella multocida* (e.g., doxycycline)

2. **Anti-rabies prophylaxis**
   a. **Influencing factors.** The decision to administer anti-rabies prophylaxis depends on a variety of factors, such as the:
      (1) **Type of exposure** (e.g., lick vs. bite)
      (2) **Species of the animal** suspected of carrying rabies
      (3) **Circumstances of the bite** (e.g., provoked versus unprovoked)
      (4) **Vaccination status** of the animal and the patient
      (5) **Presence of rabies in the locality**
   b. **Measures** include the following:
      (1) **Human rabies immune globulin (HRIG)** should be administered to provide passive immunization. Although HRIG is preferred, equine anti-rabies serum may also be used. The dose is divided in half; one half is injected around the bite, and the other half is injected systemically (intramuscularly).
      (2) **Human diploid cell vaccine (HDCV)** should be administered on days 0, 3, 7, 14, and 28. The possibility of using the vaccine to prevent disease after exposure derives from the long incubation period of rabies, which allows induction of a protective immune response before the onset of disease.

E. Control and prevention

1. **Control.** The incidence of rabies has decreased considerably because of a series of measures aimed at reducing the population of infected animals. Measures include the following:
   a. Intensive immunization of companion and domestic animals
   b. Control of stray domestic animals
   c. Population reduction of wildlife reservoirs
   d. Introduction of live, attenuated rabies virus in the habitat of wild animals
   e. Strict quarantines on animal importation

2. **Prevention.** Effective and safe human vaccines are available, including HDCV, which is produced in a human diploid cell line. The old vaccines prepared from infected nervous tissue caused neuroparalytic accidents, probably as a result of a cross-reactive immune reaction against nervous tissue antigens present in the vaccine. Such reactions are not seen with HDCV, which is also more immunogenic than the old vaccines, and fewer injections are required for effective immunization. The vaccine is given prophylactically to individuals with high risk of occupational exposure (e.g., veterinarians).

II. CORONAVIRUSES

A. General properties. Coronaviruses are enveloped +RNA viruses with helical symmetry. Coronaviruses owe their name to the fact that their outer surface has club-shaped glycoprotein spikes that give the virus a crown-like appearance (Latin *corona,* crown).

B. Epidemiology

1. Coronavirus infections are **most common in children.** Frequency of infection increases during the **winter, early spring,** and **spring** months.
2. **Transmission.** Coronaviruses are acquired by the **respiratory route.**

C. Pathogenesis and clinical disease

1. **Pathogenesis.** The virus causes disease at the portal of entry, and the incubation period is estimated to last 2–5 days. Reinfections are common and are related to the following two factors:
   - **a.** The virus is antigenically heterogeneous (four different antigenic groups have been defined) and viruses from more than one group can cause disease.
   - **b.** Protective immunity depends on the synthesis of mucosal antibodies. Mucosal immunity is short-lived and the incubation period is too short for a secondary response to be mounted in time to prevent reinfection.
2. **Clinical disease.** Coronaviruses were first isolated from the respiratory tract of people with common colds. The viruses are found in the stool, but whether they play a significant role in gastrointestinal disease is unknown.
   - **a. Subclinical infections** probably account for half of all coronavirus infections.
   - **b. Clinical infection.** The patient presents with symptoms of upper respiratory tract infection and a low-grade fever. The disease is usually self-limiting and the prognosis is excellent.

D. Diagnosis. Because of the mildness of the disease and the lack of specific therapy, coronavirus infections usually are clinically classified as "acute upper respiratory infections of probable viral etiology." Etiologic diagnosis may be considered for epidemiologic reasons, and can be established by isolation in tissue culture or by serology.

E. Therapy is supportive.

F. Prevention. No vaccine is available.

III. CALICIVIRUSES.

Human pathogenic caliciviruses include the Norwalk virus, Norwalk-like agents, and hepatitis E virus (HEV; see Chapter 38). The Norwalk agent was named after Norwalk, Ohio, where it was first discovered during the investigation of an outbreak of acute gastroenteritis in a public school. Other similar viruses were subsequently described, forming the group designated as Norwalk-like agents.

A. General properties. Caliciviruses are naked viruses with an icosahedral capsid. Their genome consists of +RNA.

B. Epidemiology. Caliciviruses are spread by the **fecal-oral route.**

C. Pathogenesis and clinical disease

1. **Pathogenesis.** The caliciviruses infect the small intestine. The infection is associated with villous atrophy and diarrhea. Infected individuals develop antibodies, but resistance is transient and reinfection can occur.

TABLE 37-1. Viruses Associated with Hemorrhagic Fever

Virus	Family	Distribution	Animal Carriers/Vectors
Yellow fever	Togavirus	Central and South America	Monkeys/mosquitoes
Marburg	Filovirus	Eastern Africa	Monkeys
Ebola	Filovirus	Sudan and Zaire	Monkeys
Lassa	Arenavirus	Western Africa	Rodents
Machupo	Arenavirus	South America	Rodents
Hantaan	Bunyavirus	Korea	Rodents

2. **Clinical disease.** These viruses are the **most common cause of viral gastroenteritis in adults.** They cause three types of epidemiologically defined syndromes—**winter vomiting, epidemic diarrhea** (in older children and adults), and **viral gastroenteritis.** After a very short incubation period (1–2 days) there is a gradual or abrupt onset of symptoms, including:
   a. **Nausea, vomiting,** or both
   b. **Myalgia** and **headaches**
   c. **Low-grade fever,** in approximately 50% of patients, mostly children (adults usually remain afebrile)
   d. **Moderate diarrhea** (4 to 8 loose, watery stools per day)

D. Diagnosis. The Norwalk-like agents are very difficult to cultivate; thus the diagnosis is essentially clinical and confirmation for epidemiological purposes is based on serological data.

E. Treatment is supportive.

F. Prevention. No vaccine is available.

IV. FILOVIRUSES include the Marburg virus and the Ebola virus.

A. General properties. Filoviruses are filamentous, enveloped, −RNA viruses with helical nucleocapsid symmetry.

B. Epidemiology

1. **Distribution and reservoirs.** The filoviruses are primarily distributed in equatorial and subequatorial Africa, and are believed to be primarily zoonotic. Monkeys are well-documented hosts.

2. **Transmission** to humans occasionally occurs, and human-to-human transmission seems to be possible. The precise route of spread has not been defined, except in some outbreaks in which transmission via contaminated blood-drawing materials (e.g., syringes) appeared to be one of the mechanisms of propagation.

C. Pathogenesis and clinical disease. The Marburg and Ebola viruses cause **hemorrhagic fevers.** Other viral causes of hemorrhagic fever are listed in Table 37-1.

1. **Pathogenesis.** Platelet dysfunction appears to be the major pathogenic factor involved. Hemorrhagic shock is responsible for the high mortality rate associated with these diseases.

2. **Clinical disease.** Common clinical features include fever, petechiae or purpura, gastrointestinal, nasal, and uterine bleeding, leukopenia, shock, proteinuria, and neurologic abnormalities.

V. ARENAVIRUSES.

ARENAVIRUSES. The arenavirus group includes a variety of viruses that infect rodents and may occasionally infect humans, such as the **lymphocytic choriomeningitis (LCM) virus** and the **Lassa fever virus.** Because of the epidemiologic association with rodents, the arenaviruses and some bunyaviruses are epidemiologically designated **roboviruses** (shortened from "rodent-borne viruses").

A. General properties

1. The arenavirus virions are **round** or **pleomorphic** and **enveloped.** The **viral RNA** is **segmented, single-stranded,** and of **negative polarity.**
2. Arenaviruses contain host-derived **ribosomal aggregates,** probably acquired during the budding process, which perform no known function. These electron-dense granules give the viruses a unique pebbly appearance when viewed under the electron microscope and are responsible for the name of this group of viruses, which is derived from the **Latin *arena,* sand.**

B. Epidemiology

1. **Reservoirs.** Arenaviruses commonly induce a chronic carrier state in rodents, their natural hosts. Transplacental transmission helps perpetuate the infection. The viruses may be isolated from the urine, blood, and organs of infected animals.
2. **Transmission.** The viruses can be transmitted to humans following inhalation or contact with materials contaminated with excretions of infected rodents. The virus can also be transmitted via a bite from an infected animal, but this is rare.

C. Clinical disease

1. The **LCM virus** usually causes a mild **influenza-like illness,** but occasionally may cause **meningitis,** characteristically associated with very large numbers of lymphocytes in the cerebrospinal fluid (CSF).
2. The **Lassa fever virus** was first isolated among Americans stationed in the village of Lassa, Nigeria. The virus can be transmitted person-to-person.
   a. **Subclinical disease.** Serologic surveys suggest that inapparent infections may be common, particularly among members of hunting tribes.
   b. **Clinical disease.** Lassa virus can cause epidemics associated with high mortality rates (36%–67%); the cause of these outbreaks is unknown. The disease is characterized by a **high fever, mouth ulcers, severe myalgia, a hemorrhagic skin rash, pneumonia,** and **heart** and **kidney damage.**
3. **Other arenaviruses.** Several arenaviruses found in South America cause **hemorrhagic fever.**

VI. BUNYAVIRUSES.

BUNYAVIRUSES. This family includes several genera of **arboviruses** (see Chapter 34), as well as the **hantaviruses.**

A. General properties.

General properties. The bunyaviruses are enveloped viruses with a segmented −RNA genome and a nucleocapsid of helical symmetry.

B. Clinical disease

1. The **Hantaan virus,** first described in the 1950s during the Korean war, causes a **hemorrhagic fever** with **acute renal failure.**
2. The **pulmonary syndrome hantavirus ("Sin Nombre" strain)** came to prominence in the early 1990s when it was associated with a syndrome characterized by **acute respiratory failure,** often fatal, which has predominantly affected Native Americans in

the western United States (the "Four Corners" region, northern California, and Nevada).

a. The main vectors are deer mice (*Peromyscus* species), but other rodents (e.g., chipmunks, rats, other species of mice) have been found to carry the virus as well. Person-to-person transmission has not been documented.

b. As of July 1995, this virus had infected 113 people in 23 states, with a mortality rate of 52%.

VII. REOVIRUSES

A. General properties and classification

1. **Structure.** Reoviruses are naked viruses, with a nucleocapsid of icosahedral symmetry. Reoviruses are unique because of their **segmented, double-stranded RNA genome.**

2. **Classification.** Reoviruses were originally classified with the echoviruses because they were isolated from the stools of healthy children. Sabin recognized that they were probably different and suggested the designation of reovirus, for respiratory enteric orphan virus. Three genera of reoviruses are pathogenic for humans:
   a. ***Reovirus***
   b. ***Orbivirus***
   c. ***Rotavirus***

B.

Reoviruses are clinically associated with diarrhea and upper respiratory infections and, rarely, with meningitis and encephalitis. They do not constitute a significant epidemiologic problem. The diagnosis is usually established clinically; cultures and serology are not done routinely.

C.

Orbiviruses are classified epidemiologically as **arboviruses.** The **Colorado tick fever virus** is the most prevalent orbivirus in the United States.

1. **Epidemiology**
   a. **Transmission.** Colorado tick fever is a zoonosis transmitted through a **tick-rodent-tick cycle** (man is accidentally infected). Humans are dead-end hosts for the virus; there is **no person-to-person transmission.**
   b. **Susceptibility.** The infection tends to be seen in people that spend time in the woods (e.g., hunters).
   c. **Distribution and incidence.** The disease occurs primarily in the western states, especially during tick season (May through July). Several hundred cases are reported each year; probably ten times that number of cases are undiagnosed.

2. **Pathogenesis and clinical disease**
   a. **Pathogenesis.** In humans, the virus is inoculated directly into the blood stream following a bite from an infected tick. The virus circulates bound to red blood cells, and a **prolonged viremia (2–4 weeks)** occurs.
   b. **Clinical disease**
      (1) Symptoms include **fever, chills, lethargy, prostration, headache, myalgia, ocular pain, nausea,** and **vomiting.** Colorado tick fever is occasionally associated with a rash and is almost always a self-limited disease.
      (2) In the very young, the disease may be hemorrhagic as a result of virus-induced thrombocytopenia. It is uncertain whether the infection is teratogenic if infection occurs during early pregnancy.

D.

Rotaviruses. When viewed using an electron microscope, rotaviruses look like a wagon wheel, hence their name (from the Latin *rota,* wheel).

1. **Epidemiology**

a. **Distribution.** There are four serotypes of this virus, with a worldwide distribution.
b. **Transmission.** The virus is usually isolated from the stools of infants and is probably transmitted by the **fecal-oral route.**
c. **Incidence** peaks during the cooler months.

2. **Pathogenesis and clinical disease**
   a. **Pathogenesis.** After infection, there is a short incubation period of 2–4 days. The virus multiplies in the gastrointestinal tract and disrupts the integrity of the intestinal mucosa, particularly the microvilli. The clinical consequence is diarrhea.
   b. **Clinical disease.** Rotavirus infection is the **most common nonbacterial cause of diarrhea in infants.** It can also cause diarrhea in adults. In children, the diarrhea lasts for 24–48 hours and then subsides spontaneously. In infants, the major risk is acute dehydration, which may be fatal.

3. **Prevention.** Rotavirus vaccines are currently in clinical trials.

Chapter 38

Hepatitis Viruses

John Manos
Edwin A. Brown

I. INTRODUCTION.

INTRODUCTION. The hepatitis viruses (Table 38-1), a heterogeneous group of viruses with a tropism for the liver, are the major cause of viral hepatitis (see also Chapter 55). Other viruses, including Epstein-Barr virus (EBV), cytomegalovirus (CMV), herpes simplex virus (HSV), coxsackievirus B, mumps virus, and adenoviruses also infect the liver, but hepatitis is seldom the major clinical manifestation. In addition, some bacteria, parasites, fungi, drugs, and chemicals can cause hepatitis that is clinically indistinguishable from viral hepatitis.

II. HEPATITIS A VIRUS (HAV)

A. Epidemiology

1. **Transmission.** HAV is transmitted by the **fecal-oral route.** HAV is excreted in the stool of patients 2–3 weeks before, and 8–10 days after, the onset of jaundice. Patients are most infectious prior to or at the onset of jaundice. The virus particle is **resistant to degradation,** remaining infectious in the environment for weeks.
   a. **Person-to-person transmission** can cause outbreaks in places where personal hygiene may be substandard (e.g., **institutions for the mentally handicapped, day care centers).**
   b. **Fecal contamination of a single source** (e.g., **water, shellfish)** can lead to sudden epidemics of hepatitis A.
2. **Distribution and incidence.** Infection by HAV is common on a global scale, especially in areas with poor sanitation. Over 23,000 cases of hepatitis A were reported to the Centers for Disease Control (CDC) in 1994. Because of underreporting, the actual number of cases is probably eight to ten times higher than this figure.
3. **Mortality rate.** The mortality rate is **less than 0.1%** and is usually associated with fulminant HAV infection (hepatic necrosis leading to a loss of hepatic function).

B. Clinical disease.

Clinical disease. HAV causes an acute, highly contagious form of hepatitis previously referred to as **infectious hepatitis.**

1. **Subclinical infection.** The majority of hepatitis A cases in children are subclinical and many symptomatic cases are anicteric and undiagnosed. Most infections in adults are symptomatic.
2. **Clinical infection.** The **incubation period** ranges from **2–6 weeks.**
   a. The **pre-icteric stage** is characterized by nonspecific, flu-like symptoms of anorexia, nausea, vomiting, and malaise.
   b. The **icteric stage** is characterized by hyperbilirubinemia, jaundice, hepatomegaly, right upper quadrant tenderness, and raised serum levels of liver enzymes such as alanine aminotransferase (ALT) and aspartate aminotransferase (AST).

C. Laboratory diagnosis.

Laboratory diagnosis. Although the diagnosis of hepatitis is based on clinical data and the results of tests reflecting liver function and inflammation (e.g., serum bilirubin, ALT, and AST levels), the identification of the causative agent is based on **serologic tests** that detect antibodies to HAV. The finding of IgM anti-HAV antibodies indicates current or

TABLE 38-1. The Hepatitis Viruses

Virus	Classification	Nucleic Acid	Envelope
Hepatitis A virus	Picornavirus	Single stranded + RNA	No
Hepatitis B virus	Hepadnavirus	Incomplete circular double-stranded DNA	Yes
Hepatitis C virus	Flavivirus	Single stranded + RNA	Yes
Hepatitis D virus	Unclassified	Circular single stranded − RNA	Yes
Hepatitis E virus	Calicivirus	Single stranded + RNA	No

recent infection, while the finding of IgG anti-HAV antibodies (without IgM antibodies) indicates past exposure to the virus.

D. Treatment. There is no specific treatment for acute viral hepatitis; therapy is **supportive. Immune serum globulin (ISG)** preparations (which contain anti-HAV antibodies) administered soon after exposure may prevent or ameliorate the disease.

E. Immunity after HAV infection is usually lifelong, infrequently waning in the elderly. Relapses occur, but chronic carriers of HAV have not been detected. In the United States, the prevalence of antibody to HAV increases with age, ranging from 11% in children younger than 5 years of age, to 74% in adults over 50 years of age. This high prevalence in older adults may reflect infection in the distant past when the level of sanitation was lower, rather than suggesting continuous exposure to HAV. In developing countries with inadequate sanitation, HAV infection occurs in childhood.

F. Prevention. An effective **killed virus vaccine** is available.

III. HEPATITIS B VIRUS (HBV).

Because HBV infections may become chronic, hepatitis B is considered a more serious disease than hepatitis A. Patients who fail to mount an effective immune response can carry the virus in an infectious form for life.

A. General properties

1. **Structure.** HBV was discovered by electron microscopic examination of infected hepatic tissue and was originally designated the **Dane particle.** HBV is 42 nm in diameter and has:
   - **a.** A lipid-containing **outer envelope,** which contains **hepatitis B surface antigen (HBsAg)**
   - **b.** An **inner protein core,** made up of **hepatitis B core antigen (HBcAg),** that surrounds the viral nucleic acid
   - **c.** A **genome** of circular double-stranded DNA, with an incomplete positive strand
   - **d.** A **DNA polymerase,** which also functions as a reverse transcriptase
2. **Associated antigens**
   - **a. HBsAg.** The envelope of HBV is unique because it is 70% protein. This protein, HBsAg, is strongly immunogenic.
     - **(1)** HBsAg tends to associate with itself to form 22-nm **spherical** or **rod-like particles** that **circulate in the serum** of infected patients.
     - **(2) Defective particles** were demonstrated electron microscopically in blood samples from patients with acute HBV infection and chronic carriers. Described as circular or filamentous aggregates 22 nm in diameter, they are noninfectious aggregates of surface antigen released into the circulation as a replication by-product. The original HBV vaccine was made by purifying these aggregates.

b. **Hepatitis B e antigen (HBeAg)** is not part of the virus particle. HBeAg is translated from RNA that contains the pre-core and core (HBcAg) regions. After translation, the protein is truncated at the carboxy terminus and then released from the infected cell.
   (1) HBeAg modulates the host immune response to HBV and is an important indicator of transmissibility.
   (2) Point mutations in the precore region that prevent translation of HBeAg produce mutant strains. Although these mutant strains of HBV were originally found in patients with fulminant hepatitis, the transition from HBeAg-positive to HBeAg-negative status has been shown to occur in chronically infected patients without severe disease.

B. Classification. Four antigenic strains of HBV (ayw, adw, ayr, adr) have been identified. **All strains cause the same clinical disease.** The significance of serologic typing of HBV is both epidemiologic (e.g., to trace the source of a particular outbreak) and medical–legal (e.g., to help prove or dismiss allegations against a suspected carrier).

C. Epidemiology

1. **Transmission.** HBV is found in blood and blood by-products, tears, saliva, semen, urine, feces, breast milk, synovial fluid, and cerebrospinal fluid (CSF) in acutely affected patients as well as in carriers.
   a. **Blood** and **blood by-products** are the most important vehicles of **parenteral transmission.**
   b. **Saliva** and **semen** are involved in **venereal transmission.**

2. **Prevalence**
   a. It is estimated that in the United States, 3%–5% of adults have been infected with HBV, and that 300,000 new cases of hepatitis B infection occur annually.
   b. Seven to ten percent of patients infected with HBV become chronic carriers. (This statistic corresponds to a 0.3%–0.5% prevalence of chronic HBV infection of adults in the United States.) The likelihood of becoming a carrier is greater in individuals who experienced a mild or subclinical (anicteric) infection.

3. **Incidence.** Acute hepatitis B is rarely diagnosed in children younger than 14 years of age. The incidence peaks in the 15- to 19-year-old age group.

4. **Susceptibility.** Populations at risk for HBV infection include:
   a. **Healthcare workers**
   b. **Institutionalized individuals**
   c. **Intravenous drug users**
   d. **Hemophiliacs**
   e. **Renal dialysis patients**
   f. **Infants born to HBsAg-positive mothers**
   g. **Sexual partners of HBV carriers**
   h. **Individuals with multiple sexual partners** (homosexual or heterosexual)

D. Pathogenesis and clinical disease

1. **Pathogenesis.** The **incubation period** ranges from 40–180 days.

2. **Clinical disease**
   a. **Acute**
      (1) **Subclinical infections** are more common than clinical infections. In subclinical infections, liver function studies may show elevated liver enzymes.
      (2) **Clinical infections** vary in severity. Hepatitis B tends to be more insidious in onset than hepatitis A, and the severity of the disease is related to the viral dose—the greater the inoculum, the more severe the disease. In broad terms, the clinical infection can be divided into two major categories:
         (a) **Anicteric infection** is characterized by nonspecific symptoms such as malaise and anorexia. Dark urine or bilirubinemia may occur, even though the patient is not icteric. Transaminases are usually elevated. The

complete blood count (CBC) often remains normal or it may show moderate lymphocytosis with atypical lymphocytes. Generally, these patients remain undiagnosed.

(b) **Icteric infection.** The patient, after complaining of malaise and anorexia, develops jaundice. The symptoms may progress or improve at the time that jaundice becomes evident. Once the patient is jaundiced, the diagnosis of hepatitis B is readily made using serologic tests.

(3) **Complications.** The immune response causes complications in approximately 10%–20% of patients hospitalized for the treatment of hepatitis B.

(a) Patients may develop a **serum sickness–type syndrome** characterized by joint pain, hives, urticaria, and maculopapular rashes secondary to the formation of HBsAg antigen–antibody complexes.

(b) Patients may develop **polyarteritis nodosa** or **membranous glomerulonephritis,** disorders believed to be manifestations of systemic vasculitis secondary to the deposition of soluble immune complexes.

b. **Chronic.** Carriers are defined as those individuals in whom HBsAg has been detectable for at least 6 months. Of the infected individuals who become chronic carriers, the majority (approximately 7% of HBV-infected individuals or 75% of carriers) develop chronic, persistent hepatitis B, while the remaining 3% of infected individuals develop chronic active hepatitis.

(1) **Persistent hepatitis B**

(a) Patients with persistent hepatitis have a smoldering disease. They remain clinically well but are potentially infectious. Their liver enzymes may be slightly elevated.

(b) Persistent hepatitis B can lead to terminal liver failure. It is believed that the progression of liver damage is often mediated by an immune reaction triggered by persistent viral infection of the hepatocyte.

(2) **Chronic active hepatitis.** Patients are more likely to be symptomatic and to have flare-ups of hepatitis.

(3) **Complications.** Chronic hepatocellular inflammation and necrosis from chronic HBV infection is associated with cirrhosis and hepatocellular carcinoma.

(a) **Cirrhosis.** Chronic carriers, especially those with chronic active hepatitis, may develop cirrhosis. At least 5000 deaths per year can be attributed to HBV-induced cirrhosis.

(b) **Hepatocellular carcinoma.** There is a strong association between chronic HBV infection and hepatocellular carcinoma, particularly in South Africa and China. Other cofactors, in addition to HBV infection, contribute to the development of hepatocellular carcinoma. Approximately 1200 deaths per year can be attributed to HBV-induced hepatocellular carcinoma in the United States.

E. Diagnosis

1. **Immunofluorescent staining** of infected hepatocytes demonstrates HBV core protein in the nucleus of the host cell and infectious Dane particles in the cytoplasm.

2. **Detection of viral DNA** in tissue samples is a more sensitive and modern approach to diagnosis.

3. **Serology.** For clinical purposes, the diagnosis is based primarily on serological data.

a. Antigenic structures and specific antibodies currently used in the diagnosis of HBV are listed in Table 38-2.

b. The patterns on the **HBV profile** vary according to whether the disease is acute or chronic and whether the infection is active or not (Figure 38-1).

(1) To diagnose a **recent infection,** the **HBsAg, IgM anti-HBcAg,** and **anti-HBsAg** titers should be requested. In those patients who clear the infection, serum levels of HBsAg will rise and then fall when the immune system responds to the infection. Antibody to HBsAg may not be detected for weeks as a result of the formation of antibody–antigen complexes. During this period, known as the "window period," only IgM anti-HBcAg is detectable.

TABLE 38-2. Markers for Hepatitis B Virus (HBV) Infection

Antigen	Antibody
Dane particle	
DNA polymerase	
HBsAg*	anti-HBsAg*
HBcAg	anti-HBcAg*, IgM anti-HBcAg*
HBeAg*	anti-HBeAg*

Anti-HBcAg = anti-hepatitis B core antigen antibody; *anti-HBeAg* = anti-hepatitis B e antigen antibody; *anti-HBsAg* = anti-hepatitis B surface antigen antibody; *HBcAg* = hepatitis B core antigen; *HBeAg* = hepatitis B e antigen; *HBsAg* = hepatitis B surface antigen; *Igm anti-HBcAg* = anti-hepatitis B core antigen IgM antibody.
* Used in routine serological tests.

(2) The finding of **HBeAg** in a patient with other markers of chronic infection is considered evidence of active viral replication. These individuals are highly infectious.

F. Treatment. No specific treatment for acute hepatitis B is available, so therapy is supportive. Research has focused on the treatment of chronic carriers because of the high rate of complications associated with chronic infection.

1. α-Interferon (IFN-α). Attempts to eliminate the HBV carrier state by administering IFN-α have received much attention.

a. Fewer than 50% of carriers respond to this treatment.

(1) Those that respond lose the HBV markers (i.e., HBV DNA, HBeAg, and HBsAg) and eventually develop anti-HBsAg antibody. In one study, half of those responding to IFN-α therapy remained HBsAg-negative after 5 years.

(2) Pretreatment variables associated with a positive response to IFN-α therapy include elevated serum ALT, low amounts of HBV DNA, and a short duration of disease.

b. The use of IFN-α is associated with serious side effects, such as psychosis, depression, and thyroid disease.

2. Lamivudine, a nucleoside analog used in the treatment of HIV-positive patients, has been shown to suppress chronic HBV infections. The use of this drug by itself or in combination with IFN-α for the treatment of chronic HBV infection is currently being investigated.

G. Prevention

1. Passive immunization has been practiced with **hepatitis B immune globulin (HBIg).** Administration is indicated for the following individuals:

a. Nonimmune individuals accidentally exposed to potentially infectious materials from an individual known to be HBsAg-positive

b. Individuals in intimate contact with an individual known to be infectious

c. Neonates born to HBsAg-positive mothers

2. Active immunization is possible with recombinant vaccines **(Recombivax B, Engerix B),** produced in cultures of genetically engineered *Saccharomyces cerevisiae.*

a. Indications. Prophylactic immunization is recommended for all individuals with a high risk of infection and for all newborns.

b. Schedule

(1) Adults receive two doses 1 month apart followed by a booster at 6 months.

(2) Newborns receive the first immunization at birth and repeated doses at 1 and 6 months of age. If the mother is HBsAg-positive, the child receives HBIg along with the first vaccine dose at birth.

c. Escape mutants. Children born to HBsAg-positive mothers and administered

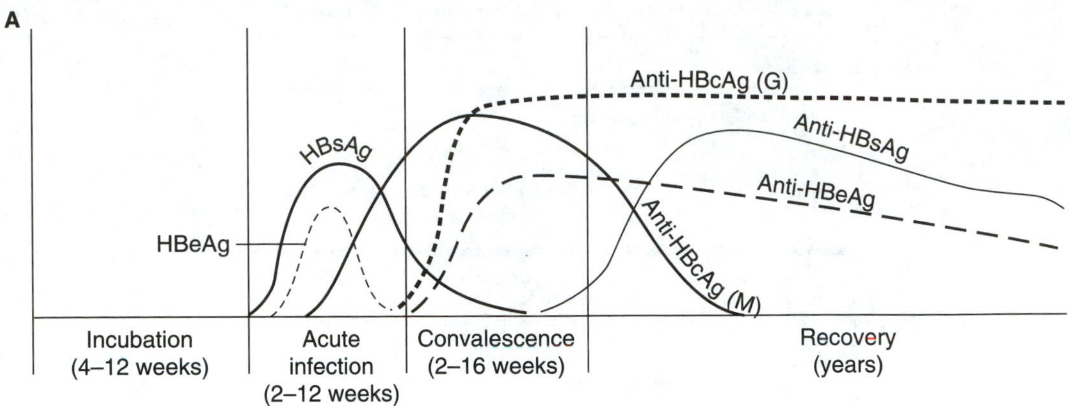
A
Anti-HBcAg (G)
Anti-HBsAg
HBsAg
Anti-HBeAg
HBeAg
Anti-HBcAg (M)
Incubation
(4–12 weeks)
Acute
infection
(2–12 weeks)
Convalescence
(2–16 weeks)
Recovery
(years)

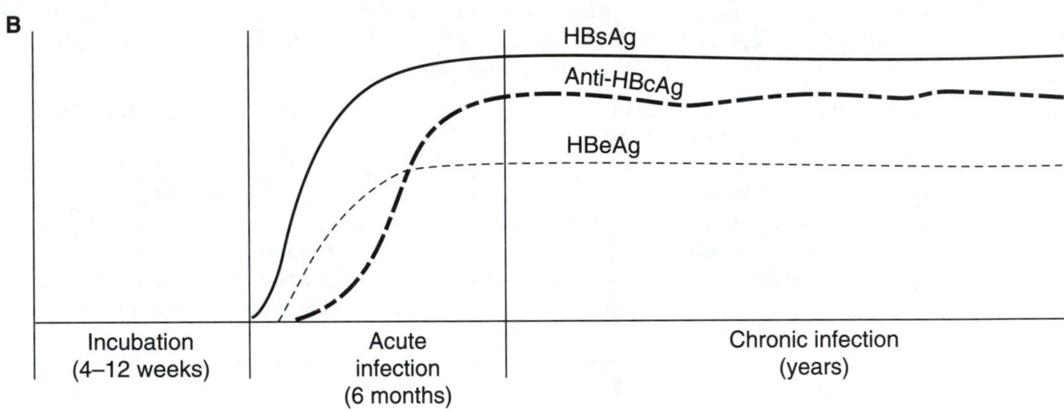
B
HBsAg
Anti-HBcAg
HBeAg
Incubation
(4–12 weeks)
Acute
infection
(6 months)
Chronic infection
(years)

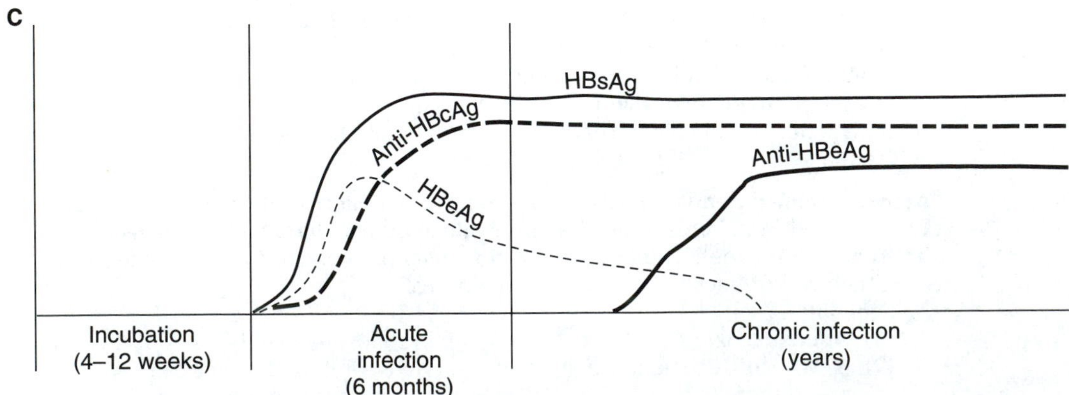
C
HBsAg
Anti-HBcAg
Anti-HBeAg
HBeAg
Incubation
(4–12 weeks)
Acute
infection
(6 months)
Chronic infection
(years)

HBIg and vaccinated against HBV at birth occassionally become infected with HBV. Most of these infants were infected *in utero;* however, strains have also been isolated from infected infants that lack the common "a" determinant, the major target antigen of the vaccine response. The immune globulin and the vaccine-induced antibodies have led to the selection of these mutant strains.

IV. HEPATITIS C VIRUS (HCV).

HEPATITIS C VIRUS (HCV). After the development of serologic tests for hepatitis A and hepatitis B, a third type of hepatitis was discovered in recipients of blood products. It was demonstrated that these cases of hepatitis were not caused by HSV, CMV, EBV, or coxsackieviruses. The existence of a new hepatitis virus was suspected when cytoplasmic tubular structures were observed in liver cells of chimpanzees infected with the serum of patients with proven non-A, non-B hepatitis. A gene library was constructed from viruses collected from the livers of animals with non-A, non-B hepatitis and, after expression in an *Escherichia coli* system, it was possible to identify proteins that were recognized by antibodies present in the serum of patients with non-A, non-B hepatitis.

A. General properties

1. **Structure.** HCV is an enveloped virus measuring approximately 35–50 nm in diameter. It contains single-stranded, linear, **positive-sense RNA** surrounded by a protein capsid.

2. **Classification.** HCV is a member of the Flavivirus family, which includes the yellow fever virus, another hepatotropic virus.

B. Epidemiology

1. Initially, HCV was defined as the major cause of post-transfusion hepatitis. When serologic surveys were applied to larger groups of patients, it was found that HCV was transmitted among intravenous drug users and was also involved in community-acquired non-A, non-B hepatitis. The mode of transmission in the community is still not understood.

2. HCV and HBV share similar epidemiological characteristics, with the exception that vertical and sexual transmission are much less common with HCV.

C. Clinical presentation.

Clinical presentation. Most infections caused by HCV are subclinical; however, over 70% of patients who are infected become chronic carriers and a significant percentage of these individuals develop **chronic hepatitis.** Most patients who are chronically infected are asymptomatic until the sequelae of chronic hepatitis intervene (i.e., cirrhosis, hepatocellular carcinoma).

FIGURE 38-1. Serologic profiles seen in acute and chronic HBV infection. (*A*) Serologic profile of a patient with acute hepatitis B who does not develop chronic hepatitis. Four to twelve weeks postinfection, hepatitis B surface antigen (*HBsAg*) is detected in the patient's serum. Shortly thereafter, an IgM response to hepatitis B core antigen (HBcAg) appears [*anti-HBcAg (M)*]. As the host's immune response mounts, HbsAg levels decrease and anti-HBsAg levels increase. The time during which neither HBsAg nor anti-HBsAg is detectable is called the "window period." After several weeks, the IgM anti-HBcAg level declines and is replaced by IgG anti-HBcAg [*anti-HBcAg (G)*]. (*B*) Serologic profile of a patient with chronic hepatitis B. After infection, HBsAg is found in the patient's serum, but instead of HBsAg being cleared and anti-HBsAg developing as seen when the HBV infection resolves, HBsAg continues to be present. An immune response to HBcAg is detectable shortly after infection (*anti-HBcAg*). Hepatitis B e antigen (*HBeAg*) is present at approximately the same time as HBsAg and is found throughout the course of chronic hepatitis. (*C*) Serologic profile of a patient undergoing late seroconversion. In some cases of chronic hepatitis B, seroconversion from HBeAg to anti-HBeAg occurs months to years after infection. These patients continue to have detectable HBsAg present in their serum and are at risk for developing hepatocellular carcinoma, but are less infectious than patients who have HBeAg.

D. Laboratory diagnosis and screening

1. **Enzyme immunoassay (EIA).** The antigens most frequently recognized in patients with non-A, non-B hepatitis became the basis for the immunoassays used to screen for hepatitis C.
   a. The HCV EIA is performed by all blood banks in an attempt to exclude chronic HCV carriers. However, because hepatitis viruses have been identified for which there are no screening tests, it is safer to exclude blood whenever there is evidence of liver inflammation.
   b. Although useful for screening, the HCV EIA has a poor positive predictive value when used to diagnose hepatitis C in the low-risk blood donor pool. In acutely infected individuals, the production of detectable antibody is delayed; therefore, it may be several weeks or even months before the EIA becomes positive. During this time, the patient is viremic and highly infectious but remains seronegative.

2. **Recombinant immunoblot assay (RIBA)** is used to confirm the diagnosis. In patients without obvious risk factors, the highly specific RIBA is performed to test for false-positive EIA results.

3. **Anti-HbcAg testing.** Epidemiologic evidence suggests that HCV carriers are often HbsAg negative but anti-HbcAg positive. For this reason, Blood Donor Centers continue to test donated blood for this "surrogate" marker since donors who are positive are more likely to be carriers of HCV or other yet unidentified hepatotropic viruses than donors who are negative.

E. Treatment

Treatment is supportive in patients with acute hepatitis C. There have been attempts at using **IFN-α** to treat patients with chronic HCV infections. Decreased hepatic inflammation, as measured by a reduction in serum ALT levels, was observed in 40%–70% of the treated patients, but over half of the patients relapsed when the IFN-α therapy was stopped.

F. Prevention

1. **Passive immunization** with **ISG** is **not effective.** Because of concerns about HCV transmission, the Food and Drug Administration (FDA) removed all HCV EIA–positive serum from the ISG preparation.

2. **Active immunization. No vaccine** is available.

V. HEPATITIS D VIRUS (HDV, DELTA VIRUS)

HEPATITIS D VIRUS (HDV, DELTA VIRUS) is a defective RNA virus that is found only in individuals infected with HBV.

A. General properties

General properties. The HDV genome is a small, circular, single-stranded RNA molecule, with no sequence similarity to HBV DNA. HDV particles have an HBsAg-rich outer envelope coded for by HBV. Because HDV depends on HBV for its replication and transmission, it is referred to as a **defective virus.**

B. Epidemiology

Epidemiology. Two modes of human infection with HDV have been defined:

1. **Simultaneous infection (coinfection) with HBV** is most common in recipients of blood products and intravenous drug abusers. If the donor is infected with HBV and HDV, the recipient can become infected with both. Fewer than 5% of those infected develop chronic HDV infection. However, an individual who develops a chronic HBV infection is likely to become an HDV carrier.

2. **HDV superinfection** of an HBV carrier is most often seen in intravenous drug users. Infection usually induces an acute hepatitis as a result of HDV replication in the

liver. More than 70% of patients superinfected with HDV become chronic carriers of HDV and are at high risk for developing chronic active hepatitis.

C. Pathogenesis and clinical disease

1. **Pathogenesis.** When injected into HBsAg-positive carrier chimpanzees, HDV multiplies to extremely high titers and often induces a severe hepatitis, either chronic or fulminant.
2. **Clinical disease**
   a. **HDV/HBV coinfection** produces a clinical syndrome similar to that seen with acute HBV infection.
   b. **HDV superinfection** often produces a severe, acute hepatitis and can be fatal. Chronic delta hepatitis is a severe disease associated with greater morbidity and mortality rates than chronic hepatitis B alone. Sixty to seventy percent of patients chronically infected with HDV develop cirrhosis and the majority of these patients die of liver disease.

D. Laboratory diagnosis.

EIAs and **radioimmunoassays (RIAs)** have been developed to diagnose acute and chronic HDV infections.

1. **IgM anti-HDV antibody** is the first marker to develop 10–15 days after the onset of disease. It is detected transiently in those who recover but may persist in chronically infected individuals.
2. **IgG anti-HDV antibody** appears in 2–11 weeks and is transient in those who clear the infection.

E. Prevention.

Because HDV can only replicate in an HBV-infected individual, HDV infection can be prevented by **immunization against hepatitis B** or **prophylaxis with HBIg.**

VI. HEPATITIS E VIRUS (HEV)

A. General properties.

HEV is a naked, icosahedral **RNA virus** measuring 27–38 nm in diameter.

B. Classification.

The virus is monotypic and has been classified as a calicivirus.

C. Epidemiology.

HEV is similar epidemiologically to HAV.

1. **Distribution.** HEV has been identified as a cause of endemic or epidemic hepatitis. Epidemics have been reported in third-world countries on the Indian subcontinent and in Africa and South America.
2. **Transmission.** HEV is transmitted by the **fecal-oral route** from person to person. Viral particles can be demonstrated electron microscopically in fecal material from infected patients and the virus has been isolated from the bile and feces of infected chimps and humans. **Water contamination** is the usual mechanism of spread in epidemics.
3. **Prevalence.** Men are affected more often than women.

D. Pathogenesis and clinical disease

1. **Pathogenesis.** The incubation period is 2–6 weeks.
2. **Clinical disease**
   a. Infected humans show biochemical and hematologic evidence of **mild liver disease.** Recovery is usually complete; however, the case fatality rate is high (approximately 20%) in women who contract the disease during the third trimester of pregnancy.
   b. HEV infections **do not become chronic.**

E. Diagnosis is usually clinical, supported by changes in serum liver enzyme levels. Serologic diagnostic methods are not commercially available.

F. Treatment is supportive.

VII. OTHER HEPATITIS VIRUSES.

Hepatitis viruses continue to be discovered. Recent evidence suggests that there are at least three more viruses that cause hepatitis. These viruses, GB-A, GB-B, and GB-C, are flavivirus-like and are distantly related to HCV. Information is limited, but they appear to be blood-borne agents that cause chronic hepatitis.

PART VI

MYCOLOGY

Chapter 39

Overview of Mycology

Arthur Di Salvo

I. CHARACTERISTICS AND CLASSIFICATION OF FUNGI

A. General characteristics. The organisms in the kingdom Fungi are **eucaryotic cells** that lack chlorophyll. Members of the kingdom Fungi have cell walls and filamentous structures and produce spores, or conidia. These organisms usually grow as **saprophytes** and decompose dead organic matter.

B. Classification. There are nine classes of fungi and 100,000–200,000 species, depending on how they are classified. Most of the 150–200 species that are pathogenic for humans belong to one of two classes:

1. **Deuteromycetes** (Fungi Imperfecti) have no recognizable form of sexual reproduction. Most pathogenic fungi belong to this group.
2. **Zygomycetes** reproduce sexually.

II. MORPHOLOGY (Table 39-1)

A. Yeasts are **unicellular** organisms that reproduce by budding or fission. Each yeast cell usually contains a single nucleus.

B. Filamentous fungi (hyphae) are **multicellular structures** with branching, tubular cells. Hyphae without septa are coenocytic (nonseptate). Masses of hyphae are called **mycelia;** the terms "hyphae" and "mycelia" are commonly used interchangeably.

C. Dimorphic fungi occur both as yeasts and as mycelia, depending on the environmental conditions:

1. In the parasitic or pathogenic form (seen in tissue, in exudates, or in cultures on enriched medium incubated at 37°C), dimorphic fungi are yeasts.
2. In nature or when grown at 25°C, dimorphic fungi exist as mycelia. Conversion to the yeast form appears to be essential for the pathogenicity of dimorphic fungi.

III. STRUCTURE.

Fungi are more similar to mammalian cells, which are also eukaryotic, than to bacterial cells, which are prokaryotic. The phylogenetic relation between fungi and humans makes antimycotic therapy difficult, because drugs that inhibit the synthesis of DNA, RNA, or protein in fungi may have the same effects on human cells.

A. Cell walls. Fungi, unlike eukaryotic mammalian cells, possess a rigid cell wall composed of chitin, glucans, mannans, and complex polysaccharides.

B. Cell membranes

1. **Types.** Fungi have a **cell membrane** that encloses the cytoplasm, **vacuoles, microtu-**

TABLE 39-1. Morphologic Classification of Medically Important Fungi

Group	Examples
Filamentous fungi	Dermatophytes
	Zygomycetes
	Malassezia furfur
	Fonsecaea species
	Phialophora species
	Madurella species
	Pseudallescheria boydii
	Aspergillus species
Yeasts	*Candida* species
	Cryptococcus neoformans
Dimorphic fungi	*Blastomyces dermatitidis*
	Histoplasma capsulatum
	Coccidioides immitis
	Paracoccidioides brasiliensis
	Sporothrix schenckii

bules, reticular endothelium, mitochondria, and other structures, and a **nuclear membrane,** which surrounds the true nucleus. Prokaryotes (bacterial cells) lack membrane-bounded organelles and a true nucleus.

2. **Composition.** Fungal membranes contain **ergosterol,** whereas mammalian cell membranes contain cholesterol. The membranes of prokaryotes, with the exception of *Mycoplasma,* do not contain sterols. This difference in membrane composition is the basis for the fungal sensitivity to the major antimycotic agent, amphotericin B.

IV. PATHOGENESIS.

The establishment of mycotic infection usually depends on the size of the inoculum and the resistance of the host. The severity of infection depends mostly on the host response to the organism.

A. Determinants of pathogenicity

1. **Toxin production.** Most common pathogenic fungi do not produce toxins.
2. **Physiologic alterations.** Many pathogenic fungi show physiologic modifications (e.g., increased metabolic rate, modified metabolic pathways, modified cell wall structure) that enhance their ability to invade tissue. The significance of these modifications as well as the mechanisms that cause them are not well understood.
3. **Thermotolerance.** Most pathogenic fungi are thermotolerant and can resist the effects of the active oxygen radicals released during the respiratory burst of phagocytes.

B. Clinical manifestations of disease

1. **Hypersensitivity reactions.** Fungal antigens can cause allergic reactions in the host.
2. **Toxicosis**
   a. **Mycotoxicosis** is caused by the ingestion of feeds and food products contaminated by toxin-producing fungi. The toxins are by-products of fungal metabolism on the substrate.
   b. **Mycetismus** is caused by the ingestion of fungi containing preformed toxin (e.g., mushroom poisoning).
3. **Infection** results from direct invasion of tissues and organs. Mycotic infection can be classified in several ways. A system based on target tissue is the most practical ap-

proach to classification. It must be noted, however, that the boundaries between these types of infections are frequently blurred, particularly in immunocompromised patients in whom mycotic agents usually not associated with systemic infection may disseminate well beyond their usual target organs.

a. **Superficial (cutaneous) mycoses** are confined to the outer layers of the skin, nail, or hair. The fungi involved are called **dermatophytes.**
b. **Subcutaneous mycoses** are confined to the subcutaneous tissue and only rarely spread systemically. They usually form deep, ulcerated skin lesions and have a protracted clinical course. The infection commonly involves the lower extremities because the causative organisms are soil saprophytes that are introduced through trauma to the feet or legs.
c. **Systemic mycoses** involve the viscera and become widely disseminated. The fungi that cause systemic mycoses have specific predilections for various organs.

V. EPIDEMIOLOGY

A. Transmission. Most of the fungi that cause systemic infections normally grow as saprophytes but can infect incidental hosts (i.e., humans and other animals) who are exposed to fungal elements or spores. Therefore:

1. Most mycotic diseases are not communicable from person-to-person.
2. Epidemic outbreaks may occur, but these are caused by a common environmental exposure, not communicability.

B. Incidence of infection. Because fungal diseases are not reportable diseases, the incidence and prevalence are not well defined; however, it is known that the incidence of mycotic infections is increasing rapidly. Contributing factors to the increased incidence include:

1. The growing population of immunocompromised patients
2. The increased use of invasive surgical techniques

Chapter 40

Diagnosis and Treatment of Fungal Diseases

Arthur Di Salvo

I. DIAGNOSIS

A. Clinical diagnosis of mycotic infection requires awareness of possible exposure to fungal habitats. A complete patient history, including occupation, avocation, and travel history, is essential to develop a differential diagnosis.

B. Laboratory diagnosis

1. **Microscopic examination of patient samples**
   a. **Potassium hydroxide (KOH) test.** Microscopic examination of skin scrapings mounted in KOH, which dissolves keratin and cellular material but does not affect fungi, is a simple and fast way to detect dermatophytes.
   b. **Direct immunofluorescence** can be used to identify fungi in fixed tissue sections.
   c. **Gomori methenamine silver (GMS) stain** stains fungal cells black in tissue sections. Conventional histologic stains, such as hematoxylin and eosin (H&E), may not stain some fungal cells.

2. **Detection of fungal antigens. Latex agglutination tests** (see Chapter 10 III A 2) are available for the detection of cryptococcal antigens.

3. **Culture and isolation**
   a. **Culture media.** Pathogenic fungi are usually grown on **Sabouraud dextrose agar** (at a slightly acidic pH of 5.6, which does not favor bacterial growth). Cycloheximide, penicillin, streptomycin, or another inhibitory antibiotic is often added to further prevent bacterial or saprophytic fungal contamination.
   b. **Technique.** Two cultures of clinical material are incubated separately at room temperature (25°C) and body temperature (37°C) to reveal dimorphism (see Chapter 39 II C 2).
   c. **Identification** of the isolated organisms is based on the following criteria:
      (1) **Macroscopic characteristics** (e.g., the width of the mycelium, septation, branching, pigmentation, spore or conidia production)
      (2) **Microscopic morphology** of the growing organisms
      (3) **Biochemical reactions**
      (4) **Nucleic acid probes** have been developed for the specific identification of the fungi that cause the most common systemic mycoses (i.e., *Blastomyces dermatidis, Coccidioides immitis, Cryptococcus neoformans, Histoplasma capsulatum*).
         (a) **Technique.** Ribosomal RNA is extracted from the culture, and single-stranded DNA probes labeled with chemiluminescent compounds are added. If one of the four target organisms is present in the culture, the corresponding DNA probe hybridizes with the RNA, allowing easy detection of the complex.
         (b) **Advantages.** The test requires minimal fungal growth (usually achieved in less than 5 days) and can be applied to mycelial or yeast forms of fungi. (Identification of dimorphic fungi by classic techniques requires a time-consuming conversion step.)

4. **Indirect methods based on the host immune response**
   a. **Skin testing (dermal hypersensitivity testing),** which was once a popular diagnostic tool, is now discouraged because the skin test may cause false-positive results in serologic tests. Skin tests are now used most often to evaluate a patient's immunity and to construct an exposure index in epidemiological studies.
   b. **Serologic tests** have been used, with variable success, for the diagnosis of several

fungal diseases. A major problem is the poor immunogenicity of many fungal cell wall components. The most common tests are based on **latex agglutination** (which usually detects IgM antibodies) and **complement fixation** (which usually detects IgG antibodies).

(1) **Disadvantages.** Complement fixation tests have several disadvantages, one of which is that cross-reactive antibodies may yield false-positive results. Antibodies are often not detectable until 1–3 months after the onset of infection.

(2) **Advantages.** Serologic tests are semi-quantitative, so antibody titers can be monitored over time to assess the evolution of disease.

II. ANTIFUNGAL THERAPY

A. General principles

1. Host defense mechanisms are often inadequate for the eradication of fungal pathogens because mammalian cells lack enzymes capable of degrading the cell wall polysaccharides of fungi.

2. Most antifungal compounds interfere with the biosynthesis of ergosterol or with its integration into the cell membrane (Figure 40-1). However, because cholesterol (found in mammalian cells but not fungi) is structurally similar to ergosterol, antifungal agents can produce serious side effects in the host.

B. Agents

1. **Polyenes**
   a. **Amphotericin B** is usually the drug of choice for most systemic fungal infections. In spite of its toxicity, it continues to be used because it is more efficient than other, less toxic compounds.
      (1) **Mechanism of action.** Amphotericin B has a greater affinity for ergosterol in the fungus cell membranes than for the cholesterol in the host cell membranes. When the drug binds to ergosterol, it causes **disruption of the cell membrane.** The resultant increased permeability causes leakage of cytoplasmic contents and cell death. At therapeutic dosages, amphotericin B is **fungicidal.**
      (2) **Administration.** Amphotericin B is usually given intravenously for extended periods (as long as 2–3 months).
      (3) **Side effects** may be severe and include fever, chills, hypotension, headache, nausea, thrombophlebitis, kidney damage, and anemia secondary to bone marrow depression.
   b. **Nystatin**
      (1) **Mechanism of action.** The mechanism of action of nystatin is identical to that of amphotericin B, but it is clinically effective only against *Candida albicans.*
      (2) **Administration.** Nystatin is administered as a topical ointment (or orally, for treatment of candidiasis of the gastrointestinal tract). Nystatin is not absorbed when administered orally and cannot be given intravenously, so it cannot be used to treat systemic candidiasis.

2. **Azoles (imidazoles and triazoles).** The clinical use of this group of antifungal agents, which includes **ketoconazole, itraconazole,** and **fluconazole,** has expanded considerably in recent years.
   a. **Indications.** These compounds are effective for the treatment of mucocutaneous candidiasis, dermatophytosis, and some systemic fungal infections.
   b. **Mechanism of action.** The azoles block the enzyme that converts lanosterol into 14-demethyllanosterol during the synthesis of ergosterol. At the recommended dosages, the azoles are **fungistatic.**

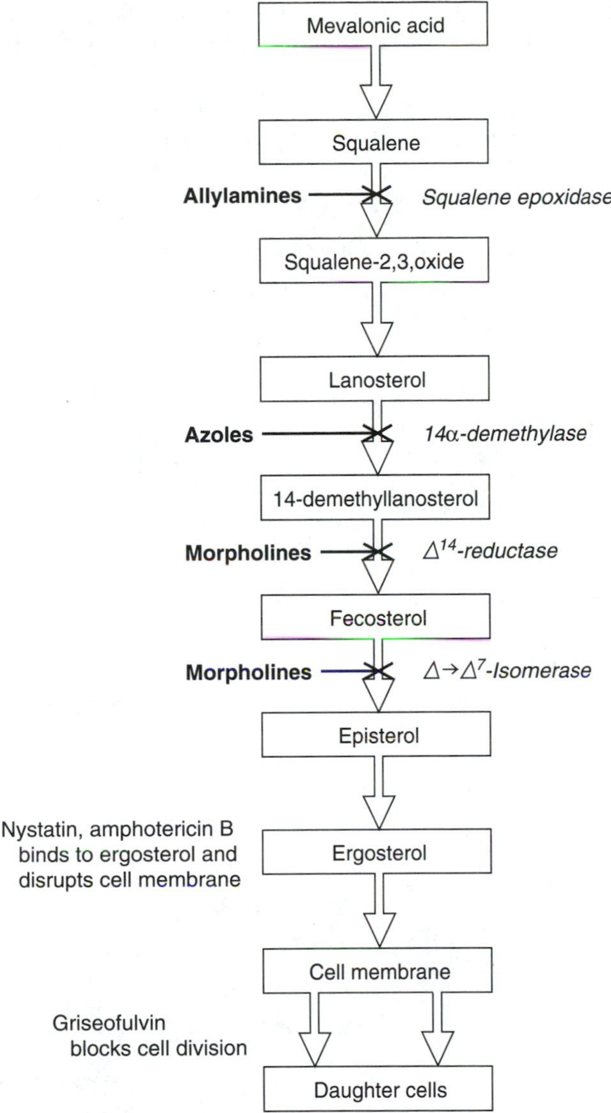

FIGURE 40-1. Mechanisms of action of the most common antifungal agents. (Modified with permission from Gupta AK, Shear NH, Sauder DN: New antifungal agents. *Curr Opin Primary Care Med* 1:34–41, 1994.)

c. **Administration.** These drugs are administered as ointments and creams for topical use and orally for disseminated skin infections and systemic infections.

d. **Side effects.** The azoles are not as toxic as amphotericin B. Nausea and other symptoms of gastrointestinal toxicity, headache, and skin rash are the most common side effects; androgen and cortisol metabolism may be affected as well.

3. **Griseofulvin** is a slow-acting drug that is used for severe skin and nail infections.
   a. **Mechanism of action.** Griseofulvin inhibits microtubule formation and prevents the formation of the mitotic spindle, thus interfering with chromosomal separation during cell division. The drug accumulates slowly in the stratum corneum of the skin, forming a barrier that prevents fungal penetration and growth.
   b. **Administration.** Griseofulvin is administered orally for extended periods (up to 1 year for the treatment of nail infections).

4. **5-Fluorocytosine** is a nucleotide analog that inhibits RNA and DNA synthesis. 5-Fluorocytosine is mainly used in association with amphotericin B to treat cryptococcosis and is administered orally.

5. **Allylamines (naftifine, terbinafine)** are selective for fungi.
   a. **Mechanism of action.** The allylamines inhibit ergosterol synthesis by preventing the oxidation of squalene.
   b. **Administration.** These compounds can be administered topically or orally and may offer an alternative to griseofulvin for the treatment of nail infections.
   c. **Side effects** are usually related to gastrointestinal intolerance.

6. **Morpholines** (e.g., **amorolfine)** interfere with ergosterol synthesis by inhibiting the conversion of fecosterol into episterol. Amorolfine is available in topical preparations and is used to treat dermatophytoses.

C. Resistance to antimycotic agents. Acquired resistance of *C. albicans* and other fungi to the azoles has been reported with increasing frequency, particularly in patients treated with these drugs for extended periods of time (e.g., patients with AIDS).

Chapter 41

Dermatophytes and Filamentous Fungi

Arthur Di Salvo

I. CUTANEOUS MYCOSES

A. Dermatophytoses

1. Etiology

- **a.** ***Trichophyton*** (21 species) infect **skin, hair,** and **nails,** and occasionally cause subcutaneous infections in immunocompromised individuals. *T. rubrum* is the most commonly identified dermatophyte in the United States.
- **b.** ***Microsporum*** (17 species) infect **skin** and **hair,** but not nails. On a global scale, *M. canis* is one of the most common dermatophyte species infecting humans, but its prevalence in the United States has decreased significantly over the last 20–25 years.
- **c.** ***Epidermophyton floccosum*** infects **skin** and **nails** but not hair.

2. Epidemiology

- **a. Habitat and modes of transmission.** Dermatophytes can be classified according to their habitat.
  - **(1) Anthropophilic** dermatophytes are usually associated with humans only; transmission is **person-to-person** by close contact or through contaminated objects (e.g., combs).
  - **(2) Zoophilic** dermatophytes (e.g., *M. canis*) are usually associated with animals. Transmission to humans occurs by close **contact with animals** (e.g., cats, dogs, cows) or contaminated animal products.
  - **(3) Geophilic** dermatophytes are usually found in the soil and are transmitted to humans by direct **exposure to soil** or by exposure to infected animals.
- **b. Distribution.** Most dermatophytes occur worldwide, but some species are geographically limited.

3. Clinical disease. The classic manifestation is generically designated **ringworm (tinea).**

- **a. Tinea corporis** is characterized by small lesions that can occur anywhere on the body.
- **b. Tinea pedis ("athlete's foot")** is an infection of the toe webs and soles of the feet. Tinea pedis is the most common fungus infection in humans.
- **c. Tinea unguium (onychomycosis)** is a difficult-to-treat infection of the nails.
- **d. Tinea capitis** is characterized by scalp lesions and commonly affects children.
- **e. Tinea cruris ("jock itch")** is an infection of the groin, perineum, or perianal area.
- **f. Tinea barbae** is ringworm of the bearded areas of the face and neck.

4. Laboratory identification

- **a.** ***Trichophyton*** species require 2–3 weeks to grow in culture and demonstrate a variety of colors. The conidia are large (macroconidia), smooth, thin-walled, septate (with up to 10 septa), and pencil-shaped (4–8 μm wide by 10–50 μm long). Identification requires special techniques, including biochemical assays.
- **b.** ***Microsporum*** species can be easily identified on the scalp because infected hairs appear bright green when illuminated with an ultraviolet Wood's light. Other dermatophytes do not exhibit this characteristic. Like all dermatophytes, *Microsporum* grow slowly in culture. The macroconidia are thick-walled, multicellular, echinulate (spiny), and spindle-shaped (7–10 μm by 30–160 μm).
- **c.** ***Epidermophyton floccosum.*** In culture, the colony may be white, yellow, or olive in color and is usually readily identified by the presence of multiple, smooth-walled, club-shaped macroconidia measuring 7–12 μm by 12–20 μm.

5. Treatment

a. **Topical therapy. Tolnaftate, clotrimazole,** and **miconazole** are usually successful for eradicating fungal skin infections. *T. rubrum* is often resistant to therapy.
b. **Oral therapy.** Oral antifungal agents may be indicated in extensive infections or infections that prove refractory to topical therapy. For some infections, particularly those involving the nails, the drug of choice is **griseofulvin,** which must be administered for several months. **Allylamines** (e.g., **naftifine, terbinafine)** may offer an alternative to griseofulvin, but their efficacy has not yet been fully established.

6. **The "id" reaction.** Patients infected with a given dermatophyte may show a typical cutaneous lesion, often on the hands, from which no fungi can be recovered or demonstrated. It is believed that the hand lesions, which often occur on the dominant hand, are secondary to immunologic sensitization to a primary (and often unnoticed) infection located somewhere else. These secondary lesions will not respond to topical treatment but will disappear if the primary infection is successfully treated.

B. Tinea versicolor

1. **Etiology.** Tinea versicolor is caused by ***Malassezia furfur,*** an organism that does not belong to the dermatophyte family, but causes skin infections catalogued under the general designation of tinea. *M. furfur* normally only infects the skin.
2. **Clinical disease.** Infection is characterized by blotchy depigmentation of the infected skin that may be accompanied by itching. The discoloration is caused by the inhibition of tyrosinase (an enzyme involved in the synthesis of melanin) by fungal lipids rich in C14 and C19 dicarboxylic acids.
3. **Epidemiology.** Up to 25% of the general population may be infected by *M. furfur* at any one time.
4. **Diagnosis** is usually possible by direct microscopic examination of potassium hydroxide (KOH)-treated skin scrapings, which typically shows intertwined mycelia and budding yeasts (commonly described as "spaghetti and meatballs").
5. **Treatment** is with **ketoconazole.**

II. SUBCUTANEOUS MYCOSES

A. Chromomycoses are subcutaneous infections caused by pigment-producing, filamentous fungi.

1. **Etiology.** Three species are most frequently involved: ***Fonsecaea pedrosoi, F. compacta,*** and ***Phialophora verrucosa.***
2. **Epidemiology**
   a. **Habitat.** The normal habitat of these fungi is soil and decaying vegetation.
   b. **Distribution.** The fungi that cause chromomycosis have worldwide distribution and are particularly abundant in areas with warmer climates.
3. **Pathogenesis and clinical disease**
   a. **Pathogenesis.** In tissue, the fungus forms **sclerotic bodies,** which are golden-brown in color, 4–14 μm in diameter, and frequently located in giant cells. The sclerotic bodies are the reproductive forms; they divide by fission and induce a granulomatous reaction. The species of the infecting organism cannot be determined by the appearance of the sclerotic body.
   b. **Clinical disease.** The lesions, which develop in subcutaneous tissue over a period of several years, can be flat or verrucous (wart-like).
4. **Laboratory identification.** No serologic tests are available to aid in the diagnosis. The identification of the species responsible for a case of chromomycosis is based on culture and isolation.

a. These organisms are called **dematiaceous fungi** because they grow as black colonies. The pigment accumulates in the mycelial cell wall (in culture and in tissue).
b. The fully developed fungus in culture shows black, long, septate and branching hyphae with terminal conidia.

5. **Treatment** is by **surgical excision.** Extensive lesions are treated with surgery plus amphotericin B or itraconazole. The therapeutic outcome is not encouraging.

B. **Mycetoma** is the term used to describe tumoriform infections caused by filamentous bacteria (e.g., actinomycetes; see Chapter 19) and some filamentous fungi. The term **eumycotic mycetoma** designates tumors caused by true fungi, as opposed to those caused by actinomycetes.

1. **Etiology.** The three most common species of true fungi involved in mycetoma formation are ***Madurella mycetomatis, Exophiala jeanselmei,*** and ***Pseudallescheria boydii.*** *E. jeanselmei* and *P. boydii* are the most common causes of mycetoma in the United States.

2. **Epidemiology**
   a. Organisms are associated with the **soil,** and the infections, acquired by **direct inoculation,** are predominately localized to the feet and legs.
   b. *P. boydii* can also be acquired by **inhalation of spores,** and most cases of pseudallescheriasis in the United States are seen as a pulmonary disease, not as a mycetoma.

3. **Clinical disease.** The mycetomas are characterized by swelling (tumefaction), abscess formation, and draining sinus tracts.

4. **Diagnosis**
   a. **Suitable specimens** for culture include the purulent exudates from draining sinuses and tissue biopsy specimens. Granules (0.5–2.0 mm in width and a variety of species-specific colors) are found in the draining exudate.
   b. **Culture and isolation.** The agents of mycetoma are all filamentous fungi that require 7–10 days for visible growth on the culture media and several more days for specific identification based on colonial morphology, conidia formation, and biochemical reactions. The species cannot be identified in fixed and stained tissue sections.
   c. **Serologic tests.** A good serologic test (with a specificity of 95% and a sensitivity of 90%) is available only for the diagnosis of pseudallescheriasis.

5. **Treatment**
   a. **Surgical excision** is recommended for eumycotic mycetomas; the surgery may be as extensive as amputation of an extremity.
   b. **Medical management** requires prolonged administration (1–3 years) of antimycotic agents such as ketoconazole. Therapeutic results are not encouraging.

III. MYCOSES CAUSED BY OTHER FILAMENTOUS FUNGI

A. **Zygomycosis (mucormycosis, phycomycosis)** is an opportunistic infection often seen in patients with uncontrolled diabetes.

1. **Etiology.** Most cases of zygomycosis are caused by three genera of fungi: ***Rhizopus, Mucor***, and ***Absidia***.

2. **Epidemiology.** These organisms have a worldwide distribution and are commonly isolated from soil samples, food, organic debris, decaying vegetables in the refrigerator, and moldy bread.

3. **Pathogenesis and clinical disease**
   a. **Pathogenesis.** The infection usually starts in the paranasal sinuses and extends to the roof of the mouth and nose. The fungus tends to invade blood vessels, where

it causes thrombosis and infarction, and enters the brain through the cribriform plate. Once infection involves the brain, death follows in a few days.

b. **Clinical disease.** The infection typically presents as cotton-like growths (fungal colonies) on the roof of the mouth or the nares. The typical patient is a diabetic patient under care for other reasons related to the diabetes (e.g., diabetic coma).

4. **Diagnosis** is usually clinical and must be immediate to allow initiation of therapy as quickly as possible. Confirmation can be obtained by culturing material collected from the patient's nose.
   a. Culture reveals a rapidly growing mold (visible in 24–48 hours) with nonseptate, ribbon-like hyphae 10–15 μm wide. The species are identified by morphology in culture.
   b. A KOH preparation of patient specimens may reveal similar findings.
   c. An immunodiffusion test is available, but therapy must be initiated before serologic results can be obtained.

5. **Treatment** involves controlling the diabetes and administering amphotericin B.

B. **Aspergillosis** is the term used for human infections caused by *Aspergillus* species.

1. **Etiology.** Several hundred species of *Aspergillus* have been identified, but three are most frequently involved as the cause of aspergillosis in the United States: ***A. fumigatus, A. niger,*** and ***A. flavus.***

2. **Epidemiology.** *Aspergillus* has a worldwide distribution. Organisms are commonly found in soil, food, paint, air vents, and even disinfectant.

3. **Clinical disease.** *Aspergillus* species can invade almost any tissue in the body, but most commonly cause disease of the respiratory system. There are three primary types of pulmonary aspergillosis:
   a. **Allergic manifestations** (e.g., asthma) can result from hypersensitivity to the organism.
   b. **Invasive disease,** with propagation of the fungus through the lung parenchyma, is usually seen in immunocompromised individuals, particularly children with chronic granulomatous disease or patients treated with cytotoxic or immunosuppressive drugs. Patients undergoing heart surgery are also predisposed to these infections.
   c. **Aspergilloma (fungus ball)** is characteristically seen in cavities formed by a previous bout of pulmonary tuberculosis. A crescent-shaped air pocket that partially surrounds a round mass of hyphae in the cavity visualized radiographically is pathognomonic. Aspergillomas are usually noninvasive.

4. **Diagnosis.** Although radiographs and clinical history may strongly suggest aspergillosis, the diagnosis must be confirmed.
   a. Because *Aspergillus* can invade the bronchus, chains of conidia are formed in the air space and they can be seen in the sputum.
   b. The diagnosis is most often confirmed by examining surgical specimens for mycelia that are wide (3–6 μm), septate, and dichotomously branching at 45° angles. The tissue reaction is usually granulomatous. Giant cells, neutrophils, and eosinophils may be present.
   c. Serologic diagnosis can also be useful, particularly in cases of allergy or disseminated infection. The double immunodiffusion test uses *Aspergillus* extracts as the antigen. Multiple precipitin bands (three or more) are usually associated with severe disease.

5. **Treatment** depends on the type of disease.
   a. Allergic conditions are treated symptomatically, by avoiding exposure (which may be difficult) and by desensitization protocols.
   b. Aspergillomas are usually surgically excised
   c. Antimycotic therapy with amphotericin B is usually reserved for patients with invasive disease. Itraconazole may be an effective therapy for aspergillosis.

Chapter 42

Yeasts and Dimorphic Fungi

Arthur Di Salvo

I. INFECTIONS CAUSED BY YEASTS.

There are many species of yeasts that can be pathogenic for humans; only two genera (*Candida* and *Cryptococcus*) are discussed here.

A. Candidiasis is the generic designation given to a wide spectrum of infections caused by many species of the genus *Candida*. The most common pathogenic species is ***C. albicans***, which is an endogenous organism.

1. **Epidemiology**
   a. **Distribution.** *Candida* species are found worldwide, particularly *C. albicans,* which is a common commensal. *C. albicans* is present in 40%–80% of healthy people as part of the normal intestinal flora.
   b. **Factors predisposing to infection.** Infections with *Candida* usually occur when a patient has some alteration in cellular immunity, normal flora, or normal physiology.
      (1) **Impaired cellular immunity** or **neutropenia** predisposes a patient to systemic fungal infections.
      (2) **Prolonged antibiotic therapy** destroys the balance of normal flora, allowing endogenous *Candida* to overgrow and disseminate through the blood stream.
      (3) **Invasive procedures,** such as the placement of artificial heart valves or indwelling catheters, produce alterations in physiology and predispose toward *Candida* infections.
2. **Clinical disease**
   a. **Superficial candidiasis.** The most common forms of candidiasis involve the skin and mucosae, particularly in patients receiving broad-spectrum antibiotics.
   b. **Candidemia** is the dissemination of *Candida* through the blood stream. Immunocompromised patients [particularly those with specific defects of cell-mediated immunity (CMI) to *C. albicans*] are likely to develop **disseminated skin and mucosal infections** or **organ infections** (e.g., pneumonia, endophthalmitis, kidney infections).
   c. **Endocarditis** is seen in patients with implanted artificial valves.
3. **Diagnosis**
   a. **Superficial candidiasis** is usually suspected on clinical grounds, and the diagnosis can be strengthened by a positive Gram stain or by examination of a potassium hydroxide (KOH) preparation of skin or mucosal scrapings.
   b. **Systemic infections** are more difficult to detect. Diagnosis requires isolation of the organism. Specimens are chosen based on the presentation of the disease (e.g., blood, vaginal discharge, urine, feces, or material from mucocutaneous lesions).
      (1) **Histology**
         (a) In a tissue section, *C. albicans* may appear as yeasts, pseudohyphae (3–5 μm in diameter), or a combination of both. The **pseudohyphae** are yeast cells with a single bud (3–4 μm in diameter) that remain attached to the parent cell, then elongate and bud again. Pseudohyphae, which are a hallmark of *C. albicans,* resemble true hyphae, but a slight constriction remains where each bud begins.
         (b) The inflammatory reaction is usually suppurative.
         (c) Chronic lesions may contain giant cells.
      (2) **Culture.** *C. albicans* usually grows in 24–48 hours on most bacterial and fungal media. The organism is 5–10 μm in diameter. Under certain conditions (in serum at 37°C), within 2–3 hours, *C. albicans* will produce germ tubes that are nonseptate, mycelia-like elongations of the yeast cell. The species can be identified by the morphology of the pseudomycelium and the chlamydospores

that form in subcultures on cornmeal agar, by carbohydrate assimilation tests, and by fermentation tests.

(3) **Serology.** Assays based on detecting specific antibodies or *Candida* antigens in body fluids are not clinically useful because they cannot distinguish between normal colonization and infection, or between fungemia and systemic infection.

4. Treatment

a. Superficial candidiasis

(1) **Cutaneous** and **oropharyngeal infections** are treated by topical application of creams and ointments containing **nystatin** or **ketoconazole,** both of which are equally effective. A nystatin suspension is effective for oropharyngeal candidiasis.

(2) **Esophageal candidiasis** is usually treated by oral administration of **clotrimazole, ketoconazole,** or **fluconazole.**

(3) **Vaginal candidiasis.** Oral **ketoconazole** or **fluconazole** (in addition to vaginal suppositories and creams) is recommended for the treatment of vaginal candidiasis, to reduce the probability of continuous reinfection from an intestinal source.

b. Candidemia. The drug of choice is **amphotericin B.** If an artificial heart valve or indwelling catheter is the source of infection, the foreign object must be replaced. Drug therapy alone will not suppress the organism if the infected foreign body remains in the host.

B. Cryptococcosis is caused by ***Cryptococcus neoformans.*** This distinctive encapsulated yeast is 5–10 μm in diameter (excluding the capsule) and reproduces by budding. The single buds are characteristically narrow at the base.

1. Epidemiology

a. Distribution. *C. neoformans* is ubiquitous, with worldwide distribution.

b. Reservoirs and transmission. Pigeon and chicken droppings are a common source of this yeast, which is easy to recover from abandoned buildings. However, a definite epidemiologic link between exposure to pigeon droppings and a specific human infection has yet to be established. Transmission is believed to be by inhalation.

c. Factors predisposing to infection. Infection is probably determined by the resistance of the host, as suggested by the fact that cryptococcosis is frequently seen in immunocompromised individuals.

2. Determinants of pathogenicity

a. The **antiphagocytic polysaccharide capsule** is the major virulence factor.

b. Melanin production may also be a virulence factor. The pigment is deposited in the cell wall, where it may protect the organism from oxidants released by phagocytic cells.

3. Clinical disease

a. Cryptococcal meningitis is the most common clinical presentation of cryptococcosis. The infection may be subacute or chronic, and the disease has a prolonged evolution of several months. The patient's symptoms may initially include vision problems and headache, followed by progressive changes in mental status that lead to nuchal rigidity, coma, and death unless adequate treatment is instituted.

b. Skin and lung infections. The incidence of pulmonary disease has increased in recent years. In some cases, a tumoriform lesion **(cryptococcoma)** may form in the mediastinum.

4. Diagnosis

a. Examination of cerebrospinal fluid (CSF) is the basis for the rapid diagnosis of cryptococcal meningitis.

(1) Protein levels are usually increased; glucose levels are decreased; and leukocyte numbers are increased (mainly because of an increase in mononuclear cells).

(2) The **India ink test,** which detects the extensive capsule of the organism, has been largely replaced by the **latex agglutination test** for antigen, which is more sensitive and more specific.

(a) The antigen detection test can be performed longitudinally to follow the evolution of disease. As the patient improves, the CSF antigen titer decreases. Conversely, an increasing titer indicates that the patient is not responding to therapy.

(b) The latex agglutination test for the detection of cryptococcal antigen can also be used on serum.

b. **Histopathology.** The inflammatory response may be absent or variable. When the reaction is granulomatous, the cryptococci are seen within giant cells.

(1) *C. neoformans* cells can be visualized with the **hematoxylin and eosin (H&E) stain** or the **Gomori methenamine silver (GMS) stain.** A special dye, **mucicarmine,** stains the polysaccharide capsule bright red; this appearance is diagnostic of cryptococcal disease.

(2) **Direct immunofluorescence** using fluorescein-labeled anti-*C. neoformans* antibody can also be used to definitively identify this yeast in formalinized tissue samples.

c. **Serology.** An indirect immunofluorescence test that measures the binding of antibody in serum to fixed *C. neoformans* yeast cells does not discriminate between acute infection and past exposure.

d. **Culture** is the most specific approach to diagnosis.

(1) CSF, biopsy material, and urine are the preferred samples for isolation of this yeast. *C. neoformans* can be isolated from the urine of immunocompromised patients with central nervous system (CNS) or systemic infections, even in the absence of urinary tract symptoms.

(2) Colonies of *C. neoformans* are creamy, white, and mucoid (because of the capsule). Growth is usually visible in 24–48 hours. Because this yeast is sensitive to cycloheximide, the initial plating medium must be free of this antibiotic.

(3) Identification of the organism is based on urease production, carbohydrate assimilation, or by direct immunofluorescence using a fluorescein-labeled anti-*C. neoformans* antibody.

5. **Treatment**

a. **Initial treatment.** The drugs of choice to treat cryptococcus infection are a combination of **amphotericin B** and **5-fluorocytosine (5-FC),** which act synergistically. 5-FC is administered orally and is less toxic than amphotericin B, but if it is used by itself, relapses are frequent. Dual medication increases the efficiency of therapy and allows a reduction of the dose of amphotericin B, thereby reducing toxicity.

b. **Prevention of relapses.** Patients with disseminated disease and immunocompromised patients are usually placed on maintenance therapy with oral **fluconazole** (which readily penetrates the spinal fluid) to prevent relapses.

II. INFECTIONS CAUSED BY DIMORPHIC FUNGI

A. **Blastomycosis** is an acute or chronic infection caused by ***Blastomyces dermatitidis.*** This organism exists as a yeast in tissues or when cultured at 37°C. In nature, or when cultured at room temperature on Sabouraud dextrose agar, it appears as a white, cottony mold (mycelium).

1. **Epidemiology**

a. **Distribution.** *B. dermatitidis* is found in the eastern half of North America and sporadically in other parts of the world.

b. **Reservoirs and transmission.** *B. dermatitidis* can be isolated from soil that contains organic debris (rotting wood, animal droppings, plant material). People collecting firewood, tearing down old buildings or pursuing other outdoor activities are at risk for infection. The lungs are the portal of entry.

2. **Clinical disease.** Blastomycosis presents primarily as pulmonary or cutaneous disease, but may affect bone, the prostate, and other organs as well. Blastomycosis causes a suppurative and granulomatous reaction that develops slowly. Hence the disease usually follows a subacute or chronic course.
   a. The **cutaneous lesions** may be primary (and are usually self-limiting) or secondary (as a manifestation of systemic disease).
   b. Patients with **pulmonary infections** often present with nonspecific respiratory symptoms. Over time, weight loss, fever, productive cough, and night sweats may become apparent. Chest radiographs show obvious pulmonary disease. Not infrequently, the clinical picture is interpreted as pulmonary tuberculosis that cannot be confirmed by examination or culture of the sputum for *Mycobacterium tuberculosis.*

3. **Diagnosis** requires awareness on the part of the physician. Visualization of the yeast cells in adequate clinical samples is a quick way to establish a preliminary diagnosis. Isolation in culture is essential to confirm the diagnosis. The specimens chosen for analysis depend on the manifestations of the disease: skin scrapings or pus from skin lesions; sputum in cases of pulmonary disease; or biopsy tissue from any lesion. Occasionally, the organism can be isolated from urine if the prostate is infected.
   a. **Microscopic examination**
      (1) **KOH preparation.** A typical cutaneous lesion shows central healing with microabscesses at the periphery. A pus specimen may be obtained by nicking the top of a microabscess with a scalpel. The purulent material is smeared on a microscope slide, treated with KOH, and examined microscopically. *B. dermatitidis* appears as a round yeast cell with a double wall and often with a single bud.
      (2) **Histopathology.** The organism is readily seen in tissue sections stained by the H&E or GMS method. A double wall and a single bud with a wide base are pathognomonic of blastomycosis. The cells are 8–12 μm in diameter.
   b. **Culture.** Samples submitted for culture are incubated at 25°C and 37°C. Like all dimorphic fungi, *B. dermatitidis* can be converted to the mycelial form when incubated at room temperature, and the mycelial form can be converted to the yeast form when incubated at 37°C. Identification of the cultured organism can be accomplished in several ways:
      (1) **Microscopic examination**
         (a) A *Blastomyces* culture takes 2–4 weeks to grow at room temperature on Sabouraud dextrose agar. It appears as a white, cottony mold (mycelium). The mycelia and the fruiting bodies (microconidia) are visible using a microscope. However, *B. dermatitidis* cannot be identified by its microconidia, which are indistinguishable from those of many other saprophytes and pathogens.
         (b) At 37°C, the yeast form grows in about 7–10 days when cultured on enriched medium. It appears as a tan, butter-like, soft colony. Microscopic examination shows typical yeast cells, 8–12 μm in diameter, with a thick wall and a single bud with a wide base.
      (2) **Exoantigen test.** This test is a more rapid means of identifying the mycelial form of dimorphic fungi. In this double immunodiffusion reaction, an aqueous extract of a 7- to 10-day-old mycelial culture is precipitated against a known, standardized antiserum. A precipitin band is formed where the antigen and the specific antiserum meet. This test is 100% specific with the proper antiserum.
      (3) **Nucleic acid probes** allow rapid and highly specific identification of *B. dermatitidis* cultures.
   c. **Serology.** Two serologic tests in general use that detect antibodies to *B. dermatitidis* are generally used to diagnose blastomycosis.
      (1) **Immunodiffusion precipitin test.** This test is positive 2–3 weeks after the onset of symptoms in approximately 80% of patients with blastomycosis, and its specificity is close to 100%. A positive test indicates recent or active disease.
      (2) **Complement fixation test.** This test takes 2–3 months to become positive. Although both the sensitivity and the specificity of the complement fixation test

are poor, the quantitative results can be used to monitor patient response to therapy.

4. **Treatment. Amphotericin B,** the drug of choice, must be administered intravenously for several weeks. **Ketoconazole** has also been used for patients with a mild form of disease.

B. **Histoplasmosis** is a disease of the reticuloendothelial system caused by ***Histoplasma capsulatum.*** The yeast form is small, slightly oval, and 5–6 μm in diameter in clinical samples or in cultures at 37°C. In nature or on Sabouraud dextrose agar at room temperature, the organism grows as a white, cottony mycelium.

1. **Epidemiology**
   a. **Distribution.** *H. capsulatum* has worldwide distribution, and histoplasmosis is one of the most common fungal infections in the eastern United States, particularly along the Ohio-Tennessee-Mississippi River valley.
   b. **Reservoirs and transmission.** *Histoplasma* grows in moist soil, especially in blackbird roosts, chicken houses, and caves with abundant bat guano. The disease can be contracted by occupational exposure (e.g., by farmers and gardeners using chicken manure as fertilizer, workers harvesting bat guano from caves or clearing blackbird roosts, and so on). Inhalation of aerosolized particles contaminated with the organism is the most common mode of transmission.

2. **Pathogenesis.** The inhaled organism tends to be taken up by alveolar macrophages, but it behaves as a facultative intracellular organism (i.e., it can survive and proliferate inside phagocytic cells). The infection can then spread to other organs of the reticuloendothelial system, such as the bone marrow, lungs, liver, and spleen.

3. **Immunity.** Patients exposed to *H. capsulatum* develop cell-mediated immunity (CMI) to this fungus, as evidenced by positive skin tests after intradermal injection of histoplasmin. Epidemiological surveys have shown that many individuals in high-prevalence areas develop immunity without ever showing clinical symptoms of histoplasmosis.

4. **Clinical disease.** Many individuals exposed to *H. capsulatum* remain asymptomatic or have mild symptoms of respiratory disease. When clinical histoplasmosis develops, it generally occurs as acute pulmonary, chronic pulmonary, or disseminated disease.
   a. **Pulmonary disease** is the most common form in adults and recovery is generally complete with adequate treatment. Patients with pulmonary disease first notice a cough that may be dry initially, but eventually becomes productive. The sputum may be purulent or bloody. As the disease becomes chronic, patients lose their appetite, lose weight, and complain of night sweats. The clinical picture suggests pulmonary tuberculosis, but the chest radiograph usually shows bilateral interstitial infiltrates, which are not commonly seen in tuberculosis and are typically associated with histoplasmosis.
   b. **Disseminated disease** is most common in children. Hepatosplenomegaly is the primary sign. If untreated, the disseminated form of disease is usually fatal.
   c. **Ocular histoplasmosis,** a clinical entity frequently diagnosed by ophthalmologists in endemic areas, is apparently a hypersensitivity reaction and not a true retinal infection.

5. **Diagnosis.** Clinical specimens sent to the laboratory depend on the presentation of the disease. Sputum or biopsy material is appropriate for patients with pulmonary disease. Gastric washings are also a source of *H. capsulatum* in patients with pulmonary disease, because the sputum is frequently swallowed.
   a. **Histopathology.** In disseminated disease, *H. capsulatum* can be easily detected in lung biopsies and bone marrow aspirates. The organism can also be detected in peripheral blood.
      (1) **Blood** and **bone marrow specimens** can be stained with the **Giemsa** or **Wright's stain.** Yeast cells, 5–6 μm in diameter, are seen intracellularly, either inside tissue phagocytes or inside circulating polymorphonuclear leukocytes or monocytes in the peripheral blood.

(2) **Tissue specimens.** In tissue sections, *H. capsulatum* can be readily visualized by the **H&E** or **GMS stains.** The inflammatory reaction is generally granulomatous, with giant cells. Necrotic centers and calcification are sometimes seen.

b. **Culture** is the most specific approach to diagnosis.

(1) Samples cultured on Sabouraud dextrose agar yield a white, cottony mycelium after 2–6 weeks at room temperature. As the colony ages, it becomes tan. *Histoplasma* has a very distinct spore called a **tuberculate macroconidium** (8–14 μm in diameter).

(2) When cultured at 37°C, the yeast form appears, forming whitish-tan colonies. The cells are small (5–6 μm) and oval. However, these characteristics are not diagnostic. To confirm the diagnosis, it is necessary to convert the yeast form to the mycelial form or to perform an exoantigen test. Nucleic acid probes have been found to be rapid, highly specific and sensitive for the confirmation of *H. capsulatum* infection.

c. **Serology**

(1) **Latex agglutination tests** using latex particles coated with an antigenic fungal extract detect predominantly IgM antibodies, which arise early in the disease (in the first 2 weeks) and gradually fade in about 3 months.

(2) **Complement fixation tests** are performed separately with antigens prepared from the yeast form and from the mycelial form of the fungus. For unknown reasons, some patients react to one form and not the other, while other patients react to both.

(a) **Disadvantages** of complement-fixation tests include the fact that they cross-react with other fungal infections and the 2- to 3-month delay between infection and the appearance of detectable antibody.

(b) **Advantages.** The quantitative results allow evaluation of patient response to therapy.

(3) **Immunodiffusion test.** This test produces two significant precipitin bands, H and M. An H band or H and M bands together indicates active disease, while an M band alone may indicate active disease, past infection, or a recent skin test. (Skin testing with histoplasmin may trigger a humoral immune response that yields a positive complement fixation test or an M band in the immunodiffusion test.)

6. **Treatment.** The drug of choice is **amphotericin B.** Mild cases of pulmonary histoplasmosis can be treated with **ketoconazole.**

C. **Coccidioidomycosis** is caused by ***Coccidioides immitis.*** In tissue, the morphologic form is called a **spherule.** In nature, or when incubated at 25°C on Sabouraud dextrose agar, the fungus grows as a white, cottony mold.

1. **Epidemiology**

a. **Distribution.** The ecological niche of *C. immitis* is the Sonoran desert region, which includes the deserts of the southwestern United States (California, Arizona, Nevada, New Mexico, and Texas) and northern Mexico. Coccidioidomycosis is also endemic in limited areas of Central and South America.

b. **Reservoirs.** Desert soil, particularly archaeological middens, and rodent burrows are sources of *C. immitis.* Pottery, cotton, and other dust-laden products from the endemic region also serve as fomites for distribution of the fungus.

c. **Transmission.** The disease is acquired by the inhalation of spores. Windstorms, earthquakes, archaeological digs, and other activities that promote dust formation favor human infection. Significant disease outbreaks can occur.

d. **Mortality.** For unknown reasons, the mortality rate is approximately 25 times higher in dark-skinned ethnic groups, including Mexicans, Filipinos, and African-Americans.

2. **Life cycle.** The organism can multiply in two life cycles.

a. The **saprophytic (mycelial) cycle** is completed in the soil. **Arthroconidia,** chains of barrel-shaped spores (**arthrospores**) 2–3 μm wide by 4–6 μm long, form in alternating cells of the mycelium. When released, the spores develop into new mycelia.

b. The **parasitic (spherule) cycle** is initiated when a human or animal inhales arthroconidia. The arthroconidia are trapped in the alveolar space, where they become round and enlarge into multinucleated spherules (30–60 μm in diameter). The spherules segment into uninucleated endospores. When the spherule is mature, the wall ruptures, releasing the endospores. The parasitic cycle continues as each endospore develops into a spherule. With repeated cycles, the opportunities for direct extension, penetration into the blood stream, and systemic dissemination increase.

3. **Clinical disease.** The clinical presentation ranges from mild or asymptomatic respiratory disease to severe meningitis.
   a. **Pulmonary coccidioidomycosis** may be a mild influenza-like respiratory illness that heals spontaneously or it may progress to a severe pneumonia.
      (1) The patient with primary pulmonary coccidioidomycosis presents with the typical symptoms of a pulmonary fungal disease: fever, cough, chest pain, dyspnea, hemoptysis, and weight loss.
      (2) The clinical picture is similar to that of pulmonary tuberculosis, which can lead to misdiagnosis. A chest radiograph may not help in the differential diagnosis, because patients with coccidioidomycosis may show cavitary lesions.
   b. **CNS infection** with *C. immitis* is common. In this respect, *C. immitis* is unique; other fungi rarely affect the CNS. The early symptoms are subtle and include headache, nausea, and emotional disturbances. Progression to nuchal rigidity, stupor, and death follow unless treatment is initiated. Eosinophilia is the hallmark of the pleocytosis.
   c. **Intraocular coccidioidomycosis.** In contrast to retinal histoplasmosis, which is a hypersensitivity reaction, intraocular coccidioidomycosis is a true infection. Spherules have been demonstrated in the tissue.

4. **Diagnosis.** Clinical specimens submitted to the laboratory for diagnostic work include sputum, pus from skin lesions, gastric washings, CSF, and skin biopsy samples.
   a. **Direct examination** of a KOH preparation of sputum or properly stained tissues reveals spherules (30–60 μm in diameter) filled with endospores (3–5 μm in diameter). The finding of spherules and endospores is pathognomonic for coccidioidomycosis.
   b. **Culture**
      (1) On Sabouraud dextrose agar at room temperature, mycelial colonies grow in 2–3 weeks and develop arthrospores.
      (2) Cultures at 37°C form spherules only under special conditions.
      (3) Nucleic acid probes allow rapid and specific identification of *C. immitis* cultures.
   c. **Histopathology.** The spherules and endospores found in tissue stain readily with the H&E or GMS stain.
      (1) Spherules and endospores are diagnostic for coccidioidomycosis.
      (2) The inflammatory reaction is both purulent and granulomatous. Recently released endospores incite a polymorphonuclear response. As the endospores mature into spherules, cells of the acute reaction are replaced by lymphocytes, plasma cells, epithelioid cells, and giant cells.
   d. **Serology**
      (1) **Complement fixation test.** Complement-fixing antibodies develop in approximately 1 month. A titer of greater than 1:128 usually indicates extensive dissemination.
         (a) The quantitative results of the complement fixation test allow assessment of the patient's response to treatment.
         (b) Other systemic fungal diseases may result in cross-reactions.
      (2) **Latex agglutination test.** Latex-agglutinating antibodies develop in approximately 2 weeks. The latex agglutination test is reliable and is the easiest test to perform in a diagnostic laboratory.
      (3) **Immunodiffusion test.** The immunodiffusion test is 100% specific for *C. immitis* and has a sensitivity of approximately 85%.

(4) **Enzyme immunoassay (EIA).** An EIA test that screens for both IgG and IgM antibodies has recently become available.

5. **Treatment. Amphotericin B** is the drug of choice, but the azole derivatives are being used more frequently.

D. **Paracoccidioidomycosis** is caused by ***Paracoccidioides brasiliensis,*** a dimorphic fungus with a characteristic yeast form that ranges in size from 5–15 μm and has multiple buds.

1. **Epidemiology**
   a. **Distribution.** This disease occurs from the south of Mexico to Central and South America. It is particularly prevalent in Brazil.
   b. **Reservoirs.** The ecological niche of this organism is probably the soil.
2. **Pathogenesis and clinical disease**
   a. **Pathogenesis.** Dissemination occurs hematogenously and via the lymphatic system. The incubation period may be as long as 10–20 years. Female hormones appear to protect women from developing clinical disease.
   b. **Clinical disease.** Paracoccidioidomycosis is a chronic granulomatous disease of the mucous membranes (especially the intestinal mucosa), the skin, and the pulmonary system. Lymphoid tissue is frequently involved as well. A common triad of symptoms seen in the endemic area is **pulmonary lesions, an edentulous mouth,** and **cervical lymphadenopathy.**
      (1) *P. brasiliensis* invades the mucous membranes of the mouth, forming white plaques in the buccal mucosa and causing the teeth to fall out as a result of chronic inflammation of the gums.
      (2) The pulmonary disease follows the same clinical pattern as most fungal infections of the lungs, and can also be misdiagnosed as pulmonary tuberculosis.
3. **Diagnosis**
   a. **Clinical diagnosis.** Diagnosis may be complicated in patients who do not live in endemic areas because of the prolonged time between infection and the emergence of symptoms. Because so much time has elapsed, the patient may not realize that time spent in a part of the world where *P. brasiliensis* is prevalent is relevant to his current disorder.
   b. **Laboratory diagnosis.** The clinical material that should be submitted for laboratory examination depends on the symptoms and includes sputum, biopsy material, pus, and crust from the lesions.
      (1) **Direct examination** of a KOH preparation of sputum or crust from one of the lesions may reveal yeasts with a thin cell wall and multiple narrow-based buds. The cells may vary in size from 2–30 μm.
      (2) **Culture**
         (a) Culture on Sabouraud dextrose agar at room temperature yields dense, white mycelial colonies after 2–3 weeks. The conidia are not diagnostic.
         (b) When cultured at 37°C, whitish-tan, thick yeast colonies slowly develop. Cells in culture are larger (40–50 μm in diameter) and are surrounded by multiple narrow-based buds, 2–5 μm in size. This configuration, classically described as a **"captain's wheel,"** is diagnostic of paracoccidioidomycosis.
      (3) **Histopathology.** The inflammatory reaction is not consistent. Areas of neutrophils, granulomas, or necrosis may be seen. *P. brasiliensis* is readily seen in tissue sections stained with the H&E and GMS stains.
      (4) **Serology.** The best serologic test for detection of antibodies to *P. brasiliensis* is the **immunodiffusion test.** It is more than 99% specific and almost 85% sensitive. Given the long evolution time of this disease, the test is diagnostically useful.
4. **Treatment.** The drug of choice is **amphotericin B;** some of the azole derivatives have been reported to be useful.

E. **Sporotrichosis** is a chronic infection caused by *Sporothrix schenckii,* a dimorphic fungus whose yeast form is usually round (4–8 μm in diameter) but can assume a fusiform morphology in tissues.

1. **Epidemiology**
   a. **Distribution.** The organism is found worldwide.
   b. **Reservoirs.** *S. schenckii* is a saprophyte, growing on decaying vegetation, soil, sphagnum moss, and timbers. In the United States, forest employees accounted for 17% cases of sporotrichosis; gardeners and florists, 10%; and other soil-related occupations, 16%.

2. **Pathogenesis and clinical disease**
   a. **Pathogenesis**
      (1) Infection is contracted by abrasion, usually a thorn prick on the hand. (For this reason, sporotrichosis is also called rose grower's disease.) A pustule develops at the site and then ulcerates.
      (2) The infection initially affects subcutaneous tissues, progresses from the subcutaneous tissues to the lymphatic system, and usually stops at the regional lymph nodes draining the site of infection.
   b. **Clinical disease**
      (1) Sporotrichosis is usually a **chronic infection of the cutaneous or subcutaneous tissue** that tends to suppurate, ulcerate, and drain. As the disease progresses up the lymphatic chain, satellite abscesses form along the tract of the vessels, which can also ulcerate and release large amounts of pus before healing.
      (2) **Primary pulmonary disease** caused by *S. schenckii* is rare but has been diagnosed more frequently in recent years.

3. **Diagnosis**
   a. **Clinical diagnosis.** A patient history that suggests exposure to *S. schenckii* is very important, as in most other fungal diseases.
   b. **Laboratory diagnosis.** Samples sent for laboratory examination depend on the infection and include pus from abscesses, biopsy material of subcutaneous or organ lesions, or sputum in cases of pulmonary infection.
      (1) **Direct examination.** The organisms are usually sparse in pus or other clinical material. Therefore, KOH mounts are not diagnostically useful.
      (2) **Histopathology**
         (a) The inflammatory reaction in tissue is both pyogenic and granulomatous.
         (b) The organisms are difficult to visualize with the H&E stain but are readily seen with the GMS stain.
         (c) In tissue, the yeasts are round, oval, or cigar-shaped. It is sometimes possible to observe a characteristic tissue reaction **(Splendori reaction),** in which yeast cells are surrounded by amorphous eosinophilic "rays" forming an asteroid body.
      (3) **Culture.** Definitive diagnosis usually depends on culture.
         (a) At room temperature, *S. schenckii* colonies develop in 3–5 days and initially are white and very membranous. As the colonies age for 2–3 weeks, they become black and leathery.
         (b) Microscopically, *S. schenckii* forms a delicate, thin conidiophore. The pyriform conidia are 3 μm by 6 μm in size and are arranged in a cluster around the tip of the conidiophore, which resembles a daisy.
      (4) **Serology.** No serologic tests are commercially available.

4. **Treatment.** The cutaneous form of sporotrichosis is best treated with saturated iodides (e.g., **potassium iodide**) administered orally. For the systemic forms of disease, **amphotericin B** is the drug of choice. **Itraconazole** is also effective.

Chapter 43

Opportunistic Mycoses

Arthur DiSalvo

I. ETIOLOGY.

ETIOLOGY. For the most part, fungi are organisms of low virulence and tend to infect humans with compromised immune systems. **For the immunocompromised host, there is no such thing as a nonpathogenic fungus.** The fungi most frequently isolated from immunocompromised patients are saprophytic (i.e., from the environment) or endogenous (i.e., commensal). The most common are *Candida* species, *Cryptococcus neoformans, Aspergillus* species, and *Mucor* species.

II. PREDISPOSING CONDITIONS.

PREDISPOSING CONDITIONS. A variety of clinical conditions have been shown to predispose for the acquisition of opportunistic fungal infections (Table 43-1).

A. Functional compromise of the immune system

1. **Primary immunodeficiency,** especially when cell-mediated immunity (CMI) is affected, predisposes a patient to opportunistic mycoses.
2. **Secondary immunodeficiency**
   a. **AIDS.** Virtually all patients with AIDS will have a fungal infection sometime during the course of disease.
   b. **Malignancies** (e.g., leukemias, lymphomas, Hodgkin's disease) are often associated with a more or less profound compromise of the immune system, either intrinsically or as a consequence of therapy (see II B 6). Systemic fungal infections are a major cause of death in these patients.
   c. **Chronic, debilitating disease** can cause immunodeficiency and predispose a patient to fungal infection.

B. Therapeutic measures

1. **Transplantation.** Organ and bone marrow transplantation are associated with profound iatrogenically-induced immunosuppression.
2. **Open heart surgery** is often associated with infections by *Aspergillus* species. The ubiquitous aspergilli are thought to be introduced from the air during surgery.
3. **Indwelling catheters.** Urinary and intravenous catheters are frequently associated with fungal infections, particularly by *C. albicans.*
4. **Artificial heart valves** can be colonized by a variety of infectious agents, including *Candida* species.
5. **Whole body irradiation therapy** profoundly depresses the immune system.
6. **Therapy with cytotoxic drugs, corticosteroids,** or **immunosuppressive drugs** can predispose to fungal infection.
7. **Administration of broad-spectrum antibacterial** agents can shift the equilibrium of the normal flora in favor of endogenous fungi.

C. Other conditions

1. **Severe burns** destroy the epithelial barrier that normally prevents infection. Extensive burns are associated with immune dysfunction.
2. **Diabetes** creates favorable conditions for fungal growth (i.e., high glucose levels). Genitourinary infections are particularly common.

TABLE 43-1. Clinical Conditions and Associated Opportunistic Mycoses

Clinical Condition	*Cryptococcus neoformans*	*Candida albicans*	*Candida (Torulopsis) glabrata*	*Zygomycetes*	*Aspergillus*
Immunosuppression	√	√	√	. . .	√
Diabetes mellitus	√	√	√	√	. . .
Tuberculosis	√	. . .	. . .	. . .	√
Lymphomas	√	. . .	. . .	. . .	. . .
Hodgkin's disease	√	. . .	. . .	. . .	. . .
Leukemias	. . .	. . .	. . .	√	√
Severe burns	. . .	. . .	. . .	√	. . .
Intravenous drug abuse	. . .	. . .	. . .	. . .	√
Hyperalimentation	. . .	√	√	. . .	. . .
Catheterization	. . .	√	√	. . .	. . .
Corticosteroid therapy	√	√	. . .	√	√
Cytotoxic drug therapy	. . .	. . .	√	. . .	. . .
Antibiotic therapy	. . .	√	. . .	. . .	. . .

3. **Tuberculosis.** Disseminated disease is associated with depression of CMI (anergy).
4. **Illicit intravenous drug use.** Contaminated drugs or paraphernalia can lead to infection.

III. CLINICAL DISEASE.

In immunosuppressed patients, common fungal infections may have an unusual presentation.

A. Aggressive systemic dissemination of fungi usually associated with localized infections

may occur. For example:

1. In normal hosts, *Malassezia furfur* causes a benign and self-limited skin disease (tinea versicolor), but in immunocompromised patients, the same organism may cause a rash and fungemia. Disseminated systemic infections are a particular problem in infants receiving parenteral fat emulsions for nutrition, because *M. furfur* requires long-chain fatty acids for growth.
2. In immunocompromised patients, aspergillosis is frequently disseminated.
3. Blastomycosis tends to become disseminated in immunocompromised patients. In patients with AIDS, up to 40% have central nervous system (CNS) involvement, as compared with 3%–10% among patients who do not have AIDS.

B. Aberrant organ affinity

1. *Candida* species are usually part of the normal flora in the lower gastrointestinal tract. In immunocompromised patients, the organism can invade the esophagus and even disseminate systemically to the liver and heart valves.
2. *Cryptococcus neoformans,* which in most cases infects the meninges, frequently causes pulmonary and cutaneous infections in immunocompromised individuals.
3. *Sporothrix schenckii* may cause pulmonary or disseminated disease in immunocompromised patients.

C. Anomalous geographic distribution.

Cases of coccidioidomycosis and histoplasmosis can occur in severely immunocompromised patients outside the endemic areas, without recent travel history or known exposure to fomites from those areas.

D. Abnormal growth and abnormal histopathologic reactions

1. In typical infections with dimorphic fungi, the tissue forms predominate in histopathologic sections (e.g., spherules in coccidioidomycosis). However, in severely immunocompromised patients who contract the infection, mycelial forms are often seen in tissue.
2. Whereas the normal host reaction to fungal invasion is usually pyogenic or granulomatous, the severely immunocompromised host shows tissue necrosis with little or no evidence of inflammation.

IV. **DIAGNOSIS** of an opportunistic fungal infection requires a high index of suspicion and fine clinical judgment.

A. The diagnosis may be complicated for the following reasons:

1. Patients present with atypical signs and symptoms.
2. A fungus normally considered a saprophyte or contaminant is recovered from the patient.
3. A systemic infection may be caused by a fungus outside its known endemic area.

B. The physician must rule out clinical situations that may not require specific therapeutic measures, such as:

1. Normal colonization by fungi (e.g., the isolation of *C. albicans* from the stool)
2. Transient fungemia (often seen in patients receiving parenteral nutrition or with central lines), which usually disappears when the parenteral alimentation is stopped or the central line removed

V. **TREATMENT.** In general, therapy of mycotic diseases is difficult, and in immunocompromised patients, the results are dismal.

A. **Treatment of infections.** Therapy must be prompt and aggressive. Innovative formulations (e.g., liposomal amphotericin B) and new compounds (e.g., the echinocandidins) are being investigated with the hope of reducing toxicity.

B. **Chemoprophylaxis.** Because of the difficulty of treating mycoses and the fact that relapse and mortality rates are considerably increased in immunocompromised patients, chemoprophylaxis is extremely important. In 1995, the Centers for Disease Control (CDC) recommended guidelines for the prevention of the four major opportunistic mycotic infections (candidiasis, coccidioidomycosis, cryptococcosis, and histoplasmosis) in HIV-positive patients. After a course of induction therapy (usually with amphotericin B) the patient should receive lifelong maintenance therapy as follows:

1. Candidiasis and cryptococcosis: fluconazole
2. Histoplasmosis: itraconazole
3. Coccidioidomycosis: fluconazole; alternatively, itraconazole or ketoconazole

PART VII
PARASITOLOGY

Chapter 44

Diagnosis and Treatment of Parasitic Infections

Lisa L. Steed
Eric R. James

I. OVERVIEW. Parasites are organisms that live in or on a host that provides physical protection and nourishment. Although some bacteria and fungi could be defined in this way, the term parasite is usually applied to **protozoans (single-celled organisms)** and **helminths (worms, multicellular organisms).**

A. Protozoa. The major protozoan parasites of humans are grouped within three main phyla:

1. **Sarcomastigophora**
   a. **Rhizopoda (amoebae).** Genera include *Entamoeba, Acanthamoeba,* and *Naegleria.*
   b. **Zoomastigophorea (flagellates).** Genera include *Giardia, Dientamoeba, Trichomonas, Leishmania,* and *Trypanosoma.*
2. **Ciliophora (ciliates).** *Balantidium* is the only genus in this group that is pathogenic for humans.
3. **Apicomplexa** includes the **sporozoa.** Major genera include *Plasmodium, Babesia, Toxoplasma, Isospora, Pneumocystis carinii**, *and Cryptosporidium.*

B. Helminths. Most of the medically important helminth parasites are found in three main groups of organisms:

1. **Nematodes (round worms)**
2. **Cestodes (tape worms)**
3. **Trematodes [flatworms (flukes)]**

II. DIAGNOSIS OF PARASITIC INFECTIONS. Identification of parasites is based on morphologic criteria and depends on proper specimen collection and adequate fixation. Incorrectly submitted specimens may lead to misidentification of parasites or false-negative results.

A. Macroscopic and microscopic detection

1. **Stool samples**
   a. **Specimen collection**
      (1) For optimum detection of gastrointestinal parasites, stool specimens must be collected on alternate days for a total of three specimens within 10 days. Occasionally, six specimens will need to be collected within 14 days to adequately rule out amoebiasis.
      (2) Care should be taken to avoid contaminating the sample with water or urine, which kill protozoa. In addition, if barium sulfate, mineral oil, bismuth, nonabsorbable antidiarrheal medications, or antimalarial agents have been administered, stool samples cannot be collected for examination until at least 7 days after administration of these substances.

* *Pneumocystis carinii* has been reclassified as a fungus. However, because most available information has been obtained by parasitologists, *P. carinii* will be discussed in Chapter 45.

(3) Liquid stools submitted within 30 minutes of collection or soft/semiformed stools submitted within 1 hour of collection can be examined directly for protozoan trophozoites (the active, motile form of the organism). Trophozoites in stools disintegrate rather than encyst and will be missed if the stool is not examined quickly or preserved as soon as collected. Stools that cannot be examined within these time limits must be preserved with adequate fixatives to maintain protozoan morphology and prevent further development of helminth eggs and larvae.

b. Examination

(1) Macroscopic examination

(a) Occasionally, adult *Ascaris lumbricoides* or *Enterobius vermicularis* or tapeworm proglottids may be seen within the stool.

(b) Blood and mucus, which may harbor amoebae, are easy to detect.

(c) Substances that will render the specimen unacceptable, such as barium sulfate, can also be seen.

(2) Microscopic examination entails a direct wet mount, a stool concentrate, and a permanently stained smear. Together, these examinations are known as a **stool for ova and parasites (O&P).**

(a) Direct wet mount. The use of direct wet mounts is limited to liquid stools submitted within 30 minutes of collection or soft/semiformed stools submitted within 1 hour of collection.

(i) A small amount of stool and a drop of saline are mixed on a microscope slide to form a suspension. (Liquid stool does not require saline.) The suspension is covered with a glass cover slip and examined for trophozoites.

(ii) This procedure is repeated using stool and a weak iodine solution to stain the parasites. Blood and mucus, if present, are also examined. Helminth eggs and larvae and protozoan cysts may also be detected, although these are usually seen after concentration procedures.

(b) Concentration procedures allow detection of small numbers of parasitic cysts as well as helminth eggs and larvae. Stools are most often concentrated by sedimentation.

(i) A drop of sediment and a drop of saline are mixed on a microscope slide, covered with a cover slip and examined.

(ii) A drop of sediment is also mixed with a drop of weak iodine solution to stain the parasites, covered with a cover slip, and examined. Iodine kills trophozoites, but enhances the visibility of nuclei and glycogen vacuoles in cysts.

(c) Permanently stained smears allow definitive identification of protozoa. Several staining techniques are available; the **trichrome stain** and the **iron-hematoxylin stain** are the most commonly used stains.

2. Blood samples

a. Specimen collection. Smears are prepared with fresh blood from the finger or earlobe or from venous blood collected in ethylenediaminetetraacetic acid (EDTA) anticoagulant. Several blood specimens may be required to make the diagnosis.

b. Examination. Automated hematology instruments will not detect parasitized red blood cells. Both thick and thin blood smears must be made for optimum detection of parasites.

(1) Thick smears are used to screen larger amounts of blood; the red blood cells are lysed during the Giemsa staining procedure, causing the stained parasites to stand out more clearly.

(a) Parasites stain bluish purple with reddish nuclei.

(b) At least 200 to 300 fields are examined to detect light parasitemia.

(2) Thin smears provide definitive species identification; the red blood cells remain intact during Giemsa staining.

3. Tissue samples. Specimen collection and preparation depends on the suspected parasite and on the type of specimen to be examined.

a. Skin biopsies should be submitted for routine histology.

b. **Lymph nodes, splenic tissue, liver aspirates, bone marrow,** or **cerebrospinal fluid (CSF)** can demonstrate intracellular forms of *Trypanosoma* and *Leishmania.*
   (1) Part of the material is examined as a direct wet mount and part of the material is prepared as a smear and stained with Giemsa stain prior to examination.
   (2) Tissue may also be prepared for routine histology.
c. **"Skin snips"** (thin horizontal slices of epidermis) are submitted for detection of *Onchocerca volvulus.* The "skin snips" are incubated in saline to allow emergence of the microfilariae.

4. **Sputum samples.** The specimen is examined as a direct wet mount (with and without iodine) or as a permanently stained smear.

B. Culture. *Trypanosoma* amastigotes and trypomastigotes, *Toxoplasma gondii* trophozoites, and *Leishmania* amastigotes can be cultivated from specimens inoculated onto specialized media. Specimens, especially those from skin, should be collected with extreme care to avoid bacterial contamination. Culture techniques are performed only by specialized microbiology reference laboratories and the Centers for Disease Control (CDC).

C. Serology. Serologic techniques are available for the diagnosis of toxoplasmosis, amoebiasis, leishmaniasis, Chagas' disease, malaria, trichinellosis, schistosomiasis, cysticercosis, and hydatid disease (echinococcosis).

III. TREATMENT OF PARASITIC INFECTIONS

A. General principles. Protozoa and helminths are eukaryotes. Their biochemical pathways are often considerably different from those of bacteria but similar to those of the human host. Therefore, most antibacterial agents are ineffective against parasites, and potential targets for antiparasitic agents are limited. The number of good antiparasitic agents is relatively small and some of the drugs of choice have been in use for decades.

B. Antiprotozoal agents

1. **Drugs used for the treatment of amebiasis, trichomoniasis, cyclosporiasis, and giardiasis**
   a. **Metronidazole** is a nitroimidazole.
      (1) **Indications.** Metronidazole is effective against *Trichomonas, Entamoeba, Giardia,* and *Balantidium.*
      (2) **Mechanisms of action.** Several mechanisms of action for metronidazole have been proposed.
         (a) Ultrastructurally, metronidazole appears to disrupt the internal membranes of protozoa. The anaerobic metabolism of protozoa causes the production of an acid metabolite, a hydroxy metabolite, and (through ferredoxin or flavodoxin enzymes) reduced nitro radical anions. Reduced metronidazole may then generate superoxide, leading to cellular damage.
         (b) Reduced metronidazole interacts with nucleotides, inhibiting the formation of DNA and RNA.
         (c) Metronidazole may inhibit glucose metabolism.
   b. **Quinacrine hydrochloride**
      (1) **Indications.** Quinacrine hydrochloride is effective against *Giardia.*
      (2) **Mechanism of action.** Quinacrine hydrochloride is thought to bind between the two strands of DNA, preventing RNA transcription.
   c. **Iodoquinol**
      (1) **Indications.** Iodoquinol is indicated for asymptomatic amoebiasis and *Dientamoeba fragilis* infections.
      (2) **Mechanism of action.** The mechanism of action of iodoquinol is currently unknown.

d. **Amphotericin B**

(1) **Indications** include primary amoebic meningoencephalitis, central nervous system (CNS) infection by *Acanthamoeba* species, and leishmaniasis.

(2) **Mechanism of action.** Amphotericin B appears to react with cholesterol in the cell membrane, increasing membrane permeability and causing the organism to lose low molecular weight compounds, including amino acids and glucose.

e. **Propamidine isethionate**

(1) **Indications.** Propamidine isethionate has recently become the preferred treatment, usually in combination with neomycin, for acanthamoebic keratitis.

(2) **Mechanism of action.** Propamidine isethionate binds nonintercalatively to DNA, but it has not been proven that this is its mechanism of action against *Acanthamoeba.*

2. **Drugs used for the treatment of trypanosomiasis**

a. **Nifurtimox**

(1) **Indications.** Nifurtimox is effective against *Trypanosoma cruzi,* the causative agent of Chagas' disease.

(2) **Mechanism of action.** Nifurtimox acts chiefly through the generation of superoxide and other free radicals and oxidants. *T. cruzi* lacks catalase and glutathione peroxidase, enzymes that detoxify hydrogen peroxide. Therefore, hydrogen peroxide produced by superoxide dismutation is available to react with superoxide to produce hydroxyl radicals. Hydroxyl radicals are potent oxidants capable of damaging a range of cellular targets, including membranes, proteins, and DNA.

b. **Allopurinol**

(1) **Indications.** Allopurinol is used in the treatment of Chagas' disease, and is also effective for treating leishmaniasis.

(2) **Mechanism of action.** Allopurinol has many diverse pharmacologic activities. Its antiparasitic action is generally ascribed to the fact that as an isomer of hypoxanthine, a purine, allopurinol reduces the rate of purine synthesis.

c. **Suramin**

(1) **Indications.** Suramin is used in the treatment of early African trypanosomiasis. (The drug does not cross the blood–brain barrier; therefore, it is ineffective in advanced disease.) In addition, it is used as a macrofilaricide in onchocerciasis.

(2) **Mechanism of action.** Blood stream forms of the African trypanosomes do not rely on mitochondrial respiratory enzymes. Rather, they use glycerol 3-phosphate oxidase and glycerol 3-phosphate dehydrogenase to regenerate nicotinamide adenine dinucleotide (NAD). Suramin blocks the action of these two enzymes, preventing reduced nicotinamide adenine dinucleotide (NADH) oxidation and resulting in diminished adenosine triphosphate (ATP) synthesis. Suramin appears to have a similar mechanism of action against *Onchocerca.*

d. **Melarsoprol**

(1) **Indications.** Because it crosses the blood–brain barrier, melarsoprol is useful in the treatment of late-stage African trypanosomiasis with CNS involvement.

(2) **Mechanism of action.** Melarsoprol is an organic arsenical that inhibits glycerol 3-phosphate oxidase.

e. **Eflornithine**

(1) **Indications.** This drug is used increasingly against African trypanosomiasis.

(2) **Mechanism of action.** Eflornithine inhibits ornithine decarboxylase, an enzyme essential to polyamine synthesis. Interference with polyamine synthesis leads to destabilization of DNA and interruption of its replication. The differential effect on the parasite is thought to occur because of the parasite's rapid rate of reproduction and greater need for polyamines (as compared with the host).

3. **Drugs used in the treatment of leishmaniasis. Pentavalent antimonials,** such as **sodium stibogluconate** and **meglumine antimonate,** are the drugs of choice for the treatment of leishmaniasis. These compounds are reduced to their trivalent forms

after administration to a patient. In this state, they inactivate sulfhydryl (-SH) groups in proteins and interfere with enzymes involved in glycolysis and the tricarboxylic acid (TCA) cycle.

4. Drugs used in the treatment of malaria

a. Chloroquine

(1) Indications. Chloroquine, an aminoquinoline, is still recommended for the treatment of uncomplicated malaria.

(2) Mechanisms of action. Two modes of action have been proposed for this drug (and for the related compound quinine, effective against *Plasmodium* and *Babesia*).

(a) Ferriprotoporphyrin, a compound produced by the parasite from hemoglobin, is capable of parasite lysis. However, normally, ferriprotoporphyrin is harmlessly sequestered within the parasitized erythrocyte. Following conjugation with chloroquine, ferriprotoporphyrin is released, enabling it to lyse the intracellular parasite.

(b) Chloroquine is strongly basic. The drug, initially able to diffuse into the *Plasmodium* food vacuole, becomes protonated and nonpermeant in the acidic environment. It neutralizes the pH of the food vacuole, rendering the lysosomal enzymes nonfunctional and resulting in starvation of the parasite.

b. Fansidar (sulfadoxine–pyrimethamine)

(1) Indications. Fansidar is indicated for the treatment of complicated chloroquine-resistant malaria.

(2) Mechanism of action. Fansidar is a combination of two folate cofactor inhibitors. Sulfadoxine inhibits dihydropteroate synthetase, which converts pteridine and *p*-aminobenzoic acid (PABA) to dihydropteric acid, the precursor of dihydrofolic acid. Pyrimethamine inhibits dihydrofolate reductase, which prevents production of tetrahydrofolate from dihydrofolate. Ultimately, the synthesis of thymine from uracil is interrupted. Synergistic inhibition at two sites in the folate pathway provides more efficient interruption of DNA synthesis.

c. Primaquine is an 8-aminoquinoline.

(1) Indications. Primaquine is particularly effective for eliminating *Plasmodium vivax* hepatic hypnozoites.

(2) Mechanisms of action

(a) It has been suggested that primaquine interferes with mitochondrial oxidation by disrupting ubiquinone, which acts as an electron carrier in the mitochondrial respiratory chain.

(b) Superoxide, hydrogen peroxide, and redox-active labile metals are generated by the oxidative activity of primaquine in erythrocytes and may also play a role in the antimalarial action of this drug.

(c) It has been suggested that primaquine may interrupt pyrimidine synthesis.

d. Proguanil

(1) Indications. Proguanil is used as a malaria prophylactic.

(2) Mechanism of action. Proguanil is metabolized to cycloproguanil, a dihydrofolate reductase inhibitor.

e. Qinghaosu (artemisinin) is a sesquiterpene lactone extracted from *Artemisia,* an herb used for centuries in China to treat patients with malaria. Several derivatives (e.g., arteether, artemether, arteflene, artesunate) have similar modes of action. These compounds contain a bridged endoperoxide that reacts with iron in the malaria-infected erythrocyte to generate free radicals, which lead to the oxidation of membrane protein thiols.

5. Drugs used in the treatment of toxoplasmosis

a. Pyrimethamine is a dihydrofolate reductase inhibitor that interferes with DNA synthesis. This drug is usually used in combination with sulfadiazine and spiramycin or clindamycin in the treatment of toxoplasmosis.

b. Trimethoprim–sulfamethoxazole is discussed in III B 6 a.

6. Drugs used in the treatment of *Pneumocystis carinii* infections

a. Trimethoprim–sulfamethoxazole

(1) Indications. Trimethoprim–sulfamethoxazole is the drug of choice against *P.*

carinii and is also used to treat *Toxoplasma, Plasmodium,* and *Isospora* infections.

(2) **Mechanism of action.** Trimethoprim–sulfamethoxazole has a mechanism of action similar to that of Fansidar [see III B 4 b (2)]. Sulfamethoxazole inhibits dihydropteroate synthetase and trimethoprim, like pyrimethamine, inhibits dihydrofolate reductase.

b. Pentamidine

(1) **Indications.** Pentamidine is the alternative to trimethoprim–sulfamethoxazole for the treatment of *Pneumocystis,* and is also a second-line drug for leishmaniasis and for African trypanosomiasis.

(2) **Mechanism of action.** This compound is a diamidine and is thought to act by binding to A-T–rich regions of DNA. It may also disrupt ribosomal RNA synthesis.

7. Antibacterial compounds with antiparasitic properties

a. Agents and indications

(1) **Doxycycline** is the drug of choice for *Balantidium,* and also has activity against *Plasmodium.*

(2) **Clindamycin** and the **tetracyclines** have activity against *Babesia, Plasmodium,* and *Entamoeba.*

b. Mechanism of action

(1) These antibacterial agents are thought to exert antiparasitic effects chiefly by altering the intestinal flora, resulting in an environment that is unfavorable for the parasites. In the case of *Entamoeba,* these agents also control secondary bacterial invasion of the intestinal wall.

(2) When direct action of these antibiotics against intracellular protozoa has been demonstrated, it is thought to be by inhibition of protein synthesis through mechanisms similar to the agent's antibacterial mechanisms.

C. Anthelmintic agents

1. Drugs used for the treatment of nematode infections

a. Benzimidazoles (mebendazole, thiabendazole)

(1) Indications

(a) **Mebendazole** is the drug of choice for most enteric nematodes (*Enterobius, Trichuris, Ascaris,* and hookworm). It is also useful against some related tissue nematodes (*Capillaria philippinensis, Strongyloides,* and *Trichinella*).

(b) **Thiabendazole** is the drug of choice for *Capillaria hepatica, Strongyloides,* and the parasites responsible for visceral and cutaneous larva migrans.

(2) Mechanisms of action

(a) Mebendazole

(i) This drug disrupts microtubule formation, affecting the functioning of the helminth's gut cells and the ability of the parasite to obtain nutrients.

(ii) It also inhibits glucose transport. This mechanism of action is unique to mebendazole among the benzimidizoles and may be the main mode of action against *Trichinella* muscle-stage larvae, which obtain nutrients transcuticularly.

(b) **Thiabendazole.** In addition to its ability to disrupt microtubules, thiabendazole also inhibits fumarate reductase, a key enzyme in anaerobic respiration.

b. Ivermectin

(1) **Indications.** Ivermectin is a broad-spectrum anthelmintic. It is the drug of choice for onchocerciasis and is prophylactic against heartworm. It has some effect against *Ascaris, Strongyloides,* and *Wuchereria.*

(2) **Mechanism of action.** Ivermectin binds at, or close to, glutamate-gated chloride channels in nematodes, interrupting neuromuscular activity. Ivermectin has also been reported to nonspecifically interfere with the binding of retinol to the parasite's retinol-binding protein, although whether this contributes to parasite death is not known.

c. **Pyrantel**

(1) **Indications.** Pyrantel has efficacy against enteric nematodes (e.g., *Ascaris,* hookworm).

(2) **Mechanism of action.** This drug causes a ganglion-stimulating type of neuromuscular paralysis in these helminths, resulting in their rapid expulsion from the host intestine.

d. **Diethylcarbamazine citrate (DEC)**

(1) **Indications.** DEC is the drug of choice for lymphatic filariasis and loiasis, and is also effective against those nematodes causing visceral and cutaneous larva migrans.

(2) **Mechanism of action**

(a) DEC activates muscle cholinergic receptors in the worm, causing depolarization and muscle paralysis. Cells of the immune system are then assumed to attack and kill the parasite. This is thought to be the main mechanism of action against L3, L4, and adult worms.

(b) Against microfilariae, DEC appears to facilitate access of phagocytic cells to surface antigens on the worm. DEC may even act directly on the phagocytes. In a nonimmune host, DEC has no effect on microfilarial numbers, indicating that a competent immune response is essential to the effectiveness of DEC.

2. **Drugs used for the treatment of cestode and trematode infections**

a. **Praziquantel**

(1) **Indications.** Praziquantel is the drug of choice against most important trematodes and cestodes, with the exception of *Fasciola.*

(2) **Mechanisms of action**

(a) Praziquantel binds and inhibits the antioxidant enzyme glutathione-S-transferase (GST), which has been shown to play an important role in the ability of trematodes and cestodes to survive within their hosts. Praziquantel is only effective *in vivo* in immunocompetent hosts, indicating that it may only partially inactivate the antioxidant defense of the parasite, allowing phagocytes and other immune cells to complete the job of killing.

(b) Other effects of praziquantel—disruption of the tegument in trematodes and some cestodes and paralysis in cestodes—have not been explained.

b. **Niclosamide**

(1) **Indications.** Niclosamide has potent activity against many cestodes, including *Diphyllobothrium, Taenia,* and *Dipylidium.* It is poorly absorbed through the host gut, reducing toxicity to the host.

(2) **Mechanisms of action.** The drug appears to have several modes of action.

(a) It uncouples oxidative phosphorylation and electron-transport reactions in mitochondria. ATP production is inhibited and glucose uptake is suppressed.

(b) In *Dipylidium,* niclosamide rapidly causes paralysis. The adult cestodes are no longer able to maintain their attachment to the intestinal wall and are destroyed as they pass through the gastrointestinal system.

c. **Bithionol**

(1) **Indications.** Bithionol is the drug of choice for fascioliasis and is highly effective against paragonimiasis and some cestode infections.

(2) **Mechanisms of action.** Like niclosamide [see III C 2 b (2)], the main mode of action of this compound is the uncoupling of oxidative phosphorylation. In *Paragonimus,* bithionol has been shown to interrupt glycolysis, the TCA cycle, and succinate oxidation.

d. **Albendazole** is the drug of choice for hydatid disease and neurocysticercosis. The primary modes of action are similar to the other benzimidazoles [see III C 1 a (2)].

D. Resistance to antiparasitic agents. Parasites generally reproduce rapidly and sooner or later develop resistance to the drugs used to treat them. Resistance has developed most noticeably in *Plasmodium* species, which are now almost universally resistant to chloroquine.

Chapter 45

Medical Protozoology

Eric R. James

I. INTRODUCTION.

INTRODUCTION. Parasites are transmitted in three major ways: fecal-oral transmission, vector transmission, and direct penetration (Figure 45-1). In general, transmission is favored by poor sanitation environments or by an abundance of vectors and reservoirs. Therefore, a great deal of success in control of parasitic diseases can be achieved by simple public hygiene measures.

II. AMOEBAE

A. *Entamoeba histolytica*

1. **General characteristics.** The parasite exists in two forms—a feeding trophozoite form (20–30 μm in diameter) and a resistant cyst form (10–20 μm).
   a. **Trophozoites** usually have one locomotor pseudopodium, a prominent nucleus, and food vacuoles. They can be found in fresh stools.
   b. **Mature infective cysts.** The trophozoites encyst in the cecum or colon. The cyst contains an organism with four nuclei and reduced or absent chromatoidal bars and glycogen deposits.
2. **Epidemiology**
   a. **Distribution.** *E. histolytica* is a cosmopolitan intestinal parasite, affecting 10% of the world's population (ranging from <1% in developed nations to >50% in some tropical regions).
   b. **Transmission.** The disease is transmitted via the **fecal-oral route;** contaminated vegetables or water are a common source of infection.
   c. **Reservoirs.** There are no known animal reservoirs; however, asymptomatic human carriers can act as reservoirs.
3. **Pathogenesis and clinical disease**
   a. **Pathogenesis.** Certain strains of *E. histolytica* are more virulent than others. Virulence is related to the secretion of a potent cysteine proteinase, which assists the parasite in digesting the extracellular matrix and in invading tissue.
      (1) **Noninvasive.** Most infections remain localized to the intestine, with minimal invasion of the mucosa. This is usually the behavior of the parasite in individuals with normal immune systems.
      (2) **Invasive.** In immunocompromised patients and pregnant women, the infection is more likely to be invasive.
         (a) **Intestinal wall.** The trophozoites penetrate the intestinal epithelium and produce **granulomatous ulcers (amebomas)** in the mucous membrane and submucosa. These ulcers contain active, rapidly dividing trophozoites. Intestinal perforation and peritonitis may ensue.
         (b) **Extraintestinal sites.** Invasion is not limited to the intestinal wall. Trophozoites may enter mesenteric blood vessels and be carried to extraintestinal sites, principally the **liver.** Hepatic amebiasis usually results in a single abscess in the upper right lobe. **Lung** and **brain** abscesses are seen occasionally.
   b. **Clinical disease**
      (1) **Asymptomatic infection** is common.
      (2) **Symptomatic infection**
         (a) **Uncomplicated intestinal infection.** The most common symptoms of uncomplicated intestinal infection are diarrhea, cramps, and flatulence.

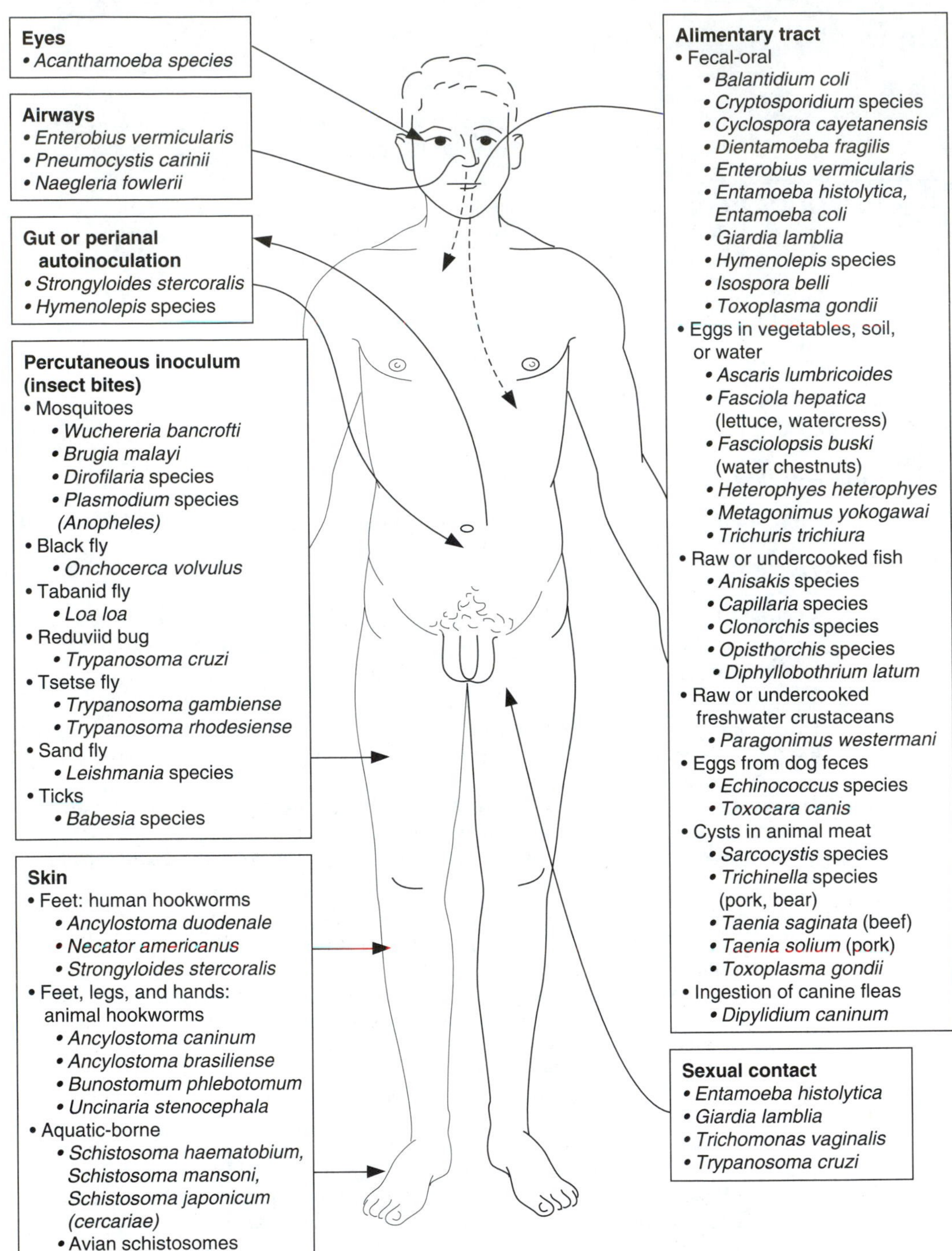

Eyes
• Acanthamoeba species
Airways
• Enterobius vermicularis
• Pneumocystis carinii
• Naegleria fowlerii
Gut or perianal autoinoculation
• Strongyloides stercoralis
• Hymenolepis species
Percutaneous inoculum (insect bites)
• Mosquitoes
• Wuchereria bancrofti
• Brugia malayi
• Dirofilaria species
• Plasmodium species (Anopheles)
• Black fly
• Onchocerca volvulus
• Tabanid fly
• Loa loa
• Reduviid bug
• Trypanosoma cruzi
• Tsetse fly
• Trypanosoma gambiense
• Trypanosoma rhodesiense
• Sand fly
• Leishmania species
• Ticks
• Babesia species
Skin
• Feet: human hookworms
• Ancylostoma duodenale
• Necator americanus
• Strongyloides stercoralis
• Feet, legs, and hands: animal hookworms
• Ancylostoma caninum
• Ancylostoma brasiliense
• Bunostomum phlebotomum
• Uncinaria stenocephala
• Aquatic-borne
• Schistosoma haematobium, Schistosoma mansoni, Schistosoma japonicum (cercariae)
• Avian schistosomes
Alimentary tract
• Fecal-oral
• Balantidium coli
• Cryptosporidium species
• Cyclospora cayetanensis
• Dientamoeba fragilis
• Enterobius vermicularis
• Entamoeba histolytica, Entamoeba coli
• Giardia lamblia
• Hymenolepis species
• Isospora belli
• Toxoplasma gondii
• Eggs in vegetables, soil, or water
• Ascaris lumbricoides
• Fasciola hepatica (lettuce, watercress)
• Fasciolopsis buski (water chestnuts)
• Heterophyes heterophyes
• Metagonimus yokogawai
• Trichuris trichiura
• Raw or undercooked fish
• Anisakis species
• Capillaria species
• Clonorchis species
• Opisthorchis species
• Diphyllobothrium latum
• Raw or undercooked freshwater crustaceans
• Paragonimus westermani
• Eggs from dog feces
• Echinococcus species
• Toxocara canis
• Cysts in animal meat
• Sarcocystis species
• Trichinella species (pork, bear)
• Taenia saginata (beef)
• Taenia solium (pork)
• Toxoplasma gondii
• Ingestion of canine fleas
• Dipylidium caninum
Sexual contact
• Entamoeba histolytica
• Giardia lamblia
• Trichomonas vaginalis
• Trypanosoma cruzi

FIGURE 45-1. Portals of entry for major human parasitic infections.

(b) **Amebic dysentery.** When the parasite invades the intestinal wall and ulcers develop, patients present with fever, profuse diarrhea that contains blood and mucus, and severe abdominal pain.

(c) **Hepatic amebiasis** is accompanied by peripheral eosinophilia and is fatal if untreated. When extraintestinal abscesses are involved, the symptoms depend on the organ and on the size and location of the abscess.

4. Laboratory diagnosis

a. Microscopic examination

(1) **Stool samples.** The presence of **quadrinucleated cysts** or **trophozoites containing ingested erythrocytes** in wet mounts or fixed and stained preparations of stool (or sputum) is diagnostic.

(2) **Mucosal scrapings** obtained by sigmoidoscopy can be used as an adjunct to the conventional ova and parasite (O&P) workup in cases of suspected amoebiasis.

(a) Six or more areas of the mucosa should be sampled for accurate results.

(b) Examination may involve a direct wet mount, a permanently stained smear, and immunostained smears (using either immunofluorescent or immunoenzymatic techniques).

(3) **Lung, liver** or **brain biopsy samples** submitted for routine histology and Giemsa-stained touch preparations will reveal *E. histolytica* when the infection has caused extraintestinal abscesses.

b. Serology. Tests for anti-*E. histolytica* antibodies assist in diagnosing **extraintestinal infections.**

5. Treatment

a. Pharmacologic therapy

(1) **Metronidazole** is the **drug of choice** for patients with symptomatic intestinal and extraintestinal amebiasis. In patients with extraintestinal amebiasis, metronidazole is administered parenterally.

(2) **Paromomycin** is used when metronidazole is not effective.

(3) **Antibacterial agents** may be indicated for patients with **complicated intestinal amebiasis** because these patients are at significant risk for secondary infection of the intestinal ulcerations.

b. Supportive measures include **oral rehydration** and **electrolyte replacement.** In patients with severe intestinal hemorrhaging, **blood transfusion** may be necessary. **Surgery** is required when intestinal perforation has occurred.

6. Control and prevention

a. Treatment of **asymptomatic carriers** is controversial, but administration of **iodoquinol** has been suggested as a way to avoid dissemination by carriers.

b. Improving basic hygiene and sanitation practices is the most effective way of controlling outbreaks of amebiasis, because *E. histolytica* thrives in conditions where standards of sanitation and hygiene are poor.

B. *Acanthamoeba* species

1. General properties. ***Acanthamoeba* spp.** are free-living amoebae which, as trophozoites, have numerous characteristically pointed pseudopodia.

2. Epidemiology. *Acanthamoeba* are found in soil and lakes. Infection of the eye by contaminated contact lenses is the most common mode of infection.

3. Pathogenesis and clinical disease

a. Pathogenesis. *Acanthamoeba* species inhabit the immunologically privileged sites (i.e., the **eye** and **brain).** The organism may directly invade the nasal mucosa and gain access to the brain, or it may enter the body through dermal abrasions.

b. Clinical disease

(1) **Ulcerative keratitis.** Feeding trophozoites produce opacification and an ulcerative keratitis, which, if untreated, leads to perforation and loss of the eye.

(2) **Primary amoebic meningoencephalitis.** *Acanthamoeba* species can cause meningoencephalitis, although this presentation is more common with *Naegleria fowleri* (see II C).

4. **Laboratory diagnosis**
   a. **Corneal scrapings** or **biopsy** are used to detect *Acanthamoeba* species using routine histology, staining with calcofluor white, or culture (not widely available).
   b. **Cerebrospinal fluid (CSF)** is submitted in cases of suspected amoebic meningoencephalitis. Motile amoebae can be seen in stained or unstained CSF.

5. **Treatment** is difficult and protracted because the drugs of choice, **propamidine isethionate, polyhexamethylene biguanide,** and **clotrimazole,** kill the trophozoites slowly and do not affect the cysts. After apparent cure, residual cysts (which are extremely resistant to adverse conditions) can hatch and reactivate the infection. **Amphotericin B** is used in cases of meningoencephalitis.

C. *Naegleria fowleri*

1. **Epidemiology.** *N. fowleri* thrives in warm water at lower oxygen tensions. It is often found in the mud at the bottom of puddles, ditches, and lakes. The infection is acquired by accidental inhalation of contaminated water while swimming or playing.

2. **Pathogenesis and clinical disease**
   a. **Pathogenesis.** After the flagellated trophozoite is inhaled, it penetrates the lamina cribrosa to enter the brain.
   b. **Clinical disease.** *Naegleria fowleri,* which reproduces more rapidly than *Acanthamoeba,* causes a considerably more serious form of **primary amoebic meningoencephalitis.** The patient starts complaining of headache and fever and deteriorates rapidly into a deep coma. The disease is almost always fatal; death occurs within 4–7 days of the development of symptoms.

3. **Laboratory diagnosis.** The finding of trophozoites in the CSF is diagnostic.

4. **Treatment. Amphotericin B** and **miconazole** have been used to treat some cases successfully.

D.

Entamoeba gingivalis is closely related to *E. histolytica* but is regarded as nonpathogenic, although it is associated with periodontal disease. *E. gingivalis* trophozoites live in the gingival margins, where they eat tartar-scavenging bacteria and epithelial cells. This organism may occasionally ingest erythrocytes, but not lymphocytes (this is the characteristic that distinguishes *E. histolytica* in the sputum of patients with a lung abscess from *E. gingivalis*). *E. gingivalis* does not form a cyst, and is believed to be transmitted by kissing or sharing of eating and drinking utensils.

E.

Entamoeba hartmanni was formerly classified as the small nonpathogenic race of *E. histolytica.* Morphologically similar to *E. histolytica, E. hartmanni* does not ingest host cells.

F.

Entamoeba coli inhabits the same niche as *E. histolytica*, but is usually bigger both as a trophozoite (measuring more than 25 μm in diameter) and as a cyst (17 μm diameter). *E. coli* trophozoites do not ingest erythrocytes and do not invade tissues; therefore, this species is regarded as a nonpathogenic commensal. The **cyst** has **eight nuclei** (versus the four of *E. histolytica*). This organism has been estimated to infect more than 19% of the United States population.

G.

Entamoeba nana and ***Iodamoeba butschlii*** are considered nonpathogenic, although these organisms may cause chronic, fulminating diarrhea in some patients. The trophozoites and cysts of both organisms are smaller than those of *E. histolytica.*

III. FLAGELLATES

A. *Giardia lamblia (intestinalis)*

1. **General properties**
   a. *G. lamblia* exists as a trophozoite (8 × 14 μm) and a cyst (11 μm long). The trophozoite is bilaterally symmetrical with two prominent nuclei and four pairs of fla-

gella originating from basal bodies between the nuclei. The organism is flattened with a concave ventral adhesive disc used for attachment to the surface of intestinal epithelial cells.

b. Reproduction is by asexual longitudinal division.

2. Epidemiology

a. Distribution. *G. lamblia* is a cosmopolitan parasite, common in temperate latitudes and in developed countries, as well as in the tropics. Endemic foci of a more pathologic variety of *Giardia* have been identified in St. Petersburg (Russia), Mediterranean areas, and regions of Central Asia.

b. Transmission is by the **fecal-oral route.** The source of infection may be infected human carriers or wild animals that act as reservoirs of infection and contaminate water with the cysts passed in their feces.

(1) Drinking contaminated water is the usual mode of infection. In the United States, hikers often acquire this parasite after drinking mountain stream water contaminated by infected beavers ("beaver fever"). *Giardia* trophozoites encyst as the feces dehydrate during their passage through the large intestine. Cysts are passed in the feces and may survive in water up to 3 months. Following ingestion by a new host, excystation occurs in the duodenum and the life cycle of the parasite begins again.

(2) Giardiasis occasionally occurs in outbreaks, often affecting preschool-aged children in daycare centers and their immediate families.

3. Pathogenesis and clinical disease

a. Pathogenesis. The parasite inhabits the small intestine. Coating of the distal villi with many trophozoites is thought to lead to malabsorption, particularly of lipids and lipid-soluble vitamins (e.g., vitamin A). Damage to the villi is also associated with the infection, but the trophozoites do not penetrate the mucosa and, in immunocompetent individuals, the disease usually resolves spontaneously within 4 weeks. Hypogammaglobulinemia (particularly IgA deficiency) and achlorhydria predispose to the development of symptomatic disease.

(1) Heavy infection causes a general disaccharidase deficiency, resulting in lactose intolerance that usually resolves after treatment.

(2) In extreme cases, severe dehydration may be life-threatening.

b. Clinical presentation. Symptoms vary with the age and immunologic status of the host and the strain of *Giardia.*

(1) Symptomatic children usually present with watery diarrhea.

(2) Older patients may present with nausea, anorexia, explosive, watery, "fermenting" stools, flatulence, a low grade fever, abdominal distention, and gastric cramps. Stools are foul smelling but without pus or blood.

4. Laboratory diagnosis

a. Microscopic examination

(1) Stool samples. Because cysts are shed intermittently, several specimens may be required to diagnose infection. The presence of cysts or trophozoites in the stool specimen is diagnostic. (Trophozoites are more likely to be seen if the stools are watery.) Stains, such as iodine or trichrome, aid in the microscopic examination.

(2) Duodenal contents may also be examined for *G. lamblia.*

b. Serology. *G. lamblia* can also be detected by one of several enzyme immunoassays (EIAs) or by a fluorescent monoclonal antibody stain.

c. Enterotest. An alternative to microscopic examination of stool samples is the Enterotest, or **"string test."** A string is taped to the patient's face and a gelatin capsule attached to the string is swallowed. After the capsule has dissolved and the string has reached the duodenum (approximately 4 hours later), the string is retrieved and examined for parasites. With the advent of the *Giardia* antigen test, the use of the Enterotest has sharply declined.

5. Treatment

a. Metronidazole and **quinacrine hydrochloride** are the drugs of choice. Quinacrine has a higher cure rate but is more toxic.

b. **Furazolidone** may be preferred for pediatric patients.
c. **Tinidazole** is also relatively effective.
d. **Erythromycin** and **mepacrine** have been shown to be active against *Giardia* in recent studies.

6. **Prevention**
   a. **Boiling, filtering,** or **adding iodine to water** in endemic areas where the water supply may be contaminated is recommended. The cysts resist chlorine treatment.
   b. In daycare centers, **frequent hand washing by staff, separation of diaper changing areas** from areas of other activities, and **separation of feeding areas** are all essential preventive measures.

B. ***Dientamoeba fragilis*** is a flagellate that used to be considered an ameba. Although it is classified with the flagellates based on ultrastructure and immunologic characteristics, *D. fragilis* does not possess a flagellum and moves slowly by extending a single flat pseudopodium.

1. **Epidemiology**
   a. **Distribution.** *D. fragilis* is distributed worldwide.
   b. **Life cycle.** The life cycle of this organism is not well understood. No cyst stage has been described, and the trophozoites are not resistant to gastric secretions.
   c. **Reservoirs.** No reservoirs or vectors have been identified, although it has been suggested that the trophozoites may be transported to new human hosts in the eggs of *Trichuris trichiura* (whipworm).
2. **Pathogenesis and clinical disease.** *D. fragilis,* which does not invade the intestinal wall, produces a relatively mild chronic intestinal disturbance. Fibrosis of the intestinal wall (particularly the appendix) has been reported.
3. **Laboratory diagnosis.** Trophozoites (usually binucleate) are visible in fecal preparations.
4. **Treatment. Iodoquinol** and **tetracycline** are effective against this parasite.

C. ***Trichomonas* species**

1. ***Trichomonas hominis*** (*Pentatrichomonas hominis*) is an intestinal parasite that is sometimes associated with diarrhea.
2. ***Trichomonas tenax*** is found in the oral cavity, where it is associated with periodontal disease.
3. ***Trichomonas vaginalis*** is found in the genitourinary tract and infection is frequently symptomatic. The vulva and vagina are most affected.
   a. **General properties.** *T. vaginalis* exists as a trophozoite (9 × 19 μm) and does not have a cyst form. The trophozoite has a single nucleus, an axostyle, and five flagella, one of which is attached to the organism's body surface to form an undulating membrane.
   b. **Epidemiology.** *T. vaginalis* is a cosmopolitan, strictly human, sexually transmitted flagellate, occurring in 10%–25% of women. Asymptomatic males may act as reservoirs of infection for their partners.
   c. **Pathogenesis and clinical disease**
      (1) The normal vaginal environment has a pH of 3.8–4.5 with a healthy epithelial surface rich in glycogen and *Lactobacillus.* The bacilli convert glycogen to lactic acid, which maintains the pH.
         (a) *T. vaginalis* feeds on host cells (which may cause disruption of the glycogen levels) and bacteria (inducing the pH to rise). *T. vaginalis* infections thrive at pH levels that exceed 4.9.
         (b) Epithelial erosion may occur, leading to petechiate hemorrhages and metaplastic changes to the epithelium.
      (2) **Clinical disease**
         (a) Although an altered vaginal environment is common in **women** with **trichomoniasis,** not all who are infected report symptoms. Symptoms in-

clude **tenderness, hyperemia, itching,** and a **profuse, frothy, malodorous discharge** containing bacteria, pus, and trophozoites. Heavy infections may cause dysmenorrhea and dysuria.

(b) Although infections are **usually asymptomatic** in **men,** *T. vaginalis* may infect the urethra and bladder.

d. Laboratory diagnosis. The clinical symptoms are very suggestive, but the diagnosis can be confirmed by microscopic examination or isolation by culture.

(1) Microscopic examination. Vaginal secretions, urethral discharge, prostatic secretions, or urine sediment can be examined for *T. vaginalis.*

(a) Direct wet mount. A small amount of the specimen is mixed with a drop of saline on a microscope slide, covered with a cover slip, and examined for the jerky motility of the trophozoite or the movement of its undulating membrane.

(b) Staining. Alternatively, a smear of the specimen can be made, allowed to air dry, stained with a fluorescent monoclonal antibody, and examined.

(2) Culture. Although culture is the most sensitive method for detecting *T. vaginalis,* it is expensive and somewhat technically difficult, and therefore limited in availability.

e. Treatment

(1) Metronidazole is the drug of choice. Pessaries (particularly during pregnancy when metronidazole may be contraindicated) and acid douches are useful.

(2) In order **to prevent recurrence,** the patient's **sexual partner should be tested** for *T. vaginalis* infection **and treated** if necessary.

D. *Leishmania* species

1. General properties

a. The *Leishmania* species alternate between **two distinct forms** during their life cycle.

(1) During the **amastigote** stage, the organism is an intracellular parasite of macrophages in the human host. In amastigotes, the flagellum barely protrudes from the cytoplasm (amastigote means "without flagellum") and the organism measures 1.5–5 μm diameter.

(2) During the **promastigote** stage, the organism parasitizes the gut of sandflies. In this form, the parasite measures approximately 3 μm $\times$ 20 μm.

b. During both stages, the organism contains a prominent nucleus, a kinetoplast, a basal body, a flagellum and scant mitochondria. Metabolism is predominantly anaerobic.

2. Epidemiology

a. Distribution. Four main species (each with many strains) exist in foci throughout the tropics and subtropics. Leishmaniasis is endemic in **Central** and **South America, Africa,** the **Middle East** and **Central** and **Southern Asia,** affecting more than 12 million people.

b. Reservoirs and transmission. Female **sandflies,** of the genus *Phlebotomus* in Africa and Eurasia and *Lutzomyia* in the Americas, are the main vectors. Many animals act as reservoir hosts, principally canids and rodents, and leishmaniasis in most locations in the world is a zoonosis.

(1) The insect vector becomes infected when taking a blood meal from an infected mammalian host. The blood contains infected monocytes and macrophages with intracellular amastigotes.

(2) In the insect gut, the amastigotes are released from the macrophages. They transform into promastigotes and reproduce rapidly to fill the gut and pharynx. When the insect next takes a blood meal, the promastigotes are injected into the mammalian host.

(3) In the mammalian host, the promastigote is phagocytosed into a vacuole by a macrophage. It resists digestion and is released into the cytoplasm, where it transforms into an amastigote and starts reproducing by binary fission. Heavily parasitized macrophages rupture to release their amastigotes, which infect new macrophages through the same process.

3. **Pathogenesis and clinical disease**
   a. **Pathogenesis.** Infection and growth of the *Leishmania* organisms is under the control of the host immune system.
      (1) The establishment of infection in susceptible individuals correlates with a predominantly TH_2-type response, which is inefficient as a defense against intracellular parasites. In susceptible individuals, infected macrophages are initially activated, but not sufficiently to kill the intracellular organisms. The ineffective activation is, however, sufficient to cause inflammation. Eventually, the macrophages are destroyed. Because of the ineffectiveness of the macrophages and their eventual depletion, the lesions do not heal and the disease progresses.
      (2) In contrast, resistance to *Leishmania* is associated with the increased capacity of infected macrophages to eliminate the intracellular organisms, which is related to secretion of interferon-γ (IFN-γ) by activated TH_1-type cells.
   b. **Clinical disease** depends on the population of macrophages affected.
      (1) **Cutaneous leishmaniasis** can be caused by a variety of organisms. In Asia and Africa, *L. tropica, L. major,* and *L. aethiopica* cause what is known as **Old World cutaneous leishmaniasis (oriental sore).** In the Americas, *L. mexicana* and *L. peruviana* are the causes of **New World cutaneous leishmaniasis.**
         (a) **Symptoms** include **skin ulcers,** the number, size, and characteristics of which vary with the causative species of *Leishmania.* The ulcers are usually painless, but are often secondarily infected with bacteria. Cutaneous ulcers usually heal completely but may leave a prominent scar.
         (b) **Immunity.** After a number of outbreaks, the patient may become immune. Immunity is nonsterile and corticosteroid or immunosuppressive therapy can cause relapses.
      (2) **Mucocutaneous leishmaniasis (espundia),** caused by *L. braziliensis,* involves macrophages of the skin around the mucous membranes. Disease starts with a cutaneous lesion that enlarges to involve the **mouth, nose,** and **soft palate,** leading to severe tissue destruction and **disfigurement.**
      (3) **Visceral leishmaniasis (kala-azar)** is usually caused by *L. donovani,* which disseminates systemically and infects macrophages of the liver, spleen, bone marrow, and lymph nodes, causing **hepatomegaly, splenomegaly, lymphadenopathy,** and **anemia.** Left untreated, visceral leishmaniasis is usually fatal. Nonimmune individuals exposed to *Leishmania* organisms for the first time while traveling to areas where leishmaniasis is prevalent can develop disseminated leishmaniasis caused by species other than *L. donovani.*

4. **Laboratory diagnosis**
   a. **Microscopic examination**
      (1) **Cutaneous ulcer aspirates, scrapings,** or **biopsy specimens** are examined for leishmanial amastigotes. Active lesions should be disinfected and the central necrotic material removed prior to collection of material from the ulcer margin by aspiration, scraping, or biopsy. Several slides of the material are made and Giemsa stained.
      (2) **Spleen** and **bone marrow aspirates** are used as specimens when visceral disease is suspected. Giemsa-stained smears prepared from the **buffy coat** can also demonstrate leishmanial amastigotes.
   b. **Serology.** Positive results on EIA or indirect immunofluorescence testing demonstrate reactivity to cultured promastigotes or antigens extracted from them and support the clinical diagnosis.

5. **Treatment**
   a. The **pentavalent antimonials** (e.g., **sodium stibogluconate, meglumine antimonate)** are used to treat leishmaniasis. Resistant cases have been treated with **pentamidine** and **amphotericin B.** Proper treatment usually requires intramuscular or intravenous administration for at least 1 month.
   b. **Cytokine therapy** to activate TH_1 responses and macrophages is being considered as a possible new method of treatment.

6. **Control and prevention**
   a. **Control**
      (1) **Destruction of animal reservoirs** or their nesting sites and burrows reduces transmission to humans.
      (2) **Residual insecticide spraying** is helpful in control.
   b. **Prevention.** There is **no effective vaccine.** In Russia and Israel, live organisms injected into nonexposed cutaneous sites are used to stimulate the development of acquired immunity.

E. *Trypanosoma* species

1. ***Trypanosoma brucei rhodesiense*** and ***Trypanosoma brucei gambiense*** are subspecies of *Trypanosoma brucei brucei,* a cattle parasite responsible for nagana, a devastating disease that prevents livestock rearing in much of sub-Saharan Africa.
   a. **General properties.** The trypanosomes can exist in one of two forms.
      (1) In the **epimastigote,** the kinetoplast is centrally located near the nucleus.
      (2) In the **trypomastigote,** the kinetoplast is located at the anterior end. The flagellum runs the length of the body and forms a lateral undulating membrane. Trypomastigotes measure approximately 14 × 33 μm.
   b. **Epidemiology**
      (1) **Distribution** is focal.
         (a) ***T.b. rhodesiense*** infects humans in **eastern** and **southern Africa.**
         (b) ***T.b. gambiense*** infects humans in **western Africa.**
      (2) **Transmission**
         (a) **Insect bite.** Both the male and female **tsetse fly** (*Glossina* species) act as vectors. Fly habitats include sparsely wooded savanna and agricultural areas, and, in western Africa, riverine areas.
            (i) The tsetse fly acquires the infection with a blood meal from an infected host. Many species of wild game animals act as reservoirs of infection for *T.b. rhodesiense.* These animals appear to be unaffected by the parasite. Pigs may act as reservoirs for *T.b. gambiense.*
            (ii) The trypomastigotes transform to epimastigotes within the fly's gut and migrate to the salivary glands, where they convert back into metacyclic trypomastigotes. Metacyclic trypomastigotes are infective to humans.
            (iii) When the infected fly bites a human, the trypanosomes are injected at the site of the bite with the fly's saliva. They enter the skin, where they reproduce clonally by binary fission, and within a few days they migrate to the lymph ducts and glands and eventually enter the blood. The cycle takes over 20 days.
         (b) **Human-to-human transmission** (via tsetse flies) is thought to be the exception for *T.b. rhodesiense,* but the rule for ***T.b. gambiense.***
   c. **Pathogenesis and clinical disease.** *T.b. rhodesiense* and *T.b. gambiense* cause **African trypanosomiasis (Rhodesian sleeping sickness** and **Gambian sleeping sickness,** respectively).
      (1) **Pathogenesis.** African trypanosomiasis is associated with **waves of parasitemia,** each wave representing the emergence of a single clone of parasites expressing a **variant surface glycoprotein (VSG).** The surface antigen changes with each parasitemic wave. As host antibodies (specific to the VSG) kill off one wave of parasites, a new dominant clone carrying a different VSG emerges **(antigenic variation).** The parasite genome contains a battery of genes capable of coding for VSGs. By the time the host has successfully mounted an antibody response capable of eliminating the dominant clone, a new variant clone has already emerged.
         (a) New parasitemic waves occur approximately every 7–10 days.
         (b) It is estimated that the VSG gene repertoire is extensive enough to allow the parasite to vary its surface antigens without repeat for at least 40 years.

(2) **Clinical disease**

(a) A **chancre** (a necrotic erythematous nodule) appears at the site of the tsetse fly bite. Biopsies of the chancre reveal rapidly dividing parasites.

(b) The patient experiences **cervical lymphadenopathy, recurrent high fevers** (which correlate with the waves of parasitemia), **headaches,** and, sometimes, a **rash.**

(c) Eventually, the patient develops **hepatic** and **renal damage, myxedema, pericardial inflammation** and **effusion, muscle tremors, epileptiform convulsions,** and **coma.** In Gambian sleeping sickness, CNS symptoms take several years to develop, but in Rhodesian sleeping sickness, CNS manifestations develop in only 3–6 months, leading to death in 6–9 months if the disease is untreated.

d. **Laboratory diagnosis.** Definitive diagnosis is made by demonstration of trypomastigotes in stained blood, lymph node aspirates, or CSF smears. (In African trypanosomiasis, only trypomastigotes are found in infected humans.)

(1) Blood for trypanosome examination is best collected during febrile episodes.

(2) Thick and thin blood smears are used for detection of trypanosomes. Giemsa-stained smears prepared from the buffy coat can also demonstrate trypanosomes.

e. **Treatment**

(1) **Suramin** is the traditional drug of choice, but it can be highly toxic. Patients should be carefully monitored during treatment.

(2) **Melarsoprol** is used to treat advanced disease with CNS involvement.

(3) **Eflornithine,** an ornithine decarboxylase inhibitor, is becoming the new drug of choice.

f. **Control and prevention**

(1) **Control.** Attempts at control have traditionally included selective spraying of the nighttime resting sites of tsetse flies and clearing of tsetse habitats with careful wildlife management.

(2) **Prevention.** Because of its apparently almost limitless capacity for varying the antigen on its surface, the prospects for a vaccine to protect against African trypanosomiasis look bleak. Currently, research is focusing on identifying less variable immunogenic components (e.g., in the flagellar pocket) that could be exploited as vaccine targets.

2. ***Trypanosoma cruzi***

a. **Epidemiology**

(1) **Distribution.** *T. cruzi* is widespread in **Central** and **South America** and infects approximately 25 million people. Occasional localized outbreaks have been reported in Texas and California.

(2) **Reservoirs.** *T. cruzi* infects most mammals; **opossums** and **armadillos** are the main reservoirs of infection.

(3) **Transmission**

(a) **Insect bite. Triatomine bugs** of several genera, including *Panstrongylus* and *Rhodnius,* act as vectors. The metacyclic trypomastigotes develop in the hindgut of triatomine bugs. The bite wound is contaminated with infected feces deposited as the bugs take their blood meal. In the mammalian host, trypomastigotes (measuring approximately 20 μm in length) enter the blood and many other types of cells, where they escape destruction, transform into amastigotes, and commence multiplication.

(b) **Blood transfusion.** Parasites can also be transmitted by blood transfusion, the predominant mode of transmission in urban areas.

(c) **Sexual** and **congenital transmission** of *T. cruzi* have also been reported.

b. **Pathogenesis and clinical disease.** *T. cruzi* causes **Chagas' disease.**

(1) **Acute disease.** Lesions and inflammation occur at the bite site, which is frequently near the eyes (**Romaña's sign**) or mouth.

(2) **Intermediate stage.** Acute disease is followed by an intermediate stage in which the infection becomes generalized. The symptoms are suggestive of sys-

temic disease and include **fever, adenopathy, splenomegaly, electrocardiogram changes suggestive of myocarditis, edema,** and **leukocytosis.**

(3) **Chronic stage.** *T. cruzi* amastigotes are found in many tissues as intracellular pseudocysts, particularly in the heart muscle and ganglion cells of the esophagus. Many cross-reacting antigens between *T. cruzi* and human heart and nerve tissue have been characterized. It is possible that autoimmune reactions to these tissues, triggered by parasite antigen, may play a role in the development of chronic Chagas' disease. Progressive destruction of host tissues can lead to the following conditions.

(a) **Apical aneurysm** of the heart and **congestive heart failure** can occur as a result of heart muscle loss and alterations in conduction. Chagas' disease is the leading cause of heart disease in Latin America.

(b) **Megaesophagus** and **megacolon** can be caused by loss of tone secondary to the destruction of nerve ganglia involved in the autonomic control of these organs.

c. Laboratory diagnosis

(1) **Microscopic examination.** During the acute and intermediate stages of disease, infection can be demonstrated by finding trypomastigotes in stained blood smears and amastigotes in biopsy material.

(2) **Serologic tests** are used for diagnosis in the chronic stage of disease, when parasites are difficult to detect.

(3) **Xenodiagnosis.** When standard methods of diagnosis are inconclusive, the following methods can be used:

(a) Laboratory-reared triatomine bugs can be allowed to feed on the patient suspected of having Chagas' disease; subsequent dissection of the bugs will reveal parasites in the hindgut.

(b) Injection of the patient's blood into a surrogate rodent host may lead to detectable parasitemia.

d. Treatment

(1) **Allopurinol** and **nifurtimox** are the drugs of choice. Both drugs must be administered for several months. Because nifurtimox produces severe side effects, patients are often reluctant to complete the course of treatment.

(b) An inhibitor specific for cruzain, the major digestive enzyme of *T. cruzi* amastigotes, is being developed as a potential new chemotherapeutic agent.

e. Control

(1) Mud and thatching, traditionally used in house construction, provide ideal sites for bugs to live. Reconstruction of dwellings using concrete or brick with tin roofs helps prevent disease transmission and may represent the best long-term solution.

(2) Residual insecticide sprays and prophylactic drugs are also used.

IV. CILIATES. *Balantidium coli* is the only ciliate that is pathogenic for humans.

A. General properties.

General properties. This organism is large, and possesses a macronucleus and a micronucleus. Cilia cover its surface and are used in locomotion and in moving food toward the cytostome (mouth). The organism exists as a trophozoite (100 × 50 μm) in the lumen of the cecum and colon and as a cyst (60 × 40 μm), which is passed in feces.

B. Epidemiology

1. **Distribution.** *B. coli* is an extremely common parasite of pigs. Although its distribution is cosmopolitan, it rarely causes disease in humans. It is usually a disease associated with pig farming.

2. **Transmission** is by the **fecal-oral route.** Cyst-contaminated food is the usual source. The cysts hatch in the small intestine, where the parasite multiplies and completes its life cycle.

C. Pathogenesis and clinical disease

1. **Pathogenesis.** *B. coli* feeds principally on starch but also will ingest bacteria, erythrocytes, and epithelial cells. **Mucosal invasion** results in hyperemia and local hemorrhage with ulceration, which may lead to dissemination to other sites.
   a. **Malnourishment** seems to predispose to mucosal invasion by *B. coli,* because glycogen levels are reduced in these individuals.
   b. **Concurrent infection with** *Trichuris* (whipworm), a worm that burrows into the gut epithelium, may encourage tissue invasion by *B. coli.*

2. **Clinical disease.** *B. coli* causes **balantidiasis.**
   a. **Most infections are asymptomatic.**
   b. When parasite burdens are heavy, **dysentery** and **colitis** may develop, accompanied by **nausea, vomiting, fever,** and **headache.** Death as a result of *B. coli* infection is extremely rare, but may occur following perforation of ulcers and peritonitis.

D. Laboratory diagnosis is usually confirmed by microscopic identification of trophozoites or cysts in feces.

E. Treatment. Metronidazole and doxycycline are the drugs of choice.

V. SPOROZOANS

A. *Plasmodium* species.
Four species of *Plasmodium* parasitize humans—***P. falciparum, P. vivax, P. malariae,*** and ***P. ovale***—and are responsible for **malaria.**

1. **Epidemiology**
   a. **Incidence.** *Plasmodium* species cause more than 250 million infections and 1–2 million deaths per year, primarily in infants and nonimmune adults.
   b. **Distribution.** Malaria is endemic in over 100 countries in the **tropics** and **subtropics** and was also formerly present in many temperate regions, including the United States and Europe. Malaria eradication in temperate zones occurred during the 1940s and 50s through the use of insecticides, principally DDT.
   c. **Transmission.** Females of over 60 species of **mosquitoes** of the genus *Anopheles* are the vectors of *Plasmodium.*

2. **Life cycle**
   a. **Inoculation.** Human infection commences when **sporozoites** are injected along with mosquito saliva during blood feeding.
   b. **Exoerythrocytic cycle.** The sporozoites enter the circulatory system and are carried to the liver, where they penetrate hepatocytes.
      (1) Over the next 6–14 days, each parasite, now a **trophozoite,** grows and divides into numerous **merozoites,** which form a cluster **(schizont)** within an infected liver cell.
      (2) In *P. vivax* and *P. ovale* malaria, some organisms remain dormant in the liver as **hypnozoites** for up to 1 year before undergoing schizogony and causing relapses.
   c. **Erythrocytic cycle.** The infected liver cells rupture, releasing merozoites, which penetrate erythrocytes.
      (1) The merozoite, contained within a parasitophorous vacuole formed by the invagination of the erythrocyte's surface membrane, becomes a **trophozoite** and starts digesting hemoglobin.
      (2) The young (ring-stage) trophozoite matures and multiplies inside the erythrocyte to form a **schizont** containing 6–12 **merozoites.** (In *P. vivax* infection, 12–24 merozoites are contained within the schizont.)
      (3) The erythrocyte eventually bursts to release the merozoites. This erythrocytic

cycle is repeated approximately every 48 hours (or 72 hours in the case of *P. malariae* infection).

d. A small number of mature trophozoites develop into male or female **gametocytes.** The gametocytes are ingested by mosquitoes with their blood meal and continue their sexual cycle in the mosquito midgut.

(1) After leaving the erythrocyte, the male gametocyte exflagellates (i.e., it divides into 8 microgametes) and fertilization of the female macrogamete occurs.

(2) The resulting ookinete burrows through the midgut wall and becomes an oocyst. The oocyst grows to contain thousands of **sporozoites** and ruptures in 10–20 days. The released sporozoites migrate to the salivary glands of the mosquito, completing the cycle.

3. Pathogenesis and clinical disease. Ten to fourteen days after the erythrocytic cycle begins, the parasite numbers reach a density that induces the onset of symptoms. Fever and chills, diarrhea, headache, and sometimes pulmonary and cardiac symptoms are typical. *P. vivax* malaria tends to follow a chronic course with periodic relapses, whereas *P. ovale* malaria is generally mild. *P. malariae* malaria is less severe than *P. falciparum* malaria, but it may cause nephrotic syndrome in children following glomerular deposition of immune complexes.

a. Fever. The pathogenesis of fever in malaria is unclear. Fever **coincides with red blood cell lysis,** and is likely to be caused by the release of interleukin-1 (IL-1) and tumor necrosis factor-α (TNF-α) by macrophages activated during the processing of red blood cell debris.

(1) In the early stages of infection, the febrile episodes are irregularly timed because red blood cells are lysed almost continuously.

(2) With time, the erythrocytic asexual cycle becomes synchronous and periodic febrile episodes become obvious, coinciding with the lysis of infected red blood cells. The periodicity is 48 hours for *P. falciparum, P. vivax,* and *P. ovale* infections (tertian malaria) and 72 hours for *P. malariae* infections (quartan malaria).

b. Anemia. Destruction of erythrocytes leads to anemia and enlargement of the liver and spleen. *P. vivax* and *P. ovale* preferentially invade reticulocytes, while *P. malariae* parasitizes old erythrocytes. Because of the repeated hemolytic crises, anemia may become severe, and the patient complains of **extreme fatigue** and **weakness.**

c. Large-scale intravascular lysis of red blood cells is seen in ***P. falciparum*** malaria. Its pathogenesis is unclear, but may result in part from the **infection of erythrocytes** and in part from a **hypersensitivity reaction to quinine.** Quinine–antibody complexes are adsorbed to the erythrocyte surface, leading to complement activation and lysis.

(1) Massive hemoglobinuria (blackwater fever), a consequence of intravascular hemolysis, can lead to **acute tubular necrosis** and **renal failure.**

(2) Cerebral malaria. In *P. falciparum* malaria, late-stage schizonts elaborate proteins that are expressed on the erythrocyte surface. The proteins promote aggregation to other noninfected erythrocytes and adhesion to capillary endothelial cells, constricting capillary blood flow and causing **anoxia, ischemia,** and **numerous small hemorrhages.** When this happens in the brain, it can be rapidly fatal, depending on the extent of the ischemic lesions.

d. Immunity gradually develops. If the patient survives, episodes become less severe. The balance between infection and host resistance is very obvious in *P. malariae* malaria, which may persist subclinically for many years, showing recrudescences when the patient becomes immunologically compromised.

4. Laboratory diagnosis

a. Microscopic examination. A clinical diagnosis of malaria is best confirmed by demonstration of the parasites in a Giemsa-stained blood smear. Because each species has distinct morphologic characteristics during the erythrocytic cycle, microscopic examination of the smear allows determination of the causative organism.

(1) Banana-shaped intraerythrocytic gametocytes identify *P. falciparum* infection.
(2) Enlarged erythrocytes with intracellular, coarse, brick-red stippling (Schüffner's dots) are characteristic of *P. vivax* infection.
(3) Schüffner's dots in oval-shaped red blood cells are characteristic of *P. ovale* infection.

b. **Serology** may assist diagnosis of light infections.

5. **Treatment**

a. **Pharmacologic therapy.** The chemotherapy of malaria is complex and constantly changing. The CDC in Atlanta, Georgia, maintains a hotline [(404) 332-4555] with information about the latest recommended drugs and dosages for the treatment of malaria.
(1) **Chloroquine** is the drug of choice for uncomplicated malaria in areas without resistance. Chloroquine resistant malaria is found in most areas of falciparum malaria, and also in many areas of vivax malaria.
(2) **Quinine** is usually the preferred alternative when chloroquine therapy fails. It is also the drug of choice for complicated, severe malaria and cerebral malaria.
(3) **Fansidar** is another commonly used alternative, although a significant number of patients experience Steven-Johnson type exfoliative dermatitis as a side effect.
(4) **Primaquine** is used for *P. vivax* and *P. ovale* infections to eradicate the hypnozoites, as well as for treating relapses of *P. vivax* and *P. ovale* malaria.
(5) **Clindamycin, trimethoprim-sulfamethoxazole, mefloquine, halofantrine,** and **qinghausu** are also used in various regimens. **Desferrioxamine,** an iron chelator, is being investigated clinically.

b. **Supportive measures** include administration of antipyretics during febrile crises, transfusion for severe hemolytic anemia, and dialysis for acute renal failure.

6. **Host factors that influence susceptibility to malaria**

a. **Duffy-negative individuals are naturally resistant to infection with** *P. vivax. P. vivax* invasion of erythrocytes is mediated through interaction with Duffy Fy group antigens, which are absent from the red blood cells of many Africans and most African-Americans.

b. **Glucose-6-phosphate dehydrogenase (G6PD) deficiency.** Trophozoites do not develop effectively in red blood cells deficient in G6PD because the parasite is unable to use the hexose monophosphate shunt as an energy source.

c. **Hemoglobinopathies.** Abnormal hemoglobins do not support parasite growth. This increased resistance to malaria appears to account for the high incidence of individuals with sickle cell trait in Africa.

7. **Control and prevention**

a. **Control** entails **elimination of mosquito breeding sites** through residual insecticide spraying, improvements in land drainage, and removal of standing water, particularly in inhabited areas. **Insecticide-impregnated bed nets** are now being used increasingly in control campaigns.

b. **Prevention**
(1) **Prophylactic chemotherapy.** The prophylactic of choice is **proguanil,** occasionally with chloroquine. Long-term use of antimalarials as prophylactics can produce serious side effects.
(2) **Vaccination.** Several vaccines are under development.
(a) The first widely tested vaccine (Spf66) is a synthetic polypeptide construct that contains epitopes of antigens present on sporozoite- and erythrocytic-stage parasites. This vaccine has achieved a moderate reduction in new infections during field trials in Colombia, Tanzania, and Gambia.
(b) Vaccines using other candidate molecules, including an antigametocyte vaccine aimed at breaking transmission to the mosquito, are also being developed.

B. *Babesia* species

1. Epidemiology

a. **Transmission.** *Babesia* species are normally parasitic in wild and domestic animals. *Babesia divergens* infects ungulates and *Babesia microti* infects rodents. Both parasites are transmitted by **ticks** and both produce disease in humans.
   (1) Ticks become infected when taking a blood meal containing infected erythrocytes.
   (2) The parasite is transmitted transovarially to the tick's offspring, enabling the next generation of ticks to infect mammalian hosts.

b. **Incidence and distribution.** Human infection with *Babesia* is rare, but cases have been reported in Africa, southern Europe, and parts of New England, particularly Nantucket Island, Massachusetts, and Shelter Island, New York.

2. Pathogenesis and clinical disease

a. **Pathogenesis.** Vermicles (similar to the sporozoites of *Plasmodium*) are inoculated into the host via the tick's saliva during feeding. The vermicles penetrate host erythrocytes, where they develop into trophozoites, then into schizonts. Eventually, the infected erythrocytes rupture, releasing merozoites into the blood stream.

b. **Clinical disease. Babesiosis (piroplasmosis)** is a **hemolytic disease** similar to malaria but without an exoerythrocytic cycle.
   (1) Disease caused by *B. divergens* can be severe, even fatal, in splenectomized and debilitated patients. (Most patients are older than 50 years of age.)
   (2) *B. microti* causes a self-limiting febrile disease characterized by fatigue and anorexia.

3. Laboratory diagnosis.
Detection of intraerythrocytic forms in stained thin blood smears confirms the clinical diagnosis.

4. Treatment

a. ***B. microti* infections. Clindamycin,** in association with **quinine,** is the treatment of choice.

b. ***B. divergens* infections.** Experience in treating *B. divergens* infections is limited. Chloroquine and other antimalarials are ineffective.

5. Prevention.
To prevent infection, tick-infested areas should be avoided, and ticks should be removed from clothing and from pets.

C. *Toxoplasma gondii*

1. Epidemiology

a. **Distribution.** Exposure to *T. gondii* occurs in all regions of the world. More than 40% of the population of the United States is seropositive, and similar seropositivity levels have been found in other countries.

b. **Hosts.** *T. gondii* is an obligate intracellular parasite widespread among wild and domestic animals.
   (1) **Cats** are the **definitive hosts.**
   (2) Other commonly infected mammals (including humans) and birds serve as **paratenic hosts.** Only asexual reproduction occurs in paratenic hosts; however, both definitive and paratenic hosts can act as reservoirs for human infection.
   (3) Cockroaches, flies, and earthworms can serve as noninfected **transport hosts.**

c. **Transmission**
   (1) **Ingestion of contaminated food** is a common mode of transmission.
   (2) **Transplacental.** In humans, *T. gondii* can cross the placenta to infect the developing fetus. Transplacental transmission occurs at a rate of approximately 1 infection per 2700 live births and can result in stillbirth, microcephaly, hydrocephaly, chorioretinitis, or visceral disease. Manifestations are most severe when the infection occurs during the first trimester.

d. **Susceptibility.** Those most at risk of infection are **meat handlers, hunters, anyone who eats raw** or **undercooked meat** (including chicken), **pregnant women,** and **young children.**

2. **Life cycle. Infection in the cat** commences with ingestion of oocysts containing **sporozoites** or meat infected with muscle pseudocysts containing **bradyzoites.** Both sporozoites and bradyzoites are infective.
   a. They invade the epithelial cells of the cat's intestine, where they become **trophozoites.**
   b. The trophozoites multiply by schizogony into **merozoites.**
   c. Released merozoites may then penetrate other tissue cells and repeat the cycle, or they may develop through four defined stages in the gut epithelium into female or male **gametes.**
      (1) **Fertilization** of a macrogamete by a microgamete occurs within the host cell. Sporogonic replication leads to an oocyst that contains two sporocysts, each of which contains four sporozoites.
      (2) **Mature oocysts are passed in the cat's feces** and can remain infective in the environment for many months.
3. **Pathogenesis and clinical disease**
   a. **Pathogenesis.** Paratenic hosts, including humans, become infected by ingesting oocysts in contaminated food or bradyzoites or tachyzoites in meat products of other infected animals.
      (1) The infective forms emerge in the small intestine, penetrate the mucosa, and enter a range of host cell types. In macrophages, the replicating intracellular forms are known as **tachyzoites.**
      (2) As immunity to the infection develops, asexual replication and invasion of host cells slows. Infected cells form **pseudocysts** that contain numerous bradyzoites surrounded by a thick wall. These pseudocysts persist for years, particularly in immunologically privileged sites (e.g., the CNS and retina). Immunosuppressive therapy, stress, and immunocompromising infections (e.g., HIV) can cause reactivation of the tissue cysts or render the individual particularly susceptible to primary infection.
   b. **Clinical disease** is termed **toxoplasmosis.**
      (1) Most infections are asymptomatic or produce a mild, nonspecific illness. Occasionally, more acute symptoms resembling those of mononucleosis, aseptic meningitis, hepatitis, myocarditis, or pneumonia occur. Febrile illness may be prolonged but recovery is usually spontaneous.
      (2) In HIV-positive patients, spastic paralysis, blindness, myocarditis, and death may follow reactivation of *T. gondii* when the patient develops clinical AIDS.
4. **Laboratory diagnosis**
   a. **Serology.** Serologic assays for toxoplasmosis are the most common parasitic serology tests and are the method of choice for diagnosing the infection. Both **indirect fluorescent antibody** and **EIA for IgM and IgG antibodies** are offered in many hospital and state health department laboratories.
      (1) A positive IgM antibody titer indicates early primary infection and a rising IgG antibody titer indicates an active infection.
      (2) The antibody response usually peaks 4–8 weeks postinfection.
   b. **Microscopic examination.** Confirmatory diagnosis may be made by identifying *Toxoplasma* in stained sections of biopsy material. Giemsa-stained smears prepared from the buffy coat will also demonstrate *T. gondii* trophozoites.
5. **Treatment**
   a. **Pyrimethamine, sulfadiazine,** and **spiramycin** administered together for 3–4 weeks is the recommended treatment. Administration of **folinic acid** intramuscularly to prevent hematologic toxicity from pyrimethamine is also recommended.
   b. **Trimethoprim-sulfamethoxazole** and **clindamycin** may also be effective, although none of the recommended drugs is effective against tissue cysts.
   c. Toxoplasmic encephalitis in patients with AIDS requires more aggressive therapy. Corticosteroids may be given concomitantly to reduce ocular inflammation when present.
6. **Control and prevention**
   a. **Control** is difficult because of the diversity of animal reservoirs. A live vaccine that employs a genetically engineered strain of *T. gondii* that fails to produce

oocysts is being developed for use in cats and may help to reduce transmission, particularly to pregnant women and small children.

b. Prevention

(1) Pregnant women and small children should avoid close contact with cats and their litter boxes.

(2) Deep freezing of meat kills the parasite.

D. *Isospora* species

1. Epidemiology

a. *Isospora belli* is transmitted by the **fecal-oral route.**

b. *Isospora (Sarcocystis) hominis* infection is acquired by eating **raw** or **undercooked meat.**

2. Clinical disease

a. In healthy individuals, *I. belli* and *I. hominis* cause transient infections of the intestinal epithelium, with mild, self-limiting diarrhea. *I. hominis* can infect extraintestinal tissues, particularly muscle, causing minimal symptoms.

b. In patients with AIDS, *Isospora* infections may progress to a chronic severe disease.

3. Laboratory diagnosis. Diagnosis of *I. belli* relies on the demonstration of oocysts in feces. *I. belli* cysts are acid-fast. The oocysts are oval and contain two spherical sporoblasts. Extraintestinal *I. hominis* can be visualized in a muscle biopsy as a spindle-shaped or cylindrical-cyst up to 1 cm in diameter.

4. Treatment. Trimethoprim-sulfamethoxazole is the drug of choice.

E. *Cryptosporidium parvum*

1. Epidemiology. *C. parvum* is a cosmopolitan and common parasite of domestic livestock.

a. Transmission occurs via **ingestion of oocysts.** Human infections usually occur when drinking supplies become contaminated with farm runoff, as in the 1993 outbreak in Milwaukee that affected an estimated 400,000 people.

b. Life cycle. Trophozoites live in the epithelial cells of the crypts and the villi of the intestine and grow into schizonts. The schizonts rupture the host cell, releasing merozoites that penetrate epithelial cells. Following fertilization of a macrogamete by a microgamete, an oocyst is produced and passed via the feces.

2. Clinical disease. Cryptosporidiosis was recognized first as an infection of the immunocompromised, but in recent years it has also been detected in outbreaks affecting previously healthy individuals. In normal hosts, *C. parvum* causes watery, profuse **diarrhea** without blood that is usually self-limiting. In HIV-positive individuals, *C. parvum* is a major cause of chronic diarrhea.

3. Laboratory diagnosis

a. Stool samples. Smears of a fresh or formalin-fixed, concentrated stool are stained with a modified acid-fast (Kinyoun) stain or with a fluorescent monoclonal antibody.

b. Intestinal, gallbladder, or **biliary tree biopsies** may be submitted for detection of *Cryptosporidium* species. The techniques used for detection of this parasite in stool apply to biopsied material as well. Giemsa-stained biopsies will also demonstrate the parasite.

c. Sputum samples. Formalin-fixed sputum or other respiratory specimens may reveal oocysts.

4. Treatment. The drug of choice is **spiramycin. Clindamycin** has also been used effectively.

F. *Cyclospora cayetanensis*

1. Epidemiology

a. Incidence. *Cyclospora* appears to be distributed worldwide and is a common cause of "traveler's diarrhea," but its incidence and prevalence in the United States are unknown.

b. **Transmission.** Infection appears to be acquired by ingestion of oocysts in water or with contaminated fruits (e.g., strawberries) or vegetables.

2. **Clinical disease.** Pathogenesis is related to host immune status.
   a. **Immunocompetent individuals** develop a watery diarrhea with low-grade fever and abdominal cramps. Relapses are common.
   b. In **immunocompromised patients** the parasite produces a prolonged diarrhea.

3. **Laboratory diagnosis.** *Cyclospora* oocysts are detected in stool samples.
   a. Fresh or formalin-fixed stool smears are stained with the modified acid-fast (Kingoun) stain. Parasites stain similarly to *C. parvum* but are larger (8–10 μm).
   b. Parasites autofluoresce when viewed under ultraviolet illumination.

4. **Treatment.** Trimethoprim–sulfamethoxazole is curative after 1 week of treatment. Immunocompromised patients require a longer course of trimethoprim–sulfamethoxazole.

VI. *PNEUMOCYSTIS CARINII*

A. Epidemiology

1. **Incidence.** Knowledge of the epidemiology of this parasite is poor. *P. carinii* infection must be common, however, because neonates start to show seropositivity between the ages of 1 and 2 years, and by the age of 5 years, 75% of children have developed antibodies to *P. carinii.*

2. **Transmission.** The infection is acquired by the **respiratory route.** Immunocompetent individuals appear to control the infection quickly, but some remain subclinically infected and act as carriers. In such individuals, the parasites occur as a trophozoite (measuring 2–8 μm in length) in the alveoli. The trophozoites are located in an extracellular matrix attached to epithelial cells. After passing through a precystic stage, the trophozoites develop into cysts that are released in the sputum.

B. Clinical disease.

The pathogenicity of this organism is closely related to the functional state of the host immune system.

1. In **immunocompetent individuals,** the infection is **asymptomatic.**

2. In **immunocompromised patients** (particularly those with AIDS or other severe immune deficiency disorders), *P. carinii* causes an interstitial pneumonia. ***P. carinii* pneumonia (PCP)** is the **most common cause of death in patients with AIDS.** Dyspnea, fever, and a nonproductive cough are the usual symptoms; mild anemia and hypoxia may occur.

C. Laboratory diagnosis.

P. carinii cysts can be detected in a variety of specimens. Induced sputum specimens are acceptable, but bronchoalveolar lavage specimens or biopsied lung tissue are preferred.

1. Smears are stained with the Gomori methenamine silver stain, Giemsa stain, or with a fluorescent monoclonal antibody. Silver-stained *P. carinii* organisms appear as dark brown or black cysts containing two to eight sporozoites.

2. Multiple specimens may be required to confirm infection.

D. Treatment and prevention

1. **Trimethoprim-sulfamethoxazole** is the drug of choice both for treatment and long-term prophylaxis (in HIV-positive patients).

2. **Pentamidine** (administered intramuscularly or via an inhaler) is an alternative for patients who fail to respond to trimethoprim-sulfamethoxazole therapy or develop side effects from it.

Chapter 46

Medical Helminthology

Eric R. James

I. NEMATODES (ROUNDWORMS)

A. Introduction

1. **General properties**
   a. **Morphology and anatomy.** Nematodes have an anterior mouth and posterior anus and range from 90 μm to 1000 mm in length. They are cylindrical with a thick surface tegument; their shape is maintained by a positive hydrostatic pressure that limits movement to a sinusoidal snake-like motion.
   b. **Life cycle and reproduction**
      (1) All nematodes hatch from eggs as first-stage larvae (L1) and metamorphose by molting through second-, third-, and fourth-stage larvae (L2, L3, and L4) to become adult worms. Life cycles range from simple (e.g., ingestion of the egg is followed by development from egg to adult in the intestine) to complex (e.g., involving tissue migration or intermediate hosts or vectors).
      (2) All species are diecious but some can reproduce by parthenogenesis.

B. Intestinal nematodes

1. ***Enterobius vermicularis*** **(pinworm)**
   a. **General properties.** *E. vermicularis* is a small, white roundworm. Females average 10 mm in length, males, 3 mm. The worm has a direct life cycle with no tissue migration phase.
   b. **Epidemiology**
      (1) **Distribution.** *E. vermicularis* is cosmopolitan, though this helminth is most common in temperate areas.
      (2) **Incidence and prevalence.** More than 1 billion cases occur worldwide. Peak prevalence is in the 5- to 6-year-old age group; 30%–40% of affected children are white, and 10%–15% are black. Adults are more refractory, indicating that resistance may occur with age (possibly by acquired immunity).
      (3) **Transmission.** Eggs are deposited in a sticky secretion on the perianal skin by nocturnally wandering female worms. Eggs also contaminate bed clothes and can be aerosolized during bed making. Infection occurs via **ingestion** or **inhalation of eggs.**
   c. **Pathogenesis and clinical disease.** The eggs hatch in the large intestine. Worms mature in 2–4 weeks and live for 2 months. Continuous reinfection is common.
      (1) Approximately one-third of infections are **asymptomatic.**
      (2) The most common presentation is irritation and **pruritus ani.** Sometimes itching is severe, and secondary bacterial infection occurs. Occasionally, necrosis of the mucosal surface produces pain when nerve endings are exposed.
      (3) Worms often occur in the appendix and may be associated with appendicitis, but causation has not been proved. Rarely, worms **may migrate to ectopic sites,** mostly within the female genitourinary tract.
   d. **Laboratory diagnosis**
      (1) **Cellophane tape test.** *E. vermicularis* females lay their eggs on the perineum during the night. Touching the perianal skin with the sticky side of the tape will pick up the eggs; the tape is affixed to a microscope slide and examined. Eggs are oval, approximately 55 × 25 μm in size, and flattened on one side, and they contain a larva.
         (a) Specimens should be collected prior to bathing or using the toilet.
         (b) Four to six consecutive negative pinworm tape preparations are required to rule out infection.

(2) **Stool samples.** Eggs are only rarely seen in the stool, but in patients with heavy worm burdens, adult female worms may be seen in stool samples.

e. **Treatment**

(1) Single doses of **mebendazole** and **pyrantel pamoate** are highly effective. Because ongoing reinfection routinely occurs, treatment should be repeated after 10–14 days to kill the newly acquired developing adult worms.

(2) **Prevention of reinfection.** Some physicians recommend treating the patient's entire family. The eggs are not resistant to desiccation and usually only survive 6–12 hours, but they may remain viable for a few weeks in colder, more humid environments. Bed linens and towels should be washed.

2. ***Trichuris trichiura*** **(whipworm)**

a. **General properties.** *T. trichiura* is a roundworm that lives in the colon—the thinner, anterior halves of their bodies are embedded in the mucosa and the thicker, posterior ends extend into the lumen. Adult females are approximately 50 mm long. Males are 35 mm long, with a coiled tail. The worm has a direct life cycle.

b. **Epidemiology**

(1) **Distribution and prevalence.** Trichuriasis is a cosmopolitan disease, but the prevalence and intensity of infection is higher in the tropics and subtropics. In the United States, infection is most common in the southeast. Approximately 800 to 1000 million cases occur worldwide.

(2) **Transmission** occurs through **ingestion of eggs,** usually on **contaminated vegetables** or in soil.

c. **Pathogenesis and clinical disease.** Eggs are not immediately infective and require at least 2 weeks' incubation.

(1) Most infections are asymptomatic or cause minor mucosal irritation.

(2) Heavier infections are characterized by diarrhea, anorexia, nausea, mucosal hemorrhage, anemia, and rectal prolapse. Extremely heavy infections may result in death, but this is rare.

d. **Laboratory diagnosis.** Diagnosis is made by identifying eggs in feces. Eggs are oval, barrel-shaped, and have distinctive protruding polar plugs. The eggs measure approximately $50 \times 20\ \mu m$.

e. **Treatment. Mebendazole** is the drug of choice in the United States, but it is only moderately effective.

3. ***Ascaris lumbricoides***

a. **General properties.** *A. lumbricoides* is a large roundworm that usually inhabits the ileum. Females are 300×5 mm in size; males, 200×4 mm. The life cycle is indirect: adult worms in the ileum release embryonated eggs, which are passed in the feces and mature in moist soil in 10–15 days.

b. **Epidemiology**

(1) **Distribution.** *Ascaris* has a cosmopolitan distribution and is endemic to the United States (particularly the southeastern states). *A. lumbricoides* causes approximately 1 billion infections per year worldwide.

(2) **Transmission.** Infective eggs may survive years in shaded, moist, warm soil. Eggs can be ingested with vegetables or in drinking water.

c. **Pathogenesis and clinical disease**

(1) **Pathogenesis.** Eggs hatch in the duodenum, releasing L2 that penetrate the mucosa, enter the circulatory or lymph system, and migrate via the liver and heart to the lungs. The larvae molt twice in the lungs and enter the alveoli after 10 days, where they migrate into the trachea and esophagus. From the esophagus, they pass to the stomach and ileum (ectopic sites include the bile or pancreatic ducts). Adult *Ascaris* resist digestion in the intestinal tract by secreting a trypsin inhibitor.

(2) **Clinical disease.** Most infections are light and symptomless.

(a) A **transient pneumonitis** occurs during the larval migration phase. This pulmonary infiltration with eosinophilia, also known as **Loeffler's syndrome,** is characterized by fever, a dry cough, and radiograph mottling. Hypersensitive patients may experience urticaria and asthma.

(b) Adult worms may cause **nausea** and **vomiting.** Intestinal obstruction occurs in 0.2% of patients (usually small children with very heavy worm burdens).

(c) **Complications**

(i) Heavy infections can exacerbate malnutrition and contribute to vitamin A and C deficiency.

(ii) Death occurs in 0.02% of cases and is usually associated with obstruction or with hypersensitivity reactions.

d. Laboratory diagnosis

(1) The pulmonary symptoms may be attributed to *Ascaris* following detection of larvae in sputum.

(2) Gastrointestinal infection in asymptomatic patients may only be recognized after adult worms are passed or vomited. Usually, gastrointestinal infection is diagnosed by finding eggs in the feces, though a radiopaque radiograph will reveal adult worms. The eggs (60 × 45 μm) are stained brown from bile and have a bumpy (mammillated) surface.

e. Treatment

(1) **Pharmacologic treatment. Pyrantel** and **mebendazole** are 90%–100% effective. (Ivermectin used experimentally has also been effective.) **Anaphylactic shock,** resulting from the death of a large number of worms, is a risk of therapy.

(2) **Surgery** may be required for intestinal obstruction.

(3) **Supportive therapy** (e.g., administration of glucocorticoids or bronchodilators) may be advisable during the pulmonary phase of infection.

f. Control and prevention. Ascariasis is associated with poor sanitation and hygiene. Proper treatment and disposal of sewage and filtering of drinking water reduces incidence. Vegetables and hands should be washed well before meals.

4. *Necator americanus* and *Ancylostoma duodenale* (hookworms)

a. General properties

(1) Adult worms are creamy white, approximately 10 mm long, and live mostly in the jejunum. In heavy infections, they are also found in the cecum.

(2) The two species of hookworms are differentiated by their dentition: *N. americanus* has two broad cutting plates in its buccal cavity, while *A. duodenale* has two pairs of sharp teeth. The mouth and teeth are used to attach to the mucosal surface, and for sucking blood: approximately 150 μl/day/worm in the case of *A. duodenale,* and 40 μl/day/worm in the case of *N. americanus.*

(3) Adult hookworms live in the intestine and lay eggs that are passed in the feces. The eggs hatch in soil, releasing larvae (L1) that feed on soil bacteria, and molt twice to become infective filariform larvae (L3). These larvae survive 2–5 weeks in warm, moist soil.

b. Epidemiology

(1) **Distribution and incidence.** Hookworms are distributed throughout the tropics and subtropics (*N. americanus* is endemic in the southeastern United States). These worms account for approximately 800 million infections worldwide.

(2) **Transmission** is by larval penetration of skin, usually through the feet.

c. Pathogenesis and clinical disease. The larvae migrate in a pattern similar to that of *Ascaris*—from the skin hematogenously to the lungs, up the trachea, and down the esophagus to the ileum. Worms frequently change their attachment sites. Considerable blood loss can lead to a chronic hypochromic and microcytic anemia secondary to iron deficiency. Severity of symptoms depends on worm burden; most hookworm infections are effectively asymptomatic because the worm burden is low.

(1) **"Ground itch."** Pruritic inflammation at the site of penetration is followed by intense itching and serpiginous papular eruptions. The reaction may persist for several weeks and may be more severe after a second exposure. Secondary bacterial infection may occur.

(2) **Loeffler's syndrome** may occur but is less severe than in *Ascaris* infection.

The syndrome begins 1 week after infection and lasts up to 3 weeks; signs include a cough, bronchitis, and fever.

(3) **Abdominal pain** and **anemia** are symptoms of moderate to heavy infections.

d. **Laboratory diagnosis.** Anemia accompanied by the finding of blood in the feces is suggestive, and definitive diagnosis is provided by finding embryonated, thin-shelled eggs in the feces. Eggs of both species of hookworm are identical.

e. **Treatment.** Most anthelmintics (except piperazine) are moderately effective. **Mebendazole** and **pyrantel pamoate** are frequently used. Cure rates are significantly lower when *N. americanus* is the cause of infection.

f. **Control and prevention.** Proper disposal and treatment of sewage is necessary to avoid contamination of soil. Patients should be advised to wear shoes. Reinfection is extremely common in endemic areas.

5. ***Strongyloides stercoralis***

a. **General properties.** The life cycle is similar to that of the hookworms; however, *S. stercoralis* has additional free-living generations. It is thought that reproduction, both of the free-living and the parasitic females, occurs mostly by parthenogenesis.

b. **Epidemiology**

a. **Distribution.** *S. stercoralis* is a cosmopolitan parasite found throughout the tropics and subtropics. It is endemic in the southeastern United States.

b. **Transmission.** Autoinfection takes place when the eggs hatch in the rectum or perineum and filariform larvae develop locally, eventually penetrating the gut mucosa or perineal skin. Autoinfection leads to a level of infection unrelated to the initial worm burden.

c. **Pathogenesis and clinical disease**

(1) **Pathogenesis.** Adult worms burrow deep into the crypts of the intestine, causing mucosal breakdown and an increase in the number of goblet cells and mucus.

(2) **Clinical disease**

(a) In **immunocompetent patients,** up to 50% of cases are asymptomatic.

(i) Skin penetration of larvae may cause a "ground itch" in presensitized individuals that is more severe than that associated with hookworm infection.

(ii) Larvae migrating through the lungs may cause pneumonitis.

(iii) Epigastric pain, watery diarrhea, and eosinophilia accompany moderate to heavy intestinal infection.

(b) In **immunocompromised patients,** autoinfection leads to a **disseminated form of strongyloidiasis** with larvae of all stages in all organs of the body, including the heart, lungs, liver and central nervous system (CNS). **Untreated disseminated disease is fatal.**

d. **Laboratory diagnosis.** A clinical diagnosis is supported by the finding of eggs passed in feces, similar to those of hookworms. The **Harada-Mori test,** which entails incubation of feces to allow the larvae to hatch and develop, allows differentiation of *Strongyloides* infection from hookworm infection based on identification of the tail of the filariform larvae. **Duodenal contents** may be examined for *S. stercoralis* larvae as well.

e. **Treatment. Thiabendazole** is the drug of choice in the United States. **Mebendazole** is moderately effective, but less so for disseminated disease. **Ivermectin** is also effective.

f. **Control and prevention.** Proper disposal and treatment of sewage and wearing of shoes helps to control the incidence of disease.

6. ***Trichinella* species**

a. **General properties**

(1) **Appearance.** *Trichinella* species are small, roundworms. Males and females are 1 mm and 2.5 mm long, respectively.

(2) **Life cycle**

(a) Newborn larvae are born live into the tissues of the intestinal villi.

(b) The larvae penetrate the lymph or circulatory system, are carried passively to all parts of the body, and invade striated muscle cells, to become intracellular parasites.

(c) After 17 days, larvae are full-grown and a capsule has formed over each parasitized myocyte (the "nurse cell"). Muscle larvae remain dormant for as long as 5–10 years, when they die and the capsules become calcified. When a new host ingests meat containing infective larvae, the larvae are released from their capsules by pepsin and hydrochloric acid in the stomach.

b. Epidemiology

(1) Distribution. The originally described species, *T. spiralis,* has been divided into five species according to the range of hosts infected and the geographic distribution.

(a) *T. spiralis* exists as a domestic zoonosis, predominantly cycling between pigs and rats, in all regions where humans rear pigs, from North America to the Far East. It also occurs as a feral zoonosis, cycling between the major wild carnivores of North America and Eurasia.

(b) *T. nativa* is notable for its resistance to freezing, and it cycles between Arctic carnivores (Eskimos have the highest levels of human *Trichinella* infection.)

(c) *T. nelsoni* is found in Africa, south of the Sahara. Major wild carnivores and omnivores are hosts.

(d) *T. britovi* occurs in Eastern Europe and Russia.

(e) *T. pseudospiralis* is distributed worldwide, including Australasia, in carnivorous and carrion-eating birds.

(2) Incidence. Autopsy studies suggest 150,000 to 300,000 new infections are acquired annually in the United States, yet only approximately 100 cases are reported.

(3) Transmission. Trichinellosis, primarily a zoonotic disease, is sporadically acquired by humans through **consumption of infected meat** (usually pork or bear meat). In France, in the 1980s, infected horse meat caused major outbreaks of human trichinellosis.

c. Pathogenesis and clinical disease. Many cases of trichinellosis are asymptomatic and many other symptomatic cases go unrecognized or are misdiagnosed. The pathology and disease depend on the number of worms present and the stage of infection.

(1) Intestinal stage. Worms are mature 5 days postinfection and live for 2–3 weeks in the intestine before being expelled by the host immune response.

(a) Intestinal pathology includes villous atrophy and inflammation.

(b) Symptoms include nausea, vomiting, diarrhea, and abdominal pains. Very heavy infections can be fatal.

(2) Migratory stage. The migratory stage involving newborn larvae lasts 1–4 weeks. The migrating larvae cause pneumonitis, neurologic symptoms, conjunctivitis, splinter hemorrhages under the nails, and muscle tenderness.

(3) Muscle stage. The muscle stage starts approximately 3 weeks after infection and lasts up to several months.

(a) Growth and encystment of the larvae causes inflammation around the infected muscle cells and produces symptoms of muscle tenderness, spasm, and edema. Hypersensitivity reactions may occur. Eosinophilia and increased levels of IgE are pronounced during the migratory and muscle stages.

(b) Larvae only encyst in striated muscle (not the heart) and locate in those muscles used most (e.g., the tongue, diaphragm, intercostals, orbitals). Death may occur in cases of heavy parasitization of the diaphragm and intercostal muscles from cardiac and respiratory failure.

d. Diagnosis

(1) Clinical diagnosis. Trichinellosis usually affects groups of people who have shared the same food source, so epidemiologic data are important for diagnosis and management. Patients usually present with splinter hemorrhages under nails, eosinophilia, extreme muscle tenderness, and periorbital edema.

(2) **Laboratory diagnosis**

(a) **Serologic tests,** such as enzyme immunoassay (EIA), are available and can help establish a probable diagnosis.

(b) **Routine histology** reveals *Trichinella* in **muscle biopsy samples** (gluteus or triceps muscle biopsies are usually preferred).

e. **Treatment. Mebendazole** reduces the number of migrating larvae and kills encysting larvae. **Corticosteroids** should be used to reduce the intense inflammatory response in the muscles.

7. ***Capillaria philippinensis*** and ***Capillaria hepatica***

a. **Epidemiology**

(1) **Distribution**

(a) *C. philippinensis* is found in the Philippines and Thailand.

(b) *C. hepatica* is found in Central and South America, Africa, and Asia. *C. hepatica* has also been reported from Hawaii and the southern states in the continental United States. However, in the United States, capillariasis occurs mostly in travelers to, or immigrants from, the main endemic areas.

(2) **Hosts**

(a) ***C. philippinensis.*** Marine mammals are the definitive hosts. The life cycle of *C. philippinensis* is completed when the eggs are ingested by fish, where they hatch and develop into infective larvae in the muscles in 3–4 weeks.

(b) ***C. hepatica.*** **Rodents** are the definitive hosts. With *C. hepatica,* the life cycle is only completed when the rodent dies and the eggs are released into the soil.

(3) **Transmission.** Capillariasis is a zoonosis; human *C. philippinensis* infection occurs by **ingestion of raw** or **undercooked fish.**

b. **Pathogenesis and clinical disease**

(1) ***C. philippinensis.*** The adult worms of *C. philippinensis* burrow into the wall of the jejunum. Symptoms include epigastric and abdominal pain, chronic diarrhea, and borborygmi. The intestinal epithelium becomes edematous with flattened and atrophic villi, and malabsorption occurs. In patients with heavy infections, the liver becomes congested and atrophic, and anorexia, nausea, vomiting, muscle wasting, cachexia, and death may follow.

(2) ***C. hepatica***. The adult worms of *C. hepatica* live in the liver parenchyma and lay eggs in the tissues. The liver becomes enlarged and painful; granulomas surround the dead worms and egg masses. Patients usually have eosinophilia and jaundice.

c. **Laboratory diagnosis**

(1) ***C. philippinensis*** infections are diagnosed by finding **eggs in the feces.**

(2) ***C. hepatica*** infections are diagnosed by **liver biopsy.**

d. **Treatment. Mebendazole** is the drug of choice for *C. philippinensis;* for *C. hepatica,* **thiabendazole** is the drug of choice.

8. ***Anisakis marina*** **and related organisms** (e.g., *Phocanema, Pseudoteranova, Contracaecum*)

a. **Epidemiology**

(1) **Distribution** is worldwide. Human infections are common in Japan, the Netherlands, and along the West coast of the United States.

(2) **Transmission.** These worms use numerous species of marine mammals as definitive hosts and numerous species of fish as intermediate hosts. Human infection occurs via **consumption of raw** or **undercooked fish,** including fish that has been lightly pickled, salted, or smoked.

b. **Pathogenesis and clinical disease.** When the L3 is ingested by humans, it attaches to the wall of the stomach or small intestine using a tooth. The resultant ulcer and surrounding granulomatous reaction is accompanied by extreme pain. Rarely, perforation occurs, leading to peritonitis.

c. **Laboratory diagnosis** can be made using gastroscopy; the lesion is tumor-like. Evidence of the mucosal granulomatous reaction and inflammation may be seen radiographically. Diagnosis is often not made until after surgery.

d. **Treatment** entails **surgery** to remove the larva and surrounding granulomatous tissue.

e. **Prevention.** To avoid infection, fish should be cooked well before being eaten. Control in the Netherlands has been effected by routinely storing fish at −17°C before distribution.

C. Filarial nematodes

1. ***Wuchereria bancrofti*** and ***Brugia malayi***
   a. **General properties.** Adult female worms measure 100 x 0.25 mm, while males measure 40 × 0.1 mm.
   b. **Epidemiology**
      (1) **Distribution**
         (a) *W. bancrofti* occurs in Africa, India, parts of Southeast Asia, Indonesia, the Pacific islands, South America, southeast China, northern South America, and the Caribbean islands. The organism was also found in the southeastern United States until the 1920s.
         (b) *B. malayi* occurs in southern India, Southeast Asia, Indonesia, and China.
      (2) **Incidence.** Together, these parasites account for over 90 million cases of lymphatic filariasis.
      (3) **Transmission and reservoirs.** *W. bancrofti* and *B. malayi* are transmitted by mosquitoes of several genera, particularly *Culex, Aedes,* and *Anopheles.* Dogs, cats, monkeys, wild carnivores, and rodents serve as reservoirs for *B. malayi.*
   c. **Life cycle**
      (1) Adult worms can live in the mammalian host lymphatic system for up to 17 years, where they viviparously produce blood-dwelling microfilariae (pre-L1). The microfilariae are ingested by mosquitoes, penetrate the stomach wall, grow, and metamorphose through stage L2 and L3 within the thoracic flight muscles.
      (2) After approximately 10 days, the L3s migrate to the mosquito's salivary glands, proboscis, and associated structures, from which they are injected into the next host.
      (3) In humans, the L3 migrates through the deep tissues, molting to an L4 and then an adult in approximately 10 days. The adult penetrates the lymphatics after 4–12 months.
   d. **Pathogenesis and clinical disease**
      (1) **Lymphatic filariasis.** Many cases remain clinically symptomless for years.
         (a) Patients experience lymphangitis, headache, nausea, and urticaria during the early, acute stages of the disease.
         (b) Lymphatic damage—lymphadenitis, lymphedema, chyluria, hydrocele—is progressive and linked to the host immune response.
            (i) The presence of masses of adult worms causes lymph node and duct dilation, leading to **lymph retention** in the areas drained by the affected nodes and vessels.
            (ii) The immune response is specifically down-regulated early in infection. The end of immunologic anergy coincides with the disappearance of microfilariae and a rapid increase in lymph duct hyperplasia, edema, and fibrosis. Secondary bacterial infections of the skin cause it to thicken and harden, culminating in **elephantiasis.**
      (2) **Tropical pulmonary eosinophilia** occurs in a subgroup of patients and is more common in visitors from nonendemic areas. These patients do not have circulating microfilariae and respond well to therapy.
   e. **Laboratory diagnosis**
      (1) **Microscopic examination**
         (a) Definitive diagnosis is made by demonstrating microfilariae in a **thick blood smear.** Physicians must take into account that microfilariae typi-

cally exhibit **nocturnal periodicity** (i.e., they remain sequestered in the capillary beds of the deep organs during the day and appear in the peripheral circulation at night, coinciding with the biting habits of the vector mosquitoes).

(b) A **Giemsa-stained thin blood smear** is used to differentiate *W. bancrofti* microfilariae, which have no nuclei in the tip of the tail, from those of *B. malayi,* which have two prominent nuclei at the tip of the tail.

(2) **Serologic tests** (EIA) support a clinical diagnosis.

f. **Treatment**

(1) **Diethylcarbamazine citrate (DEC)** is the drug of choice, because it kills microfilariae as well as adult worms (slowly). **Ivermectin** kills microfilariae, but not adults.

(2) **Antibiotic soaps** and **topical creams** can be used to reduce the elephantiasis.

2. ***Onchocerca volvulus***

a. **Epidemiology**

(1) **Distribution.** *O. volvulus* is distributed throughout large areas of tropical Africa, and is focal in Yemen and Central and South America.

(2) **Incidence.** Approximately 20 million people are infected by *O. volvulus.* Approximately 0.5 million patients are blind and many more have severe visual impairment.

(3) **Transmission.** Black flies of the genus *Simulium* are the insect vector of this disease.

b. **Life cycle**

(1) Female worms live up to 18 years, and each produces approximately 2000 microfilariae every day. The microfilariae become disseminated in the epidermis and dermis, where they are picked up by a biting black fly.

(2) The microfilariae complete their development in the fly, molting twice in the fly's thoracic muscles within approximately 10 days; they then migrate to the mouth parts and are deposited on the skin when the black fly next bites.

(3) The larvae penetrate the skin, migrate, and develop into adult worms over the next 18 months. Adult females (up to 500 × 0.4 mm) live in subcutaneous fibrous nodules and male worms (40 × 0.2 mm) migrate between nodules.

c. **Pathogenesis and clinical disease.** *O. volvulus* causes **onchocerciasis (river blindness).** The severity of disease depends on the parasite burden and the duration of infection. Adult worms provoke little reaction while alive; disease is caused entirely by microfilariae.

(1) In the skin, a papular rash, edema, depigmentation and hyperpigmentation (leopard skin), atrophy of the yellow elastic fibers, and degeneration occur. Inguinal lymph gland enlargement leads to hanging groin.

(2) The most severe aspect of the disease is blindness, caused by invasion of the eye by the wandering microfilariae. Punctate keratitis advances to sclerosing keratitis in the anterior segment, and iritis and synechiae with mottling of the retina advancing to chorioretinitis and optic nerve atrophy occur in the posterior segment.

d. **Diagnosis**

(1) **Clinical diagnosis.** The presence of palpable subcutaneous nodules, skin lesions, or ocular changes in an endemic area is characteristic. Slit lamp examination of the eye will reveal microfilariae in the aqueous humor.

(2) **Laboratory diagnosis.** Infection is confirmed by finding microfilariae (unsheathed, measuring 300 × 8 μm) moving out of **skin snips** taken from the iliac crest or outer canthus and incubated in saline.

e. **Treatment**

(1) **Nodulectomy** to remove adult worms is recommended for head nodules, but is largely cosmetic in other parts of the body because more than 50% of the nodules are found in the deep tissues and are not palpable.

(2) **Ivermectin** is the drug of choice. It is not curative, having little effect on adult worms, but will temporarily reduce the number of microfilariae. Some side effects occur in heavily infected patients.

f. **Control and prevention**

(1) **Insecticides.** The larvae and pupae of the black fly vectors live on rocks and vegetation in fast-flowing water. Insecticides have been successful in reducing fly populations and preventing disease as part of the onchocerciasis control program implemented in west Africa.

(2) **Ivermectin.** Because insecticide resistance is becoming significant, control is moving toward mass therapy with ivermectin.

3. ***Loa loa***

a. **Epidemiology**

(1) **Distribution.** *Loa loa* is found in two large areas of west and central Africa.

(2) **Transmission.** *Loa loa* is transmitted by large **tabanid flies** similar to horse or deer flies, which acquire the worm by sucking blood from infected individuals and later depositing larvae in the skin of uninfected subjects.

b. **Clinical disease.** In **loaiasis, calabar swelling,** a mild, transient, inflammatory swelling, is characteristic and is accompanied by **eosinophilia.** Patients may experience intense **itching** and **pruritus accompanied by fever.** In chronic infections, the worms may migrate into deeper tissues and may cause neurologic symptoms.

c. **Laboratory diagnosis.** The fugitive swellings with eosinophilia and patient history are suggestive. The diagnosis is usually confirmed by finding microfilariae in blood taken during the day.

d. **Treatment. DEC** is the drug of choice because it kills adult worms and microfilariae. If the worm is visible (e.g., in the conjunctiva) a local anesthetic can be used to immobilize the worm. The worm is then surgically removed so as to avoid fragmentation, which may lead to severe, immediate hypersensitivity reactions.

4. ***Dirofilaria* species**

a. **Epidemiology.** *D. immitis,* which commonly causes heartworm infection in dogs in the United States, *D. tenuis,* a raccoon parasite found in the United States, and *D. repens,* a dog parasite common in Europe, are being implicated in an increasing number of human infections. In the United States, *D. immitis* is the most common cause of human dirofilariasis.

(1) **Distribution.** *D. immitis* is now present throughout the continental United States and is highly endemic in the Mississippi Valley, and eastern and southeastern states.

(2) **Transmission.** The life cycle is typical of filarial parasites; however, the microfilariae develop to infective larvae in the malpighian tubules of **mosquitoes,** the insect vector of this disease.

b. **Pathogenesis and clinical disease**

(1) **Pathogenesis**

(a) In humans, the infective L3 may molt to an L4.

(b) The L4 then migrates, usually lodging in the lungs (in the case of *D. immitis*) or subcutaneous tissues (in the case of *D. tenuis*). In most cases, an arteriole in the right lung is occluded causing a thrombus. The lesion that develops is inflammatory with many eosinophils. All worms found have been dead. Subcutaneous nodules or swellings may form around parasites throughout the body.

(2) **Clinical disease.** Most pulmonary cases of **zoonotic filariasis** are asymptomatic. Coughing, thoracic pain, hemoptysis, fever, malaise, chills, and myalgia may occur, however.

c. **Laboratory diagnosis.** A coin-type lesion resembling a neoplasm is seen on routine radiographs. Definitive diagnosis is made via microscopic examination of biopsied material postoperatively.

d. **Treatment.** DEC and ivermectin are used prophylactically in dogs. For humans, **surgery** is required.

5. ***Toxocara canis.*** Maturation of some species of nematodes cannot occur in human tissue, but their **larvae can cause disease.**

a. **Epidemiology**

(1) **Incidence**

(a) **Canine.** All dogs become infected with *T. canis* at some time, usually as puppies. In one study in New York state, 78% of dogs were found to be infected with *T. canis.*

(b) **Human.** Infections are most frequently reported in young children, though seropositivity rates of up to 20% have been reported in the general United States population.

(2) **Transmission.** Human infections are usually acquired by close association with pet dogs and by frequenting areas where dogs defecate (e.g. parks).

b. **Pathogenesis and clinical disease**

(1) **Pathogenesis.** When ingested by humans, the eggs hatch and the L2 undergoes an abnormal migration throughout the body. The lungs, liver, muscles, heart, brain, and eyes are invaded most frequently, but any organ may be involved. The severity of disease and symptoms are determined by the number of invading larvae and their location in the body. Granulomas form in all locations where worms die.

(2) **Clinical disease.** *T. canis,* as well as other related ascarid species of domestic animals, causes **visceral larva migrans.**

(a) **Mild disease.** Patients present with fever, liver enlargement, and eosinophilia.

(b) **Severe disease.** Manifestations include pulmonary infiltration with eosinophilia (50% of patients), and, less commonly, permanent brain damage and cardiorespiratory failure. CNS or cardiac involvement may be fatal.

(i) Symptoms include gastrointestinal disturbances, splenomegaly, behavioral changes, and seizures.

(ii) Ocular lesions are fairly numerous. Endophthalmitis occurs in 60% of patients and retinitis occurs in 10%. The retinitis is often accompanied by retinal detachment, and sometimes a unilateral fibrotic lesion that resembles a retinoblastoma.

c. **Laboratory diagnosis.** The clinical presentation, eosinophilia, and elevated liver enzymes (e.g., transaminases) are suggestive; EIA for *T. canis* antigens is usually confirmatory.

d. **Treatment.** Toxocariasis is usually self limiting in immunocompetent adults and older children, but **corticosteroid** administration may help to reduce the inflammation. **Thiabendazole** (as well as the other benzamidazoles) and **DEC** have been used successfully.

6. ***Ancylostoma caninum*** and ***Ancylostoma braziliense.*** Like *T. canis,* it is the **larvae** of *A. caninum* and *A. braziliense* and other **animal hookworms** (e.g., *Uncinaria stenocephala, Bunostomum phlebotomum*) that **cause disease.**

a. **Epidemiology.** Beaches and soil (especially warm, moist, shaded, sandy soil) are ideal habitats for the animal hookworm larvae and infection can be an occupational disease of construction workers and plumbers.

b. **Pathogenesis and clinical disease**

(1) **Pathogenesis.** Unlike the human hookworms (*A. duodenale* and *N. americanus*), these parasites fail to exit the skin and instead continue to migrate. The larvae may advance 20–50 mm per day between the dermis and epidermis.

(2) **Clinical disease.** The animal hookworms cause **cutaneous larva migrans.**

(a) A **creeping, serpiginous, erythematous, inflammatory eruption with pruriginous papules** produced by the migration of larvae is characteristic. Occurring mostly on the feet, legs, and hands, the rash may last weeks or months and be accompanied by secondary bacterial infection.

(b) **Edema** and a cellular infiltrate consisting primarily of neutrophils and eosinophils is accompanied by intense **itching.**

c. **Diagnosis.** The nature of the tunnels and accompanying symptoms differentiates cutaneous larva migrans from scabies. A biopsy obtained from the head of the tunnel in advance of the inflammation may yield the larva.

d. **Treatment.** In the United States, **thiabendazole** is the drug of choice, with DEC as an alternate. Topical corticosteroids or antibiotics may be indicated.

II. CESTODES (TAPEWORMS)

A. Introduction

1. **General properties**
   a. **Anatomy.** Cestodes **lack a digestive tract.** Adult cestodes consist of **three regions:**
      (1) A **scolex** (with suckers and possibly hooks) for attachment
      (2) An **undifferentiated neck region,** from which proglottids develop
      (3) **Mature** or **gravid proglottids,** which contain the hermaphroditic reproductive system (male organs develop before female organs)
   b. **Morphology.** New proglottids bud off from the neck region behind the scolex and remain attached as a long ribbon.

2. **Hosts.** The life cycles of cestodes are usually complex and involve one or more intermediate hosts.
   a. Typically, the eggs are passed in the feces and infections are acquired by eating the intermediate host, which contains larvae at the infective stage. Infections in humans are generally well tolerated but should be treated.
   b. Sometimes humans serve as intermediate hosts for animal tapeworms—these infections are often potentially life threatening.

B. *Diphyllobothrium latum* is the "broad fish tapeworm."

1. **General properties.** *D. latum* has short, wide proglottids and may reach a total length of 3–10 m.

2. **Epidemiology and life cycle**
   a. **Distribution.** *D. latum* is distributed throughout Europe, particularly the northern, central, and eastern regions (including Russia), as well as Japan, Chile, Argentina, and the Great Lakes area (and other lakes areas) of the United States and Canada.
   b. **Life cycle.** Eggs are passed in feces and hatch in fresh water, releasing a larva that is ingested by the first intermediate host, a small copepod. When a fish ingests the infected copepod, the larva is released, which burrows into the fish muscle. In 4 weeks, the larva becomes infective. Large carnivorous fish, by eating infected small fish, concentrate infective larvae in their muscles.
   c. **Transmission** to humans occurs through **consumption of raw** or **undercooked fish** (including lightly pickled, salted, or smoked fish).

3. **Pathogenesis and clinical disease**
   a. **Pathogenesis.** Worms mature in 3–5 weeks and can live for as long as 25 years. The adult worm attaches to the mucosal lining of the ileum or jejunum using two sucking groves (bothria) on the scolex.
   b. **Clinical disease.** *D. latum* causes **diphyllobothriasis.**
      (1) Most infections are asymptomatic. Occasionally, mechanical obstruction can cause symptoms of discomfort, nausea, vomiting, diarrhea, and weight loss.
      (2) In 2% of patients (up to 20% in northern Europe), a megaloblastic anemia develops as a result of vitamin B_{12} absorption by the parasite.

4. **Diagnosis.** Gravid proglottids burst to release eggs, or drop off and burst later in the feces. Diagnosis is based on the identification of eggs, which are oval and operculated, or proglottids in the feces.

5. **Treatment. Praziquantel** is highly effective and **niclosamide** is moderately effective. Vitamin B_{12} supplements are required for patients with anemia.

C. *Hymenolepis diminuta* and *Hymenolepis nana*

1. **General properties.** Adult *H. diminuta* worms grow to 600 mm, and adult *H. nana* worms grow to 40 mm.

2. **Epidemiology**
   a. **Definitive hosts. Rodents** are the primary definitive hosts for *Hymenolepis* species; **humans** may serve as definitive hosts as well.

b. **Transmission**

(1) ***H. diminuta*** infection occurs by ingestion of small flour beetles, which are the intermediate hosts, in **contaminated grain products.**

(2) ***H. nana*** is the only tapeworm that does not require an intermediate host.

(a) **Fecal-oral route.** Eggs are passed in feces.

(b) **Autoinfection** with *H. nana* is also common—the egg hatches prematurely in the intestine, liberating a larval onchosphere that burrows into the villi, reemerging 4 days later to develop into an adult worm.

c. **Susceptibility.** In the United States, these tapeworms primarily infect institutionalized children.

3. **Pathogenesis and clinical disease**

a. **Pathogenesis.** The adult attaches to the gastrointestinal mucosa using four sucking disks and a hooked rostellum.

b. **Clinical disease.** Most cases of **hymenolepiasis** are asymptomatic.

(1) **Gastrointestinal symptoms** (e.g., nausea, vomiting, pain, and diarrhea) occur in patients with heavy worm burdens (i.e. more than 2000 worms).

(2) **Epileptiform fits** may be associated with allergic responses to the released antigens of the worms.

4. **Laboratory diagnosis** is based on the demonstration of eggs in fecal smears.

5. **Treatment. Praziquantel** is the drug of choice.

D. ***Taenia saginata*** and ***Taenia solium.*** *T. saginata* is called the beef tapeworm because cattle are the intermediate host; similarly, *T. solium* is known as the pork tapeworm.

1. **Epidemiology**

a. **Distribution.** Both *T. saginata* and *T. solium* are globally distributed in all regions where beef or pork are eaten. However, infection rates are low in the United States, and *T. solium* is usually only found in the Southwest.

c. **Life cycle.** Eggs are passed in feces and must be transported to pasture to reach the intermediate host. After the egg hatches in the host's intestine, the **onchosphere** (embryo) emerges from the egg and penetrates a blood vessel. The onchosphere migrates to, and penetrates, striated muscle, where it becomes a **cysticercus** surrounded by a fibrous capsule derived from the host. Cysticerci may lie dormant for many years.

d. **Transmission**

(1) Humans are the definitive host for both species; ingestion of cysts in raw or undercooked meat is the source of infection.

(2) Humans can also serve as an intermediate host for *T. solium.* The larval form of *T. solium* is acquired by ingesting *T. solium* eggs (fecal-oral transmission) or following the passage of proglottids from the intestine into the stomach during vomiting.

2. **Clinical disease**

(1) **Taeniasis**

(a) *T. saginata* preferentially attaches to the wall of the ileum and can grow to lengths of 5–20 m, while *T. solium* preferentially attaches to the wall of the jejunum and grows to lengths of 2–10 m.

(b) Infections are usually subclinical. Adult tapeworms may cause nausea, abdominal pains, weight loss and diarrhea.

(2) **Cysticercosis** is a more serious condition. It results from dissemination of *T. solium* larvae, which encyst in the muscles and other tissues (e.g., the CNS). **Neurocysticerosis** usually develops years after infection, when the brain cysts die and induce an intense inflammatory reaction. CNS symptoms resemble those caused by cerebral tumors, meningitis, and encephalitis, and include intracranial hypertension and behavioral changes.

3. **Laboratory diagnosis**

a. The clinical diagnosis is supported by the detection of gravid proglottids in the feces and is confirmed by finding eggs (round, approximately 40 μm diameter, and containing an onchosphere with hooks) in the feces.

b. Radiographs and serology (EIA), and sometimes a biopsy, are required to diagnose cysticercosis.

4. **Treatment**
   a. **Praziquantel** is the drug of choice for treating *Taenia* infections in adults; **niclosamide** is also highly effective.
   b. In patients with cysticercosis, higher doses of **praziquantel** are recommended with coadministration of **corticosteroids** to reduce the inflammation that results from death of the cysticerci. **Albendazole** is the recommended treatment for neurocysticercosis. **Surgery** may be necessary in some cases.

E. ***Dipylidium caninum*** is a common tapeworm of dogs that can infect humans.

1. **General properties.** Adult worms are small (approximately 400 mm long).
2. **Epidemiology**
   a. **Life cycle.** Adult worms release gravid proglottids, which are independently active when passed in feces or present on the perineum. The gravid proglottids eventually disintegrate to liberate clumped packets of eggs. The eggs are then eaten by the dog flea and develop into larvae and cysticerci within the flea.
   b. **Transmission and susceptibility.** Human infections occur by inadvertent ingestion of fleas. Children with pet dogs are most frequently infected.
3. **Clinical disease.** Most cases of dipylidiasis are asymptomatic; however, abdominal discomfort and diarrhea may occur.
4. **Diagnosis** is confirmed by identification of proglottids or clusters of eggs in the feces.
5. **Treatment. Praziquantel** and **niclosamide** are suggested for treatment.

F. ***Echinococcus granulosus*** and ***Echinococcus multilocularis***

1. **Epidemiology**
   a. **Hosts.** Dogs are definitive hosts for the adult worms of the *Echinococcus* species, and herbivores serve as intermediate hosts.
      (1) A domestic cycle of transmission of *E. granulosus* between cattle or sheep and domestic dogs occurs in most areas of the world where cattle and sheep are reared, including the western United States. Feral cycles of transmission involving wild canids and wild herbivores occur as well.
      (2) For *E. multilocularis,* the life cycle principally involves foxes and small rodents.
   b. **Transmission.** While dogs, the definitive host, are infected by eating contaminated meat, humans, like the usual intermediate hosts, become infected following ingestion of eggs passed in dog feces.
2. **Pathogenesis and clinical disease**
   a. **Pathogenesis.** The eggs hatch in the intestine and the larvae are distributed by the circulation into various tissues, where they develop into hydatid cysts.
      (1) *E. granulosus* cysts are spherical with an inner germinal layer, surrounded in turn by thick cuticular and fibrous layers. Numerous brood capsules and protoscoleces bud off internally from the germinal layer; sediment in the cyst fluid is known as **"hydatid sand."**
      (2) *E. multilocularis* cysts lack a thick cyst wall and external as well as internal budding occurs, producing a multilobed cyst. Portions of the cyst may form metastatic secondary cysts in other locations.
   b. **Clinical disease** is known as **echinococcosis (hydatid disease).**
      (1) In humans, *E. granulosus* hydatid cysts take several years to develop sufficiently to cause symptoms. Symptoms depend on the size of the cyst and on its location. Cysts induce inflammation (with eosinophilia in approximately 25% of cases), leading to fibrosis and pressure on the affected organ.
         (a) Most cysts occur in the **liver** or **lungs.**
         (b) Cysts in **bone,** the **CNS, heart,** and **kidney** carry a serious prognosis. Up to 10% of all diagnosed cases are fatal.
      (2) *E. multilocularis* hydatids are also predominantly located in the **liver,** where they form a mass of cyst vesicles in a dense fibrous stroma surrounded by tis-

sue necrosis. Multilocular hydatids do not grow well in humans, may not contain protoscolices, and may become calcified early. Because the cyst walls are thin, there is little pressure on the infected organ. However, secondary cysts may spread to the **lungs, brain,** and **lymph glands.**

3. **Diagnosis**
   a. **Radiographs, ultrasound,** and **computed tomography (CT) scans** are helpful for visualizing cysts.
   b. **Routine histology.** *Echinococcus* species can be detected in aspirates or biopsies of liver or lungs, sputum, or urine. Biopsies are dangerous because accidental rupture of the cyst may cause leaks of hydatid sand, leading to the generation of numerous new cysts, as well as anaphylactic reactions.
   c. **Serology.** EIA helps to establish the diagnosis.

4. **Treatment. Albendazole** is the drug of choice. **Surgical removal of cysts** may follow successful treatment.

III. TREMATODES (FLATWORMS, FLUKES)

A. Introduction

1. **General properties**
   a. **Morphology.** The trematodes are typically **leaf shaped.**
   b. **Anatomy**
      (1) Trematodes have an **oral** and a **ventral sucker** used for attachment and movement.
      (2) They have a **blind-ending gut** and a **flame cell excretory system** ending in a posterior excretory duct.
      (3) They are **hermaphroditic,** except for the **blood flukes,** which are **diecious.**

2. **Classification.** Four major groups of trematodes affect humans: **blood flukes, liver flukes, lung flukes,** and **intestinal flukes.**

3. **Life cycle.** The life cycles of all human flukes are similar.
   a. The eggs hatch after contacting fresh water to release a **ciliated miracidium larva,** which seeks out and burrows into a specific species of **snail.**
   b. Inside the snail, two or three cycles of asexual reproduction occur culminating, in 4–6 weeks, in the release of **cercariae** into the water. Schistosome cercariae are directly infective and penetrate the skin, while the cercariae of other flukes encyst as metacercariae on vegetation or in an intermediate host.

B. *Schistosoma* species (blood flukes).

There are three main species of schistosomes pathogenic to humans—***S. mansoni, S. haematobium,*** and ***S. japonicum.*** Other less common species reported to infect humans include *S. mekongi, S. vietnamiensis, S. intercalatum, S. curasoni* and, perhaps, *S. mattheei* (a sheep parasite).

1. **Epidemiology**
   a. **Incidence.** Schistosomes, as a group, infect 200–300 million people and cause 750,000 deaths per year.
   b. **Distribution**
      (1) *S. mansoni* is found focally around the Caribbean (including the Dominican Republic and Puerto Rico), in Venezuela and Brazil, and in large areas of Africa and in Arabia.
      (2) *S. haematobium* is limited to Africa and one small focus in India.
      (3) *S. japonicum* occurs in Japan (rarely), China, Taiwan, and the Philippines.
   c. **Hosts and reservoirs.** Each species of schistosome uses a different species of **aquatic snail** as an intermediate host. Humans are essentially the reservoirs of disease, except in the case of *S. japonicum,* where rodents, ungulates, and other wild mammals can maintain infection.

d. **Transmission** is via **penetration of the dermis.** Schistosomiasis is associated with activities that involve contact with **fresh water** (e.g., fishing, washing, irrigating, recreation). Unlike most parasitic diseases, this disease has become more widespread as a result of economic improvements (e.g., dams, irrigation schemes).

2. **Pathogenesis and clinical disease**

a. **Penetration.** Cercariae that escape from the snail host are free-swimming in water and viable for a maximum of 24 hours. If they contact human skin during this time, they attach using mucus secretions from their acetabular glands, shed their tails to become schistosomula, and enzymatically and mechanically burrow through the skin and into a capillary.

(1) In previously exposed individuals, initial symptoms of infection include a **transient dermatitis** caused by cercariae penetrating through the skin.

(2) **Katayama syndrome,** an allergic reaction that occurs during migration of the schistosomula through the liver, may occur in some patients.

b. **Migration.** Schistosomula are carried via the cardiopulmonary circulation to the hepatic artery and liver. Here, they cross from the hepatic arterial system to the portal venous system and back-migrate into the mesenteric blood vessels. During this last stage of migration, considerable growth takes place, resulting in adult worms 10–20 mm in length.

c. **Reproduction.** Males and females pair up and eggs are laid in the blood vessel walls. To complete the cycle, eggs must pass through the blood vessel wall, intestinal musculature, and mucosa to reach the lumen (in the case of *S. mansoni* and *S. japonicum*) or from the vessels of the bladder and vesicle plexus into the genitourinary tract (in the case of *S. haematobium*). Symptoms begin 4–6 weeks after infection and vary according to the number of worms present. In heavy infections, the patient experiences an acute phase marked by **fever, bloody diarrhea** or **bloody urine,** and **weight loss.**

(1) ***S. mansoni*** and ***S. japonicum*** infection. If the patient survives the acute phase of infection, the disease becomes chronic and debilitating. Eggs lodge in the liver and later, in the lungs, brain, and other organs.

(a) The eggs, which contain miracidia, are encapsulated in granulomata.

(i) Periintestinal granulomata are "ejected" through the gut wall into the lumen.

(ii) Hepatic granulomata cannot be expelled from the liver. The eggs die and become fibrosed and calcified. Hepatomegaly is characteristic; as the liver tries to regenerate, it enlarges considerably. The portal pressure increases, and anastomoses and esophageal varices develop. This chronic disease is largely untreatable and patients die from **liver failure, spontaneous rupture of esophageal varices,** or **secondary complications.**

(2) ***S. haematobium*** infection. The passage of eggs across the ureter and bladder walls causes injury and hematuria. Long-term complications include:

(a) **Hydronephrosis.** With time, fibrosis and calcification of the walls of the bladder and ureters develops, blocking urine flow and leading to enlargement of the ureters and kidneys.

(b) **Bladder cancer.** In Egypt, bladder cancer is the most common cancer and is directly linked to *S. haematobium* infection.

3. **Laboratory diagnosis**

a. **Microscopic examination.** Definitive diagnosis is made by identifying the eggs in the stool or urine.

(1) ***S. mansoni*** and ***S. japonicum.*** Eggs of *S. mansoni* are oval with a large lateral spine and those of *S. japonicum* are almost round with a short lateral spine.

(2) ***S. haematobium*** is usually detected in the **urine.** A first-voided urine is concentrated and examined via a direct wet mount for eggs, which are oval with a prominent terminal spine. A 24-hour urine collection may be used if low levels of infection are suspected. A **bladder** or **rectal biopsy** may be submitted for routine histology.

b. **Serologic tests (EIA)** may be helpful when no eggs are found (e.g., in cases where the adult worms locate in ectopic sites such as the CNS, spinal vessels, or orbital vessels).

4. **Treatment.** There are at least four drugs available that will treat all forms of schistosomiasis in a single dose without serious side effects. The drug of choice is **praziquantel.** Other drugs include **metrifonate** and **niridazole** for *S. haematobium,* **oxamniquine** and **niridazole** for *S. mansoni,*and **oltipraz** for *S. japonicum.*

5. **Control and prevention**
   a. **Long-term control** is based on improvement of sanitation and patient education.
   b. **Prevention.** A recombinant vaccine for *S. mansoni* based on the parasite's glutathione-S-transferase (GST) is currently entering limited clinical trials.

C. ***Trichobilharzia, Gigantobilharzia, Heterobilharzia***, and ***Schistosomatium*** are schistosome species of birds (particularly ducks and other waterfowl) and mammals that cause transient human infections.

1. **Epidemiology.** Transmission occurs through water activities. The banks and shallow areas of any body of fresh water in the United States may be home to the snail intermediate hosts of these schistosomes.

2. **Pathogenesis and clinical disease.** Infection causes an **allergic dermatitis.**
   a. The first exposure may be asymptomatic.
   b. A second exposure results in itching, 10–30 minutes after exposure. Macules appear and vanish in 10–24 hours. After 5–14 days, papules appear and the itching returns. This reaction is associated with the death and destruction of larvae in the skin. The papules heal within 1 week, but secondary bacterial infection from scratching can occur.
   c. Following a third exposure, the response is accelerated and more intense. Papules occur within 3 days, and there may be marked urticaria.

3. **Diagnosis.** Concurrent infection of a group of patients with a common history of recent close association with fresh water is suggestive.

4. **Treatment. Topical antiinflammatory agents** and **antibiotics** may be required for cases with intense inflammation or secondary bacterial infection.

D. ***Clonorchis* species.** Human **liver fluke** infection is caused primarily by ***Clonorchis* (*Opisthorchis*) *sinensis,*** and other related species (*Opisthorchis felineus* and *Opisthorchis viverrini*), all with similar morphology and life cycles.

1. **Epidemiology**
   a. **Distribution**
      (1) *C. sinensis* occurs in Japan, Korea, China, and Vietnam.
      (2) *O. viverrini* is found predominantly in Thailand and Laos.
      (3) *O. felineus* is found in Kazakhstan, Russia, Turkey, Latvia, Lithuania, and Poland.
   b. **Hosts**
      (1) Eggs are passed in the feces and are eaten by **fresh-water snails** of specific species. The eggs hatch within the snail's gut, where the first asexual reproductive phase takes place to produce redia, which migrate into the snail's digestive gland.
      (2) Cercariae shed from infected snails penetrate the skin of **fresh-water fish,** where they encyst as metacercariae in the subcutaneous tissues and muscles.
      (3) Ingestion of metacercariae in raw or undercooked infected fish transmits the disease to its definitive hosts, which include **humans** and **fish-eating mammals** (particularly cats and dogs).

2. **Pathogenesis and clinical disease**
   a. **Pathogenesis.** The adult flukes measure 20 × 4 mm and may live as long as 20–30 years in the bile duct, gallbladder, and pancreatic duct. The worms feed on the duct epithelium and cause biliary hyperplasia, fibrosis, cirrhosis, and cholangitis. Intercurrent bacterial infection via the damaged bile duct epithelium may be fatal.

b. **Clinical disease.** More than 70% of infections are asymptomatic. Heavier worm burdens (100–1000) lead to symptoms of hepatomegaly, diarrhea, anorexia, and epigastric pain. *Clonorchis* infection is also associated with the development of cholangiocarcinoma of the bile ducts.

3. **Diagnosis** is based on the detection of small (30 μm × 15 μm), oval, operculated eggs in the feces.

4. **Treatment. Praziquantel** is the drug of choice.

E. *Fasciola hepatica* and *Fasciola gigantica*

1. **Epidemiology**
   a. **Distribution.** *Fasciola* species are cosmopolitan, found in all sheep-rearing and many cattle-rearing areas. Cases of *Fasciola* infection occasionally are reported in the western United States.
   b. **Hosts.** The definitive hosts are sheep, cattle, and other domestic and wild herbivores.
   c. **Transmission** occurs by ingestion of metacercariae on grass or vegetables, principally **watercress** and **lettuce** for humans.

2. **Pathogenesis and clinical disease.** *Fasciola* species cause **fascioliasis (sheep liver fluke disease).** The metacercariae hatch and the larvae burrow through the gut wall, penetrate the liver, and eat their way through the parenchyma to the bile ducts. The severity of disease depends on the worm burden and the duration of infection.
   a. Migration of the larvae through the liver parenchyma causes necrotic lesions. Acute disease is characterized by nausea, vomiting, fever, pruritus, and occasionally, anemia.
   b. In chronic infection, the symptoms are related to biliary duct damage. The adult worms are covered with numerous spines that abrade the bile duct wall and lead to thickening and fibrosis, cholecystitis, and cholelithiasis. Later, inflammatory, adenomatous, and fibrotic changes of the bile ducts develop. Obstructive jaundice may result from cholelithiasis or from chronic fibrosis of the bile ducts. In serious cases, biliary stasis, liver atrophy, and periportal cirrhosis may ensue.

3. **Diagnosis**
   a. **Clinical diagnosis.** An association with sheep- or cattle-rearing and a history of consumption of homegrown raw watercress or vegetables, together with fever, eosinophilia, liver enlargement, and elevated serum transaminase levels is highly suggestive.
   b. **Laboratory diagnosis.** Definitive diagnosis is made by finding large (150 × 80 μm) operculated eggs in the feces.

4. **Treatment. Bithionol** is the drug of choice.

F. *Paragonimus westermani,* a lung fluke, is the most common of approximately 32 species of *Paragonimus* that infect a wide variety of wild mammals.

1. **General properties.** These flukes measure up to 16 mm x 8 mm and occur in pairs within pulmonary cysts.

2. **Epidemiology**
   a. **Distribution.** *P. westermani* is distributed worldwide in foci, but is particularly prevalent in the coastal regions of the Far East, Africa, and South America. An estimated 1.6 million cases are reported in South Korea alone. Many wild carnivores, including, mink, bobcats, foxes, cats, tigers, badgers, weasels, dogs, wolves, monkeys, and muskrats, have been reported to be infected and could act as reservoirs of infection.
   b. **Hosts.** Several species of **aquatic snails** are potential first intermediate hosts, followed by **freshwater crustaceans** (crayfish, shrimp, crabs) as second intermediate hosts.
   c. **Transmission.** Human infections occur from ingestion of **raw** or **undercooked infected freshwater crayfish, shrimp,** and **crabs.**

3. **Pathogenesis and clinical disease.** *P. westermani* causes **paragonimiasis (lung fluke disease).** The metacercariae hatch in the intestine, burrow through the intestinal wall, and migrate through the diaphragm, reaching the lungs in 15–20 days.
   a. The disease is usually asymptomatic during the migratory phase.
   b. A fibrous capsule develops around the paired flukes, inducing chronic coughing, thoracic pain, copious brown or blood-stained viscous sputum, and hemoptysis accompanied by fever. Often tuberculosis is suspected.
   c. Ectopic brain cysts are particularly serious, causing cephalgia, convulsions, hemiplegia, paresis, and symptoms similar to those of meningitis.

4. **Diagnosis** is suspected on the basis of imaging techniques and supported by positive serology results. Without confirmatory serologies, differentiating paragonimiasis from other infections (e.g., tuberculosis) or neoplasia is difficult. Definitive diagnosis is made by finding the very large operculated eggs (100 μm × 60 μm) in the sputum or the feces.

5. **Treatment. Praziquantel** is the drug of choice. **Bithionol** is also effective.

G. ***Fasciolopsis buski*** is an **intestinal fluke.**

1. **General properties.** *F. buski* may grow as large as 80 mm × 20 mm.

2. **Epidemiology**
   a. **Distribution.** *F. buski* is found in the Far East, from India to Korea.
   b. **Transmission.** The eggs hatch in fresh water after an embryonation period of several weeks. Two stages of asexual reproduction occur in the snail intermediate host before cercariae emerge to encyst on water vegetation, particularly **red caltrop** and **water chestnut.** Human infection occurs from eating these vegetables raw.

3. **Pathogenesis and clinical disease.** *F. buski,* as well as several other species (e.g., *Metagonimus yokogawai, Heterophyes heterophyes*), cause intestinal fluke disease. Ingested metacercariae excyst in the duodenum and mature in 3–4 months in the ileum.
   a. Few symptoms occur in light infections.
   b. Heavier infections produce diarrhea, pain, anemia, edema, and even death. Ulceration and hemorrhage occur at the site of attachment of the fluke and large amounts of mucus are produced. Marked eosinophilia (more than 30% eosinophils in the white blood cell differential) is present in over one third of patients.

4. **Diagnosis.** Clinical symptoms in a patient from an endemic area with eosinophilia are suggestive. The diagnosis is confirmed by identification of eggs in the feces.

5. **Treatment. Praziquantel** is the drug of choice.

PART VIII
MAJOR INFECTIOUS DISEASES

Chapter 47

Bacteremia and Sepsis

Gerald E. Wagner
Gabriel Virella
Victor Del Bene

Case 1

An 80-year-old man is brought to the emergency room by his son, who noted that his father had become lethargic and had decreased urination over the past 4 days. The patient was homebound and over the past week had remained in bed. His medical history included several bouts of acute urinary tract obstruction and an enlarged prostate gland.

On physical examination, the patient is febrile (temperature, 103.5°F), hypotensive (95/55 mm Hg) and difficult to arouse. His mucous membranes are dry and skin turgor is poor. The urinary bladder is percussable to the level of the umbilicus. Rectal examination shows an enlarged prostate. The white blood count is 15,000/mm^3 with 20% bands and 60% polymorphonuclear (PMN) cells.

- *What is the most likely cause of this patient's problem?*
- *What diagnostic tests are indicated?*
- *Should the patient be hospitalized?*
- *Should antibiotic therapy be started, and if so, with what type of agent or agents?*
- *What is appropriate follow-up?*

Case 2

A 21-year-old male college student reports a 3-day history of fever and a 2-day history of dizziness on standing. Five days earlier, the patient had sustained a crushing injury to the lateral forefoot, resulting in an an abrasion and laceration. The area became swollen, hot, red, and tender over the next 4 days, with yellow drainage from the laceration.

Physical examination shows a temperature of 103.4°F, a blood pressure of 100/60 mm Hg lying down and 80/40 mm Hg sitting up, and a pulse rate of 100 beats/min lying down and 150 beats/min sitting up. The patient's face and trunk are flushed. Puffy edema of the face and extremities is noted. The right foot is swollen, red, and hot, and the lateral aspect of the forefoot is abraded and lacerated, with copious yellow pus exuding from the laceration. A Gram stain of the wound exudate shows Gram-positive cocci in clusters with numerous PMN cells. The white blood cell count is 15,800/mm^3 with 35% bands and 60% neutrophils.

- *What is the best diagnosis?*
- *What is the pathophysiology behind the patient's systemic signs and symptoms?*
- *What tests are necessary to confirm the diagnosis?*
- *What antibiotic treatment should the patient receive?*
- *What immediate complications are anticipated and how should they be treated?*

I. INTRODUCTION.

INTRODUCTION. The terms bacteremia, septicemia, and sepsis are often used interchangeably, but they refer to two distinct clinical conditions.

A. Bacteremia

A. Bacteremia is defined by the isolation of bacteria from the peripheral blood.

1. **Sources.** Bacteria may be introduced into the circulation by physical means (e.g., trauma), or they may be shed into the blood stream from a focus of infection.
2. **Implications**
   a. Bacteremia **may be transient and inconsequential.** Bacteria such as *Staphylococcus epidermidis, Bacteroides melaninogenicus,* and *Clostridium perfringens* frequently can be recovered from the blood of apparently healthy persons.
   b. Bacteremia **may lead to the establishment of distant foci of infection. Hematogenous dissemination** plays a major role in the pathogenesis of bacterial meningitis, bacterial pneumonia, septic arthritis, osteomyelitis, pulmonary and extrapulmonary tuberculosis, disseminated gonococcemia, enteric fever, typhoid fever, Rocky Mountain spotted fever, and syphilis.
   c. Bacteremia **may progress to septic shock** if untreated. (Septic shock may also develop without evident bacteremia). Bacteremia should be diagnosed as early as possible and immediately treated as vigorously as possible.

B. Sepsis (septicemia)

B. Sepsis (septicemia) is a systemic disease triggered by an infection and characterized by hemodynamic abnormalities and organ failure.

1. **Sources.** The severe changes in homeostasis follow the activation of the complement and coagulation systems and the release of mediators from activated host cells (particularly macrophages, PMN leukocytes, and endothelial cells). Prostration and hypotension are the early signs suggestive of sepsis.
2. **Implications.** If untreated, the condition progresses to **circulatory collapse (septic shock), disseminated intravascular coagulation (DIC), multiple organ failure,** and **death.**

II. DIAGNOSIS OF BACTEREMIA.

DIAGNOSIS OF BACTEREMIA. To confirm a diagnosis of bacteremia, bacteria must be isolated from the blood. The organisms most frequently isolated from blood cultures are listed in Table 47-1.

A. Various factors influence the successful recovery of bacteria from blood.

1. **Attention to proper technique for blood collection** is important to avoid misdiagnosis as a result of contamination by skin bacteria.
   a. The skin at the site of each venipuncture to obtain blood for culture should be thoroughly disinfected.
   b. Blood should be drawn from two different sites. (The probability of having identical contaminants in samples from different sites is very small.)
2. **Multiple samples should be taken.** The probability of obtaining a positive blood culture in a bacteremic patient increases if more than one set of samples is sent to the laboratory.
   a. Studies indicate that three blood samples taken over a 24-hour period allow for successful recovery of bacteria in 99% of patients with bacteremia, whereas the recovery rate is only 80% when only one blood culture is obtained.
   b. If the patient's status prevents blood collection over a 24-hour period, three samples should be taken over a period of several hours.
3. **Blood for culture should be drawn before initiating antimicrobial therapy.** If that is not possible, or if the patient is suspected of developing bacteremia while receiving antimicrobial therapy, cultures from blood sampled over a 24-hour period may not be positive, and additional samples must be obtained over a longer time period.

Table 47-1. Relative Frequency of Isolation of Organisms from Peripheral Blood

Organism	Frequency of Isolation
Gram-positive cocci	31%–41%
Staphylococcus aureus	7%–19%
Coagulase-negative staphylococci	6%–16%*
Enterococcal species	3%–9%*
Pneumococcus	14%–33%†
Gram-positive rods	1%
Gram-negative rods and coccobacilli	47%–61%
Escherichia coli	12%–35%
Klebsiella species	4%–17%*
Proteus species	2%–11%
Pseudomonas species	7%–13%*
Haemophilus influenzae	1%–18%†
Anaerobes	2%–17%*
Bacteroides species	3%–10%
Fungi	2%–12%*
Candida species	2%–7%*

Adapted from McGowan JE, Shulman JA: Blood stream invasion. In *Infectious Diseases.* Edited by Gorback SL, Bartlett JG, Blacklock NR. Philadelphia, WB Saunders, 1992.

* Indicated range corresponds to nosocomial infections. Much less frequently isolated from community-acquired infections.

† Indicated range corresponds to community-acquired infections. Much less frequently isolated from nosocomial infections.

B. Culture and isolation techniques

1. Ten milliliters of blood are collected from each venipuncture site in adults (less volume is collected from infants and young children).
2. One half of the blood is used to inoculate a bottle of medium in air (for aerobic bacteria), and the other is used to inoculate a bottle in an oxygen-depleted environment (for anaerobes).
3. The inoculated bottles are examined daily for 5–7 days using techniques that detect carbon dioxide released during carbohydrate metabolism.
   a. The contents of bottles found to be positive are examined by Gram staining, and, if positive, seeded in adequate media for growth and isolation.
   b. If no evidence of growth is seen at 5–7 days, the cultures are reported as negative. (If slow-growing bacterial species are suspected, the observation period may be lengthened.)

III. TREATMENT OF BACTEREMIA AND SEPSIS.

Immediate, aggressive therapy is mandatory when bacteria are isolated from the blood stream of a patient exhibiting symptoms of bacteremia or shock.

A. Bacteremia

1. **Antimicrobial therapy.** Ideally, the chemotherapeutic agent should be chosen based on the results of susceptibility tests of the bacteria isolated from the blood. Intravenous, bactericidal, **broad-spectrum antimicrobial agents** with relatively low toxicity are preferred.
   a. In most cases, therapy must be initiated before culture results are available. The **empirical choice** of an antimicrobial agent should be based on as many elements as possible, such as the results of a Gram stain of purulent material from any

focus of infection (e.g., an abscess), age and condition of the patient, and source of infection (hospital versus community).

b. Preliminary laboratory results (e.g., isolation of a Gram-positive coccus) can be used to revise the empirical choice of antimicrobial agents until the susceptibility tests are completed.

2. **Surgical excision, debridement, draining,** or other, similar, measures should be immediately employed to eliminate identifiable sites of focal infection.

B. **Septic shock.** All efforts should be made to avoid the development of septic shock, because significant morbidity and mortality rates are associated with sepsis, regardless of the therapeutic measures taken.

1. Vigorous **antimicrobial therapy** is essential.
2. **Supportive measures** (e.g., fluid replacement, administration of inotropic agents) should be instituted to counteract the profound homeostatic alterations that characterize septic shock.
3. Administration of **antagonists** to the most important mediators of septic shock or substances that block the cellular receptors for those mediators has met with limited success.
4. **Surgical excision of necrotic tissues** may be necessary.

IV. BACTEREMIC INFECTIONS AND SEPSIS

A. Gram-negative bacteremia

1. **Etiology.** Gram-negative bacteremia, with or without the classic symptoms of sepsis, is most frequently caused by members of the families Enterobacteriaceae and Pseudomonaceae.
   a. ***Escherichia coli*** is the most common etiologic agent of Gram-negative bacteremia, accounting for 35% of the cases.
   b. Other Enterobacteriaceae (***Klebsiella, Enterobacter, Proteus,*** and ***Serratia***) account for 38% of the cases.
   c. ***Pseudomonas aeruginosa*** is the etiologic agent in 12% of the cases.
2. **Origin and predisposing factors**
   a. **Origin.** The gastrointestinal tract, urinary tract, and skin are the most frequent sites of origin of the bacteria involved in Gram-negative bacteremia.
   b. **Predisposing factors** include:
      (1) Surgery (abdominal, genitourinary)
      (2) Urinary tract manipulations (e.g., catheterization)
      (3) Underlying diseases that may compromise the patient's defenses
      (4) Large blood loss as a consequence of trauma or surgery
      (5) Ischemia of the intestinal wall
3. **Incidence.** The incidence of Gram-negative bacteremia in the United States is estimated at 71,000 to 300,000 cases annually, representing approximately 1% of all patients admitted to hospitals.
4. **Pathogenesis.** The release of endotoxin (LPS) by Gram-negative bacteria as they are destroyed is the principal trigger of sepsis. Most systemic effects of endotoxin are indirect, mediated mainly through pro-inflammatory cytokines [interleukin-1 (IL-1), tumor necrosis factor-α (TNF-α), and interleukin-8 (IL-8)] released by macrophages activated by endotoxin, and through the activation of the complement and coagulation systems.
   a. **Fever, prostration,** and **negative metabolic balance** are caused mainly by IL-1 and TNF-α, acting at the hypothalamic level.
   b. Many factors may cause **hypotension.**

(1) LPS and other bacterial products can activate the coagulation and complement systems. Bradykinin and C5a are potent vasodilators.
(2) Interleukin-2 (IL-2) released by lymphocytes nonspecifically activated by IL-1 or TNF-α can greatly increase vascular permeability.
(3) Activated macrophages and PMN lymphocytes release a variety of vasodilatory compounds, including platelet-activating factor (PAF), histamine, and nitric oxide.

c. Development of **DIC** depends partly on the direct activation of the coagulation cascade by microbial factors, and partly on the activation of phagocytic cells, which promote clotting by a variety of mechanisms.
(1) IL-1 and TNF-α released by activated phagocytes increase the expression of cell-adhesion molecules (CAMs) in endothelial cells.
(2) Activated phagocytes adhere to endothelial cells and release cytokines, proteases, and superoxide, which synergistically lead to endothelial cell damage. As a result, the damaged endothelium acquires procoagulant properties.
(3) Activated phagocytes release PAF, the most potent platelet aggregator that has been characterized.

5. Clinical manifestations. The clinical manifestations of Gram-negative bacteremia are identical regardless of the species of Gram-negative bacteria causing the disease. The severity of the symptoms, however, may vary considerably among patients. In fully developed cases, the symptoms evolve over time.

a. During the bacteremic stage that precedes fully developed sepsis, typical symptoms include high fever, shaking, chills, prostration, and, occasionally, nausea and vomiting.
b. Within 3–8 hours of the onset of the initial symptoms, the patient may develop hypotension, which may evolve into shock.
c. Classic symptoms of sepsis occur only in 30%–40% of patients with Gram-negative bacteremia. In many other patients, the clinical manifestations are more subtle and may be limited to fever.

6. Special types of Gram-negative bacteremia

a. *Bacteroides* bacteremia is most frequently caused by *B. fragilis,* and rarely by *B. melaninogenicus.*

(1) Origin and predisposing factors

(a) Origin. Bacteremia caused by *Bacteroides* commonly results from an abscess or other focus of infection seeding the blood stream. Less frequently, *Bacteroides* is introduced to the blood stream through minor trauma to the oral cavity, genitourinary tract, gastrointestinal tract, or skin.

(b) Predisposing factors. Sepsis caused by *Bacteroides* occurs most frequently in debilitated patients or in people with underlying disease, particularly:
(i) Hospitalized patients recovering from abdominal or gynecologic surgery, especially if an abdominal abscess develops postsurgically
(ii) Nonhospitalized patients older than 40 years recovering from recent surgery or receiving prophylactic antibiotics in preparation for abdominal surgery
(iii) Women, following septic abortion
(iv) Chronically ill patients with infected decubitus ulcers

(2) Clinical manifestations. *Bacteroides* sepsis tends to be more protracted and less precipitous in onset than other types of Gram-negative sepsis.
(a) Sepsis usually appears as a prostrating febrile illness that develops over several days or a few weeks.
(b) Peripheral leukocytosis (sometimes exceeding 40,000/mm^3), chills, spiking fever, and the persistence of bacteria in the blood stream are characteristic.
(c) Jaundice, thrombophlebitis, and infective embolism in the lung, liver, or brain are seen in a significant percentage of septic patients.

(d) Septic shock occurs in 25%–35% of patients, usually late in the course of the disease.

b. **Clostridial bacteremia** can be caused by any of the more than 70 species of *Clostridium,* but *C. perfringens* causes more than 90% of the cases. Less virulent species, *C. septicum* and *C. ramosum*, can produce shock or fatal illness in newborns or debilitated or immunocompromised patients.

(1) **Origin.** Clostridial septicemia is assumed to originate from the colon, biliary tract, or uterus, although a site of origin is clinically apparent in only about 50% of patients.

(2) **Clinical manifestations**

(a) **Gastrointestinal source.** Clostridial sepsis developing from a gastrointestinal source is an acute, serious, febrile illness. Extensive intravascular hemolysis (caused by *C. perfringens* α-toxin), acute renal tubular necrosis (due to free hemoglobin toxicity), and hypotension are characteristic.

(b) **Septic abortion.** Sepsis developing as a consequence of infection associated with abortion usually develops within 24–72 hours. Patients may complain of severe myalgia, abdominal cramps, sharp gastrointestinal pain, nausea, vomiting, diarrhea, and foul bloody or brown vaginal discharge in addition to the usual symptoms of fever, chills, malaise, and headache.

(i) The sepsis syndrome may progress dramatically within a few hours, causing oliguria, hypotension, jaundice, intravascular hemolysis, and shock.

(ii) Septic abortion is often associated with pulmonary emboli originating from infected pelvic veins (septic phlebitis).

c. **Meningococcemia** is most often caused by *Neisseria meningitidis* serogroups A and B. *Neisseria* bacteremia usually leads to meningitis, which may develop without symptoms of sepsis, but it may also be associated with a severe form of sepsis, particularly in children and young adults.

(1) **Meningococcemia** is associated with fever, malaise, weakness, nausea, vomiting, chills, headache, myalgia, and arthralgia. Petechial hemorrhages are the most characteristic finding on physical examination.

(2) **Waterhouse-Friderichsen syndrome** is a particularly serious form of fulminating meningococcemia that carries a high mortality rate.

(a) The patient presents with a high fever (e.g., as high as 105.8°F) of sudden onset, chills, nausea, vomiting, myalgia, weakness, and headache.

(b) Widespread petechial hemorrhages appear suddenly and may coalesce into large purpuric areas. DIC is prominent and ischemic necrosis of the skin and internal organs (e.g., adrenals) develops rapidly.

(c) Hypotension and shock develop precipitously and the prognosis in these patients is poor; both mortality and morbidity rates are high.

B. Gram-positive bacteremia

1. **Etiology.** Various Gram-positive bacteria are associated with bacteremia, with or without sepsis. Sepsis is most likely to develop in patients infected with group A staphylococci, viridans streptococci, and *Streptococcus pneumoniae.*

2. **Pathogenesis.** Staphylococci and streptococci release exotoxins that can bind to major histocompatibility complex-II (MHC-II) molecules on macrophages. The bound exotoxins interact with T lymphocytes having the appropriate receptors. Because cross-linking of MHC-II molecules and T cell receptors stimulates large numbers of T lymphocytes and macrophages, the exotoxins are known as "superantigens."

a. The cytokines released by activated phagocytes and lymphocytes produce the same effects described for Gram-negative sepsis (see IV A 4). Thus, many clinical features of Gram-positive septic shock are indistinguishable from those of Gram-negative septic shock.

b. Some exotoxins, particularly toxic shock syndrome toxin-1 (TSST-1), can be directly toxic to endothelial cells, which can contribute to increased vascular permeability and shock.

c. *S. pneumoniae* does not secrete exotoxins, but cell wall peptidoglycan and capsular polysaccharide, which can activate macrophages and the coagulation and complement systems, may be the factors that induce sepsis.

3. **Special types of Gram-positive bacteremia**
   a. **Staphylococcal bacteremia** is most frequently caused by coagulase-positive *Staphylococcus aureus.* Coagulase-negative staphylococci (i.e., *S. epidermidis* and *S. saprophyticus*) occasionally cause bacteremia (0.1% of diagnosed cases, and probably many more undiagnosed cases).
      (1) **Origin**
         (a) ***S. aureus*** in the blood stream usually originates from an infectious focus, such as a **cutaneous abscess** or a **furuncule.** Minor trauma to the skin may also cause staphylococcal bacteremia.
         (b) ***S. epidermidis*** and ***S. saprophyticus.*** Virtually all cases of bacteremia caused by coagulase-negative staphylococci result from **contaminated intravenous catheters, cannulae, hydrocephalic shunts,** or the **paraphernalia used in intravenous drug abuse.**
      (2) **Clinical manifestations** of staphylococcal bacteremia correlate with the source of the bacteria, the primary foci of infection, and dissemination of the bacteria.
         (a) ***S. aureus.*** The disease usually progresses slowly, with no specific symptoms suggestive of sepsis.
            (i) The most common result is the establishment of **infection at a distant site.**
            (ii) Rarely, bacteremia caused by *S. aureus* follows a **fulminant** course, evolving rapidly into septic shock, which may be fatal in 24–48 hours. **Staphylococcal toxic shock syndrome** (**TSS**) results from the systemic effects of TSST-1 released from infectious foci. Staphylococcal TSS was originally reported in women who used high-absorbency tampons during the menstrual cycle, but the syndrome can also develop in men and nonmenstruating women (see Chapter 12 I E 3 c).
         (b) ***S. epidermidis.*** Bacteremia caused by *S. epidermidis* is more insidious and less dramatic than that caused by *S. aureus.* Transient, asymptomatic bacteremia caused by *S. epidermidis* is probably a daily occurrence. In individuals with artificial heart valves, however, *S. epidermidis* is the most common cause of early **prosthetic valve endocarditis.**
   b. **Streptococcal bacteremia**
      (1) **Origin.** The source of infection may be difficult to determine. Surgical procedures and nonpenetrating minimal trauma are often the only apparent possible sources of bacteria.
      (2) **Pathogenesis.** The strains responsible produce pyrogenic exotoxins A, B, or both, which are closely related to erythrogenic toxin and perhaps to TSST-1. These toxins induce the massive release of cytokines from activated macrophages and lymphocytes.
      (3) **Clinical manifestations. Streptococcal toxic shock syndrome** [see Chapter 12 II B 2 a (9)] may occur in association with group A β-hemolytic streptococcus bacteremia.
         (a) The onset may be unremarkable, such as a sore throat and low-grade fever, or an infection of the soft tissues that is not initially cause for alarm. In many cases, pain [localized to a limb or mimicking peritonitis, pelvic inflammatory disease (PID), pneumonia, acute myocardial infarction, or pericarditis] and fever are the initial symptoms.
         (b) Unique to streptococcal sepsis is the development of an **exanthem** that frequently evolves into hemorrhagic bullae as part of toxic epidermal necrolysis.
         (c) Symptoms of sepsis and shock, such as high fever and profound hypotension, develop rapidly and may progress to DIC, adult respiratory distress syndrome, acute renal failure, and myocardial depression (in part because of cardiomyopathy mediated by streptococcal exotoxins). In pa-

tients with initial soft-tissue infection, the development of septic shock is often associated with purulent, eventually necrotizing, fasciitis and myositis.

Case 1 Revisited

The elderly patient with urinary tract obstruction and obtundation most likely has Gram-negative bacteremia, probably caused by *E. coli* originating from the urinary tract.

Blood samples for culture should be drawn immediately. A urinary catheter should be inserted and an aliquot of urine sent for analysis, culture, and antibiotic susceptibility.

The patient should be hospitalized, because he is most likely bacteremic and shows signs of severe dehydration and shock, which strongly suggest sepsis.

The patient should be given antibiotics, in addition to fluids and, possibly, pressor agents. In an elderly man with a urinary tract infection, *E. coli* and enterococci are often isolated simultaneously from the peripheral blood, so the antibiotic regimen must cover both possibilities. A combination of a β-lactam and an aminoglycoside antibiotic should be used.

Within 1–2 days, when blood culture and urine culture results are available, the antibiotic regimen should be reassessed to be sure it is appropriate for treating the organism or organisms isolated and cost effective. Plans for long-term prevention of a recurrent obstruction and infection must be formulated.

Case 2 Revisited

In the case of the college student with the foot injury, the best diagnosis is sepsis and shock due to staphylococcal wound infection, specifically, TSS. The Gram stain is consistent with *S. aureus.*

The toxin produced in the wound by staphylococci (TSST-1) is liberated into the blood stream. TSST-1, a "superantigen," activates large numbers of macrophages and T lymphocytes. The cytokines released by these cells affect the temperature center of the hypothalamus, causing fever. Cytokines also cause dilation of the peripheral capillaries (which results in decreased total peripheral resistance and hypotension) and disrupt the capillary permeability barrier (which results in loss of intravascular fluid into the tissue space in all parts of the body). As a consequence of these changes, the patient develops hypotension, and, if not properly treated, may develop shock, which is characterized by poor organ perfusion. Poor organ perfusion can lead to multi-organ failure and, eventually, death.

Cultures of the wound pus and at least two sets of blood cultures are indicated. Antibiotic-susceptibility tests should be performed on the organisms obtained. If *S. aureus* is cultured, it can be tested for TSST-1 production.

Immediate treatment in a hospital should include a semisynthetic anti-staphylococcal penicillin administered intravenously. The wound in the right forefoot requires immediate treatment, including wound incision, drainage, and debridement.

Because of decreased peripheral resistance and increased capillary permeability, the need to administer a large amount of intravenous fluid should be anticipated. Vasopressor agents that increase the total peripheral resistance may be indicated if primary surgical, antibiotic, and intravenous fluid therapies are not immediately successful.

Chapter 48

Pneumonia

Gerald E. Wagner
Victor Del Bene

Case 1

A 20-year-old man presents with a 4-day history of sudden-onset fever, chills, rigors, and cough. He is producing large amounts of rust-colored sputum, which has been blood-tinged for 1 day. He has pain in the left knee. His medical history is unremarkable except for heavy alcohol intake. His health-insurance plan has a heavy deductible, so he did not seek treatment promptly.

Physical examination reveals an ill-appearing man with a temperature of 103°F. His skin is warm and dry. There is dullness to percussion, increased tactile and vocal fremitus, tubular breath sounds over the right posterior lower lung field and a loud, high-pitched, diastolic murmur over the sternum. The patient's left knee is swollen, tender, red, and hot.

- □ *What is the differential diagnosis?*
- □ *What is causing this disease?*
- □ *What is the pathophysiology of the heart murmur and left knee arthritis?*
- □ *What diagnostic tests should be performed?*
- □ *When should therapy be started and what drugs should be used?*

Case 2

An 80-year-old woman in a nursing home complains of a 3-day history of a "cold" characterized by rhinorrhea, mild sore throat, nasal congestion, and watery eyes. Her temperature has been as high as 104°F. She has a nonproductive, constant cough. Physical examination shows a moderately anxious elderly woman with a temperature of 102°F, warm and dry skin, and poor turgor. Chest examination reveals expiratory wheezes and rales in both posterior bases. Laboratory results reveal leukocytosis (10,000/mm^3) with 50% neutrophils and 5% bands.

- □ *What is the differential diagnosis?*
- □ *How should the diagnostic possibilities be tested?*
- □ *What therapy is available?*

I. INTRODUCTION

A. Nomenclature. Several terms are used to designate different clinical and radiologic appearances of lung infections.

1. **Pneumonia** (sometimes used as a broad term for infection of the lungs) specifically refers to infections involving the lung parenchyma and the air spaces, which often show consolidation due to inflammatory exudate.

2. **Bronchitis** designates infections of the bronchial mucosa, without involvement of the lung parenchyma; when the parenchyma is involved, the infection is called **bronchopneumonia.**

3. **Pneumonitis** refers to interstitial inflammation, which is often caused by viral infections or toxic compounds.

4. **Lobar pneumonia** is characterized by consolidation of lung parenchyma within the anatomic boundaries of a lobe.

B. Causes of lung infections. Bacteria, viruses, fungi, and parasites can infect the lungs. Some organisms (such as *Streptococcus pneumoniae* and *Mycoplasma pneumoniae*) may cause lung infections even in previously healthy individuals; some (such as *Pneumocystis carinii* and some viruses) may cause lung infections only in immunocompromised individuals; and others (such as respiratory syncytial virus) may infect the lungs of young children with incompletely developed immune systems.

II. BACTERIAL PNEUMONIA,

caused by a variety of bacteria, is acute and abrupt in onset. The inflammatory process results in consolidation of the lung, reflected by dullness on percussion, increased air sounds on auscultation, and opacity in the chest radiograph.

A. Pneumonia caused by *S. pneumoniae* (pneumococci). Pneumococcal pneumonia is the most common form of bacterial pneumonia, accounting for approximately 80% of cases.

1. **Etiology.** Any of the more than 80 serotypes of *S. pneumoniae,* commonly referred to as the pneumococci, can cause pneumonia, although 14 capsular types cause the vast majority of cases in the United States. The pneumococci are indigenous to the upper respiratory tract in 30%–40% of the population.

2. **Epidemiology.** The incidence of pneumococcal pneumonia is low in healthy people; at least 75% of patients have an underlying illness.
   a. **Predisposing factors**
      (1) Disease occurs most frequently in the very young, the elderly, and people with compromised immunologic defenses.
      (2) Patients who have difficulty clearing upper respiratory secretions because of increased volume of the secretions or poor laryngeal reflexes during sleep are more susceptible to infection.
   b. The **mortality rate** is approximately 10%, even among patients who receive adequate chemotherapy based on *in vitro* sensitivity testing; most deaths occur among patients with underlying disease.

3. **Pathogenesis.** The pathogenesis of pneumococcal pneumonia is not completely understood.
   a. **Infection**
      (1) Infection probably occurs by aspiration of upper respiratory tract secretions containing pneumococci rather than by inhalation of bacteria into the lungs.
      (2) It is not known whether virulent pneumococci are spread by aerosolization or by direct contact.
   b. **The pneumonic process**
      (1) The outpouring of fibrinous edema fluid, erythrocytes, and leukocytes into alveolar spaces is the initial response to pneumococcal multiplication.
      (2) Bacterial components and complement split products increase capillary permeability and stimulate chemotaxis of neutrophils into the alveolar spaces. The polysaccharide capsule of *S. pneumoniae* has antiphagocytic properties and prevents complement activation, so complement-mediated lysis and opsonization are not efficient mechanisms for bacterial disposal.
      (3) Pneumococci rapidly proliferate at the leading edge of infection. **Consolida-**

tion occurs at the center of the infectious focus because of leukocyte activity and coagulating exudates.

(4) Eventually, antibodies to the capsular pneumococcal polysaccharide are formed. These antibodies bind to the capsule and activate complement, overriding the anticomplement activity of the pneumococci. The bacteria become opsonized and are then engulfed by macrophages and neutrophils.

(5) Healing occurs as macrophages remove alveolar debris, dead pneumococci and neutrophils, erythrocytes, and fibrin fragments. Pulmonary function returns to normal within a few weeks despite the intense inflammatory response; necrosis of the lung is rare.

4. **Clinical manifestations.** A history of rhinorrhea, pharyngitis, and cough of several days' duration is common in patients with pneumococcal pneumonia.

 a. **Symptoms**

  (1) The onset of disease is sudden, with **fever** (temperature typically 103.5°F), **pleuritic chest pain,** and a **hard, shaking chill** accompanied by teeth chattering as the temperature rises. Repeated rigors are uncommon.

  (2) **Cough** and **sputum** production intensify with time, and the sputum is typically rust colored due to alveolar hemorrhage.

  (3) The symptoms are severe and are usually accompanied by **prostration** within 48 hours.

 b. **Physical findings**

  (1) The patient typically is perspiring and warm, with **tachycardia** and **tachypnea.** Cool, vasoconstricted skin is a sign of imminent cardiovascular collapse.

  (2) **Fine rales (crackles)** are present on auscultation before signs of consolidation become evident.

 c. **Chest radiograph**

  (1) In classic lobar pneumonia, the chest radiograph shows single lobar consolidation. In contrast, bronchopneumonia, *P. carinii* pneumonia, and viral pneumonias tend to be bilateral or form abscesses (which usually show air–fluid levels).

  (2) A variety of bacteria and noninfectious pulmonary conditions (e.g., pulmonary embolism, lung carcinoma) may cause radiologic images similar to those of lobar pneumococcal pneumonia, and infections caused by *S. pneumoniae* may not show typical images on the chest radiograph.

5. **Diagnosis.** The visualization of large numbers of lancet-shaped Gram-positive cocci arranged in pairs in conjunction with macrophages and neutrophils in sputum smears suggests pneumococcal pneumonia, but the diagnosis must be confirmed by isolation of *S. pneumoniae.*

 a. Positive cultures from **expectorated sputum** are difficult to interpret because of possible contamination with *S. pneumoniae* or other organisms from the normal oropharyngeal flora.

 b. Positive **blood** cultures are truly confirmatory, but only approximately 30% of patients with pneumococcal pneumonia are bacteremic.

 c. **Pleural fluid,** if present, should be obtained by thoracocentesis, examined by Gram stain, and cultured.

6. **Treatment**

 a. **Antimicrobial therapy.** Pneumonia has historically been treated with large doses of intravenous **penicillin G.** Resistance to penicillin is increasing, so empiric therapy is now started with a **third-generation cephalosporin.** If β-lactam antibiotics are not indicated, **vancomycin** is used.

 b. **Supportive therapy** is essential to sustain the vital functions of the patient while antimicrobial therapy is given time to act.

7. **Immunoprophylaxis.** Immunization with polyvalent vaccine containing capsular polysaccharides from the 14 most virulent strains of *S. pneumoniae* significantly reduces the incidence of disease in susceptible adult populations. Like other polysaccharide vaccines, the vaccine is less effective in children, generally ineffective in infants

younger than 2 years of age, and variably effective in other at-risk individuals, such as immunocompromised or asplenic patients.

B. Pneumonia caused by other pyogenic cocci

1. **Etiology.** *Staphylococcus aureus, Streptococcus pyogenes,* other *Streptococcus* species, and *Neisseria meningitidis* occasionally cause pneumonia. These pneumonias are usually secondary to:
   a. Other infections that may depress the immune system, such as viral influenza
   b. The introduction of infectious agents directly into the blood stream, such as occurs in intravenous drug abusers
   c. A variety of predisposing conditions, such as very young or old age
2. **Clinical manifestations** of pneumonia caused by these pyogenic cocci vary little from those of pneumococcal pneumonia (see II A 4), except for pneumonia caused by *S. aureus,* which is often characterized by considerable destruction of lung tissue.
3. **Diagnosis** is confirmed by culture and identification of the etiologic agent from sputum, blood, pleural fluid, or lung tissue obtained by transbronchial or open-lung biopsy.
4. **Treatment**
   a. **Antimicrobial therapy** is initially based on the probable cause of the pneumonia and later revised according to the results of susceptibility tests of the culture isolates.
   b. **Supportive treatment** should also be given.

C. Pneumonia caused by Gram-negative bacilli

1. **Etiology.** ***Klebsiella pneumoniae, Escherichia coli,*** and ***Pseudomonas aeruginosa*** are the principal causes of Gram-negative bacillary pneumonia, but other Gram-negative rods may cause pneumonia in some circumstances.
   a. ***Haemophilus influenzae*** is a common cause of pneumonia in children younger than 5 years and in adults older than 60 years.
   b. ***Legionella pneumophila*** infects individuals who are elderly, debilitated, immunocompromised, or have predisposing conditions, such as chronic bronchitis.
2. **Epidemiology.** Gram-negative bacillary pneumonia accounts for approximately 10% of all cases of bacterial pneumonia.
   a. The **incidence** of Gram-negative bacillary pneumonia is highest among immunocompromised individuals whose upper respiratory tract is colonized by Gram-negative aerobic rods; these patients have acute or chronic illness. Gram-negative bacillary pneumonia occurs frequently in hospitalized patients, nearly 50% of whom have oropharyngeal colonization (in contrast to only 5% of healthy individuals). About 25% of these patients develop pneumonia; lung infection is probably caused by aspiration of oropharyngeal secretions.
   b. **Predisposing factors.** Alcoholics, drug abusers, and other people subject to periods of unconsciousness and decreased laryngeal reflexes are susceptible.
   c. The **mortality rate** is approximately 50%, even with adequate antimicrobial therapy. Debilitated patients with *P. aeruginosa* pneumonia have a mortality rate of 80%.
3. **Clinical manifestations** are similar to those of pneumococcal pneumonia: fever, chills, and a productive cough.
   a. **Highly mucoid** and **bloody sputum**—described as **"currant jelly"**—can be seen in *K. pneumoniae* infections.
   b. **Cavitation of the lung, hypotension, delirium,** and **shock** are common.
   c. **Radiologic findings** include evidence of nonspecific lung injury ranging from peribronchial effusion to dense unilobar consolidation of the upper lobe.
4. **Diagnosis.** Culture and identification of the etiologic agent confirms the diagnosis. The best specimens for differentiating between bacteria colonizing the upper respiratory tract and those causing pneumonia are aseptically obtained transtracheal or transthoracic aspirates and transbronchoscopic lung biopsy specimens.

5. **Treatment.** Antimicrobial agents and supportive measures are necessary for the treatment of Gram-negative bacillary pneumonia. The selection of antimicrobial agents should be based on the results of susceptibility tests of isolated organisms.
   a. **Cephalosporins** combined with **aminoglycosides** are often used empirically to initiate therapy.
   b. **Quinolones** are indicated for the treatment of pneumonia caused by *P. aeruginosa* and *Proteus* species.

D. **Pneumonia caused by *Mycoplasma pneumoniae* (atypical pneumonia)** is highly infectious and frequently occurs in epidemics.

1. **Etiology.** *M. pneumoniae* is a small, pleomorphic bacterium without a cell wall. For this reason, it does not stain with conventional bacteriologic stains.
2. **Epidemiology**
   a. *M. pneumoniae* is distributed worldwide.
   b. The lungs are the primary target organ in approximately 10% of infected people.
   c. With close contact, such as in a family, the infection spreads quickly by dissemination of contaminated respiratory droplets. Fifty percent of infected people develop clinical pneumonia.
3. **Clinical manifestations.** *Mycoplasma* pneumonia develops slowly.
   a. The initial symptom is usually a nonproductive cough that eventually produces a watery to mucoid sputum. The cough lasts approximately 2 weeks in untreated patients.
   b. A temperature of 100°F–103°F, headache, chills, rhinorrhea, chest pain, malaise, and generalized myalgia are common.
   c. Physical, radiologic, and laboratory findings resemble those of viral pneumonia (see III D).
   d. Most patients recover without complications or sequelae.
4. **Diagnosis**
   a. **Isolation.** The diagnosis is best confirmed by isolating *M. pneumoniae* on appropriate media.
   b. **Serologic tests** are often used instead of isolation, because not many clinical laboratories are equipped to grow and identify *Mycoplasma.*
      (1) **Cold agglutinins** develop in approximately 50% of patients. These are nonspecific, cross-reactive antibodies that agglutinate human red blood cells with the I antigen. A high titer of cold agglutinins is good evidence of infection and justifies appropriate antibiotic therapy.
      (2) The presence of *Mycoplasma*-specific IgM antibodies is a better indication of *Mycoplasma* pneumonia than the presence of cold agglutinins.
5. **Treatment. Tetracycline** or **erythromycin** is the drug of choice. Antibiotic therapy decreases the severity and duration of the disease but does not immediately eliminate the bacteria from the upper respiratory tract.

E. **Pneumonia caused by *Mycobacterium tuberculosis* and related organisms** is discussed in Chapter 18 II.

III. VIRAL PNEUMONIA

A. **Etiology.** A variety of viruses can infect the lungs. Most often, viruses cause interstitial pneumonitis, but the term "viral pneumonia" is most commonly used to designated viral infection of the lungs.

1. Common etiologic agents include respiratory syncytial virus, adenovirus, parainfluenza virus, and influenza virus A and B.

2. Less common etiologic agents include herpes viruses, rhinoviruses, rubeola virus, echoviruses, coronaviruses, and coxsackieviruses.

3. Viral pneumonia may also occur as a complication of viral syndromes that as a rule do not affect the lungs.
   a. Cytomegalovirus (CMV) pneumonia typically is seen in patients with leukemia, lymphoma, or tissue transplants. Primary CMV pneumonia occurs in neonates and immunocompromised adults.
   b. Varicella (chickenpox) pneumonia secondary to the skin rash occurs in children.

B. Epidemiology

1. **Incidence**
   a. Viral pneumonia is estimated to affect approximately 0.1% of the population each year (the incidence is difficult to determine because it is not a reportable disease and some patients never seek medical attention.)
   b. The incidence in children younger than 5 years is more than four times that of the overall population; respiratory syncytial virus is the most common etiologic agent in this age group.

2. **Predisposing factors.** Age and immunologic status play important roles in the type and severity of disease.
   a. The incidence is highest in patients with underlying disease that affects cell-mediated immunity (CMI).
   b. Hospitalized patients, organ transplant recipients, the very young, and the elderly are prime candidates for infection.

3. **Transmission.** Viral pneumonia is spread by droplet inhalation; coughing and sneezing are the primary means of transmission. Hand-to-hand contact may also spread the infection.

4. **Seasonal variation.** Viral pneumonia is most common in midwinter and spring, in part because of "population closeness," which facilitates transmission.

C. Pathogenesis. The **primary foci of infection** is usually in the cells of the upper respiratory tract. The infection may spread to the lungs via contaminated mucous secretions or by hematogenous or lymphatic dissemination.

D. Clinical manifestations

1. **General features**
   a. **Symptoms**
      (1) Initially, the patient experiences nasal congestion, coryza, and eye discomfort. Variable symptoms of sore throat and hoarseness are followed by headache, fever, chills, malaise, myalgia, and a nonproductive cough. Nonspecific symptoms become more severe as the pneumonia progresses; prostration may occur suddenly.
   b. **Physical examination findings** are not usually specific or remarkable; **chest radiographs** show bilateral interstitial inflammation.

2. **Specific features**
   a. **Influenza A virus pneumonia** is the most common pneumonia in adults.
      (1) Symptoms and physical examination findings
         (a) The disease begins abruptly with fever (temperature of 102°F–104°F), malaise, and prostration.
         (b) Coughing is generally nonproductive, but small quantities of bloody sputum may be produced as the disease progresses.
         (c) Chest pain is substernal; rales and rhonchi are typical auscultatory findings.
      (2) Laboratory findings
         (a) White blood cell counts are elevated, frequently to more than 10,000/mm^3, with a marked left shift.
         (b) Chest radiographs show diffuse—often bilateral—bronchopneumonia.

(c) Changes in blood gases and pH indicate the severity of infection.

b. **Respiratory syncytial virus pneumonia** is most serious in the very young, although it also occurs in the elderly.

(1) **Symptoms**

(a) The most prominent clinical manifestations are fever, dyspnea, and wheezing with intercostal retraction.

(b) Children younger than 1 year tend to develop **bronchiolitis,** whereas children 4–5 years of age commonly develop **bronchopneumonia.**

(c) Rales and rhonchi are present, cough is variable, and sputum is scanty.

(2) **Laboratory findings.** White blood cell counts and differential counts are not specific. Chest radiographs show bilateral bronchopneumonia.

c. **Adenoviral pneumonia** usually occurs in military recruits and children; it seldom occurs in civilian adults. In children, the disease is usually bilateral, causes significant impairment of gas exchange in the alveoli, and may be fatal. Complications, such as bronchiectasis and chronic pulmonary disease, are seen only in children.

(1) **Symptoms.** The pneumonic syndrome produced by adenovirus types 1, 2, 3, and 7 is indistinguishable from bacterial pneumonia in its symptoms and physical findings, although some features are more characteristic of adenovirus pneumonia—pharyngitis, rhinitis, rales, nausea, and vomiting are common features of adenoviral pneumonia and are not usually seen in bacterial pneumonia.

(2) **Laboratory findings.** White blood cell counts may be as high as 30,000/mm^{3,} but two-thirds of patients have leukocyte counts within normal limits.

d. **Measles (rubeola) pneumonia** occurs in 7%–50% of patients with measles, usually in children younger than 6 years. Generally, pneumonia develops within 5 days of the appearance of the rash; primary measles pneumonia (appearing without a preceding rash) is a severe, often fatal disease that affects immunologically compromised people.

(1) **Rales** and **rhonchi** on chest examination are generally the only abnormal findings.

(2) **Radiographic evidence of interstitial pneumonia** is common.

E. Treatment. In most cases, the treatment of patients with viral pneumonia is supportive. In some cases, however, treatment may be indicated:

1. Young children with pneumonia caused by **respiratory syncytial virus** may benefit from **ribavirin** administration.
2. Immunocompromised patients with pneumonia caused by **CMV** are treated with **ganciclovir.**

F. Complications. Bacterial superinfection is a major cause of morbidity and mortality in patients with viral pneumonia. Bacterial superinfections should be treated with antibacterial agents chosen according the results of antimicrobial susceptibility testing.

IV. FUNGAL PNEUMONIA. *P. carinii* pneumonia is a major cause of morbidity and mortality in immunocompromised patients, particularly those with AIDS.

A. Etiology. *P. carinii* has been identified in humans and other mammals with symptomatic or asymptomatic infection. Its life cycle is unknown.

B. Epidemiology

1. Asymptomatic infection appears to be common during the first 2 years of life. The disease is occasionally endemic or intermediately epidemic in **premature** or **malnourished infants.**
2. *P. carinii* is the most common cause of sporadic interstitial pneumonia in **immunocompromised patients.**

a. Approximately half of patients with **AIDS** develop *P. carinii* pneumonia.
b. Other predisposing factors include prolonged use of corticosteroids in **patients with lymphoproliferative malignancies, organ grafts,** and **autoimmune diseases.** The corticosteroids may activate latent infections in these patients.

C. **Clinical manifestations** vary greatly, in part because of concomitant infections with other agents (e.g., 25% of the patients are infected with CMV). As a rule, initial symptoms progress rapidly over a period of a few days; however, frank pneumonia and respiratory distress develop gradually.

1. **Symptoms**
   a. Early symptoms are nonspecific and include fever (temperature of 102°F–104°F) and shaking chills. A nonproductive cough develops in fewer than half the patients. Shortness of breath may be the only patient complaint.
   b. Respiratory distress, indicated by tachypnea, nasal flaring, and eventually cyanosis, develops gradually if the patient is not treated or does not respond to therapy.
2. **Physical examination findings.** Chest auscultation is remarkable for the absence of findings.
3. **Laboratory findings**
   a. Chest radiographs typically show diffuse patchy infiltrates in both lungs.
   b. The most consistent finding in blood chemistry is hypoxemia. Lymphopenia and hypoalbuminemia are often present.

D. **Diagnosis** requires demonstration of *P. carinii* in the lung. **Bronchoalveolar lavage samples** are usually preferred, but if they yield negative results, **transbronchial biopsy specimens** may be used.

1. Silver stains reveal typical multinucleated cysts. Giemsa stain or toluidine O may also reveal the cysts. Direct immunofluorescence can be used to detect the organism in lung tissue.
2. Cultures for bacteria, mycobacteria, other fungi, and viruses should be started, to rule out concomitant infections.

E. **Treatment. Trimethoprim–sulfamethoxazole** is the drug of choice. **Pentamidine** is recommended for patients who cannot tolerate or who do not respond to trimethoprim–sulfamethoxazole.

F. **Prophylaxis.** Severely immunocompromised patients respond poorly to therapy. For this reason, prophylaxis with **trimethoprim–sulfamethoxazole** is recommended for patients at risk (e.g., HIV-positive individuals).

Case 1 Revisited

The 20-year-old patient has bacterial pneumonia complicated by alcoholism and delay in seeking health care.

Acute onset of a febrile disease with rigors, pulmonary symptoms, signs of lung consolidation, and rust-colored sputum suggest *S. pneumoniae* as the cause. Because of the history of heavy alcohol abuse, which can be associated with immunocompromise, one must consider the possibility of a Gram-negative pneumonia (most likely involving *K. pneumoniae*). A history of bouts of unconsciousness or seizures would raise the possibility of a necrotizing pneumonia caused by aspiration of anaerobes from the mouth.

The heart murmur may be the result of endocarditis following bacteremia, which may also be the cause of infectious arthritis of the left knee.

Gram stains and cultures of sputum, joint fluid, and blood should be obtained. Gram-positive, lancet-shaped diplococci and large numbers of leukocytes (particularly neutrophils) in the sputum can confirm a diagnosis of *S. pneumoniae* pneumonia. The aortic heart valve and the left knee have probably been infected by this organism, which is often found in the blood stream of patients with pneumonia; therefore, joint fluid and blood cultures would most likely yield the same organism.

Intravenous administration of a third-generation cephalosporin should be initiated promptly. If the organism is later found to be susceptible to penicillin G, penicillin, which is much less expensive, should be used.

Case 2 Revisited

In an elderly nursing-home patient in the fall or early winter, the most likely diagnosis is influenza virus pneumonia. Primary bacterial pneumonia or bacterial superinfection of viral pneumonia should be considered in the differential diagnosis.

The diagnosis can be made on the basis of epidemiologic data and laboratory tests. If other patients in the nursing home have similar signs and symptoms, influenza viral pneumonia is most likely. Chest radiographs would show bronchopneumonia rather than consolidating lobar pneumonia. Blood cultures would be negative for bacteria, and Gram stain and culture of sputum would reveal the normal oropharyngeal flora. Knowledge of the prevalent strains of influenza virus circulating in the community at the time can be obtained from the county or state health department and may help elucidate the diagnosis and influence therapeutic and prophylactic measures.

If the prevalent virus is an influenza A virus, and if the nursing home patients and staff had not been vaccinated that year or had received a vaccine that did not protect against the virus spreading in the community, the patient should be treated with amantadine or rimantadine. Amantidine and rimantidine could also be administered prophylactically to other elderly patients and to staff members.

Chapter 49

Meningitis and Encephalitis

George M. Johnson
Gerald E. Wagner
Gabriel Virella

Case 1

A 5-day-old boy born at 37 weeks' gestation is brought to his pediatrician because of inconsolable crying, refusal to feed, and occasional vomiting that began within the past 6 hours. The pregnancy had been uncomplicated and the delivery uneventful. The patient had no problems as a newborn and was discharged with his mother 36 hours after delivery. His mother was not ill, and no other family members were ill.

On examination, the baby appears listless but is irritable when handled or moved. His breathing is shallow, and his respiratory rate is 70 respirations/min. His temperature is 96.4°F, his pulse rate is 160 beats/min, and his blood pressure is 72/54 mm Hg. His anterior fontanel is full but not bulging. He has no rash, but his hands and feet are pale, blotchy, and cool to touch. His chest radiograph is normal. A complete blood count reveals a white blood cell count of 12,400/mm^3 with 61% polymorphonuclear leukocytes and 5% bands.

- □ *What is the most likely diagnosis?*
- □ *What additional diagnostic tests are indicated?*
- □ *What is the appropriate next step?*
- □ *What organisms are most likely to cause this infection?*
- □ *Is this child's disease contagious?*

I. INTRODUCTION. Numerous infectious agents affect the nervous system. Some organisms release neurotoxins or cause degenerative lesions of poorly understood pathogenesis. Other agents directly infect the nervous system, including the meninges or the brain.

A. Meningitis is inflammation of the meninges.

1. **Bacterial meningitis** is defined as meningitis with evidence of pathogenic bacteria in the cerebrospinal fluid (CSF).
2. **Aseptic meningitis** is defined as meningitis without the usual evidence of pathogenic bacteria in the CSF.

B. Encephalitis is inflammation of the parenchyma of the brain.

C. Meningoencephalitis is inflammation of the brain and meninges.

II. BACTERIAL MENINGITIS is an acute, life-threatening infection. The mortality rate is approximately 10%–15% (depending on the bacteria involved), even with appropriate

Table 49-1. Bacteria Involved in Childhood Meningitis at Different Ages

Neonatal (<1 month)	Infant (1 month–2 years)	Preschool Age (2–5 years)	School Age (5–12 years)	Adolescent (12–18 years)
*Escherichia coli**	*S. pneumoniae*	*S. pneumoniae*	*Streptococcus pneumoniae*	*S. pneumoniae*
Group B *Streptococcus*	*N. meningitidis*	*N. meningitidis*	*Neisseria meningitidis*	*N. meningitidis*
Klebsiella species	*Haemophilus influenzae* type B	*H. influenzae* type B	*H. influenzae* type B	. . .
Listeria monocytogenes	. . .	. . .	. . .	. . .
Group D streptococci	. . .	. . .	. . .	. . .

* Strains with K1 capsular antigen are most common.

antimicrobial therapy. The incidence of disease decreases with age; the prevalence of a particular etiologic agent is also related to the patient's age.

A. **Etiology.** Bacteria most commonly associated with meningitis are encapsulated and have high affinity for specific receptors in the choroid plexus or the meninges.

1. More than 80% of cases of bacterial meningitis beyond the neonatal period are caused by *Streptococcus pneumoniae, Neisseria meningitidis,* and *Haemophilus influenzae* type b.
   a. Eighteen of the more than 80 recognized serotypes of *S. pneumoniae* are responsible for 90% of cases of pneumococcal meningitis.
   b. Four serogroups (A, B, C, and Y) of *N. meningitidis* cause most cases of meningococcal meningitis, which can affect both children and young adults. *N. meningitidis* can cause epidemic outbreaks, particularly in overcrowded conditions (e.g., in military barracks, day care centers).
   c. The frequency of meningitis caused by *H. influenzae* type b has decreased considerably since the introduction of the *H. influenzae* type b conjugate vaccines.

2. The remaining 20% of cases are caused by various pathogenic and opportunistic bacteria, including *Listeria monocytogenes,* Gram-negative enteric rods, *Staphylococcus aureus, Streptococcus pyogenes, Staphylococcus epidermidis,* and *Mycobacterium tuberculosis.*

B. **EPIDEMIOLOGY**

1. **Age dependence**
   a. **Meningitis in children.** Table 49-1 lists the bacteria that most often cause bacterial meningitis in children of different ages.
   b. **Meningitis in older children, adolescents,** and **adults** is considerably less common and is most often caused by *N. meningitidis* or *S. pneumoniae.*
   c. **Meningitis in the elderly** is most often caused by *S. pneumoniae.*

2. **Predisposing factors** include those related to the organism and those related to the host.
   a. **Bacterial factors**
      (1) Organisms with **polysaccharide capsules** resist phagocytosis and are poorly immunogenic in children younger than 2 years.
      (2) Bacteria have **surface antigens** (e.g., the K1 antigen of *Escherichia coli*) that are tropic for the meninges.

b. Host factors

(1) Gender. For unknown reasons, meningitis is more prevalent in men than in women (1.7:1 ratio).

(2) Prematurity, prolonged or **difficult delivery,** and **maternal infection** contribute to meningitis in the neonate. Immaturity of the immune system in the neonate and increased opportunity for exposure to pathogenic bacteria play a role.

(3) Age. The risk of contracting bacterial meningitis is greatest between birth and 5 years of age, with peak incidence in the first month of life.

(4) Congenital immunodeficiencies predispose to meningitis.

(a) Agammaglobulinemia and functional asplenia (e.g., sickle cell disease) increase the susceptibility to encapsulated bacteria.

(b) Complement deficiencies (particularly of the terminal components C5–C9) predispose to *N. meningitidis* meningitis.

(c) Cell-mediated or combined immunodeficiencies predispose to *L. monocytogenes* and viral meningitis.

(5) Acquired immunodeficiencies increase the susceptibility to opportunistic organisms (e.g., in AIDS patients) and to encapsulated bacteria (e.g., in patients who have undergone splenectomy).

(6) Poor sanitation, lack of access to preventive care, and **overcrowding** are predisposing factors.

(7) Exposure of the cranial vault or spine (e.g., congenital, post-traumatic, or surgical) facilitates direct penetration of bacteria into the meningeal space.

C. Pathogenesis

1. Bacterial access to the meninges or subarachnoid space

a. Bacteremic spread of organisms from the nasopharynx or other foci of infection accounts for most cases of bacterial meningitis.

b. Direct invasion

(1) Bacteria may directly invade the meningeal space from a contiguous focus of infection (e.g., sinusitis, mastoiditis, skull and vertebral osteomyelitis, possibly otitis media).

(2) Interrupting the integrity of the CSF space allows ascending invasion by pathogenic bacteria. Loss of CSF integrity may be congenital (e.g., dermoid sinuses, meningomyeloceles), traumatic (e.g., penetrating injury or basilar skull fracture), or surgical (e.g., CSF shunt).

2. Release of bacterial products. Once infection is established, bacteria replicate and release toxic compounds (e.g., endotoxin, teichoic acids, and peptidoglycan).

a. These bacterial products cause changes in vascular permeability and perfusion both directly and through activation of leukocytes. Activated leukocytes release a variety of proteases and inflammatory mediators [e.g., tumor necrosis factor-α (TNF-α), interleukin-1 (IL-1), interleukin-8 (IL-8), and platelet activating factor (PAF)].

b. Complement split products, generated by leukocyte and bacterial proteases, and certain cytokines (e.g., IL-8) are chemotactic for neutrophils and other granulocytes and cause massive influx of these cells into the meningeal space.

c. The cumulative effects of toxic and vasoactive compounds released by bacteria and leukocytes include interstitial edema, increased intracranial pressure, decreased cerebral blood flow, and subsequent damage to the brain. In addition, systemic effects of the same compounds may develop (see Chapter 47 IV A 4).

D. Clinical manifestations vary considerably depending on the virulence of the organism and the age of the patient.

1. In **neonates,** the signs of meningeal irritation (nuchal rigidity and Brudzinski's and Kernig's signs) are infrequent and are often minimal when found. Early signs include temperature instability, irritability, poor feeding, and vomiting.

2. In **children 1–18 months of age,** signs and symptoms are often nonspecific and in-

Table 49-2. Characteristics of Cerebrospinal Fluid in Different Types of Meningitis

Type of Meningitis	Leukocytes/ mm^3 (Range)	Predominant Cell Type	Glucose Concentration	Protein Levels	Microbiological Tests
Bacterial	0–60,000	Neutrophils	Very low (< 5–20 mg/dl)	Elevated	Positive*
Viral	0–1000	Mononuclear cells†	Normal (65–70 mg/dl)	Normal to slightly elevated	Negative
Tuberculous	25–500	Mononuclear cells	Low (20–40 mg/dl)	Elevated	Negative
Fungal	0–1000	Mononuclear cells	Low	Elevated	Negative‡

* Including Gram stain, culture, and rapid diagnostic tests for bacterial antigens.
† Neutrophils may predominate in early stages.
‡ India ink tests, fungal cultures, and agglutination tests for fungal antigens may be positive.

clude fever, irritability, drowsiness, vomiting, poor feeding, crying when handled, bulging fontanels (due to increased intravascular pressure), and febrile seizures.

3. In **older children and adults,** the severity of the symptoms varies.
   a. Nearly all patients have fever, headache, and nuchal rigidity.
   b. The most common finding is a stiff neck characterized by pain and resistance on flexion.
   c. Neurologic findings may include Brudzinski's and Kernig's signs.
   d. Seizures, vomiting, lethargy, drowsiness, and irritability on movement are common signs. Confusion, agitated delirium, and stupor occur less frequently.
   e. Coma, when it develops, is a poor prognostic sign.

E. Diagnosis

1. **Lumbar puncture.** A rapid and thorough examination of the CSF is important to confirm a diagnosis of meningitis.
   a. A lumbar puncture is not without risk in a patient with suspected meningitis because of the elevated intracranial pressure. Rapid withdrawal of CSF when the pressure is elevated can cause herniation of the cerebellar amygdala and death.
   b. Lumbar puncture is contraindicated when signs of significantly increased intracranial pressure (retinal changes, altered pupillary responses, and hypertension with bradycardia) are present. A computerized tomography (CT) scan can be obtained to better evaluate the risks.
2. **CSF findings** (Table 49-2)
   a. The **white blood cell count** is elevated (typically 500–10,000/mm^3), with a predominance of neutrophils and other granulocytes. However, these findings may be absent early in the disease.
   b. **Glucose levels** are low (typically < 40 mg/dl, less than half of the level of serum glucose).
   c. **Protein levels** are high, but it needs to be considered that normal levels vary considerably with age (120–150 mg/dl in premature babies, 10–120 mg/dl in term infants, and < 45 mg/dl after 3 months.
   d. A positive **Gram stain** or positive results in **latex agglutination tests** for *S. pneumoniae, N. meningitidis,* and *H. influenzae* can allow a rapid diagnosis.
   e. **Cultures**
      (1) **Bacterial cultures** should always be requested. One-quarter to one-half of children with bacterial meningitis have received antibiotics prior to admission, which may cause sterile CSF cultures. However, **it is very rare for all CSF parameters to be normalized by prior treatment.**
      (2) **Viral cultures** may also be indicated during the peak enterovirus season (late summer to early fall), or during an epidemic of viral meningitis.

Table 49-3. Recommendations for Initial Antimicrobial Treatment of Meningitis in Different Age Groups

	Neonates (< 1 month)	**Infants (1–3 months)**	**Children (> 3 months)**	**Older Children, Adults**
Most commonly involved organisms	Group B *Streptococcus;* Gram-negative bacilli; *Listeria monocytogenes*	Group B *Streptococcus;* Gram-negative bacteria; *Streptococcus pneumoniae; Neisseria meningitidis; Haemophilus influenzae*	*S. pneumoniae; N. meningitidis; H. influenzae*	*S. pneumoniae*
Recommended antibiotic	Ampicillin plus an aminoglycoside	Ampicillin plus an aminoglycoside or third-generation cephalosporin	Third-generation cephalosporin	Third-generation cephalosporin*

* Plus additional antibiotics for resistant or tolerant strains of *S. pneumoniae.*

3. **Other findings.** The **complete blood count** usually shows leukocytosis and neutrophilia. Other findings may reflect concomitant sepsis or involvement of other organs.

F. Treatment

1. **Antibiotic therapy**
   a. **Empiric therapy.** Early treatment is of paramount importance. Because different bacteria are involved in different age groups, the recommendations for initial empiric treatment vary (Table 49-3).
   b. **Definitive antibacterial therapy** is based on the results of antibiotic susceptibility tests. In neonates, the lumbar puncture should be repeated until the CSF is sterile, and again at the end of therapy. In older infants and children, repeated lumbar punctures are not necessary.
2. **Adjunctive therapy** includes:
   a. **Dexamethasone** for children older than 2 months, to reduce the inflammatory component of meningitis
   b. **General supportive care** (maintenance of ventilation, oxygenation, perfusion, and hydration, and nutritional support)

G. Prevention

1. **Isolation.** Patients with meningitis caused by *H. influenzae* or *N. meningitidis* should be isolated for 24 hours after initiation of antibiotic therapy, because the disease caused by these bacteria is highly contagious.
2. **Prophylactic antimicrobial therapy**
   a. Antimicrobial agents should be administered to **close contacts of patients with meningitis** caused by *H. influenzae* or *N. meningitidis.* **Rifampin** is the preferred antibacterial agent. Treatment should begin as soon as the diagnosis is made.
   b. Prophylactic antimicrobial therapy administered **during labor and delivery** to a woman colonized with group B streptococci can reduce the incidence of early-onset infection with group B streptococci in the newborn.
3. **Immunoprophylaxis**
   a. **The *H. influenzae* type b conjugate vaccine** is effective and is recommended as part of the routine immunization schedule for all children.
   b. ***N. meningitidis* vaccines** are available and are recommended in outbreaks.

Table 49-4. Infectious Causes of Aseptic Meningitis

Bacteria*	*Mycobacterium tuberculosis,* bacteria originating from brain abscess, epidural abscess, acute or subacute bacterial endocarditis; *Bartonella henselae* (cat scratch disease)
Viruses	Enteroviruses, mumps, lymphocytic choriomenigitis, Epstein-Barr virus, arboviruses, varicella-zoster virus, herpes simplex virus, HIV, influenza A and B viruses, adenovirus, measles virus, rubella virus, cytomegalovirus, parainfluenza virus, and other viruses
Rickettsiae	*Rickettsia rickettsiae* (Rocky Mountain spotted fever), *Rickettsia prowazecki* (typhus), *Coxiella burnetii* (Q fever), *Ehrlichia chafeensis*
Chlamydia	*Chlamydia psittaci*
Spirochetes	*Treponema pallidum, Borrelia burgdorferi, Leptospira interrogans*
Mycoplasma	*Mycoplasma pneumoniae, Mycoplasma hominis,* and *Ureaplasma urealyticum*
Fungi	*Candida albicans, Cryptococcus neoformans, Coccidioides immitis, Histoplasma capsulatum, Blastomyces dermatidis*
Protozoa	*Toxoplasma gondii, Plasmodium falciparum, Naegleria fowlerii,* Acanthamoeba, *Trichinella spiralis*
Nematodes	*Toxocara, Baylisacaris procyonis, Angiostrongylus cantonensis*
Cestodes	*Taenia solium, Echinococcus granulosus*

* Partially treated meningitis may present as an aseptic meningitis.

(1) Both bivalent (A and C) and quadrivalent vaccines (A, C, Y, and W135) are available, but only serogroup A is immunogenic in children younger than 2 years.

(2) The quadrivalent vaccine is not indicated for general preventive use except for military personnel and patients with asplenia or deficiencies of the terminal complement components (C5–C9).

c. ***S. pneumoniae*** **vaccine.** A vaccine for the most prevalent serotypes of *S. pneumoniae* is available and is recommended for individuals at risk, such as those with asplenia.

H. Prognosis

1. **Average mortality rates** for bacterial meningitis are **10%–15%.** Meningitis mortality rates are 6.5% for *H. influenzae,* 12% for *N. meningitidis,* and 28% for *S. pneumoniae.*

2. Up to 50% of the survivors have some **neurologic sequelae,** and in 10%, the sequelae are severe.
   a. **Neurosensory hearing loss** is the most common neurologic problem and has been associated with low CSF glucose.
   b. Other sequelae include **retardation, spasticity, behavioral disorders,** and **paresis.**

III. ASEPTIC MENINGITIS.

Historically, aseptic meningitis was the term for an illness with acute onset, clinical signs of meningitis, white blood cells but no bacteria in the CSF, and a short and benign course. This illness was most likely enteroviral meningitis. Aseptic meningitis is most commonly caused by a viral agent, especially an enterovirus, when the disease occurs in epidemics (summer and fall). Aseptic meningitis can also result from a wide variety of infectious (Table 49-4) and noninfectious causes.

A. Viral meningitis

1. **Etiology**
   a. The **enteroviruses** (coxsackieviruses A and B, echovirus, numbered enteroviruses, and poliovirus) are the most common causes of viral meningitis in the United States.
   b. **Mumps virus** used to be a relatively frequent cause of viral meningitis, but the frequency of its involvement has decreased with vaccination.
   c. **Herpes simplex virus (HSV), rubella, cytomegalovirus (CMV), rabies virus,** the **arboviruses,** and many other viral agents also may cause meningitis.

2. **Epidemiology**
   a. Enterovirus infections commonly occur in late summer and early fall; mumps virus infections typically occur in late winter and early spring.
   b. Viral meningitis is principally a disease of the young; it rarely occurs after age 40.

3. **Clinical manifestations.** Signs and symptoms of viral meningitis develop gradually over a few days to a week.
   a. Patients usually complain of a sore throat, fever, anorexia, malaise, and myalgia.
   b. More indicative symptoms develop with time, including lethargy, vomiting, severe headache, and stiff neck.
   c. Physical findings include fever and nuchal rigidity, with or without Brudzinski's or Kernig's sign.

4. **Diagnosis.** As in bacterial meningitis, the diagnosis is usually confirmed by the examination of CSF obtained by lumbar puncture (see Table 49-2).
   a. The opening pressure may be elevated.
   b. The **number of leukocytes** is moderately increased, typically to 100–500 cells/mm^3; counts over 1000/mm^3 are rarely observed.
      (1) Early in viral meningitis, granulocytes predominate.
      (2) In a repeat CSF examination 6–12 hours later, mononuclear cells generally predominate.
   c. The CSF **glucose concentration** is usually normal.
   d. The CSF **protein concentration** may be normal or moderately elevated.
   e. Identification by **cell culture** of a specific virus as the causative agent is successful in about 25%–30% of cases.

5. **Treatment** for most cases of viral meningitis is symptomatic and supportive. In an otherwise healthy individual, hospitalization is not absolutely required when the diagnosis of viral meningitis is unequivocal.

6. **Prognosis.** The prognosis for viral meningitis is good; death is exceptional, and complications, if any, are mild and usually reversible.

B. Tuberculous meningitis. This disease is characteristically a chronic or subacute meningitis.

1. **Etiology.** The vast majority of cases are caused by *Mycobacterium tuberculosis.* The organism infects the central nervous system (CNS) and meninges during the bacteremia that accompanies primary infection or reactivation. Meningitis usually results from reactivation and subsequent expansion of these initial infectious foci at a later date.

2. **Clinical manifestations.** The illness typically has an insidious onset with moderate constitutional symptoms and gradual progression.
   a. Low-grade fever, headache, and altered mental status are the most common early symptoms.
   b. Fever, protracted headache, confusion, lethargy, meningeal signs, and cranial nerve palsies are commonly found later on physical examination. The disease can accelerate, with development of stupor and coma progressing to more severe neurologic involvement (seizures, hemiparesis, and hemiplegia). Hydrocephalus may develop.

c. Untreated tuberculous meningitis is fatal, with death usually occurring within 5–8 weeks of the onset of symptoms.

3. **Diagnosis**
   a. **Clinical diagnosis** requires a high index of suspicion. Evidence of active infection elsewhere is variable (20%–70% of patients).
   b. **Laboratory diagnosis**
      (1) A **tuberculin skin test** may be positive in up to 80% of patients.
      (2) **CSF evaluation** is critical (see Table 49-2). The opening pressure is often elevated. Laboratory findings typically show elevated protein levels (100–500 mg/dl), low glucose levels (< 45 mg/dl in 80% of patients), and mononuclear pleocytosis (100–500 cells/mm^3 in most patients). Positive stains for acid-fast bacilli are useful because they can be obtained rapidly, although they are not very sensitive.
      (3) **CSF cultures** are positive in about 75% of cases, although multiple CSF samples may be needed to obtain a positive culture. Detectable growth of *Mycoplasma* requires more time than growth of pyogenic bacteria in culture.
   c. **Other diagnostic modalities**
      (1) **Cranial CT** or **magnetic resonance imaging (MRI)** scans are generally indicated because of the high incidence of hydrocephalus associated with tuberculous meningitis.
      (2) **Chest radiographs** may reveal hilar adenopathy, miliary pulmonary disease, and upper lobe infiltrates or cavitary lesions. Most children and 50% of adults have pulmonary lesions.

4. **Treatment**
   a. **Antimicrobial therapy.** When clinical suspicion is high, therapy should begin before proof of infection is obtained. Therapy for tuberculous meningitis generally requires three or four agents and must be altered if resistant bacteria are responsible for the infection.
      (1) The major antituberculous agents are isoniazid, rifampin, pyrazinamide, streptomycin, and ethambutol.
      (2) The duration of therapy is 2 months using three to four agents, followed by at least 7–10 months using two to three drugs.
   b. **Corticosteroids** are generally indicated in patients with rapidly deteriorating mental status, increased intracranial pressure, cerebral edema, stupor and coma, and focal neurologic findings.
   c. **Surgical shunting** is used to treat hydrocephalus that results from tuberculous meningitis.

C. Fungal meningitis. Fungi are relatively uncommon etiologic agents of meningitis, but the frequency of fungal meningitis is increasing with increasing numbers of immunocompromised patients.

1. **Etiology.** Most fungi that cause systemic and opportunistic mycoses can infect the CNS; some fungi show a distinct predilection for meningeal tissue. Most fungi that cause meningitis infect the CNS by hematogenous dissemination from primary foci of infection in the lungs.
   a. The most common causative agents are *Cryptococcus neoformans* and *Coccidioides immitis.*
   b. Other agents include *Histoplasma capsulatum, Blastomyces dermatitidis,* and *Candida* species.

2. **Epidemiology** of *C. neoformans* and *C. immitis* is discussed in Chapter 42.

3. **Clinical manifestations** of fungal meningitis vary with the extent of meningeal involvement and usually differ from those of acute bacterial meningitis (fungal meningitis has more subacute and chronic presentations). Development of hydrocephalus is much more common in fungal meningitis than in bacterial meningitis.
   a. **Cryptococcal meningitis** can be subacute or chronic. Patients develop symptoms of meningoencephalitis, sometimes with symptoms suggesting a space-occupying lesion in the brain.

(1) **Disease course.** The disease can last from a few days (when the disease follows a rapid, precipitous evolution) to years. Generally, however, the disease follows a subacute course with progressive deterioration over a period of weeks to months.

(2) **Symptoms.** The most common symptom is frontal headache of increasing severity. Additional symptoms are fever, weight loss, nausea, vomiting, and mental and visual aberrations.

(3) **Physical findings** include cranial nerve dysfunction, positive Brudzinski's and Kernig's signs, and increased intracranial pressure. Skin lesions, bone lesions, lymphadenitis, and other visceral lesions occur in approximately 10% of patients.

b. Coccidioidal meningitis is a granulomatous disease of the CNS that is usually fatal if untreated.

(1) **Disease course.** Meningitis may be the first recognizable evidence of coccidioidomycosis, because the primary pulmonary disease is usually asymptomatic and undiagnosed. Meningitis occurs at least 3–6 months after primary infection. Relapses are relatively common; they occur most frequently 1–2 years after apparent resolution of disease.

(2) **Symptoms.** Most symptoms are nonspecific (headache, fever, weakness, confusion, mental and behavioral abnormalities, stiff neck, diplopia, ataxia, and vomiting).

(3) **Physical findings.** Skin lesions at the nasolabial fold are common.

4. Diagnosis. An early diagnosis allows early treatment and better prognosis. Unfortunately, the diagnosis may be difficult, because the CSF may appear normal and smears and cultures may be negative. Many fungi can be isolated from the CSF only rarely, and many fungi require days to weeks to grow and be identified. Exclusion of other types of meningitis often assumes a major role in the diagnosis of fungal meningitis.

a. Patient history

(1) **Cryptococcal meningitis** should always be suspected in people with compromised cell-mediated immunity (CMI) who develop symptoms of meningitis.

(2) **Coccidioidal meningitis** should be suspected in patients with the appropriate symptoms who also have:

(a) Past or concurrent coccidioidomycosis at other sites

(b) A history of travel to areas where coccidioidomycosis is endemic, or exposure to fomites from such areas

b. CSF examination shows moderate leukocytosis (50–500 cells/mm^3) with mononuclear cells predominating. Protein levels are usually elevated, while the glucose levels vary between 20% and 50% of the blood levels (see Table 49-2).

(1) **Cryptococcal meningitis** can be diagnosed by several techniques.

(a) Microscopic examination of an India-ink preparation of the CSF sediment demonstrates encapsulated yeast cells in 50% of non-AIDS cases and in more than 75% of AIDS-related cases.

(b) CSF culture and identification of cryptococci can confirm the diagnosis in more than 95% of cases.

(c) Detection of the capsular antigen of *C. neoformans* in CSF by a latex-agglutination test is a sensitive and rapid technique. Positive results are obtained in 94% of cases; however, patients with rheumatoid factor can yield false-positive results.

(2) **Coccidioides meningitis** is difficult to diagnose.

(a) Microscopic examination of the CSF is usually negative.

(b) Approximately 70% of patients have negative CSF cultures.

(c) Serodiagnosis can be made by demonstrating complement-fixing antibodies in the CSF. Only approximately 70% of patients have detectable complement-fixing antibody titers on the first examination, but as the disease progresses, nearly all patients develop complement-fixing antibodies in the CSF.

5. **Treatment**
   a. **Amphotericin B** by itself or with **5-fluorocytosine** is classically used to treat fungal meningitis. Treatment of coccidioidal meningitis requires intrathecal administration of amphotericin B.
   b. **Fluconazole** has been approved for treatment of cryptococcal meningitis in AIDS patients and appears to be the drug of choice for chronic suppressive therapy in these patients.
   c. **Itraconazole** is also effective for cryptococcal meningitis. Fluconazole together with itraconazole may be effective for coccidioidal meningitis.

D. Parasitic meningoencephalitis

1. **Primary amebic meningoencephalitis**
   a. **Etiology.** Primary amebic meningoencephalitis can be caused by *Acanthamoeba* species and by *Naegleria fowlerii,* which causes a considerably more serious form of the disease.
   b. **Epidemiology** is discussed in Chapter 45.
   c. **Clinical manifestations.** The initial symptoms are headache and fever, which quickly develop into a deep coma. Primary amebic meningoencephalitis is almost always fatal within 4–7 days of the development of symptoms.
   d. **Diagnosis.** The finding of trophozoites in the CSF is diagnostic.
   e. **Treatment.** Treatment is **usually unsuccessful. Amphotericin B** has been most frequently used to treat this disease.

2. **Cerebral toxoplasmosis**
   a. **Epidemiology**
      (1) **Prevalence.** *Toxoplasma gondii* is prevalent worldwide.
      (2) **Transmission.** Persons most at risk of infection are meat handlers, hunters, and anyone who eats raw or undercooked meat.
         (a) Humans are usually infected by ingesting oocysts in contaminated food or bradyzoites or tachyzoites in meat products from infected animals.
         (b) Handling litter boxes of infected cats is also a common way to acquire the infection, particularly in the United States.
      (3) **Predisposing factors.** *T. gondii* pseudocysts persist for years, particularly in immunologically privileged sites such as the CNS and retina. **Immunosuppressive therapy, stress,** and **immunocompromising infections** (e.g., HIV) can reactivate the tissue cysts.
   b. **Clinical manifestations**
      (1) Reactivation in the eye results in chorioretinitis, which leads to blindness.
      (2) Reactivation in the brain leads to encephalitis. The symptoms of encephalitis, such as headaches, dizziness, and spastic paralysis, may be difficult to evaluate in patients with AIDS, who can suffer from a variety of brain infections and abnormalities.
   c. **Diagnosis**
      (1) Diagnosis is usually based on **serologic assays.** A positive IgM antibody titer indicates a primary infection, and an increasing IgG antibody titer indicates an active infection. However, in immunocompromised patients, serologies may not be helpful.
      (2) **Staining.** Identification of *Toxoplasma* in stained sections of biopsy material is not affected by compromise of the immune system and is often used to confirm the diagnosis.
   d. **Treatment. Pyrimethamine** with **sulfadiazine** and **spiramycin** is the treatment of choice. **Trimethoprim-sulfamethoxazole** and **clindamycin** have also been used with some success. **Corticosteroids** may be given concomitantly to reduce ocular inflammation, if present.
   e. **Prevention** is difficult, due to the diversity of animal reservoirs. HIV-positive patients and patients receiving immunosuppressive or cytotoxic drugs should avoid close contact with cats and their litter boxes. Deep freezing of meat kills the parasite.

IV. VIRAL ENCEPHALITIS

A. Etiology. Numerous agents, including many of the bacteria that cause meningitis, can also cause encephalitis, usually meningoencephalitis. The bacteria that cause cat-scratch disease and Lyme disease can also cause encephalitis, but encephalitis is most often caused by a wide variety of viruses. Arbovirus, enterovirus, HSV, and rabies virus are the most common causative agents.

B. Epidemiology

1. Arbovirus infections predominate in the summer, during mosquito season.
2. Rabies is also more frequent during the warm months, when opportunities for transmission increase.

C. Clinical manifestations. Signs and symptoms are not very different from those of viral meningitis (see III A 3) and include fever, anorexia, malaise, severe headache, vomiting, lethargy, and coma. Dramatic signs of cerebral dysfunction are the major differentiating feature of viral encephalitis.

D. Diagnosis. The confirmation of encephalitis varies considerably depending on the cause.

1. The diagnosis of rabies and HSV encephalitis is usually achieved by visualization of typical cellular changes or by demonstration of viral antigens by direct immunofluorescence in brain biopsies.
2. The diagnosis of most other types of encephalitis is confirmed by serology.

E. Treatment

1. **HSV encephalitis** can be treated effectively with **acyclovir.** Therapy must be initiated as early as possible to be effective.
2. **Other viral causes.** There is no effective therapy for encephalitis caused by other viruses.

F. Prognosis. The prognosis is much poorer than that for viral meningitis.

1. **Mortality rates** vary from 20%–70%, depending on the causative agent. Undiagnosed rabies encephalitis has a mortality rate of virtually 100%.
2. **Sequelae** are common, but their frequency varies with the age of the patient and the agent responsible for the infection. Frequent sequelae include:
   a. Mental or intellectual dysfunction or mental retardation
   b. Neuromotor difficulties, including spasticity, seizures, and deterioration of specific neural functions such as vision or hearing

Case 1 Revisited

The clinical presentation of this child suggests meningitis or sepsis. Neonates have the highest risk of bacterial meningitis. However, in this age group, the clinical presentation of any major infection is generally nonspecific.

A lumbar puncture to obtain samples for cerebrospinal fluid (CSF) analysis and a blood sample is indicated. The CSF and blood samples should be cultured; in addition, the CSF can be Gram stained. Analysis of the baby's CSF reveals a leukocyte count of 950 cells/mm^3 with 90% polymorphonuclear leukocytes, a glucose level of 25 mg/dl, and a protein level of 190 mg/dl. The CSF Gram stain is negative, except for the detection of group B streptococcal antigen. Culture of the CSF is positive for group B streptococcus (*Streptococcus agalactiae*). Serum chemistries are normal except for a low carbon dioxide tension, indicative of a mild acidosis.

This infant should be admitted to the hospital because the risk of serious infection, especially meningitis, is high. Empiric antibiotic therapy directed at the most likely bacterial etiologies of meningitis in this age group should be started after cultures are obtained.

Group B streptococci, *Escherichia coli,* other enteric Gram-negative bacilli (e.g., *Klebsiella*), *Listeria monocytogenes,* and, rarely, group D streptococci (enterococci) are the most likely causative agents of meningitis in neonates.

This infant would not be considered contagious, but routine hand-washing by personnel caring for the patient is recommended to prevent spread to other infants. Isolation and cohorting with other infected or colonized infants is recommended only during nursery outbreaks.

Chapter 50

Degenerative Brain Diseases Caused by Viruses and Unconventional Agents

Jean-Michel Goust

Case 1

A 12-year-old girl is found at 3 A.M. walking barefoot in the snow and is brought to the emergency room. The girl knows her name, but is confused regarding time and place and is unable to give her address and phone number. Her medical history is unremarkable. Her parents say that they entered the United States 3 years ago, but are vague regarding previous immunizations. The girl is well-nourished but unable to follow simple commands. She exhibits postural abnormalities, and frequently extends and rotates her hands and forearms. Her pupils are symmetric and responsive to light; there is no papilledema. Her muscle tone is diffusely increased with brisk reflexes. Screens for alcohol and drugs are negative. An emergency electroencephalogram (EEG) shows diffuse abnormalities, suggesting an encephalopathic process. Magnetic resonance imaging (MRI) reveals many hyperintense abnormalities in both hemispheres. A cerebrospinal fluid (CSF) sample is obtained by lumbar puncture. Analysis reveals that the CSF is clear and contains 40 lymphocytes/μl. The total protein is 140 mg/dl, and glucose and sodium levels are normal. No bacteria or fungi are detected. Anti-measles hemagglutinin antibodies are positive (1280 in the serum and 10,240 in the CSF).

- *What is the most likely diagnosis in this patient?*
- *How can the diagnosis be confirmed?*
- *What is the prognosis for this young patient?*
- *How could this disease have been prevented?*

Case 2

A 22-year-old homosexual man is brought to a neurologist because he is becoming blind following a febrile illness with lymphadenopathies and weight loss. Neurologic examination shows bitemporal hemianopsia with visual acuity at 20/200 as a result of cortical blindness. His mental status is sluggish. MRI of the brain reveals extensive deep white matter loss, predominantly in the occipital areas. The patient is HIV-positive with a $CD4^+$ cell count of 80 cells/mm^3.

- *What is the most likely diagnosis?*
- *What should be done to confirm the diagnosis?*
- *What type of therapy should be instituted?*

I. INTRODUCTION.

The degenerative diseases of the brain are usually characterized by slow irreversible progress, often with partial remissions followed by exacerbations. For many diseases, the causative agent is unknown, but viral infections have been implicated in a heterogeneous group of diseases that includes **subacute sclerosing panencephalitis (SSPE), progressive multifocal leukoencephalopathy (PML),** and **tropical spastic paraparesis.** Unconventional agents (prions) have been implicated in the pathogenesis of **Creutzfeldt-Jacob disease** and related conditions.

II. SUBACUTE SCLEROSING PANENCEPHALITIS (SSPE)

A. Etiology. SSPE is caused by a **persistent infection** with **measles virus.** The strains of measles virus associated with SSPE appear to be genetically abnormal, causing persistent infection and long-term degenerative changes in the brain.

B. Epidemiology. SSPE can affect children or adults of any age.

C. Pathogenesis. The persistent production of viral proteins and nucleic acids without the production and export of viral particles eventually overloads and destroys the infected glial cells.

1. **Host factors.** A major factor in the pathogenesis of SSPE is an imbalanced immune response to measles virus.
   - **a.** Very high antibody titers against measles virus nucleocapsids and hemagglutinins are detected in the serum and cerebrospinal fluid (CSF) of patients with SSPE. In the CSF, the antibodies are seen as multiple homogeneous bands of IgG, suggesting a clonally restricted immune response to a small number of antigenic determinants.
   - **b.** A specific cell-mediated response is suggested by heavy perivascular cuffing of lymphocytes in the central nervous system (CNS) lesions. $CD8^+$ T cells able to kill measles virus–infected fibroblasts can be isolated from patients with SSPE.
2. **Viral factors.** Cloning and sequencing of SSPE-associated strains show a number of mutations in the genes for the M (matrix) and F (fusion) proteins. These mutations cause premature termination of transcription or translation of unstable proteins.
   - **a.** The M protein is critical for viral assembly; abnormal M protein can account for the absence of progeny budding from infected brain cells.
   - **b.** The introduction of a stop codon in the gene for the F glycoprotein results in diminished exposure of this viral antigen on the cell surface. Consequently, the virus is not as likely to spread from cell to cell by formation of syncytia. In addition, the low level of expression of viral antigens on the cell membrane allows the virus to remain shielded from immune attack.

D. Clinical manifestations. SSPE evolves slowly but steadily, with progressive deterioration of brain function, until a state of decerebration develops and death ensues, months to years after the onset of symptoms.

E. Diagnosis. The diagnosis of SSPE can be suspected when high levels of antibodies to measles nucleocapsid antigens are detected in the serum and CSF. Additional supporting evidence is provided by the demonstration of a very strong, ongoing intrathecal immune response characterized by the production of IgG. Oligoclonal bands, indicating heterogeneity, are visible when the CSF is separated using isoelectric focusing. Magnetic resonance imaging (MRI) of the brain shows extensive lesions in the deep white matter, often associated with atrophy. However, none of these tests is pathognomonic. The diagnosis must be established beyond any doubt by **brain biopsy,** if only to rule out a treatable cause for the patient's symptoms.

F. Treatment and prognosis. There is no effective therapy. SSPE is relentless, irreversible, and fatal.

Table 50-1. Characteristics of Subacute Sclerosing Panencephalitis (SSPE) and Progressive Multifocal Leukoencephalopathy (PML)

	SSPE	**PML**
Age range	2–30 years	Adults
CNS abnormalities	Gray and white matter	Gray and white matter
Infected cells in CNS	Neurons and oligodendrocytes	Astrocytes and oligodendrocytes
Inflammatory cells in CNS	Abundant	Few or none
Demonstration of virus in brain biopsies by EM	Never	Always
Recovery of virus from brain tissue	Measles*	Papovavirus (JC strain)
Antibodies in serum and CSF	Very high†	Low or absent
Preexisting immunocompromise	None	Always‡
Prognosis	Fatal	Fatal

CSF = cerebrospinal fluid; CNS = central nervous system; EM = electron microscopy.
* By co-culture with permissive cell lines.
† Intrathecal immune response against the virus.
‡ PML is only seen in immunosuppressed patients.

G. Prevention. Although the strains of SSPE-associated measles virus have distinct genomic abnormalities, they share enough antigens with the wild-type measles virus for the **measles vaccine** to be effective prophylaxis for SSPE. Since the introduction of measles vaccination, SSPE has become almost extinct, but it essential to maintain a high level of immunity to measles virus in the population to prevent the reemergence of SSPE.

III. PROGRESSIVE MULTIFOCAL LEUKOENCEPHALOPATHY (PML) shares some of the features of SSPE, but also has unique characteristics (Table 50-1).

A. Etiology. PML is caused by the **JC virus,** one of the few papovaviruses that are pathogenic for humans. Although the JC virus is prevalent in the general population, the virus is normally latent in kidney cells. It has also been found in the bone marrow.

B. Predisposing factors. PML is seen only in immunosuppressed patients in whom the depression of immune functions seems to allow the spread of the previously latent virus. Patients with AIDS, Hodgkin's disease, and chronic lymphocytic leukemia, and patients iatrogenically immunosuppressed as a consequence of the administration of cancer chemotherapy or post-transplantation immunosuppressive regimens are susceptible.

C. Pathogenesis. Because most immunosuppressed individuals do not develop PML, and also because the brain does not normally contain JC virus genomes, viral-dependent factors must determine the activation of an asymptomatic infection by the JC virus and subsequent development of PML.

1. In normal carriers of the JC virus, the viral genome remains unintegrated during the latency period. When the immune system becomes functionally depressed, the virus enters a phase of active replication and disseminates by the hematogenous route.
2. The JC virus shows marked neurotropism and tends to infect predominantly glial cells (astrocytes and oligodendrocytes).
   a. This cell specificity is a function of the enhancer/promoter element of the viral genome, which seems to be specifically transactivated by a cellular factor specifically produced in glial cells.

b. Mutations in the JC virus enhancer/promoter element could play a key role in determining increased affinity for the cellular transactivator in glial cells, therefore increasing the CNS tropism of JC viruses and explaining why only some patients develop the disease.

D. **Clinical manifestations.** PML occurs only in immunosuppressed adults. Frequently, the first complaint is of decreased vision, related to hemianopsia or cortical blindness. After a few weeks, hemiparesis, then quadriparesis, develop. Confusion heralds the onset of the final phase; coma and death occur shortly thereafter.

E. **Diagnosis**

1. The CSF is usually normal.
2. MRI of the head shows extensive destruction of the white matter without evidence of inflammation.
3. **Needle brain biopsy** is necessary to rule out a treatable opportunistic infection. It can also confirm the diagnosis if nuclear inclusion bodies are visualized in the oligodendrocytes.

F. **Treatment and prognosis.** Intrathecal administration of β-interferon has been shown to slow the progression of PML in some patients. Whatever the underlying disease, PML is invariably fatal. Survival after the diagnosis of PML in full-blown AIDS does not exceed 4–6 weeks.

G. **Prevention.** No vaccine is available.

IV. DEGENERATIVE RETROVIRAL DISEASES OF THE CNS

A. **Progressive spastic paraparesis** is one of the clinical presentations associated with infection by human T lymphotropic virus-I (HTLV-I).

1. **Epidemiology.** Once the HTLV-I DNA becomes integrated into the host DNA, it can remain latent for 20–30 years without creating any health problem in more than 95% of carriers.
   a. Circulating antibodies may be detected in up to 30% of the population in endemic areas (southern Japan, the Caribbean).
   b. In the continental United States, South Carolina is an area of relatively high prevalence, with a seropositivity rate of 0.3%.
   c. One out of 7000 HTLV-I–infected individuals develops a slowly progressive spastic paraparesis.
2. **Pathogenesis.** HTLV-I isolated from patients with T-cell leukemia is indistinguishable from HTLV-I isolated from patients with spastic paraparesis, even at the level of the DNA sequence; therefore, the same virus associated with a malignant process in some patients causes a progressive neurological disorder in others. The host response may play an important role in determining the outcome of HTLV-I infection.
3. **Clinical manifestations**
   a. **Symptoms.** HTLV-I–associated myelopathy typically is characterized by stiffness and weakness of both lower extremities and bladder incontinence. In most patients, the disease spares the upper extremities and the cranial nerves.
   b. **Physical examination findings.** Examination of the lower extremities reveals increased muscle tone, very brisk reflexes often associated with ankle or patellar clonus, a bilateral Babinski reflex, and relatively mild alteration of proprioception.
4. **Diagnosis.** The brain and spinal cord usually appear normal on MRI. Detection of anti–HTLV-I antibodies in the patient's serum supports the diagnosis. Confirmation usually requires demonstration of:

a. An intrathecal anti–HTLV-I immune response
b. the HTLV-I genome in the patient's peripheral blood using polymerase chain reaction (PCR) studies
c. Lymphocytes in the CSF

B. **AIDS-associated dementia** is a relatively common manifestation of HIV infection (see also Chapter 57).

1. **Pathogenesis.** HIV infects the immune and the nervous systems at about the same time (i.e., very early in the disease).
   a. The microglial cells are the main target for HIV in the CNS.
   b. HIV infection of the CNS is nonlytic. The effects on brain function are probably a consequence of metabolic changes associated with viral replication.

2. **Treatment.** Both the IQ and positron emission tomography (PET) scan of infected patients improve during treatment with **zidovudine (azidothymidine, AZT),** suggesting that the brain function changes may be reversible, at least temporarily.

V. DEGENERATIVE DISEASE CAUSED BY UNCONVENTIONAL AGENTS include **kuru, Creutzfeldt-Jakob disease,** and **Gerstmann-Sträussler disease.**

A. Introduction

1. **Kuru,** first reported in New Guinea in 1957, is a progressive, fatal, neurologic disorder. Kuru was seen only in members of the Fore tribe. The tribe members became infected by eating the brains of the deceased (a form of ritualistic cannibalism). The infectious nature of the disease was proven by Gajdusek and his coworkers, who succeeded in transmitting kuru to chimpanzees using extracts of patients' brains. When cannibalism was abandoned by the Fore tribe, the disease disappeared.

2. **Creutzfeldt-Jakob disease** is a chronic degenerative disease of the CNS characterized by progressive dementia with abnormal movements. It has a worldwide distribution and appears to be mostly sporadic.

3. **Gerstmann-Sträussler disease** appears to be an inherited disease, transmitted as an autosomal dominant trait.

B. Epidemiology

1. **Creutzfeldt-Jacob disease.** Gajdusek and his colleagues, following up on their observations with kuru, succeeded in transmitting Creutzfeldt-Jakob disease to chimpanzees using brain extracts from patients. Accidental proof of the infectivity of Creutzfeldt-Jakob disease was provided over the years by several cases of human-to-human transmission:
   a. From infected patients to neurosurgeons
   b. From patient to patient following the use of insufficiently sterilized brain electrodes
   c. Through corneal and dura mater grafts
   d. Through pituitary extracts

2. **Gerstmann-Sträussler disease.** Because it is possible to induce disease in animals using brain extracts from patients with Gerstmann-Sträussler disease, this genetic disease may also be caused by an infectious agent.

C. **Etiology.** The nature of the infectious agent or agents responsible for Creutzfeldt-Jacob disease, Gerstmann-Sträussler disease, and kuru has puzzled scientists for years. No viral particles have ever been detected in brain tissues of patients or animals with these diseases. The unusual characteristics of the infectious agent involved in Creutzfeldt-Jakob disease, which is the best characterized of the unconventional agents affecting humans,

Table 50-2. Properties of the Agent Responsible for Creutzfeldt-Jakob Disease

Classic "Viral" Properties	Atypical Physicochemical Properties	Atypical Biological Properties
Excluded by 0.1-μm filters	Not inactivated by ribonucleases, deoxyribonucleases, or ultraviolet irradiation	Very long incubation period (months to years; 30 years is common)
Titrable by LD^{50}*	Does not contain nucleic acid	Causes disease with slow, relentless progression
Inactivated at 212°F	Not inactivated by formaldehyde or glutaraldehyde	Degenerative histopathology limited to neurons: affected cells lack inclusion bodies; no evidence of inflammatory response
		No interferon production
		Not sensitive to interferon
		No change in the clinical course by immunosuppression
		No alteration of T and B cell functions

* Dilution of an infectious preparation to cause death in 50% of the animals injected.

are listed in Table 50-2. Creutzfeldt-Jacob disease appears to be caused by a totally new type of infectious agent, consisting mainly of proteins and called a **prion.** These small proteinaceous infectious particles contain an abnormal isoform of a cellular protein that is a major and necessary component.

1. **Structure.** Structural studies of prions have used material from sheep suffering from scrapie, a spontaneous degenerative brain disease with strong similarities to Creutzfeldt-Jacob disease. A protein designated **prion (PrP) 27-30** was identified in the brains of infected animals.
2. **Replication.** The mechanism of prion replication is unknown. It has been speculated that prions may serve as templates for the formation of protein crystals, and that the accumulation of mutated products causes metabolic alterations that eventually kill the neurons.

D. Pathogenesis

1. Normal cells have a membrane protein related to the prion proteins (known as PrP^{c}). This protein has a protease-resistant core that is disease-specific (PrP^{sc}) and appears to be derived from PrP 27-30 following removal of the terminal amino acids by partial proteolysis. PrP^{sc} remains almost exclusively intracellular and polymerizes into amyloid rods. By remaining intracellular and being protease resistant, PrP^{sc} does not induce any type of immune response.
2. Abnormal versions of PrP are linked to the development of neuronal degenerative diseases.

E. Clinical manifestations.

Clinical manifestations. The CNS pathology of all three diseases is almost identical: a spongiform encephalopathy with amyloid plaques and astrocytic reaction, with virtually no inflammatory response around the degenerative areas. Only the neurons are affected by a degenerative process.

F. Prevention

1. Tissues should not be collected for transplantation from patients suffering from unexplained dementia.

2. Prions resist inactivation by some of the classic disinfection methods and tissue-fixation agents but can be inactivated by autoclaving at 250°F, 15 psi for 120 minutes.

Case 1 Revisited

The combination of clinical symptoms and laboratory data suggests that this teenager with a doubtful immunization history has SSPE.

Although the findings of antibodies to the measles virus nucleocapsid, oligoclonal IgG bands in the CSF, and atrophy of the white matter on MRI are highly suggestive of the diagnosis, a stereotactic needle biopsy of the left frontal area is necessary to confirm the diagnosis.

SSPE is invariably fatal. The patient will experience progressive deterioration of brain function, until death occurs, months to years after the onset of symptoms.

Vaccination against measles protects against SSPE. This disease would be eradicated if the policy of mandatory measles vaccination were strictly enforced.

Case 2 Revisited

Neurologic disease may be the presenting symptom in a patient with AIDS. Once the diagnosis of AIDS is established, the neurologic symptoms are easier to interpret as suggestive of PML, although other neurologic diseases seen in AIDS patients should also be considered. The results of the MRI study, however, strongly support the diagnosis of PML.

Given the extremely poor prognosis of the degenerative diseases of the brain, brain biopsy is usually done to establish the diagnosis beyond any doubt.

There is no known treatment for PML; the clinical course is associated with progressive deterioration and death.

Chapter 51

Urinary Tract Infections

Gerald E. Wagner
Gabriel Virella
Victor Del Bene

Case 1

A 24-year-old woman with a 1-day history of burning of the urethra at urination, suprapubic pain, and frequent voiding of small amounts of urine makes an appointment with her primary care physician. She tells the doctor that when she has the urge to urinate, she must urinate promptly or she experiences "dribbling" of urine. She has noted her urine to be cloudy and red-tinged. She is sexually active.

Physical examination reveals a temperature of 99°F and tenderness to palpation in the midline of the abdomen superior to the pubic bone.

- *What is the diagnosis and physiopathology of this patient's condition?*
- *Are urine analysis and blood cultures indicated?*
- *If so, what would you expect to find on urinalysis and culture?*
- *Should a complete blood count be obtained?*
- *What is the best treatment for this patient?*
- *What advice and follow-up recommendations would you give to this patient?*

I. INTRODUCTION

A. Outpatient medicine. Urinary tract infections are among the most common infectious diseases seen by primary care physicians in an ambulatory setting. Community-acquired urinary tract infections are considerably more prevalent in women, and only a minority of cases present a significant therapeutic problem.

B. Inpatient medicine. Hospitalized patients also develop urinary tract infections, usually as a consequence of urethral catheterization. These infections, which usually involve debilitated hosts and pathogens resistant to multiple antibiotics, raise considerable therapeutic problems.

II. INFECTIONS OF THE URETHRA, BLADDER, AND RENAL PELVIS

A. Epidemiology. Most cases of urinary tract infection occur in ambulatory, non-hospitalized people who are otherwise healthy. Various factors predispose to urinary tract infection:

1. **Gender.** Women are 30 times more likely than men to develop urinary tract infections, partly owing to anatomic factors that facilitate contamination of the perineal area and upward invasion of the bladder by the intestinal flora.

a. The incidence of urinary tract infection in women appears to increase linearly with age. Urinary tract infection is diagnosed in approximately 1% of school-aged girls, and the incidence peaks at about 10% in women older than 60 years.
b. Men rarely develop urinary tract infections; the incidence peaks at about 1% in men older than 60 years. Obstruction of urinary flow due to prostatic hypertrophy plays an important pathogenic role in this age group.

2. **Anatomic abnormalities.** Abnormalities in the anatomy of the urinary tract, especially those resulting in obstruction or reflux and incomplete voiding of urine, predispose to urinary tract infections. Congenital anatomic abnormalities are the most common predisposing cause of recurrent urinary tract infections in young children.

3. **Mechanical factors**
   a. **Catheters, probes,** and **swabs** may introduce microorganisms into the urethra and bladder, causing infection.
   b. **Sexual intercourse** can have similar effects.
   c. **Improper use of tampons, douches,** and **vaginal swabs** may inoculate the tip of the urethra with the indigenous vaginal flora.
   d. Obstruction of urinary flow by **kidney stones** is an important predisposing factor.

4. **Metabolic factors**
   a. Disorders such as **diabetes** significantly increase the risk of urinary tract infection, probably because of the increased sugar content of the urine. The incidence of urinary tract infection in diabetic men is approximately the same as in healthy women (i.e., 30 times higher than in healthy men).
   b. Metabolic abnormalities that increase the formation of kidney stones increase the risk of urinary tract infection.

5. **Hospitalization.** Patients with indwelling urinary catheters frequently develop urinary tract infections despite the use of aseptic techniques and disinfection. The risk of infection increases with the duration of catheterization.

B. Etiology

1. **Common causative agents**
   a. **Enterobacteriaceae** indigenous to the gastrointestinal tract cause the vast majority (about 80%) of urinary tract infections.
      (1) ***Escherichia coli*** accounts for 50%–85% of cases, and ***Klebsiella pneumoniae*** is responsible for another 8%–13%.
      (2) ***Staphylococcus saprophyticus*** and **group D streptococci (enterococci)** are the only Gram-positive enteric bacteria that commonly cause urinary tract infections.
   b. **Opportunistic bacteria,** such as ***Proteus, Serratia,*** and ***Pseudomonas*** species, are frequently the cause of urinary tract infections in hospitalized patients. These organisms are usually resistant to the most common antibacterial agents.

2. **Infrequent causative agents**
   a. **Bacteria. *Staphylococcus aureus, Corynebacterium,*** and **lactobacilli** occasionally are isolated from infected urine but often are secondary to other syndromes.
   b. **Yeasts. *Candida*** species may be isolated from the urine of diabetic women or patients with indwelling catheters. The presence of the yeast usually represents only saprophytic colonization of the urethra. Ascending candidiasis of the urinary tract is rare; repeated isolation of *Candida* may indicate pyelonephritis secondary to disseminated candidiasis.
   c. **Viruses. Adenovirus type 2** is the apparent cause of acute hemorrhagic cystitis in children.

C. Clinical manifestations.

Symptoms depend on whether the infection is in the lower urinary tract (urethritis and cystitis) or in the upper urinary tract (acute nonobstructive pyelonephritis).

1. **Urethritis.** Characteristic symptoms include dysuria (i.e., pain or burning sensation during urination), frequent urination, and urgency of urination.

2. **Cystitis**
   a. Characteristic symptoms include suprapubic pain and tenderness, frequency of urination caused by diminished bladder capacity, and occasional hematuria.
   b. Although urethrocystitis may be asymptomatic, it usually causes malodorous urine and incontinence, especially in older women.
3. **Acute nonobstructive pyelonephritis**
   a. Characteristic symptoms include flank pain, renal tenderness on palpation, fever and chills, and hematuria. The symptoms of lower urinary tract infection are usually present.
   b. Nonspecific symptoms such as nausea, vomiting, diarrhea, and constipation may confuse the diagnosis.
   c. The clinical manifestations of acute pyelonephritis may resolve spontaneously in the absence of therapy.

D. Diagnosis. The diagnosis of a urinary tract infection is confirmed by demonstrating the presence of an etiologic agent, usually a bacterium, in the urine. However, a first-time, uncomplicated cystitis in a sexually active woman is often treated without requesting urinalysis or culture.

1. **Urine samples**
   a. **Collection**
      (1) The **midstream clean-catch technique** is the most commonly used collection method. If properly executed, this technique minimizes contamination by the indigenous microbes of the urethra or vagina.
         (a) The urethral meatus and adjoining areas should be thoroughly cleaned with soap and water and dried with a sterile sponge. Disinfectant solutions should not be used because they can inhibit the growth of the etiologic agent.
         (b) After voiding is initiated, the urine sample is collected in midstream.
      (2) **Catheterization** or **suprapubic aspiration** may be necessary when the patient is unable to cooperate.
   b. **Handling.** Urine samples must be transported rapidly to the clinical laboratory to prevent overgrowth by contaminating microorganisms. Refrigeration of the sample may affect results.
2. **Urine cultures.** Quantitative urine cultures may distinguish between contamination and actual infection. The collected urine is used to inoculate a variety of media, including medium selective for Enterobacteriaceae (such as MacConkey agar) and blood agar to obtain a total bacteria count. With the proper technique and dilutions, discrete colonies—each corresponding to the growth of a single bacterium—are visible after 18–24 hours of incubation.
   a. Significant bacteriuria, indicative of a urinary tract infection, was classically defined as 10^5 or more colonies/ml of properly collected and transported urine. However, recent studies suggest that $>10^2$ bacteria/ml of urine should be considered significant.
   b. Because it is difficult to obtain rapid bacterial counts in the urine at the 10^2–10^3 level, treatment in patients with clear symptoms of urinary tract infection is often initiated without obtaining bacterial counts.
   c. Contamination is indicated by isolation of large numbers of more than one species of bacteria.
3. **Microscopic examination of uncentrifuged urine** is a rapid way to estimate the number of bacteria in the specimen.
   a. Observation of at least one bacterium per high-power field ($1000\times$) is considered equivalent to 10^5 bacteria/ml of urine.
   b. The presence of leukocytes or erythrocytes is consistent with, but not diagnostic for, urinary tract infection.
   c. Squamous epithelial cells of vaginal origin indicate improper collection of urine.

E. Treatment is intended to rapidly and completely eliminate infecting bacteria to prevent complications and early recurrences.

1. **General guidelines for antibiotic therapy of urinary tract infection**
   a. **Any antibiotic eliminated by the kidney and to which an organism is susceptible can be safely and effectively used.**
      (1) Some commonly used antibiotics, such as erythromycin, are not eliminated in the urine.
      (2) Although disk-diffusion susceptibility tests are based on average serum levels of the therapeutic agent, the level of the drug in the urine may be 10–100 times higher.
   b. **Culture and susceptibility testing** may not be necessary for uncomplicated lower urinary tract infections, but is important for pyelonephritis and complicated infections. In these cases, susceptibility testing mostly provides information to be used if the patient does not respond to empiric antibiotic therapy.

2. **Lower urinary tract infections**
   a. The proper dose of an antimicrobial agent and the duration of therapy for lower urinary tract infections are controversial.
      (1) For **uncomplicated infections with Enterobacteriaceae,** conventional therapy consists of moderate doses of a broad-spectrum antibiotic. **Amoxicillin** or **trimethoprim–sulfamethoxazole** given orally for 3–7 days is the most commonly prescribed regimen in such cases. It has been proposed that a single large dose of either amoxicillin or trimethoprim–sulfamethoxazole may be sufficient to cure uncomplicated urethritis or cystitis.
      (2) **Fluoroquinolones** are effective against ***Pseudomonas*** and ***Proteus*** species, which are often resistant to more common antimicrobial agents.
   b. A prompt response after 1–2 days of antibiotic treatment is expected in uncomplicated cystitis in women. If the symptoms persist, urinalysis, urine culture, and antibiotic-susceptibility testing are indicated.

3 **Acute pyelonephritis** is a more severe condition, with considerable potential for relapse or serious complications when adequate therapy is not instituted promptly.
   a. Either a **fluoroquinolone** or a **third-generation cephalosporin,** such as ceftriaxone, is effective and is the best choice for empiric therapy.
   b. Administration regimens of 3–10 days are successful, with slightly higher rates of cure obtained with longer administration of higher doses.

4. **Complicated UTI,** in which infection is associated with anatomic or functional abnormalities of the urinary tract, is also effectively treated with **fluoroquinolones.**

F. Complications

1. **Bacteremia** and **septic shock.** Urinary tract infection is the major source of Gram-negative rods in the blood stream.
   a. In patients with urinary tract abnormalities and underlying disease, bacteremia and septic shock are serious and frequently fatal complications of urinary tract infections.
   b. Performing a urologic procedure on a patient with a urinary tract infection can introduce microorganisms into the circulation.
   c. Renal or perirenal abscesses as a sequelae of urinary tract infection can cause bacteremia.

2. **Severe kidney damage** resulting from papillary necrosis has been described in patients recovering from acute pyelonephritis.

3. **End-stage chronic pyelonephritis** as the result of a urinary tract infection is rare.

III. PROSTATITIS is a term that refers to inflammatory conditions of the prostate that are usually infectious in origin.

A. Etiology

1. **Bacterial prostatitis** may be acute or chronic. The most common etiologic agents of urinary tract infections (i.e., ***E. coli, Klebsiella,*** and ***Proteus***) and ***Pseudomonas*** com-

monly cause prostatitis as well. *Streptococcus faecalis* and *Staphylococcus epidermidis* are less common causes of bacterial prostatitis.

2. **Nonbacterial prostatitis**
   a. **Bacteria.** Nonbacterial prostatitis (i.e., prostatitis with negative bacterial cultures) may actually be caused by **anaerobic bacteria, *Mycoplasma,*** and ***Chlamydia.***
   b. **Parasites** (e.g., *Trichomonas vaginalis*) and **fungi** (e.g., *C. albicans*) rarely cause prostatitis.
   c. **Viruses.** There is no compelling evidence that viruses cause prostatitis, although many cases of symptomatic disease occur following viral infections of the upper respiratory tract.

B. Clinical manifestations

1. **Acute bacterial prostatitis**
   a. **Symptoms** include fever, chills, and other symptoms of systemic involvement. The characteristic symptoms of lower urinary tract infection are present; nonspecific complaints such as anorexia and myalgia also are common.
   b. **Physical examination findings.** The prostate is swollen, firm, indurated, warm to the touch, and very tender.

2. **Chronic bacterial prostatitis** is more subtle in clinical presentation. The patient usually has a history of recurrent urinary tract infection.
   a. **Symptoms.** This syndrome is unique for its absence of specific symptoms until the patient complains of cystitis.
   b. **Laboratory findings.** The patient has significant bacteriuria and pyuria during the symptomatic phase of disease.
   c. **Physical examination findings.** The prostate is usually small and firm; it may be tender during the symptomatic phase.

C. Diagnosis

Diagnosis of prostatitis is made on the basis of clinical manifestations and culture results. Accurate diagnosis of the type of prostatitis is essential for effective therapy.

1. **Bacterial prostatitis.** Diagnosis of acute and chronic bacterial prostatitis is generally straightforward.
   a. In **acute bacterial prostatitis,** urinalysis typically shows significant bacteriuria and a large number of leukocytes, particularly granulocytes.
   b. In **chronic bacterial prostatitis,** the microscopic characteristics of expressed prostatic secretions may be diagnostically useful.

2. **Nonbacterial prostatitis** is a diagnosis of exclusion. Negative cultures on conventional media do not detect infection caused by *Mycoplasma* and *Chlamydia* species.

D. Treatment

1. Prostatitis is best treated with trimethoprim–sulfamethoxazole because trimethoprim penetrates prostatic tissue well. The **fluoroquinolones** are the best choice for patients resistant or allergic to trimethoprim.

2. If the patient is severely ill with an acute form of the disease, parenteral administration of **cephalosporins, aminoglycosides,** or both may be required.

E. Complications

1. **Pyelonephritis** is a common complication of bacterial prostatitis when antimicrobial therapy is delayed.

2. Other complications are the same as those of any severe urinary tract infection (see II F).

3. No direct evidence supports a role for bacterial prostatitis in carcinoma.

Case 1 Revisited

This young woman has the classic symptoms and signs of cystitis, commonly called "honeymoon cystitis" because of its occurrence after intercourse. The responsible organism is likely to be a variety of *Escherichia coli* that expresses adhesion factors, allowing it to colonize the urogenital mucosa. This organism was most likely colonizing the vaginal mucosa when vaginal intercourse caused its migration to the urethra, where it multiplied, eventually reaching the bladder. Inflammation of the mucosae of the bladder and urethra causes exaggerated stimulation of the superficial bladder nerves, producing the symptoms described by the patient.

In a patient with a first-time, uncomplicated cystitis that occurred following sexual activity, laboratory studies such as urinalysis and culture may not be necessary prior to instituting treatment with antimicrobials. Blood cultures are certainly not indicated because bacteremia is rare in cases of uncomplicated cystitis and the patient has no signs or symptoms that would suggest bacteremia or sepsis.

Urinalysis in this patient is likely to be abnormal, showing pyuria (leukocytes in the urine) and hematuria. Bacteria would likely be detected on a Gram stain of the urinary sediment, and culture would likely yield over 10^5 colonies of *E. coli*/ml of urine.

A complete blood count is not indicated, because an increase in peripheral blood leukocytes is rarely seen in patients with cystitis and, if present, would not change the diagnosis or treatment.

Oral administration of trimethoprim—sulfamethoxazole for 3 days would be an adequate regimen for this patient.

After 3 days, the patient should return to the physician for a follow-up evaluation. At that time, her symptoms should be gone and she should remain symptom-free thereafter. The patient should be advised to empty her bladder after intercourse to prevent colonization of the urethra.

Chapter 52

Gastroenteritis and Food Poisoning

Gabriel Virella
Edmund Farrar

Case 1

A healthy 4-year-old boy fell acutely ill with fever, nausea and vomiting, abdominal cramps, and loose stools. On the third day, malaise and bloody diarrhea developed, and he was given an oral antibiotic. On the fifth day, he became pale and lethargic and was admitted to the hospital. He lives in a suburb and attends a child-care facility, but no other children there, and no family members, are ill. Meals are consumed at home and occasionally at restaurants. There are no sick pets in the home and no other animal exposures. On admission, the boy's vital signs are as follows: temperature, 101°F; pulse rate, 130 beats/min; respiration rate, 35 breaths/min; and blood pressure 80/40 mm Hg. The boy is awake but lethargic. Head and neck examination reveals pale mucosae. There is moderate diffuse abdominal tenderness without masses or rebound tenderness. Skin turgor is reduced. Rectal exam shows maroon, liquid feces. There is minimal urine output, as measured by an indwelling catheter.

- □ *What is the meaning of bloody diarrhea?*
- □ *Is the infection localized to the gastrointestinal tract or disseminated?*
- □ *How can the lethargy, paleness of mucosae, reduced skin turgor, and reduced urinary output be interpreted?*
- □ *What is the causative agent?*
- □ *What was the most likely source of infection?*
- □ *Should this patient be treated with antibiotics?*

Case 2

A previously healthy 55-year-old businessman is admitted to the emergency service at 2:00 A.M. with nausea, vomiting, and profuse watery diarrhea. His vital signs showed tachycardia (120 beats/min), blood pressure of 120/60 mm Hg, and a temperature of 98.3°F. He is given intravenous fluid replacement and shows progressive improvement. He is discharged by noon the next day. At 3:00 A.M. on the same morning, another patient is brought to the hospital. Both had attended the same wedding. A quick check of area emergency rooms reveals that ten other wedding guests have also sought medical care for similar symptoms. The parents of the bride report that several other guests have fallen ill but have not been taken to the hospital.

- □ *What is the most likely cause of this outbreak of diarrheal disease?*
- □ *How could the diagnosis be confirmed?*
- □ *How could the source of the outbreak be traced?*
- □ *How should the patients be treated?*

I. INTRODUCTION

A. Definitions

1. **Diarrhea** is the excretion of more than 200 g of stool/day. The stool usually has a loose consistency, and the frequency of excretion increases. Diarrhea can be caused by bacteria, viruses, or parasites. There are two basic types of diarrhea:
   a. **Profuse secretory diarrhea,** characterized by the frequent passage of watery stools, is usually caused by the secretion of **exotoxins** or by **viral infection** of the intestinal mucosa.
   b. **Dysentery** is characterized by the frequent passage of stools with low volume that contain mucus and pus, and by abdominal cramps and pain during defecation (tenesmus). Dysentery and bloody diarrhea are usually caused by the release of **cytotoxins** or by the **invasion** of the mucosa by bacteria or protozoa.

2. **Gastroenteritis** is an infection (acute or chronic) of the gastrointestinal tract that includes diarrhea and symptoms of gastric irritation (e.g., nausea, vomiting, epigastric pain). Bacteria and viruses are the most common etiologic agents.

3. **Enterocolitis** is an infection of the lower gastrointestinal tract that does not produce symptoms of gastric irritation.

4. **Food poisoning** is a type of acute gastroenteritis in which the ingestion of a single meal can be identified as the vehicle for infection. Bacteria and bacterial toxins are most commonly implicated in classic cases of food poisoning.

B. Prevalence

1. Acute gastroenteritis is one of the most common forms of infectious disease.

2. The prevalence of particular causative agents depends on the **age of the patient,** the **season of the year,** and **socioeconomic factors.** For example, in the United States, rotaviruses are the most common cause of diarrhea in infants, particularly in the colder months, while in older individuals these viruses are rarely implicated as causes of acute gastroenteritis. Cholera and typhoid fever, very prevalent in underdeveloped and developing countries, are rarely diagnosed in industrialized nations.

C. Clinical presentation. Diarrhea, vomiting, abdominal pain, and fever, in different combinations, are the most common clinical symptoms of acute gastroenteritis.

1. Fever in a patient with gastroenteritis usually means that the causative agent is invasive. The invasion can be limited to the intestinal mucosa, extend to the submucosa, or spread systemically through the circulation (bacteremia).

2. Profuse, watery diarrhea usually indicates the effects of a toxin.

II. INFECTIOUS DIARRHEA AND GASTROENTERITIS

A. Epidemiology. There are two main modes for transmitting infectious agents that cause diarrhea and gastroenteritis.

1. **Fecal-oral transmission** may involve:
   a. Direct person-to-person transmission (usually involving crowding and poor personal hygiene; seen in jails, mental institutions, and day care centers)
   b. Contamination of meat, poultry products, or seafood during processing
   c. Contamination of food during or after cooking

2. **Food-borne transmission** may involve distribution to consumers of meat, poultry products, seafood, or vegetables that have been contaminated before processing (e.g., by a zoonotic organism).

B. Pathogenesis of bacterial diarrhea

1. Colonization and proliferation

a. Infectious diarrhea may result from:
- **(1)** Multiplication of an organism in the gastrointestinal tract
- **(2)** The mobilization of host defense mechanisms in an attempt to eliminate the invading infectious agent

b. All diarrhea-producing bacteria adhere to intestinal mucosal cells. Adherence is usually mediated by surface proteins such as fimbriae (colonization factors) and non-fimbrial adhesins.

c. Once bacteria start proliferating in the intestine, they can:
- **(1)** Induce structural abnormalities of the mucosal cells via poorly defined mechanisms, which result in increased excretion of fluids and electrolytes
- **(2)** Release toxins
- **(3)** Invade the intestinal mucosa

2. Noninvasive bacteria

a. The most important toxin-producing enteropathogenic bacteria are:
- **(1)** *Vibrio cholerae*
- **(2)** Enterotoxigenic *Escherichia coli* (ETEC)
- **(3)** Verotoxin-producing (VTEC, EHEC, *E. coli* O157:H7)
- **(4)** *Shigella dysenteriae* type 1
- **(5)** *Clostridium perfringens*
- **(6)** *Clostridium difficile*
- **(7)** *Vibrio parahaemolyticus*
- **(8)** Some strains of *Staphylococcus aureus*

b. Toxin-producing bacteria may release **enterotoxins** or **cytotoxins.**
- **(1) Enterotoxins** (e.g., cholera toxin) produce fluid secretion by several mechanisms, including stimulation of adenylate cyclase activity. Enterotoxins produce an essentially pure biochemical lesion and have virtually no histopathologic effects on the intestinal mucosa.
- **(2) Cytotoxins** (e.g., Shiga toxin, Verotoxin, and *C. difficile* toxin) have enterotoxic as well as general cytotoxic activity.
  - **(a) Bloody diarrhea.** At the intestinal level, cytotoxin-producing bacteria cause tissue damage, leading to inflammation and blood loss.
  - **(b) Hemolytic-uremic syndrome.** Shiga toxin and the verotoxin produced by *E. coli* O157:H7 cause massive endothelial cell damage, which results in disseminated thrombosis with massive consumption of platelets and clotting factors. This, in turn, leads to thrombocytopenia and coagulopathy. These toxins also cause vasoconstriction and microangiopathic hemolytic anemia. In the kidney, the combined effects of endothelial toxicity on glomerular capillaries and hemoglobin toxicity on tubules lead to acute renal failure with uremia, hypertension, and encephalopathy. Death occurs in the most severe cases.

3. Invasive organisms (e.g., *Salmonella enteritidis, Shigella*) penetrate the bowel epithelium. These organisms stimulate an intense acute inflammatory reaction with accumulation of large numbers of polymorphonuclear (PMN) leukocytes. This direct damage to the intestinal mucosa and the accompanying inflammatory reaction results in the presence of blood, mucus, and inflammatory cells in the stool.

C. Diagnosis.

Identifying the precise cause of acute gastroenteritis is a low priority issue when the patient is only mildly ill with profuse diarrhea or vomiting and no constitutional symptoms. When an outbreak of a contagious form of diarrhea is suspected, or when the disease is severe or associated with constitutional symptoms, identification of the responsible microorganism becomes important.

1. Patient history. Clues to the causative organism may be gleaned from the **type of diarrhea, incubation time,** and **associated symptoms** (Tables 52-1, 52-2, and 52-3).

Table 52-1. Noninvasive Versus Invasive Diarrhea

	Noninvasive	Invasive (Bacterial/Parasitic)
Stool	Profuse secretory (Severe, watery)	Dysentery (blood, mucus, PMN leukocytes)
Fever	No	Yes
Systemic toxicity	No	Yes
Abdominal pain	Mild	Severe (cramping, tenesmus)
Site of infection	Small intestine	Colon

PMN = polymorphonuclear.

Table 52-2. Features of Specific Types of Noninvasive Bacterial Diarrhea

	Vibrio cholerae	*Escherichia coli*	*Clostridium perfringens*	*Bacillus cereus**	*Staphylococcus aureus*†
Incubation (hours)	12–72	24–72	6–12	3–8	1–6
Duration (hours)	48–120	24–48	12–24	12–24	6–12
Abdominal cramps	0	+	+ + + +	+ +	+ +
Vomiting	+	±	+	+ +	+ + + +

* Diarrhea can be caused by preformed toxin or by toxin elaborated in the intestine by proliferating bacteria.
† Diarrhea can be caused by ingestion of toxin-contaminated food.

2. **Laboratory diagnosis**
   a. **Fecal specimens** are preferred for the diagnosis of gastroenteritis with watery diarrhea. A simplified flow chart of the steps followed in a study of a fecal sample is shown in Figure 52-1.
   b. **Intestinal biopsy samples** may provide more information if invasive diarrhea is suspected.
   c. **Blood cultures** are indicated when constitutional symptoms are present.
   d. **Enzyme immunoassay (EIA)** may aid in the identification of viral agents or exotoxins.

Table 52-3. Features of Specific Types of Invasive Bacterial Diarrhea

	Shigella	*Escherichia coli*	*Salmonella*	*Yersinia enterocolitica*
Incubation (hours)	24–72	24–72	8–48	1–6
Duration (hours)	48–120	24–48	12–24	6–12
Abdominal pain	+ + + +	+ + + +	+	+ +
Vomiting	+ +	+	+	+ +
Fever	+ +	+ +	+ + + +	+ +

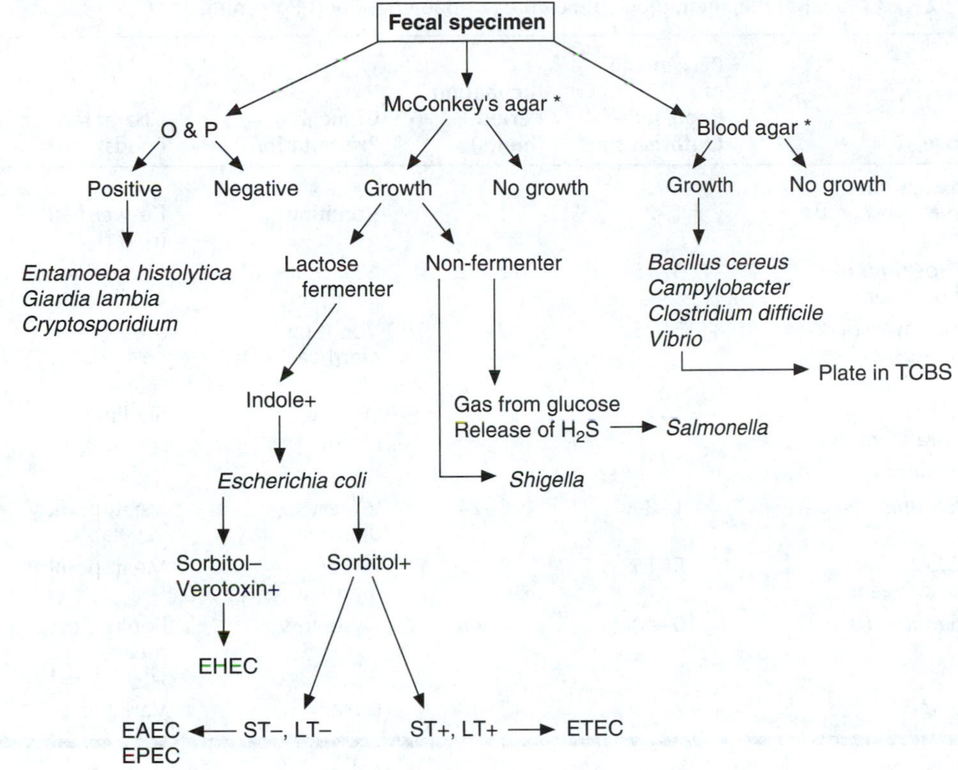

FIGURE 52-1. Simplified protocol for identifying enteropathogenic bacteria. MacConkey agar and blood agar are basic culture media that may vary according to the suspected organism. It should be noted that final identification usually requires more complete biochemical or serologic tests. *EAEC* = enteroaggregative *Escherichia coli; EHEC* = enterohemorrhagic *E. coli*; *EPEC* = enteropathogenic *E. coli*; *ETEC* = enterotoxigenic *E. coli*; H_2S = hydrogen sulfide; *LT* = heat-labile toxin; *O&P* = ova and parasites; *ST* = heat-stable toxin; *TCBS* = thiosulfate-citrate-sucrose-bile salts agar.

D. Treatment. While most cases of noninvasive diarrhea are usually self-limited and do not require specific therapy, cases of invasive diarrhea are usually more severe and require more aggressive therapy.

1. Cases of acute gastroenteritis with profuse watery diarrhea and no constitutional symptoms can be treated supportively with fluid and electrolyte administration. Oral rehydration is usually adequate in previously healthy patients. Very young children and elderly individuals may require intravenous fluid administration.
2. In cases with evidence of mucosal invasion (mucosal diarrhea, inflammatory cells in fecal samples) or with constitutional symptoms, more aggressive therapy, including antibiotics, is indicated. As in many other infectious diseases, if the patient is severely ill, empiric treatment should be initiated as soon as proper samples are collected, to be revised when the causative agent is identified and characterized.
3. Hospitalization and aggressive therapy are indicated whenever the symptoms suggest septicemia or the hemolytic-uremic syndrome.

III. FOOD POISONING

A. INTRODUCTION

1. A classic case of food poisoning has the following features:
   a. **Similar symptoms in several members of a group** sharing a meal
   b. **Acute onset** a few hours after food ingestion

Table 52-4. Clinical and Epidemiological Features of Bacterial Food Poisoning

Cause	Percentage of Reported Outbreaks	Incubation Period (hours)	Clinical Presentation	Characteristic Foods
Intoxication				
Bacillus cereus	1–2	1–6	Vomiting	Re-warmed fried rice
Clostridium botulinum	5–15	12–72	Neuromuscular paralysis	Canned foods of all types
Staphylococcus aureus	15–25	2–4	Vomiting, diarrhea	Meats, custards, salads
Vibrio parahaemolyticus	1–2	10–24	Watery diarrhea	Shellfish
Infection				
Bacillus cereus	1–2	6–24	Watery diarrhea	Meat, poultry, vegetables
Clostridium perfringens	5–15	9–15	Watery diarrhea	Meat, poultry
Salmonella	10–30	6–48	Dysentery	Poultry, eggs, meat, vegetables
Shigella	2–5	12–48	Dysentery	Variable

2. Food poisoning may be caused by:
   a. **Intoxication,** the ingestion of food containing preformed bacterial toxins
   b. **Infectious food poisoning,** the ingestion of viable infectious agents

B. Diagnosis. The type of food ingested, incubation period, and type or severity of symptoms may help establish the cause of the outbreak (Table 52-4).

1. As a rule, incubation periods of less than 12 hours indicate ingestion of **preformed toxins.**
2. Longer incubation periods indicate ingestion of **live bacteria** that must proliferate before reaching the critical mass necessary for the emergence of clinical symptoms.
3. Identification of the causative agent requires isolation of an infectious agent (e.g., in stool samples) or detection of the toxin in contaminated food.

C. Treatment. The general approach to therapy is similar to the approach for acute gastroenteritis (see II D).

1. Food poisoning by toxin-containing foods is a self-limited disease that requires **supportive therapy** only (most importantly, rehydration). Infants and elderly individuals may require more aggressive supportive therapy than previously healthy adults.
2. Administration of **antibacterial agents** is indicated only when the patient has constitutional symptoms and a live organism is suspected of causing the food poisoning. **Empiric therapy** directed against the most likely causative agents should be initiated immediately.

IV. VIRAL DIARRHEA

A. Etiology. There are two major viral causes of diarrhea in humans: the Norwalk virus and related viruses (Norwalk-like viruses) and the rotaviruses (Table 52-5).

Table 52-5. Norwalk-like Viruses and Rotavirus

	Norwalk-like Viruses	Rotavirus
Epidemiology	Epidemics in family or community; winter occurrence	Usually sporadic
Age	Older children, adults	Infants, young children
Transmission	Fecal-oral: contaminated water and shellfish	Fecal-oral
Incubation	1–2 days	1–3 days
Illness	Explosive vomiting or diarrhea; self-limited (1–2 days)	Severe diarrhea (5–8 days)
Prevalence	⅓ of epidemics in U.S.	½ of cases of severe infantile diarrhea in world
Diagnosis	Immunoassays	Immunoassays; gene probes
Virus	27-nm calicivirus	70-nm "spoked wheel" reovirus

B. Clinical manifestations. Viral diarrheas are **self-limited diseases** with no systemic invasion. Their clinical significance is directly related to the severity and duration of diarrhea or vomiting, which may result in dehydration.

C. Treatment

1. Most cases can be managed with **supportive measures** (oral fluid replenishment) on an outpatient basis.
2. Infants and debilitated patients may require **hospital admission** and intravenous administration of fluids and electrolytes.
3. No specific antiviral agents or vaccines are available for rotavirus or the Norwalk virus.

V. PARASITIC DIARRHEA

A. Etiology. Three protozoans account for most cases of infectious parasitic diarrhea (Table 52-6).

1. *Entamoeba histolytica* and *Giardia lamblia* can infect previously healthy individuals, but *Cryptosporidium* and related coccidians (e.g., *Isospora belli*) usually infect only immunocompromised individuals (e.g., patients with AIDS).
2. Rare outbreaks of diarrheal disease associated with water contaminated with *Cryptosporidium* and vegetables contaminated with *Cyclospora* have been reported.

B. Treatment entails administration of an appropriate antiparasitic agent. No effective treatment for *Cryptosporidium* infection is available.

Table 52-6. Most Common Parasitic Causes of Infectious Diarrhea

	Entamoeba histolytica	*Giardia lambia*	*Cryptosporidium*
Distribution	Worldwide; prevalent in Mexico and South America	Worldwide; prevalent in certain areas such as the Rocky Mountains, many developing countries, and the Soviet Union	Worldwide; primarily a zoonosis but also common in healthy adults and children
Disease	Amebic dysentery	Mild to moderate chronic diarrhea	Mild short-lived diarrheal disease in immunocompetent individuals; severe, relentless, life-threatening diarrhea in patients with AIDS
Complications	Abscesses (liver, lung, and brain in decreasing order of frequency)	Malabsorption	Malabsorption
Transmission	Person-to-person by fecal-oral route (contaminated water and food most frequent; sexual transmission possible)	Person-to-person by fecal-oral route (contaminated water most frequent; common in day-care centers; sexual transmission possible)	Ingestion of contaminated animal products
Diagnosis	O&P (tetranucleated cysts; erythrocyte-containing trophozoites)	O&P (typical trophozoites)	O&P (acid-fast oocysts)
Treatment	Metronidazole followed by iodoquinol	Metronidazole; quinacrine	No effective treatment

O&P = ova and parasites.

Case 1 Revisited

The bloody diarrhea strongly suggests that the patient has an intestinal infection caused by invasive or cytotoxin-producing bacteria.

The constitutional symptoms (fever, tachycardia, tachypnea, hypotension, and lethargy) suggest that the infection may be disseminated. Reduced skin turgor suggests dehydration. Paleness of mucosae and reduced urinary output suggest that the patient is anemic and has developed or is developing acute renal failure. These symptoms suggest the hemolytic-uremic syndrome. The diarrheal prodrome is associated with the majority of cases of this syndrome, but is not always present.

The precise cause of the disease can be determined only by culturing fecal material and blood. However, *E. coli* O157:H7 is the most likely cause of the hemolytic-uremic syndrome in the United States.

The fact that the child represents an isolated case of diarrhea complicates the investigation of a possible source for the infectious agent. However, a major means of *E. coli* O157:H7 transmission in recent years has been via the ingestion of undercooked hamburgers at restaurants.

For a severely ill child with symptoms of septicemia and the hemolytic-uremic syndrome, emergency admission and vigorous treatment with supportive measures and antibiotics are indicated. Supportive measures include correction of fluid and electrolyte imbalances, emergency dialysis, transfusion of packed erythrocytes, and plasmapheresis. The prognosis is guarded, but is better in patients who present with diarrhea and then develop the hemolytic-uremic syndrome than in those who do not present with diarrhea.

Case 2 Revisited

The wedding guests most likely are experiencing gastroenteritis secondary to the ingestion of food contaminated with a preformed toxin, as suggested by the short incubation time (less than 12 hours). *S. aureus* or *B. cereus* enterotoxins are the most likely causes.

To confirm the diagnosis, it would be essential to recover an enteropathogenic bacterium or its toxin from the patient. Culture of fecal samples or tests for enterotoxin can help to definitively identify the causative organism.

The source of the outbreak is most likely a food handler and can only be traced by isolating the organism from the contaminated food and testing all food handlers involved in the preparation of the meal to determine wether one of them could be the source of the infection. In the case of *S. aureus* food poisoning, this can be achieved by phage typing all isolates and determining whether one of the handlers carries *S. aureus* of the same type as the one isolated from the food. Often leftover food is not available, in which case, the source of infection can not be traced.

The treatment for toxin-induced gastroenteritis is supportive. Even if an infection is suspected, the administration of antibiotics is usually unnecessary because the infection is usually self-limiting.

Chapter 53

Infections Caused by Anaerobic Bacteria

Lisa L. Steed
Victor Del Bene

Case 1

A 33-year-old man is brought to the emergency room by his family. He has been drinking heavily and might have been unconscious for several hours. On physical examination, the patient appears stuporous, has a temperature of 103°F and has a fetid odor on his breath. Thoracic examination reveals dullness to percussion and absent breath sounds over the right posterior mid-lung field. The remaining physical examination is unremarkable.

- □ *What is the most likely diagnosis?*
- □ *What is the pathogenesis of his disease?*
- □ *What is the best treatment?*

I. GENERAL CHARACTERISTICS OF ANAEROBIC BACTERIA

A. Metabolic properties. Anaerobic bacteria are metabolically inefficient.

1. Anaerobes produce their energy by fermentation, which generates three to four molecules of adenosine triphosphate (ATP) per molecule of glucose.
2. Anaerobic metabolism produces short-chain fatty acids, methane, and hydrogen.
3. Anaerobic bacteria often require certain growth factors that they cannot produce. They tend to grow symbiotically.
4. Anaerobic bacteria cannot detoxify oxygen radicals because they lack superoxide dismutase, peroxidases, and catalase; therefore, they die if exposed to air for even a short time.

B. Physical requirements

1. Anaerobes require reduced oxygen tension (less than 10%) and elevated carbon dioxide levels (10%–30%) for optimal growth.
2. An electromotive potential of −150 to −250 mV is required for anaerobic growth. (In aerobic conditions, the electromotive potential ranges from +170 to +250 mV).

C. Distribution

1. Anaerobic organisms are found in marine sediments and deep sea water; in sand, soil, and mud (sometimes as spores, e.g., some clostridial species); and in sewage and fecal matter.
2. Body cavities in humans and other animals provide habitats for anaerobic organisms. Most anaerobes involved in mixed infections are part of the normal flora in humans.
   a. **Oral cavity.** Anaerobic Gram-positive cocci, mostly streptococci, predominate in the gingivodental sulcus, with up to 10^{12} bacteria/ml. Both *Fusobacterium nucleatum* and *F. necrophorum* can be isolated from approximately 50% of normal

adults. *Prevotella melaninogenica* and *P. oralis* can be isolated from about 40% of normal 5-year-olds and almost all teenagers. *Veillonella* species can also be isolated from the oral cavity.

b. Intestinal tract. The concentration of anaerobes in the stool is 10^{11} bacteria/g. (The concentration of *Escherichia coli* is only 10^8/g.) *Bacteroides* species predominate in two-thirds of normal adults, and *Bifidobacterium* species predominate in the remaining one-third. Among the *Bacteroides, B. thetaiotaomicron* and *B. vulgatus* are the most numerous in the intestine. *B. fragilis* is the most pathogenic, although it constitutes less than 1% of the intestinal anaerobic flora.

c. Vagina. The normal flora in a healthy woman, which can reach 10^8 bacteria/ml, is predominantly *Lactobacillus* species. Other common anaerobes are *P. melaninogenica, P. disiens,* and *P. bivia.*

II. ANAEROBIC INFECTIONS

A. Epidemiology

1. Factors predisposing to infection

a. Surgery is the underlying factor in approximately one-third of patients, closely followed by **solid tumors.** Anaerobic infections associated with malignant processes occur when the malignant tissue erodes through a mucosal surface and takes contaminating organisms with it.

b. Other factors include **immunosuppression, diabetes mellitus** (because of poor peripheral vasculature and open ulcers), **leukemia,** and **lymphomas.**

2. Incidence (Table 53-1)

a. Anaerobic cocci are found as pure cultures in about 5%–15% of infections and as mixed cultures (with other anaerobic and aerobic organisms) in about 85%–95% of infections.

b. Anaerobic bacilli cause about one-third of anaerobic infections and are often isolated as pure cultures from the site of infection. ***B. fragilis*** and ***B. thetaiotaomicron*** are the species most often isolated from infections (usually subdiaphragmatic). *B. fragilis* is the predominant anaerobe recovered from intraabdominal infections (abscesses, peritonitis) or bacteremia, although it represents less than 0.5% of the normal colonic microflora.

B. Pathogenesis.

Anaerobic infections can affect a variety of organs and tissues, including the brain, peri-oral tissues, soft tissues in any part of the body, pelvic and abdominal cavities, lungs, and liver (Table 53-2). In most instances, the infection is localized in the form of an abscess.

1. Virulence factors

a. Anaerobic cocci are seldom isolated in pure culture from the site of an infection. It is presumed that these organisms do not have potent virulence factors. The pre-

Table 53-1. Anaerobic Bacteria Most Commonly Isolated from Human Infections

Organism	Recovery (percent)
Bacteroides	34
Clostridium	20
Anaerobic cocci	18
Fusobacterium	5
Others	23

Table 53-2. Anaerobic Bacteria and the Infections Most Often Associated with Them

Organism	Infection
Spore-forming Gram-positive bacilli	
Clostridium perfringens	Gas gangrene
Clostridium difficile	Antibiotic-associated diarrhea; pseudomembranous colitis
Clostridium tetani	Tetanus
Non–spore-forming Gram-positive bacilli	
Actinomyces israelii	Actinomycoses of head, chest, or abdomen
Propionibacterium acnes	Acne vulgaris; post-cataract surgery infections
Gram-positive cocci	
Peptostreptococcus	
P. asaccharolyticus	Gynecologic and intraabdominal infections
P. magnus	Bone, joint, and intraabdominal infections
P. prevotti	Gynecologic, intraabdominal, bone, and joint infections
P. anaerobius	Gynecologic and intraabdominal infections
Streptococcus	
S. constellatus	Gynecologic and abdominal infections
S. intermedius	Human bite wound infections
S. anginosus	Gynecologic and abdominal infections
Gram-negative cocci	
Veillonella	Head, neck, dental and pulmonary infections; human bite wound infections
Gram-negative bacilli	
Bacteroides	
B. fragilis	Intraabdominal infections; bacteremia
B. thetaiotaomicron	Intraabdominal infections; bacteremia
Prevotella melaninogenica	Head, neck, dental, and pulmonary infections; human bite wound infections
Fusobacterium	
F. nucleatum	Head, neck, dental, and pulmonary infections; human bite wound infections
F. necrophorum	Peritonsillar abscesses; head, neck, dental, and pulmonary infections; human bite wound infections

cise role of anaerobic cocci isolated in conjunction with other clearly pathogenic bacteria is not well defined.

b. Anaerobic bacilli have well-defined virulence factors.

(1) Enzymes

(a) Both *Bacteroides* and *Fusobacterium* produce enzymes that contribute to their pathogenicity: collagenases, neuraminidases, DNases, heparinases, and proteases. Secretion of these enzymes allows the organisms to become locally invasive, digesting normal tissue and eventually leading to the formation of abscesses.

(b) Eighty-five percent of *B. fragilis* isolates and fifteen percent of *P. melaninogenica* isolates produce β-lactamase. *B. fragilis* engages in conjugative exchange of transposons containing β-lactamase genes without detectable plasmid carriers, a process that has also been described in enterococci.

(2) **Toxins**
   (a) **Endotoxins.** The potency of the endotoxins of different anaerobic Gram-negative bacilli is variable.
      (i) The endotoxin produced by *Bacteroides* does not contain lipid A and is thus less biologically active than classical endotoxin; therefore, *Bacteroides* species are not as likely to cause severe sepsis as other Gram-negative organisms.
      (ii) Fusobacteria have a potent endotoxin.
   (b) **Exotoxins.** The pathogenesis of *Clostridium* species depends largely on the production of endotoxins, which include cytotoxins (such as *C. perfringens* α and β toxins and *C. difficile* toxin B), enterotoxins (such as *C. difficile* toxin A), and neurotoxins (such as tetanospasmin of *C. tetani* and botulin of *C. botulinum*).

(3) **Capsules.** *Bacteroides* has an abscess-promoting and antiphagocytic polysaccharide capsule. Injection of capsular material results in massive attraction of leukocytes, forming an abscess.

(4) **Spheroplast transformation.** Fusobacteria often transform into spheroplasts that lack a cell wall. In the process, these organism release endotoxin and can cause septic shock. Their ability to survive as spheroplasts is due to lack of susceptibility to β-lactam antibiotics.

2. Host response

a. Phagocytosis. The primary host defense against anaerobic infection is the phagocytic cells, particularly polymorphonuclear (PMN) leukocytes. *Bacteroides* infections may be associated with large amounts of pus; other anaerobes cause considerably less pus formation.

b. Antibody formation. The capsular material of *B. fragilis* is immunogenic and elicits strong humoral immune responses. Unfortunately, the resulting antibodies are produced for a relatively short time and are strain-specific. Because there are many different strains of *B. fragilis,* reinfections are frequent and immunization programs are not practical.

3. Pathogenic sequence

a. Trauma decreases the blood supply, resulting in decreased oxygen tension and a reduction of the previously stable electromotive potential.

b. Contamination may come from a spore outside the body, but the bacterial source is often the normal flora from a contiguous mucosal surface such as the gingivodental sulcus, the gastrointestinal tract (especially the colon), or the vagina.

c. Proliferation

(1) Trauma and contamination together produce an area of ischemic necrosis where facultative anaerobes begin to proliferate. The facultative anaerobes further deplete the oxygen remaining in the necrotic area.

(2) Leukocytes and serum move into the area; the tissue turgor pressure increases; and the blood supply is further diminished. Consequently, the oxygen content is reduced further, and the electromotive potential continues to fall.

(3) Conditions are favorable for the growth of more fastidious anaerobes, and a mixed infection is established.

d. Selection. The chain of pathogenic events becomes a cycle in which more leukocytes are attracted to the area, turgor continues to increase, and so on, until not even the facultative anaerobes can survive, and the infection becomes completely anaerobic.

C. Etiology

1. Primary lung abscesses are usually secondary to the aspiration of material from the digestive tract.

a. The sources of contamination most often are organisms whose normal habitat is the gingivodental sulcus, such as *F. nucleatum* (recovered in over 50% of patients), *P. melaninogenica* (recovered from about 50% of patients), and peptostreptococci. Aerobic organisms, such as *Streptococcus pneumoniae, Staphylococcus*

Table 53-3. Distribution of Aerobes and Anaerobes in Specimens from Human Infections*

Organisms Cultured	Type of Specimen					
	Purulent Exudates		Blood		Other	
Anaerobes	37	79	3	3	35	85
Anaerobes + aerobes	42		0		50	
Aerobes	21		97		15	

* Values expressed as a percentage of total for each type of specimen.

aureus, Streptococcus pyogenes, and *Klebsiella pneumoniae* (the latter in nosocomial infections), are found with anaerobes in 8% of primary lung abscesses.

b. Patients with gastric disorders who aspirate their gastric contents often have lung abscesses caused by *Bacteroides fragilis* and related anaerobes and coliform bacteria.

2. **Intraabdominal infections** usually result from contamination of compromised tissue by the normal intestinal flora, usually after trauma or surgery.
   a. The main organisms recovered from the infection are *B. fragilis, E. coli,* and enterococci.
   b. Other bacteria involved include *Proteus, Klebsiella,* and *Clostridium* species.
3. **Pelvic infections** are usually secondary to the trauma of delivery or abortion and contamination by the normal vaginal flora. In cases of septic abortion, blood cultures are positive for *Peptostreptococcus* in 30% of patients, *Bacteroides* in 3% of patients, *E. coli* in 18% of patients, and other organisms in 5% of patients.

D. Clinical manifestations

1. The infection is usually close to a mucosal surface (a source of endogenous bacterial contamination), and tissue trauma (surgical or accidental) is usually evident. Deep, dirty wounds are particularly likely to be contaminated by anaerobic organisms from the soil.
2. **Tissue necrosis** and **gangrene** (a result of ischemia) are usually seen. The infected tissue usually contains large amounts of gas. On palpation, gas produces a typical sound and tactile sensation known as **crepitus.**
3. When the infection drains to the outside (spontaneously or after surgery), the **discharge is foul-smelling** as a result of the accumulation of necrotic tissue, short-chain fatty acids, and methane.

E. Diagnosis.

If routine aerobic cultures are negative but the Gram stain demonstrates the presence of bacteria, an infection by anaerobic bacteria should be suspected.

1. **Collection of specimens for anaerobic culture**
   a. Specimens must be collected by a method that **excludes air** (e.g., by using a syringe that does not contain air). Properly collected specimens, such as syringe aspirates, swabs, tissue, or bone, should be placed in an anaerobic transport device (e.g., the Port-a-Cul, a sterile tube containing agar that meets anaerobic growth requirements—reduced electromotive potential, high carbon dioxide, and low or no oxygen).
   b. Contamination by the normal flora must be avoided. For example, if an anaerobic pulmonary infection is suspected, an expectorated sputum specimen is inadequate because it may be contaminated by anaerobes from the mouth. The specimen should be obtained directly from the site of infection (e.g., by transtracheal aspiration).
   c. Table 53-3 lists the frequency of recovery of aerobic and anaerobic organisms from several types of specimens. Blood cultures are infrequently positive, partly be-

cause of the noninvasive nature of anaerobes, the widespread use of prophylactic antimicrobial agents that target anaerobes and facultative anaerobes, and the early treatment of mixed aerobic-anaerobic infections.

2. **Direct examination** of a Gram stain of material collected from a mixed anaerobic infection shows several morphotypes, such as Gram-negative bacilli, Gram-positive bacilli (which may or may not contain spores), Gram-positive cocci, and Gram-negative cocci, all on the same slide. Highly oxygen-susceptible anaerobes may die during specimen collection, transport, or initial cultivation, but can be seen on Gram staining.

3. **Culture and isolation**
   a. **Anaerobic incubation** conditions can be provided by the use of:
      (1) Sealed jars from which the oxygen has been removed and replaced with an inert gas
      (2) An anaerobic chamber, or "glove box," from which the oxygen has been removed and replaced with carbon dioxide, hydrogen, and nitrogen. Cultures are introduced into the box through an airlock, and built-in gloves allow manipulation of cultures without altering the anaerobic environment.
   b. **Identification** of anaerobic organisms uses methods similar to those used for aerobic and facultative anaerobic bacteria: Gram reaction and morphology, colony morphology, oxygen tolerance, growth requirements, biochemical characteristics, and susceptibility to antibiotics.
      (1) **Gram staining** can help in the identification of isolated organisms. For example, sporulating Gram-positive bacilli seen on the Gram stain of an isolate growing anaerobically indicate a *Clostridium* species.
      (2) **Oxygen-tolerance studies** define an organism as an anaerobe. Anaerobes have varying tolerance to oxygen. All anaerobes are susceptible to prolonged oxygen exposure during specimen collection, transport, and initial cultivation.
      (3) **Biochemical characteristics** are the predominant means of identifying an isolated anaerobe. The general principles are similar to those used to identify aerobic bacteria—the isolate is inoculated into a battery of media designed to characterize specific enzyme activities, specific substrate utilization, or generation of specific products from a given substrate. Gas–liquid chromatography of end products of fermentative metabolism provides patterns characteristic of different genera or species.
      (4) **Antimicrobial susceptibility**
         (a) Most anaerobes are susceptible to penicillin, except *Bacteroides fragilis* and sometimes *P. melaninogenica.* In most cases, susceptibility of *Bacteroides* to penicillin can be predicted accurately by the β-lactamase test.
         (b) In cases when antimicrobial treatment fails or the infection is difficult (e.g., osteomyelitis), an antimicrobial susceptibility test of the isolate is performed.

F. Treatment

1. Treatment of anaerobic infections should include **incision** and **drainage** to lower the tissue turgor pressure, raise the electromotive potential, remove large numbers of bacteria and debris, increase circulation to allow leukocyte migration to the area, and raise the oxygen tension.

2. **Systemic antibiotics** are usually chosen based on predictable susceptibility patterns, β-lactamase–test results, or susceptibility testing.

Case 1 Revisited

The patient appears to have pneumonia.

The infection was probably acquired by aspiration of oropharyngeal or gastric contents while the patient was unconscious. The aspirated material went down the trachea and the right main bronchus, into the superior segment of the right lower lobe. Along with the bacteria, the aspirate contained enzymes and cellular debris from the oral cavity. The enzymes and debris provided the initial trauma to the lung tissue and triggered an inflammatory response. As a consequence of local inflammation, the bronchioles became occluded, oxygen was depleted, and facultative anaerobes began to multiply. The accumulation of leukocytes and serum increased tissue turgor and further decreased the blood and oxygen supply. As the electromotive potential fell, even the most fastidious microorganisms could grow. The lung parenchyma became necrotic (necrotizing pneumonia), and a classic anaerobic infection developed—a putrid lung abscess, typical of alcoholics who lose consciousness.

The abscess must be drained by coughing or surgery, and the patient must be treated with systemic antibiotics. Samples from the abscess exudate should be collected for anaerobic culture. While waiting for culture results, treatment with penicillin and metronidazole should begin.

Chapter 54

Sexually Transmitted Diseases

Victor Del Bene
Gerald E. Wagner
Gabriel Virella

Case 1

A 21-year-old male college student complains of a 2-day history of dysuria and a copious urethral discharge. He has been sexually active with several female partners, and does not use condoms. There is no history of previous disease and he is unaware of disease in his sexual partners. Physical examination is unremarkable except for inflammation of the urethral meatus and free-flowing yellow, purulent discharge from the orifice. A Gram stain of an exudate smear shows numerous polymorphonuclear (PMN) leukocytes. One out of every 20 is filled with Gram-negative, bean-shaped diplococci.

- □ *What is the most likely diagnosis and what other diagnoses should be considered?*
- □ *What tests can confirm the primary diagnosis?*
- □ *What is the best approach to confirm the secondary diagnoses?*
- □ *What is the most adequate therapy for this patient?*
- □ *What sequelae should be expected from this disease in the short and long term?*
- □ *What are the public-health requirements to be followed for this patient?*

I. INTRODUCTION.

The frequency and diversity of sexually transmitted diseases has been increasing for the last decade. The responsible microorganisms include bacteria, fungi, viruses, and protozoa (Table 54-1). Hepatitis and HIV/AIDS are discussed in detail in Chapters 55 and 57, respectively.

II. EPIDEMIOLOGY

A. Gonorrhea

1. **Transmission** is normally by direct sexual contact. The bacteria die rapidly when exposed outside the body. Humans are the natural reservoir.
2. The **typical patient** is a sexually promiscuous, 20- to 25-year-old, urban man. The number of cases in sexually active adolescents has increased dramatically in the last few years. Reported cases in men outnumber those in women about 3 to 1, probably reflecting the greater frequency of asymptomatic disease among women.
3. **Incidence.** Gonorrhea is the most prevalent of the reportable sexually transmitted diseases; approximately 400,000 cases are reported yearly in the United States. Estimates of unreported cases number in the millions.

Table 54-1. The Most Common Sexually Transmitted Diseases

	Disease	Causative Agent
Bacterial	Gonorrhea	*Neisseria gonorrhoeae*
	Non-gonococcal urethritis	*Chlamydia trachomatis, Mycoplasma hominis*
	Lymphogranuloma venereum	*Chlamydia trachomatis*
	Canchroid	*Haemophilus ducreyi*
	Syphilis	*Treponemia pallidum*
	Granuloma inguinale	*Calymmatobacterium granulomatis*
Viral	Venereal warts	Papillomavirus
	Genital herpes	Herpes simplex virus
	Hepatitis B and C	Hepatitis viruses
	AIDS	HIV
	Molluscum contagiosum	Poxvirus
Parasitic	Trichomoniasis	*Trichomonas vaginalis*
	Intestinal amebiasis	*Entamoeba histolytica*
	Giardiasis	*Giardia lamblia*
Fungal	Candidiasis	*Candida albicans*

B. **Nongonococcal urethritis** is prevalent in the same population as gonorrhea.

1. **Incidence.** *Chlamydia trachomatis* is the most common cause of nongonococcal urethritis and it is believed to be the most common cause of bacterial sexually transmitted diseases in the United States. Precise incidence figures are unavailable, because this disease is nonreportable. It is estimated that *C. trachomatis* causes between 3 and 7 million new infections each year, corresponding to 30%–50% of all cases of nongonococcal urethritis.
2. *Ureaplasma* and *Mycoplasma* may cause another 30% of cases.
3. The remaining 20%–30% of cases have other causes, including herpes simplex virus (HSV) and *Trichomonas vaginalis.*

C. **Syphilis** is transmitted exclusively by sexual contact. Young, promiscuous individuals tend to be predominantly affected. The frequency of syphilis had declined until the late 1980s; since then, the frequency has been increasing. Currently, the number of cases reported in the United States is approximately 100,000 per year.

D. **Genital herpes** is caused primarily by HSV type 2 (HSV-2), which is introduced into the genital mucosa by sexual contact. Genital infection may be either symptomatic or asymptomatic.

E. **Condylomata acuminata (genital warts),** caused by several strains of papillomavirus, is a common venereal disease. Its precise frequency has not been determined, partly due to the fact that it is not a reportable disease and partly because diagnosis is difficult. The papillomavirus is transmitted by direct sexual contact. Its association with cervical carcinoma raises the possibility that this type of carcinoma may be sexually transmitted.

F. **Trichomoniasis** and **candidiasis** are common but are not usually reported, so their incidence is difficult to ascertain.

III. APPROACH TO THE PATIENT

A. **Patient history.** The physician must be tactful and nonjudgmental, but it is important to establish a good history of sexual habits and preferences (e.g., number and gender of sex partners, route of intercourse).

1. Sexually transmitted disease should be considered in any patient who seeks medical attention. Patients often avoid discussing signs or symptoms of sexually transmitted diseases because of the negative connotations these diseases carry.
   a. Itching and dysuria are among the symptoms most mentioned by patients with a sexually transmitted disease.
   b. Depending on the disease and time elapsed before the patient sees a physician, the patient may report symptoms suggesting more advanced disease, such as painful lesions, discharges, lower abdominal pain, and rash.

2. Three important points should always be considered when taking a history and ordering diagnostic tests for patients in whom sexually transmitted disease is suspected:
   a. Each patient represents at least one other person with the disease.
   b. A patient with one sexually transmitted disease is likely to be simultaneously infected with other agents capable of causing sexually transmitted disease.
   c. A patient with a history of sexually transmitted disease is likely to have other sexually transmitted diseases in the future.

B. **Physical examination** may provide clues suggesting sexually transmitted disease:

1. **Discharge** (from the urethra, vagina, or rectum)
2. **Rash** (of any type) in the genital or paragenital region, or elsewhere on the skin
3. **Ulcerative lesions** (genital areas and other areas possibly involved in sexual practices)

C. **Clinical manifestations**

1. **Discharge with pruritus or dysuria**
   a. **Vaginal discharge.** Most women normally have a minimal vaginal discharge that fluctuates throughout the month. Common microbial causes of abnormal vaginal discharge include *T. vaginalis, Candida albicans, Gardnerella vaginalis, Neisseria gonorrhoeae,* and HSV. Disease should be suspected when a smear shows large numbers of PMN leukocytes or abnormal vaginal microflora, especially if the discharge is accompanied by dysuria, dyspareunia (pain on intercourse), burning, itching, or vulvar soreness.
      (1) A thin, foamy, and foul-smelling vaginal discharge is typical of infections caused by *Trichomonas.*
      (2) Vaginitis caused by *G. vaginalis* (a facultative anaerobe) is also associated with a foul-smelling discharge.
      (3) Thick, cheesy exudates are associated with vaginal candidiasis.
   b. **Urethral discharge.** Any discharge from the male urethra (except ejaculation) is abnormal. Common causes of urethral discharge include infections with *N. gonorrhoeae, C. trachomatis,* HSV, *T. vaginalis, Candida* species, and *U. urealyticum.*
      (1) In gonorrhea, the urethral discharge is spontaneous, abundant, and purulent.
      (2) In nongonococcal urethritis, it is thin and slippery.

2. **Skin lesions**
   a. **Ulcers.** Ulcerative lesions are seen in cases of syphilis, chancroid, lymphogranuloma inguinale (donovanosis), lymphogranuloma venereum (LGV), and herpes.
      (1) The primary chancre of syphilis can be genital or extragenital. All the lesions are infectious and should not be touched with bare hands. The ulceration is usually well delimited and painless.
      (2) The ulcer of chancroid is not so well delimited and clean; it is disorganized, exudative, and painful.
      (3) Vesicular lesions (e.g., in genital herpes) that burst appear as ulcers. The patient should be asked whether the ulcers were once fluid-filled.
   b. **Granulomatous reactions,** typical of granuloma inguinale, are seen in the perineal and inguinal areas.
   c. **Rashes** can be present in several sexually transmitted diseases, including sys-

temic gonorrhea, secondary syphilis, and superficial fungal infections (e.g., candidiasis).

(1) In systemic gonococcal infection, a scant pustular rash is often visible, particularly on the toes or fingers.

(2) Secondary syphilis may be associated with a disseminated rash (one of the few that affects the palms and soles).

d. Warts are the presenting feature of condylomata acuminata and of molluscum contagiosum.

(1) **Condylomata acuminata.** The warty eruption may be exuberant on the penis and also (especially in homosexual men) on the perianal region.

(2) **Molluscum contagiosum.** The lesions are characteristically few in number and usually have an umbilicated center.

IV. LABORATORY DIAGNOSIS

LABORATORY DIAGNOSIS is usually based on the demonstration of the causative agent in adequate samples, or on serologic assays to detect an immune response to the causative agent. The samples used for diagnostic studies vary from disease to disease.

A. Urethral, vaginal, and anal exudates

Urethral, vaginal, and **anal exudates** should be examined and cultured.

1. **Gonorrhea.** In patients with gonorrhea, a Gram stain may reveal abundant pus cells (mostly neutrophils). About one in twenty of the pus cells contains large numbers of intracytoplasmic, Gram-negative, bean-shaped diplococci.
   - **a.** In men, a positive smear is sufficient for diagnosis because Gram-negative organisms do not normally colonize the urethra.
   - **b.** In women, the normal vaginal flora includes *Viellonella parvula,* which is also a Gram-negative diplococcus. For this reason, positive identification by culture or by immunofluorescence using nucleic acid probes is essential to confirm the diagnosis of gonorrhea in women. (Note that only culture provides information about antibiotic susceptibility of the causative agent.)
2. **Trichomoniasis.** A wet preparation is the best way to demonstrate *Trichomonas.*
3. **Candidiasis.** A potassium hydroxide preparation allows a fast diagnosis of candidiasis by showing typical budding yeast cells, often forming germ tubes. These can also be visualized on a Gram stain.
4. ***G. vaginalis* vaginitis.** A wet preparation or a conventional histology stain of a vaginal exudate may show "clue cells" (vaginal epithelial cells with adherent bacteria).
5. **Nongonococcal urethritis.** A smear examined by light microscopy is negative. A definitive diagnosis of *C. trachomatis* infection can be made by means of culture, antibody-based techniques, or DNA hybridization.
   - **a.** Because *C. trachomatis* is an obligate intracellular parasite, tissue-cell culture must be used to isolate it. This technique is not routinely available.
   - **b.** *C. trachomatis* (or antigens released by it) can be detected in clinical specimens by direct or indirect immunofluorescence using monoclonal antibodies to elementary bodies. Drawbacks of this technique are the subjectivity in interpretation and the requirement for a trained technician.
   - **c.** Enzyme immunoassays (EIAs) to detect lipopolysaccharide (LPS) antigens (either soluble or in the elementary-body cell wall) in urethral and cervical exudates have sensitivity levels of 90% and specificity levels of greater than 95%.
   - **d.** Rapid and simple tests of acceptable sensitivity and specificity based on DNA hybridization with *C. trachomatis*–specific gene probes are becoming increasingly popular.

B. Chancres and ulcers

Chancres and ulcers should also be examined.

1. **Darkfield microscopy** of material collected from syphilitic chancres may reveal *Treponema pallidum.*

2. A **Gram stain** of material collected from a chancroid lesion may reveal the causative agent, the Gram-negative coccobacillus *Haemophilus ducreyi.*

3. Detection of multi-nucleated giant cells on a **Tzanck preparation** of scrapings collected from the base of an ulcerated vesicle allows a diagnosis of genital herpes.

C. **Granulomatous lesions.** In a patient with granuloma inguinale, a Gram stain of material from a lesion may reveal *Calymmatobacterium granulomatis* on inflammatory cells.

D. **Rashes.** In systemic gonococcal infections, a Gram stain of the pustule fluid may reveal Gram-negative, bean-shaped diplococci ingested by PMN leukocytes.

V. TREATMENT

TREATMENT depends on the cause of the disease. In some cases, empiric treatment may be prescribed based on the common causes of a given clinical syndrome. As a rule, however, all efforts should be made to establish a precise diagnosis and to verify the susceptibility of the causative agent to the prescribed antimicrobial agents.

A. **Gonorrhea** and **nongonococcal urethritis** are difficult to distinguish clinically, and it is possible for a patient to be simultaneously infected by *N. gonorrhoeae* and by *C. trachomatis.*

1. **Gonorrhea.** Uncomplicated cases are usually treated with one of the following:
   a. **Second-** or **third-generation cephalosporin** such as ceftriaxone, which is not affected by the penicillin-specific β-lactamase produced by *N. gonorrhoeae*
   b. **Doxycycline,** which also treats *Chlamydia* and other organisms that may not be susceptible to cephalosporins (may be discontinued if the causative agent is confirmed to be *N. gonorrhoeae*)

2. **Nongonococcal urethritis.** If a diagnosis of nongonococcal urethritis is considered, there are several possible treatments. Frequently, the therapeutic response is considered indicative of whether the diagnosis was correct or not. Alternatively, the physician may collect samples to send to the laboratory and start treatment with antimicrobials while awaiting identification of the infectious agent. The most common antimicrobial agents used for treating nongonococcal urethritis are:
   a. **Erythromycin,** which is effective against *Chlamydia, Ureaplasma,* and *Mycoplasma,* but often causes symptoms of gastrointestinal intolerance
   b. **Doxycycline** or **azithromycin,** which are effective against *C. trachomatis*

B. **Syphilis** is best treated with large doses of **penicillin G.**

C. **Herpes simplex** can be treated with **acyclovir.** The precise indications, dosages, and routes of administration of this drug depend on the clinical picture.

D. **Parasitic sexually transmitted diseases** caused by *E. histolytica, T. vaginalis,* or *G. lamblia* are effectively treated with **metronidazole.**

E. **Candidiasis** can be treated with **nystatin** or **ketoconazole.** Topical ointments and suppositories are available for the treatment of vaginal candidiasis. Because a potential source of reinfection is the endogenous intestinal flora, topical treatment is often complemented by oral administration of the same antifungal agent.

VI. PREVENTION

A. Prevention of person-to-person transmission

1. Patients should be educated regarding the use of barrier contraceptives such as condoms, which prevent the transmission of most sexually transmitted diseases.

2. All of the patient's sexual partners should be notified and treated.

B. Prevention of transplacental and perinatal transmission

1. Transplacental transmission can be prevented only by preventing maternal infection. Prenatal counseling and immunization are the most effective measures.
2. Perinatal transmission of any sexually transmitted disease is best avoided by performing a cesarean section.
3. In specific cases (e.g., hepatitis B and HIV infections), immunization or treatment of the neonate may prevent or minimize infection.

VII. COMPLICATIONS

A. Pelvic inflammatory disease (PID, salpingitis) is the most common complication of gonococcal and chlamydial infection in women, occurring in approximately 15% of infected women. In some cases of gonococcal PID, the infection may propagate to the liver [Fitz-Hugh–Curtis syndrome (gonococcal perihepatitis)].

1. **Diagnosis**
   a. **Clinical diagnosis** is difficult because of the nonspecificity of the symptoms. The classic triad of fever, abdominal pain, and increased vaginal discharge is present in only about one-third of patients. Common signs include abdominal tenderness, cervical-motion tenderness, and adnexal tenderness.
   b. **Laboratory tests** show an increased white blood cell count in peripheral blood and an increased erythrocyte sedimentation rate.
   c. Confirmation of PID can be obtained in a variety of ways.
      1. **Laparoscopy** and **culdocentesis** are the most objective ways to confirm or rule out the diagnosis. Purulent material from culdocentesis should be Gram stained, examined microscopically, and cultured.
      2. Purulent endocervical discharge (10 or more white blood cells in a high-power field) supports the diagnosis. Observation of intracellular Gram-negative diplococci, positive cultures for *N. gonorrhoeae,* or positive results of tests for *C. trachomatis* or *N. gonorrhoeae* help establish the diagnosis.
2. **Complications** and **sequelae** of PID include tubo-ovarial abscess formation (usually detectable by ultrasound examination), ectopic pregnancy, and infertility.
3. **Treatment.** PID is usually treated with a third-generation cephalosporin plus doxycycline. Parenteral administration of high doses is preferred.

B. Neonatal conjunctivitis is usually the result of perinatal infection of the fetus by a mother with endocervical or vaginal infection.

1. **Gonococcal conjunctivitis** is the most common form of neonatal conjunctivitis. Infection usually becomes evident 3–7 days postpartum. Bilateral, profuse, and purulent conjunctivitis is characteristic of this syndrome.
2. **Trachoma** and **herpes simplex conjunctivitis** can also be acquired at birth.

C. Neonatal pneumonia caused by *C. trachomatis* also results from perinatal transmission.

D. Late syphilis is a multisystemic disease that may raise considerable diagnostic problems, particularly when the patient is not known to have had primary syphilis and the nonspecific screening tests are negative. The pathogenesis of late syphilis is unclear, because *T. pallidum* cannot usually be demonstrated in the characteristic degenerative lesions. The main target organs are:

1. The **central nervous system** (CNS), where late syphilis can take the form of meningovascular syphilis (with a clinical picture of chronic meningitis) or dementia
2. **Bones** and **cartilage,** which can be extensively destroyed.
3. The **heart** and **large vessels** (often the aorta and aortic valve), leading to dissecting aortic aneurysms and aortic insufficiency.

E. Congenital syphilis results from the transplacental transmission of *T. pallidum.* The infection can occur very early in pregnancy (fetuses aborted as early as the ninth or tenth week of gestation have been found to be infected).

1. **Early clinical manifestations** of congenital syphilis include abortion, stillbirth, or a variety of manifestations of disseminated syphilis in the infant.
   - **a.** Symptoms appear during the first 2–6 weeks. The initial syndrome is often snuffles, which resembles a head cold, and is followed by the development of skin rash (generally maculopapular) and mucosal lesions.
   - **b.** Hepatosplenomegaly (often associated with hyperbilirubinemia and sometimes with obvious jaundice) occurs in nearly all affected infants.
   - **c.** Skeletal abnormalities also are seen in nearly all patients on radiologic examination.
   - **d.** Enlarged lymph nodes are seen in about 50% of infected infants.
2. **Late manifestations** of congenital syphilis occur after 2 years.
   - **a.** Structural abnormalities (especially craniofacial alterations) become apparent with the development of teeth and long bones. One or several of the elements of the Hutchinson's triad (notched teeth, interstitial keratitis, and eighth-nerve deafness) are seen in approximately 75% of the affected untreated children.
   - **b.** Manifestations of obscure pathogenesis, such as keratitis, skin lesions, gummas of nasal and facial bone, periostitis, and CNS disease, occur.

F. Neonatal herpes is usually acquired perinatally, by passage through an infected birth canal, but can also be acquired during gestation, by transplacental transmission. The neonates are usually symptomatic, with either disseminated or localized disease.

1. **Disseminated disease** most likely results from transplacental transmission of the virus, and affected infants may have hepatomegaly, jaundice, bleeding diathesis, and CNS manifestations. The mortality rate in these patients is approximately 80%.
2. **Local disease** usually affects the skin, CNS, or eyes.

Case 1 Revisited

The college student most likely has urethral gonorrhea, based on the copious amount of urethral pus and the presence of Gram-negative diplococci. Other sexually transmitted diseases must be considered in the differential diagnosis, particularly nongonococcal urethritis and syphilis (both infections can occur concomitantly with gonorrhea).

Urethral gonorrhea can be confirmed by culture or by direct immunofluorescence using a fluorescein-labeled monoclonal antibody applied directly to a glass slide on which the urethral exudate has been smeared.

Nongonococcal urethritis can be confirmed by immunofluorescence using antibodies to *C. trachomatis.* Tests for nongonococcal urethritis are especially important if the patient complains of residual dysuria and thin, clear discharge after treatment for gonorrhea. Serologic tests for syphilis and an HIV-antigen test are also indicated in this patient.

The patient should be treated with a penicillinase-resistant cephalosporin.

The patient should be watched for the development of urethral obstruction (as a result of post-inflammation scarring of the urethra), persistence of milder symptoms (which would indicate that the patient may have nongonococcal urethritis as well), or the appearance of a chancre. If the first tests for syphilis and HIV are negative, the patient should be retested.

The patient should be fully informed of his diagnosis, and he should be encouraged to practice safe sex and avoid multiple partners. The county Health Department should be notified. The patient's sexual partners should be notified, treated, and counseled.

Chapter 55

Viral Hepatitis

Edwin A. Brown
Robert M. Galbraith

Case 1

Over a 1-week period, a healthy 4-year-old girl lost her appetite, complained of pains in her legs and back, and became apathetic. Her mother brought her to the clinic because of a fever of 100.1°F and mentioned that several other children at the same day care center had recently had similar symptoms. The child has not vomited or experienced diarrhea. On physical examination, the child is lethargic but awake. Mild jaundice and some tenderness over the liver are noted. There is no splenomegaly or ascites.

- □ *What is the most likely diagnosis?*
- □ *Is the infection systemic?*
- □ *Is specific therapy available?*

Case 2

A 58-year-old man visits his primary care physician because of abdominal and ankle swelling. Although previously healthy, he has noted intermittent jaundice with dark urine and light-colored stools for several months. He has become less energetic and progressively drowsy, such that he has been terminated from his job as a truck driver. He has a history of intravenous drug abuse but has been abstinent for over 25 years. He drinks a six-pack of beer every day and more on the weekends. Physical examination shows a gaunt man with jaundice, moderate ascites, and hepatosplenomegaly.

- □ *What is the most likely diagnosis?*
- □ *How can the diagnosis be confirmed?*
- □ *What is the best therapy?*

I. INTRODUCTION

A. Definitions

1. **Viral hepatitis** is viral infection of the liver that causes hepatic inflammation. The inflammation is detected by clinical symptoms of fever, nausea, malaise, and signs of jaundice and hepatomegaly; by biochemical findings of elevated liver enzymes (released from the inflamed liver parenchyma); or by liver biopsy showing inflammatory cells. Acute hepatitis is usually associated with a strong and effective antiviral response, whereas chronic hepatitis may reflect an ineffective or partial immune response with viral persistence.

a. **Acute hepatitis** refers to the initial infection with a hepatitis virus. **Fulminant hepatic failure** is caused by a severe acute infection that injures or destroys enough hepatocytes to acutely compromise hepatic function. Toxic metabolites accumulate, impairing synthetic functioning of the hepatocytes.

b. **Chronic hepatitis** refers to active disease that has been present for longer than 6 months.

(1) The extent of inflammation seen on liver biopsy can be described as:

(a) **Chronic persistent hepatitis.** Inflammation is limited to the portal tracts.

(b) **Chronic active hepatitis.** Inflammatory cells spread to the liver parenchyma, leading to hepatocyte necrosis.

(2) **Chronic carriers** are individuals who have chronic hepatitis but are asymptomatic.

2. **Cirrhosis** is the common result of chronic injury to the hepatic parenchyma. During attempts to regenerate damaged hepatocytes and supporting connective tissue, the hepatic architecture becomes disorganized, excess fibrotic tissue is produced, and nodular regeneration of hepatic parenchyma occurs.

a. The morphologic alterations result in portal hypertension, varices, and splenomegaly.

b. The loss of the synthetic and excretory functions of the hepatocytes leads to jaundice, edema, and coagulopathy.

c. Together, the destruction of hepatocytes and morphologic changes can lead to hepatic encephalopathy and ascites.

3. **Jaundice** is a yellow discoloration of the skin and sclera.

B. Epidemiology. Acute viral hepatitis is one of the most common forms of infectious disease. The main epidemiologic features of the major types of viral hepatitis are summarized in Table 55-1.

1. The **incidence** of the different types of viral hepatitis depends on patient age, socioeconomic status, level of sanitation, epidemiologic factors, the course of liver disease (acute or chronic), and associated risk factors. Geography is also important. In the United States, for example, hepatitis A, B, and C are common, hepatitis D occurs in isolated clusters, and hepatitis E is rare.

a. Approximately one-third of the population in the United States—mostly older adults—shows serologic evidence of previous infection with hepatitis A.

b. The seroprevalence of hepatitis B and C is lower, although both account for 150,000–300,000 new infections annually. There are approximately 750,000 chronic carriers of hepatitis B and 3,500,000 chronic carriers of hepatitis C.

c. Hepatitis A is the most common form of acute hepatitis in children, whereas

Table 55-1. Epidemiologic Features of Viral Hepatitis

Hepatitis Virus	Incubation Period	Clinical Presentation	Transmission Route	Risk Factors
Hepatitis A	2–6 weeks	Acute	Fecal-oral	Crowded conditions; poor hygiene; day care
Hepatitis B	2–6 months	Acute or chronic	Parenteral	IV drug abuse; sexual activity; perinatal exposure
Hepatitis C	2 weeks–5 months	Generally chronic	Parenteral	IV drug abuse; blood transfusion
Hepatitis D	1–4 months	Acute (often fulminant) or chronic	Parenteral	IV drug abuse
Hepatitis E	2–8 weeks	Acute	Fecal-oral	Untreated water

IV = intravenous.

acute hepatitis B, C, and D are more common in adults. In developing countries, the incidence of hepatitis A decreases as sanitation improves.

2. **Major risk factors**
   a. **Hepatitis A.** Risk factors include poor hygiene, close personal contact, and ingestion of shellfish.
   b. **Hepatitis B, C, and D.** Risk factors include exposure to blood or blood products, intravenous drug use, and sexual promiscuity.

C. Diagnostic tests. The prognosis and management of viral hepatitis depend on identifying the causative agent and determining whether the disease is acute or chronic.

1. **Serologic tests** include the following:
   a. **Hepatitis A virus (HAV)**
      (1) **IgM anti-HAV** is present at the onset of symptoms and is diagnostic of acute hepatitis A.
      (2) **IgG anti-HAV** indicates past infection with HAV and is not useful for diagnosing acute infection.
   b. **Hepatitis B virus (HBV)**
      (1) **Hepatitis B surface antigen (HBsAg)** is a protein in the HBV envelope. It is present in serum in both acute and chronic hepatitis B.
      (2) **Anti-hepatitis B surface antigen (anti-HBsAg)** indicates resolution of infection after acute hepatitis B, and protective immunity after vaccination.
      (3) **IgM anti-hepatitis B core antigen (IgM anti-HBcAg),** an antibody to an HBV core protein, is present in acute infection. The IgM anti-HBcAg test is the only serologic test that is positive during the window period of acute hepatitis B (1–3 months).
      (4) **IgG anti-hepatitis B core antigen (IgG anti-HBcAg)** is present for years after hepatitis B infection.
      (5) **Hepatitis B e antigen (HBeAg)** is secreted from infected hepatocytes and may inhibit the host immune response. The presence of HBeAg indicates replicating virus and thus a highly infectious person.
      (6) **Anti-hepatitis B e antigen (anti-HBeAg)** indicates that the host's immune system has responded to infection. Patients who are HBsAg- and HBeAg-positive have more ongoing viral replication and are thus more infectious than patients who are HBsAg- and anti-HBeAg-positive.
      (7) **HBV DNA.** The presence of HBV DNA in serum indicates active HBV replication.
   c. **Hepatitis C virus (HCV)**
      (1) **HCV enzyme immunoassay (EIA)** detects antibodies to several HCV antigens, indicating acute, chronic, or past infection with HCV. The HCV EIA may yield many false-positives in a low-prevalence population.
      (2) **HCV recombinant immunoblot assay (RIBA)** confirms HCV infection by detecting antibodies to individual HCV antigens. HCV RIBA is more specific than HCV EIA.
   d. **Hepatitis D virus (HDV, the delta agent)**
      (1) **IgM anti-HDV** is transiently present in co-infections and superinfections that resolve. IgM anti-HDV is often present in chronic hepatitis D (delta hepatitis).
      (2) **IgG anti-HDV** is transiently present in hepatitis D that resolves and is present in chronic HDV infections.
   e. **Hepatitis E virus (HEV).** No diagnostic tests are commercially available.
2. **Liver biopsy** is used to assess the degree of hepatic inflammation or cirrhotic changes resulting from chronic hepatitis B, C, or D. Biopsy is not useful for diagnosing acute viral hepatitis.

D. Prevention

1. **Passive immunization**
   a. **Immune serum globulin (ISG),** given prophylactically or at the time of exposure, can prevent or ameliorate hepatitis A.

b. **Hepatitis B immune globulin (HBIg)** is effective when given after exposure to HBV. HBIg can also prevent HDV infection.
c. **Gamma globulin** does not prevent hepatitis C.

2. **Vaccination**
   a. **Hepatitis A.** An effective killed vaccine for hepatitis A is available.
   b. **Hepatitis B.** An effective vaccine for hepatitis B—made of recombinant HBsAg—is available; nevertheless, about 300,000 new cases of hepatitis B occur annually in the United States. Vaccination against hepatitis B also prevents hepatitis D.
      (1) In infants born to hepatitis B carriers, administration of HBIg and vaccination against hepatitis B at birth reduce the risk of neonatal infection.
      (2) Universal administration of the hepatitis B vaccine at birth is recommended to decrease the incidence of hepatitis B in children.
   c. **Hepatitis C.** No vaccine is available to prevent hepatitis C.

3. **Behavior modification** (avoiding intravenous drug abuse and high-risk sexual practices) can lower the prevalence of hepatitis B, C, and D.

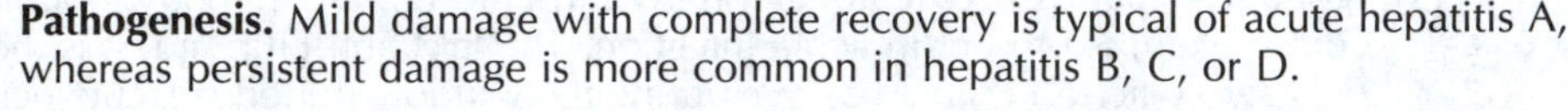

II. ACUTE VIRAL HEPATITIS

A. Pathogenesis.

Pathogenesis. Mild damage with complete recovery is typical of acute hepatitis A, whereas persistent damage is more common in hepatitis B, C, or D.

1. Liver damage is caused by the host immune response (mediated by cytotoxic T lymphocytes) to viral antigens expressed on the surface of infected hepatocytes. The hepatitis viruses are predominantly tropic for the liver, and pathogenic effects are largely confined to the liver. Extrahepatic manifestations such as polyarteritis nodosa (HBV), cryoglobulinemia (HCV), and glomerulonephritis (HBV and HCV), are caused by immune complexes containing viral antigen and antibody.
   a. HDV, an incomplete virus, requires concomitant infection with HBV to replicate.
   b. The average **incubation period** of hepatitis A is 21 days; hepatitis B, 70 days; hepatitis C, 50 days; and hepatitis E, 40 days. Because exposure frequently goes unrecognized, the physician may not be able to use incubation period as a diagnostic tool.

2. A **fulminant course** rarely occurs in hepatitis A, but is more common in hepatitis B and in cases of superinfection with HDV. Overall, fulminant hepatic failure occurs in less than 1% of patients. During fulminant hepatitis, massive necrosis of hepatocytes leads to the following secondary effects:
   a. **Tissue ischemia** and **hypoxia** caused by microcirculatory impairment, with a risk of multi-organ failure
   b. **Coagulopathy** and **hemorrhage** caused by deficient synthesis of coagulation factors in the inflamed liver
   c. **Encephalopathy** and **cerebral edema** caused by the accumulation of toxic metabolites and sodium–water imbalance
   d. **Dysfunction of the Kuppfer's cells,** the major component of the reticuloendothelial system, which increases susceptibility to other infections

B. Clinical manifestations

1. **Symptoms.** Most cases of viral hepatitis have a benign, self-limited course. Many infections are anicteric and completely unrecognized except for a "flu-like" illness.
   a. Initially, patients have nonspecific constitutional symptoms of nausea, anorexia, malaise, and abdominal pain for 7–10 days, followed by the abrupt onset of jaundice, suggesting a diagnosis of acute hepatitis. The constitutional symptoms begin to clear when jaundice appears.
   b. Approximately 10% of patients with acute hepatitis B have symptoms (fever, rash, and arthralgias) consistent with circulating immune complexes of antibody and

viral antigen. (This is the only clinical finding that allows distinction between the hepatitis viruses.)

c. Resolution occurs in 2–6 weeks in most patients, although some patients have a prolonged recovery with complaints of malaise and fatigue.

2. **Physical examination findings**
   a. Patients may have an **enlarged, tender liver.**
   b. Excretion of conjugated bilirubin turns the **urine dark,** while the lack of hepatic bilirubin excretion leads to **lighter-colored stools.**
   c. **Jaundice** is first noticed in the patient's sclera.

3. **Laboratory findings.** Routine laboratory data are usually unremarkable, although atypical lymphocytes are common.
   a. **Bilirubin.** Patients who are icteric (jaundiced) have elevated levels of conjugated bilirubin (> 2.5–3.0 mg/dl). Serum bilirubin levels may reach 5–20 mg/dl in acute disease and during exacerbation of chronic disease.
   b. **Liver enzymes.** Liver function tests assess the release of the liver enzymes **alanine aminotransferase (ALT)** and **aspartate aminotransferase (AST)** into the blood stream following hepatocyte injury. In viral hepatitis, serum ALT levels may be 10–20 times normal. ALT levels are elevated more than AST levels in viral hepatitis, whereas AST levels are elevated about twice as much as ALT levels in alcoholic hepatitis.

C. Diagnosis.

Diagnosis. Identifying the causative agent aids prognosis and allows the physician to decide whether passive immunization of individuals who may have been exposed through close contact or needle stick is indicated.

1. **Patient history**
   a. Information about **high-risk behavior** such as travel to areas of poor sanitation, intravenous drug use, or recent blood transfusion may indicate which diagnostic tests to order.
   b. Knowledge of the **incubation period** and time of probable exposure may also be helpful.

2. **Serologic tests.** A diagnosis of acute viral hepatitis is usually made by detecting antibodies to a hepatitis virus or viral antigens. The following tests are used to diagnose acute hepatitis:
   a. **HAV:** IgM anti-HAV
   b. **HBV:** HBsAg, anti-HBsAg, and IgM anti-HBcAg
   c. **HCV:** Because HCV EIA may not be positive in the first several weeks of infection, the assay may need to be repeated if all diagnostic tests are negative. Positive results should be confirmed with HCV RIBA.
   d. **HDV:** Anti-HDV may be useful in patients known to be HBV carriers.

3. **Differential diagnosis.** Acute hepatitis may be caused by other non-hepatitis viruses, particularly the herpesviruses [cytomegalovirus (CMV), Epstein-Barr virus, herpes simplex virus (HSV), and varicella-zoster virus], as well as other viruses (coxsackievirus, mumps viruses, and adenoviruses), bacteria *(Treponema pallidum, Leptospira interrogans*), toxins, and medications.

D. Treatment

1. **Typical acute viral hepatitis,** with constitutional symptoms evolving to jaundice and symptomatic improvement, can usually be managed expectantly on an outpatient basis. Liver function should be carefully monitored.

2. **Severe disease.** Hospital admission is necessary in the presence of persistently high transaminase levels, rapidly increasing bilirubin levels or prothrombin time (PT), or when acidosis develops. Treatment is essentially supportive.

3. **Fulminant hepatic failure.** When symptoms of encephalopathy suggest fulminant hepatic failure, aggressive intensive care management is essential.

III. CHRONIC VIRAL HEPATITIS

A. Etiology. HBV, HCV, and HDV cause chronic hepatitis; HAV and HEV do not.

1. **HBV.** In fewer than 10% of adults infected with HBV, the virus is not cleared, leading to chronic hepatitis. The lack of a specific or effective immune response to hepatitis B viral antigens may contribute to the chronic-carrier state (300 million people worldwide). Not surprisingly, chronic-carrier status is common in immunosuppressed patients.

2. **HCV.** Over 60% of patients with acute hepatitis C become chronically infected. Chronic hepatitis C is often detected in asymptomatic individuals when their donated blood is screened.

3. **HDV** also causes chronic hepatitis (in conjunction with HBV).

B. Pathogenesis

1. **HBV**
   - a. **Immunologically mediated hepatocellular damage.** Cell-surface expression of HBsAg and other viral antigens results in the activation of cytotoxic $CD8^+$ lymphocytes, leading to hepatocellular damage.
   - b. **Viral persistence**
     - (1) The **replicative phase** of chronic hepatitis B is characterized by viremia (detectable HBsAg and HBeAg in serum) and inflammatory changes in the liver.
     - (2) During the **nonreplicative phase** of chronic hepatitis B, HBeAg is absent and anti-HBeAg is present; HBV DNA may have integrated into the cell genome; hepatic inflammation is decreased; and viral replication is diminished. In most cases, the loss of HBeAg and the presence of anti-HBeAg signal recovery and a decrease in actively replicating virus.
   - c. **Cirrhosis** results from chronic hepatocellular damage and hepatic regeneration.
   - d. **Carcinoma.** The strong association between cirrhosis and hepatocellular carcinoma suggests that chronic hepatocellular injury and cellular regeneration promote malignant transformation. Although integrated HBV DNA is found in most cases of HBV-related hepatocellular carcinoma, the role of HBV DNA in the pathogenesis of hepatocellular carcinoma is uncertain.

2. **HCV**
   - a. **Viral persistence.** HCV probably evades the immune system through constant mutation of the dominant epitope on the envelope proteins.
   - b. **Cirrhosis** Approximately one-third of patients with chronic HCV infection develop cirrhosis 20 or more years after the acute infection.
     - (1) Alcohol appears to be a cofactor in the development of HCV-related cirrhosis. Cirrhosis is more likely to develop in alcoholics who are HCV EIA-positive than in alcoholics who are HCV EIA-negative, suggesting that many cases of cirrhosis attributed to alcohol are actually caused by chronic hepatitis C.
     - (2) Some patients also develop hepatocellular carcinoma.

3. **HDV.** Sixty percent to seventy percent of patients with chronic hepatitis D develop cirrhosis, a rate many times higher than the rate for chronic hepatitis B or C.

C. Clinical manifestations. The clinical findings do not allow clear distinction between chronic HBV, HBV/HDV, and HCV.

1. **Symptoms.** Most patients with chronic hepatitis have few, if any, symptoms until they develop cirrhosis. Some patients complain of malaise, fatigue, and loss of appetite.

2. **Physical examination findings.** Physical evidence of chronic hepatitis is usually not found until the patient develops cirrhosis.
   - a. **Stigmata** of chronic liver disease include jaundice, spider angioma, parotid enlargement, and in men, gynecomastia and testicular atrophy.

b. The **liver** may be enlarged during the early stages but is often **firm, nodular,** and **reduced in size during end-stage disease.**

3. **Laboratory findings**
   a. Patients with **chronic hepatitis B** usually have persistently elevated serum ALT. Patients with **chronic hepatitis C** characteristically have intermittent elevations of serum ALT, possibly related to the emergence of HCV mutants.
   b. In patients with **cirrhosis,** a prolonged PT or low serum albumin reflects a decrease in liver synthetic capacity. Elevated serum ammonia indicates diminished hepatic clearance. Serum bilirubin, ALT, and AST are often elevated. The serum albumin and bilirubin levels and the PT are good measures of the severity of liver disease.

D. Diagnosis

1. **Serologic tests.** Chronic viral hepatitis is diagnosed using assays similar to those used to diagnose acute hepatitis (see II D 2).
   a. **HBV.** The presence of HBsAg for more than 6 months confirms chronic hepatitis B, and the presence of HBeAg or HBV DNA indicates that the virus is actively replicating. The presence of anti-HDV in a patient with chronic HBV infection suggests co-infection with HDV.
   b. **HCV.** A positive HCV EIA with evidence of continued hepatic inflammation suggests chronic hepatitis C (there is no assay for active HCV infection). The diagnosis is confirmed using the HCV RIBA. Polymerase chain reaction (PCR) can also be used to document HCV viremia.

2. **Differential diagnosis**
   a. **Alcoholic cirrhosis.** It is important to rule out viral hepatitis in alcoholics with liver disease.
   b. **α_1-Antitrypsin deficiency, Wilson's disease, autoimmune hepatitis,** and **hepatotoxic drugs** can also cause chronic hepatitis.

E. **Complications of cirrhosis** include:

1. **Portal hypertension,** leading to edema, ascites, splenomegaly, and esophageal varices
2. **Hemorrhage,** from ruptured esophageal varices
3. **Bacterial peritonitis,** resulting from transudation and retention of fluid in the peritoneum and from the decreased ability of the cirrhotic liver to clear bacteria in the portal circulation
4. **Encephalopathy,** caused by decreased ability of the liver to detoxify cellular waste products
5. **Progressive muscle wasting**

F. Treatment

1. Although **interferon-α (IFN-α)** can be effective even in the later stages of hepatitis B and C, many patients do not respond to IFN-α therapy or relapse when therapy is discontinued. In addition, side effects of IFN-α include:
   a. Exacerbation of psychiatric disease, especially depression
   b. Exacerbation of thyroid disorders
   c. Further hepatic decompensation
   d. Thrombocytopenia

2. Management consists largely of **therapy for the complications of cirrhosis** (e.g., diuretics for fluid retention, purgation with lactulose for encephalopathy). Liver transplantation is a possibility for some patients with end-stage liver disease.

Case 1 Revisited

This child most likely has acute hepatitis A. The symptoms of mild jaundice and an enlarged, tender liver as well as the information provided by the girl's mother pertaining to the recent "epidemic" at the day care center support the diagnosis. The source of infection was most likely the fecal-oral spread of virus from an infected child to the patient. The diagnosis could be confirmed by the presence of IgM anti-HAV.

Although constitutional symptoms are present, the infection appears to be confined to the liver. The constitutional symptoms reflect nonspecific effects of liver damage and inflammatory processes triggered by circulating immune complexes and activation of immunocompetent cells. The severity of the symptoms does not correlate with or predict the subsequent clinical course. However, the possibility of acute bacterial meningitis should always be borne in mind for a lethargic child with backache and fever.

Although gamma globulin given before infection can modify or even prevent disease, no specific therapy is available once infection has occurred. The child should be managed expectantly as an outpatient, unless she is unable to eat and drink because of nausea or vomiting.

Case 2 Revisited

The duration of the intermittent jaundice and the examination findings of ankle edema, ascites, and hepatosplenomegaly suggest that the truck driver has chronic hepatitis that has progressed to cirrhosis. Chronic hepatocyte injury (from the immune response to viral antigens on the hepatocyte surface) and the accompanying inflammatory and regenerative responses lead to a poorly functioning, cirrhotic liver. The cirrhosis results in portal hypertension, which causes edema, ascites, and splenomegaly. Possible viral pathogens are HBV, HCV, and HBV/HDV co-infection.

Elevated levels of ALT, AST, or bilirubin can confirm the diagnosis of chronic hepatitis but do not identify the causative agent. A prolonged PT or a low serum albumin level can confirm that the patient has an end-stage, cirrhotic liver. Serologic testing for HBsAg and HBeAg can document chronic hepatitis B. The presence of anti-HDV would indicate HBV/HDV co-infection. A positive HCV EIA, confirmed with an HCV RIBA, can indicate chronic HCV infection. Because intravenous drug use is a risk factor for hepatitis B, C, and D, the patient may be infected with more than one hepatitis virus.

Therapy for chronic hepatitis B or C is limited to INF-α. However, in a patient with cirrhosis, therapy is less effective and may be poorly tolerated.

Chapter 56

Viral Exanthematic Diseases

Walton L. Ector

Case 1

A 9-year-old girl is brought to her pediatrician in February because of a fever that had lasted for several days and a rash that developed in the preceding 24 hours. She also has a headache, sore throat, and bothersome cough, but no gastrointestinal symptoms. No one else in the household is ill, but a classmate who had visited Mexico the previous month had just recovered from a similar illness.

On examination, the girl is alert and in mild distress. Her temperature is 102.9°F, her pulse rate is 110 beats/min, her blood pressure is 90/60 mm Hg, and her respiratory rate is 40 respirations/min. She has nonpurulent conjunctivitis with photophobia. Her posterior pharynx is injected, and the tonsillar follicles are filled with white material. The buccal mucosa is injected with scattered, raised, papular lesions. She has a papular rash on an erythematous base on her trunk, face, and arms. Her chest radiograph is normal. Her anterior and posterior cervical and suboccipital lymph nodes are enlarged. Her white blood cell count is 5600/mm^3 with a normal differential.

- ◻ *What is the most likely cause of this rash?*
- ◻ *Are any diagnostic tests indicated?*
- ◻ *Should antibiotic therapy be started?*
- ◻ *Could the disease have been prevented?*
- ◻ *Is this child's disease contagious?*

Case 2

An 18-month-old girl is brought to the emergency room with fever and a diffuse rash that had appeared 24 hours earlier. Her temperature is 104°F, and her heart rate is 180 beats/min. She has a diffuse maculovesicular rash, more pronounced in the trunk. Four vesicular lesions are visible on the soft palate. The remainder of the physical examination is unremarkable. The chest radiograph is clear; the white blood cell count is 12,000/mm^3 with a normal differential.

- ◻ *What is the most likely cause of this rash?*
- ◻ *How can the diagnosis be confirmed?*
- ◻ *Is any therapy indicated?*
- ◻ *Could the disease have been prevented?*
- ◻ *What was the most likely source of infection?*
- ◻ *Is this child's disease contagious?*

I. INTRODUCTION.

INTRODUCTION. Many viral illnesses, particularly those that affect children, cause changes in the skin or mucous membranes. Some viruses nearly always cause a skin rash (**exanthem**) or a mucosal rash (**enanthem**), such as rubeola virus (measles) and varicella-zoster virus (chickenpox). Others, such as hepatitis B virus (HBV), respiratory syncytial virus, and rhinovirus, are associated with rash so infrequently that they may not be suspected in a patient with a rash.

A. Definitions.

Definitions. Various terms are used to describe mucocutaneous lesions in viral illness:

1. **Macula** is an area of skin of any size, differing in color from surrounding skin but not elevated or depressed.
2. **Papula** is a small, circumscribed solid elevation less than 5 mm in diameter.
3. **Nodule** is a circumscribed, elevated, solid lesion 5 mm to 2 cm in diameter.
4. **Vesicles** are small, circumscribed, serum-filled elevations of skin up to 5 mm in diameter.
5. **Bullous lesions** are large (greater than 5 mm in diameter), serum filled elevations of skin.
6. **Wheals,** hard elevations of the skin caused by transient, superficial edema, are flesh-colored to pale red and last only minutes to a few hours.
7. **Ecchymosis** is a purple patch caused by extravasation of blood into the skin.
8. **Petechiae** are minute hemorrhagic spots of pinpoint to pinhead size.
9. **Ulcers** are small depressed areas of skin or mucosa caused by the superficial loss of tissue.
10. **Confluent lesions** are those that join or run together.
11. **Discrete lesions** are separate, distinct, and easy to individualize.
12. **Morbilliform (measles-like) rashes** are constituted by small red papules.
13. **Vesicular rashes** are constituted by vesicles spread all over the body.
14. **Purpura** describes the appearance of hemorrhagic areas larger than petechiae.
15. **Urticaria** is an eruption of pruritic wheals, usually of allergic origin.

B. Mechanisms of mucocutaneous reactions to viruses.

Mechanisms of mucocutaneous reactions to viruses. An understanding of the mechanisms by which viruses effect changes in the skin or mucosal areas is helpful in deciding the cause of rashes commonly seen in viral diseases.

1. Viruses may invade the epidermis, the subcutaneous tissue, or the cutaneous vascular endothelium and cause the formation of lesions due to **epithelial cell necrosis** and **associated inflammation.** These rashes are usually vesicular and include those caused by the varicella-zoster virus and herpes simplex virus (HSV).
2. Viruses may infect cells in the dermis and epidermis and trigger an **immune reaction** directed against the infected cells. The resulting rash is usually maculopapular, and the typical example is measles.
3. Systemic and mucocutaneous reactions may appear in a patient with a viral infection but without a definable immunologic reaction to the virus and without detectable virus in the affected skin area. A **cross-reactive immune reaction** may be responsible. This type of rash is exemplified by erythema multiforme and the Stevens-Johnson syndrome.
4. Urticarial rashes associated with viral illnesses are commonly seen, particularly in infants and young children. Possible mechanisms include:
   a. Direct **stimulation of mast cells** by the virus, causing release of histamine
   b. **Immediate hypersensitivity reactions** due to previous sensitization of tissue cells by antigenically similar or identical viruses

Table 56-1. Major Viral Diseases Associated with Maculopapular Rashes*

Disease	Etiologic Agent
Enteroviral infections	Echoviruses, coxsackieviruses
Roseola	Human herpes virus 6 and 7
Erythema infectiosum (fifth disease)	Human parvovirus B19
Measles (rubeola)	Paramyxovirus
Rubella (German measles)	Rubella virus
Infectious mononucleosis	Epstein-Barr virus
Cytomegalovirus infection	Cytomegalovirus
Acquired immunodeficiency	HIV-1

* Listed in order of frequency.

II. ACUTE VIRAL DISEASE WITH MACULOPAPULAR RASH (Table 56-1)

A. **Measles (rubeola)** is caused by a paramyxovirus transmitted person-to-person via the respiratory route. Measles may be the most contagious of all viral diseases. (Patients have developed measles when the only exposure has been their presence in a room occupied by a patient with measles several hours before.) Patients are contagious from the beginning of prodromal signs until 4 days after the onset of rash.

1. **Clinical manifestations**
   - a. **Prodromal symptoms** begin 10 days after exposure and include high fever of sudden onset, malaise, coryzal signs, catarrhal conjunctivitis with photophobia, and tracheal inflammation with cough. Cough is a prominent and universal symptom.
   - b. **Koplik spots** are specific for measles (see Chapter 36 II A 1 c).
   - c. The **exanthem** begins near the ears at the angle of the mandible, spreads to the face, and progresses down the trunk and down the extremities. The rash fades the same way, being seen last on the extremities. The maculopapular rash has multiple small papules on a background of erythema. The papules tend to cluster in groups called **crescents.** The erythema may become confluent, but the crescents of papules remain discrete.
   - d. **Fever** reaches its zenith as the rash erupts over a 36- to 48-hour period then begins to subside.
2. **Treatment** is usually symptomatic. Complicating bacterial infections should be diagnosed and treated with appropriate antibacterial agents.
3. **Prevention** is achieved by administering a live, attenuated virus vaccine that has proven to be highly effective.
   - a. If a nonimmune infant or adult is exposed to a patient with measles, administration of the live vaccine within 72 hours may prevent or ameliorate the disease.
   - b. Passive immunization with immune globulin given intramuscularly within 6 days of exposure also prevents the disease temporarily in nonimmune individuals.
4. **Complications** are not uncommon and can be serious. The overall mortality rate from measles in the United States since 1989 is 3 deaths per 1000 cases.
   - a. **Bacterial infections.** Probably as a consequence of the state of temporary immunosuppression that develops during the acute stage of measles, patients are susceptible to bacterial infections, such as otitis media, sinusitis, and pneumonia.
   - b. **Acute encephalitis** occurs at a rate of 0.73/1000 cases. Encephalitis results in permanent neurologic damage in approximately one-third of those patients and may cause death or permanent central nervous system (CNS) dysfunction.
   - c. **Subacute sclerosing panencephalitis (SSPE)** occurs in approximately 1 in 100,000 cases of measles, usually 7 years later, and is uniformly fatal.

B. **Atypical measles** may occur in patients who received the measles killed virus vaccine between 1963 and 1968 and are exposed to wild measles years later. Atypical measles does not appear to be contagious.

1. **Clinical manifestations.** Symptoms include fever, headache, cough, and a maculopapular rash (occasionally with some vesicles and petechial or purpuric areas) that begins on the distal extremities and spreads to the lower trunk. Antibody titers are much more markedly elevated than in regular measles.

2. **Complications.** Pneumonia is a frequent complication.

C. **Roseola (exanthem subitum)** is caused primarily by human herpesvirus-6 (HHV-6). However, some coxsackieviruses and echoviruses, particularly echovirus 16, and human herpesvirus-7 (HHV-7), also are associated with the clinical syndrome of roseola. Many cases of roseola probably occur after close exposure to adults or older children who have experienced reactivation of the virus with minimal signs.

1. **Incubation period.** The incubation period is believed to be about 9 days.

2. **Clinical manifestations**
   a. The disease usually affects children younger than 4 years and starts abruptly with **high fever** and **mild irritability.**
      (1) The patient's temperature may rise as high as 105.8°F.
      (2) Febrile convulsions occur in approximately 10% of patients. (Roseola is responsible for a large proportion of all febrile seizures in children younger than 4 years.)
   b. After 2 or 3 days, the fever abruptly starts to decrease, and a faint **maculopapular rash,** more prominent on the trunk, develops as the body temperature returns to normal.

3. **Treatment** is symptomatic. Isolation is not necessary. Secondary cases are rare.

D. **Rubella (German measles, three-day measles)** is caused by the rubella virus, a togavirus. It is transmitted person-to-person and transplacentally. Patients are contagious from 7 days before the rash to 14 days after the rash appears. Infants with congenital rubella may shed the virus for up to 1 year.

1. **Clinical manifestations**
   a. The incubation period is approximately 18 days. Symptoms include **mild fever** (seldom higher than 101°F) followed quickly by an **erythematous maculopapular exanthem** beginning on the cheeks, where the rash is most prominent, and spreading to the trunk and extremities. When fever occurs, it always peaks as the rash is erupting and disappears when the rash is fully developed. The rash fades from the face first and from the distal portions of the extremities last. There are few (if any) coryzal signs and little malaise. There is significant cervical, postauricular, and suboccipital **lymph node enlargement.**
   b. The infection is often asymptomatic (20% or more of exposed patients have increased antibody titers without a rash).

3. **Treatment** is symptomatic.

4. **Prevention.** A live virus vaccine was licensed in 1969 and has been very effective. Gamma globulin given to susceptible mothers-to-be who have been exposed to the virus may prevent fetal infection.

5. **Complications** are uncommon but include transient thrombocytopenia, encephalitis, arthritis and arthralgia (in young women), and congenital rubella syndrome (see Chapter 34 III A 2).

E. **Erythema infectiosum (fifth disease)** is caused by human parvovirus B19. The disease is moderately contagious, with the period of contagion ending approximately 1 week before the rash appears (i.e., before a diagnosis is made).

1. **Incubation period.** The interval from exposure to onset of viremia is about 5 days, but the rash does not appear until about 2 weeks later. Virus excretion lasts about 1

week after the onset of viremia, and the rash appears 1 week after viral excretion has ended.

2. **Clinical manifestations**
   a. A mild, nonspecific illness with low fever may occur during the viremic period.
   b. Approximately 80% of infected individuals develop the typical **erythematous rash** that begins on the face ("slapped cheeks" appearance). Within 24 hours, a macular or maculopapular rash appears on the trunk and extremities and quickly begins to assume a lacy or reticular pattern of erythema that is barely raised. There is no pruritus, and rarely any symptoms other than the rash. The rash usually lasts approximately 1 week, but may recur for up to 3 or 4 weeks (particularly when the skin is warmed or exposed to sunlight).
3. **Complications.** Parvovirus B19 infects hematopoietic precursor cells, causing profound **reticulocytopenia** that develops during the viremic stage and lasts about 7–10 days. Reticulocytopenia is not significant in normal patients but leads to severe problems in fetuses (profound anemia, fetal hydrops, and sometimes intrauterine death) and in children with hemoglobinopathies (e.g., sickle-cell anemia), who may develop an aplastic crisis with profound anemia.
4. **Treatment** is usually not required, except in pregnant women and patients with hemolytic anemia. In these patients, blood transfusions and intrauterine transfusions can be lifesaving.

F. **Nonspecific febrile illness with exanthem** is most commonly caused in the United States by the non-polio picornaviruses, including coxsackieviruses A and B, echoviruses, and enterovirus types 68–71. In infants and young children, some strains cause rashes in over 50% of infected patients. Other strains only rarely cause rash. Rash is less common in infected teenagers and adults, in whom nonspecific febrile illness without exanthem is the common presentation. These illnesses are transmitted person-to-person and by water and are most commonly seen in late summer and fall.

1. **Incubation period.** The **incubation period** averages 2–4 days.
2. **Clinical manifestations** are the sudden onset of **moderate fever** with few or no coryzal signs, often with headache, and sometimes with nausea and vomiting. There is usually little or no diarrhea. The **rash,** which is usually faint, maculopapular, and heaviest on the trunk, appears within 24 hours, usually beginning while fever is still present. The rash lesions remain discrete and last from 1–4 days.
3. **Treatment** is symptomatic.
4. **Complications.** Picornaviruses are frequently associated with **aseptic meningitis** and can also cause **parotitis, myocarditis in neonates,** and **pericarditis in young adults.**

III. ACUTE VIRAL DISEASE WITH VESICULAR RASH.

In general, a vesicular rash is highly suggestive of viral infection. Some viruses cause vesicles almost 100% of the time (Table 56-2), whereas others only occasionally result in vesicles. It is uncommon for infectious agents other than viruses to cause vesicular lesions, but they may be seen in Rickettsial pox, impetigo, and less commonly in other infectious diseases.

Table 56-2. Major Viruses Associated with Vesicular Rashes*

Varicella-zoster virus
Herpes simplex virus types 1 and 2
Enteroviruses (mainly coxsackieviruses)

* Listed in decreasing order of frequency.

A. **Chickenpox (varicella)** in caused by the varicella-zoster virus of the herpes family. The disease spreads person-to-person and is highly contagious from the appearance of the first lesion (which may be overlooked for 24 hours) until the last vesicle has ruptured and crusted, usually 5–6 days.

1. **Clinical manifestations**
   a. Chickenpox has a sudden onset marked by the appearance of **erythematous macules** 2–3 mm across, usually first appearing on the trunk or scalp, and spreading to the face and extremities. Nearly 50% of children have vesicles or ulcers in their mouths or throats. The initial macules develop clear vesicles in their centers within hours. These vesicles become cloudy, begin leaking fluid in the centers, then become "umbilicated" with depressed centers. **Crusting** follows rapidly and may last for several weeks. Lesions are seen in all stages at one time (in contrast to smallpox, in which all lesions are at the same stage from onset to crusting).
   b. **Fever** may be present or absent initially but always peaks as the rash fully erupts, between the third and fourth days, then quickly subsides.

2. **Treatment** is symptomatic and includes administration of antipyretic and antipruritic medications and hygienic care of the skin to avoid bacterial infection of the vesicular lesions.
   a. The use of acyclovir is controversial. It does modulate the illness if initiated within 24 hours of the onset.
   b. Treatment is particularly important in immunocompromised individuals, in whom the disease is severe.

3. **Immunity.** Placentally transferred maternal antibodies protect infants from many infectious diseases for the first 6 months of their lives; however, this is not the case for varicella-zoster virus.

4. **Prevention**
   a. An **attenuated virus vaccine** has been developed and approved by the Food and Drug Administration (FDA).
      (1) Universal vaccination of all infants at 12–18 months of age has been recommended by several medical organizations and the United States Public Health Advisory Committee on Immunization Practices.
      (2) It is also recommended that all 11- to 12-year-old children who are not immune (i.e., who have not had the disease) be vaccinated.
      (3) Vaccination of all susceptible children and adults should also be considered.
   b. Passive immunotherapy with **varicella-zoster immune globulin (VZIG)** is recommended for:
      (1) Neonates whose mothers have chickenpox erupting 5 days before to 2 days after delivery (these infants are at risk for severe chickenpox with encephalitis)
      (2) Immunocompromised patients exposed to a person with chickenpox

5. **Complications** are not common, but include bacterial cellulitis, infection of the cerebrospinal fluid (meningitis, encephalitis), Reye syndrome, giant-cell pneumonia (rare in childhood), and transient thrombocytopenia.

B. **Shingles (herpes zoster)** is also caused by the varicella-zoster virus, and is a recrudescence of an infection that has remained dormant for years in nerve cells (since the patient had chickenpox). Shingles is not uncommon in children but is more common and painful in adults. The cause for the sudden appearance of the rash of shingles in normal children is unknown.

1. **Clinical manifestations**
   a. The eruptions consist of **tough, tense vesicular lesions** in clusters along the distribution of a sensory nerve. It is unusual for more than one nerve to be involved, except in immunocompromised patients, in whom several dermatomes may be involved. The lesions last 10–28 days and may leave mild superficial scarring.

b. In children, pain is usually minimal to absent, in marked contrast to adults.

2. Treatment. Acyclovir is effective if given intravenously and is indicated in immunocompromised individuals.

3. Prevention. The incidence of zoster seems to be significantly decreased in children who have received the live, attenuated chickenpox vaccine.

4. Complications. Keratouveitis may occur if the ophthalmic branch of cranial nerve V is involved.

C. Hand-foot-and-mouth syndrome is caused by coxsackieviruses, particularly A16. The disease is highly contagious and is usually acquired from infected persons by direct contact or via water, usually in late summer or early fall.

1. Incubation period. The incubation period is usually 2–4 days.

2. Clinical manifestations

a. The disease is generally **mild in young children,** with low fever and no systemic complaints, but it may cause **more prominent malaise** and **fever in older children and adults.**

b. The rash consists of **small, superficial vesicles** on the **hands** (frequently affecting the palms) and the **feet** (affecting the soles less frequently). There are also superficial ulcers inside the lips and occasionally on the buccal mucosa. The **superficial ulcers in the mouth** seldom bother the young child but are more painful in adults. **In young children, a papular or maculopapular eruption** is seen on the **buttocks** and occasionally over the ankles and distal portion of the legs.

3. Treatment. The illness lasts only a few days, and treatment is symptomatic.

D. Herpangina is usually caused by any of several coxsackie A viruses but can also be caused by coxsackievirus B and echoviruses. The virus is transmitted person-to-person either by direct contact or via water, mainly in late summer and early fall.

1. Incubation period. The incubation period is usually 2–4 days.

2. Clinical manifestations

a. The typical case begins with **fever and headache,** sometimes with nausea and vomiting. The throat may be mildly inflamed.

b. Leukocytosis may be present early with a normal differential count.

c. By the second day, **vesicles appear on the soft palate,** usually near the tonsils. The rarity of involvement of the anterior buccal mucosa or the gums helps differentiate herpangina from herpes simplex. Herpangina also differs from herpes by its brief evolution—the lesions last only 2–4 days, while herpes lesions last 7–10 days.

3. Differential diagnosis. Early in the illness, fever, headache, sore throat, and pharyngeal inflammation (which develop before vesicles or ulcers erupt) may lead the physician to suspect streptococcal pharyngitis. The diagnosis becomes obvious after the rash develops. An elevated total peripheral white blood cell count as high as 20,000/mm^3 is not unusual and suggests a bacterial infection, but the differential count shows predominance of lymphocytes, as expected in a viral infection.

4. Treatment is symptomatic.

5. Complications are rare.

E. Herpetic gingivostomatitis is usually caused by herpes simplex virus type 1 (HSV-1). In adolescents and young adults, some cases are caused by herpes simplex virus type 2 (HSV-2). Approximately 50% of cases can be traced to contact with an older child or adult with a recent fever blister.

1. Clinical manifestations

a. The illness begins with **fever and malaise,** followed within 24 hours by **swollen red gums and ulcers** on the gums, tongue, buccal mucosa, lips, and palate.

b. The **lesions are painful,** and the patient feels irritable and restless, has difficulty sleeping, and has much difficulty eating or drinking.
c. There is a **fetid odor** to the breath, and **drooling** is copious.
d. Submental and submandibular **lymphadenopathy** is present.
e. The illness peaks in approximately 4 days, and resolution may take another week.

2. **Complications**
   a. **Dehydration** resulting from poor fluid intake may develop, particularly in infants and young children.
   b. **Kaposi's varicelliform eruption** is a severe complication that can affect patients who have atopic dermatitis. Severe vesicular eruptions occur over the areas of eczema.
   c. **Recurrence** of full-blown herpetic gingivostomatitis is rare, but in some patients, the virus remains latent in nerve cells, and the disease recurs as isolated fever blisters many times later in life.

3. **Treatment**
   a. Treatment is mostly **symptomatic** and includes administration of antipyretic drugs, topical antihistamines, and mild sedation at bedtime.
   b. A bland diet with plenty of fluids is indicated. If the patient becomes dehydrated, hospitalization and administration of intravenous fluids may be necessary.
   c. **Acyclovir** is effective against herpesvirus but must be given intravenously.
      (1) Acyclovir is seldom indicated in an immunocompetent child, but should be used in cases of generalized infection and CNS infection and in immunocompromised patients.
      (2) The efficacy of topical acyclovir ointments for therapy of common herpetic lesions has not been proven.

IV. ACUTE VIRAL DISEASE WITH URTICARIAL LESIONS.

Viruses can cause urticarial lesions to erupt. These lesions are easily mistaken for allergic reactions to foods or medications. Viruses frequently associated with urticarial reactions are listed in Table 56-3.

V. ACUTE VIRAL DISEASE WITH PETECHIAL OR PURPURIC LESIONS.

Table 56-4 lists the viruses that may cause this type of exanthem.

Table 56-3. Viruses Frequently Associated with Urticariform Rashes

Adenoviruses
Epstein-Barr virus
Coxsackieviruses and echoviruses
Hepatitis B virus
Herpes simplex virus types 1 and 2
Influenza viruses
Mumps virus

Table 56-4. Viruses Commonly Associated with Petechial or Purpuric Skin Lesions

Colorado tick fever virus
Coxsackieviruses
Cytomegalovirus (congenital infection)
Echoviruses
Lasa fever virus
Marburg virus

VI. ACUTE VIRAL DISEASE ASSOCIATED WITH ERYTHEMA MULTIFORME AND STEVENS-JOHNSON SYNDROME.

Various infectious agents and medications (particularly long-lasting sulfonamides) are associated with erythema multiforme and Stevens-Johnson syndrome (a severe form of erythema multiforme). Viruses that are occasionally associated with these eruptions are listed in Table 56-5.

A. Erythema multiforme (erythema multiforme minor)

1. **Clinical manifestations**
   a. **Rash.** Erythema multiforme has a sudden onset with the appearance of round or oval **erythematous lesions** that begin as large, raised lesions several millimeters across. These gradually enlarge, leaving flat centers that are smooth and may become dusky purplish (target or iris lesions).
      (1) The lesions **change in size and shape** (hence the designation multiforme), gradually enlarging. Two or more lesions may merge, forming areas several centimeters across.
      (2) Unlike hives, these **lesions are fixed** and do not respond to epinephrine or antihistamines. They persist for several days.
      (3) Neither blisters nor mucosal lesions are seen.
   b. **Fever** is often seen in infants.
2. **Treatment.** No specific therapy is available in cases of suspected viral etiology.
   a. If *Mycoplasma pneumoniae*, the most frequently implicated infectious agent in erythema multiforme, appears to be involved, proper antibacterial agents should be administered.
   b. If medications are suspected of causing erythema multiforme, they should be immediately suspended.

B. Stevens-Johnson syndrome (erythema multiforme major)

1. **Incubation period.** A prodromal illness with fever, malaise, sore throat, and headache commonly appears before the onset of Stevens-Johnson syndrome. In contrast, there are usually no prodromal signs, such as those that occur with erythema multiforme.
2. **Clinical manifestations.** Early skin lesions may resemble those of erythema multi-

Table 56-5. Viruses Occasionally Associated with Erythema Multiforme

Adenoviruses
Picornaviruses (coxsackie-, echo-, and polioviruses)
Epstein-Barr virus (EBV)
Herpes simplex virus types 1 and 2
Hepatitis B virus
Varicella-zoster virus

forme, but **bullous lesions** soon develop first on extremities, then on the trunk and face. **Involvement of mucous membranes** is severe and painful, with the mouth always involved and other mucosa such as the conjunctiva, anal, and vaginal areas usually involved. Large areas of **skin may become denuded with oozing.**

3. **Complications**
   a. **Dehydration** may result from lack of adequate fluid intake as well as excessive losses through denuded skin and fever.
   b. **Secondary bacterial infection** of raw skin areas can occur.
4. **Treatment.** The principles listed for the treatment of erythema multiforme apply also to the treatment of the Stevens-Johnson syndrome. In addition, supportive treatment, including fluid therapy and skin care, is indicated. Antimicrobial agents should be used in cases of secondary bacterial infection of the skin lesions. Steroids have not proved to be effective.

Case 1 Revisited

The acute onset and maculopapular rash and enanthem in the 9-year-old girl are highly suggestive of a viral infection, particularly measles. However, because the incidence of measles has declined considerably since the introduction of the vaccine, other viral infections associated with a maculopapular rash need to be considered. Differential diagnoses include streptococcal scarlet fever, which is usually associated with moderate to severe pharyngotonsillitis and a diffuse, erythematous skin rash described as fine and sandpapery due to hypertrophied pilosebaceous follicles. The tongue has a characteristic appearance, heavily coated white at first, and later red, with large, sometimes protruding, papillae (described as strawberry tongue).

The easiest way to confirm the diagnosis would be to detect a significant increase in the titer of antibodies to measles virus. However, because treatment is basically symptomatic, confirming the diagnosis is not a major clinical priority unless an outbreak is suspected. When measles is suspected, however, serologic confirmation should be done before instituting epidemic control. One case of measles in a community is now defined as an outbreak and requires strict control measures.

Antibiotic therapy should not be instituted in a patient with an uncomplicated case of measles. Antibiotics have no effect on viruses and can only promote overgrowth of resistant strains of bacteria.

Measles is spread from person to person and can be prevented by vaccination. In a child, the susceptibility to measles is likely to result from lack of vaccination or lack of response to vaccination. In young adults, immunity may have decreased owing to the lack of boosting. However, experts point to the lack of evidence for waning immunity in vaccinated patients.

The most likely source of infection in this case was the classmate who had been ill with a similar disease. Children with measles are infective from 1–2 days before the beginning of the prodromal symptoms until 4 days after the appearance of the rash. Children with measles should be isolated until not infectious.

Case 2 Revisited

The clinical picture in the infant is highly suggestive of chickenpox. The age of the patient, the type and distribution of the rash, and the elevated temperature are all typical of this viral disease.

Confirmation of the diagnosis usually relies on the evolution of the case. The diagnosis could be confirmed by histologic analysis of fluid from an unruptured vesicle [giant multinucleated cells (Tzanck cells) and lymphocytic infiltrate are characteristic] or by isolation of the virus from fluid aspirated from an unruptured vesicle.

Supportive therapy only is indicated for a patient with uncomplicated chickenpox. Careful follow-up is essential to detect evidence of pneumonia, encephalitis, or any other complication associated with chickenpox. If the evolution suggests dissemination of the infection, intravenous acyclovir is indicated. Immunocompromised children are at risk for disseminated chickenpox and should be given varicella-zoster immunoglobulin (VZIG) soon after exposure to prevent the infection, and acyclovir to avoid dissemination.

An effective live, attenuated vaccine for chickenpox is available.

The most likely source of infection is an infected sibling or an infected child in a day care center.

A patient with chickenpox is infective from the time the first lesion develops (which may be overlooked for 24 hours) until the last vesicle has ruptured and crusted, which usually takes 5–6 days.

Chapter 57

HIV and AIDS

Gabriel Virella
Salvatore Arrigo

Case 1

A 35-year-old man is seen in an outpatient clinic with a 3-month history of fatigue, loss of appetite, weight loss, fever, and night sweats. He has a cough that is worsening and has recently produced blood-tinged sputum. He is breathless on exertion and has smoked one pack of cigarettes per day for 20 years. He denies alcoholism and drug use. The patient moved 6 months ago from New Jersey to Pennsylvania. He is single, but lives with a girlfriend that came with him from New Jersey. He found a job on a poultry farm shortly after he moved, but he had to quit that job after he started feeling sick. He is now unemployed. Physical examination shows a thin and wasted male. His temperature is 37.8°C, and his respiratory rate is 22 respirations/minute. Chest auscultation is consistent with right apical consolidation. Old scars are visible on his forearms and antecubital fossa. The liver is enlarged, 2 inches below the thoracic cage, smooth, and nontender. The spleen is also enlarged and enlarged lymph nodes are palpated on the neck and groin. The remainder of the physical examination is unremarkable. The median veins of both forearms can be easily palpated and appear to be irregularly indurated.

- □ *What is the most likely diagnosis?*
- □ *What tests are indicated in this patient?*
- □ *What would be the indicated treatment for this patient at the time of presentation?*
- □ *What is the prognosis?*

I. INTRODUCTION. The acquired immune deficiency syndrome (AIDS) was first recognized in 1981–82, when the association of severe immunodepression with increased incidence of opportunistic infections and Kaposi's sarcoma in homosexual men was first noted. Testing of sera stored in blood banks has shown that the first human AIDS cases date from the 1950s and that the disease originated in Africa, then spread to Europe and the United States.

A. HIV-1. The causative agent of the syndrome is a retrovirus initially designated human T-lymphotropic virus-III (HTLV-III) or lymphadenopathy-associated virus (LAV) and now called human immunodeficiency virus (HIV). The original HIV was designated HIV-1 when a second virus, HIV-2, was found in Africa.

B. HIV-2 is less virulent, rarely causes full-blown AIDS, and is probably not spreading as widely and rapidly as HIV-1.

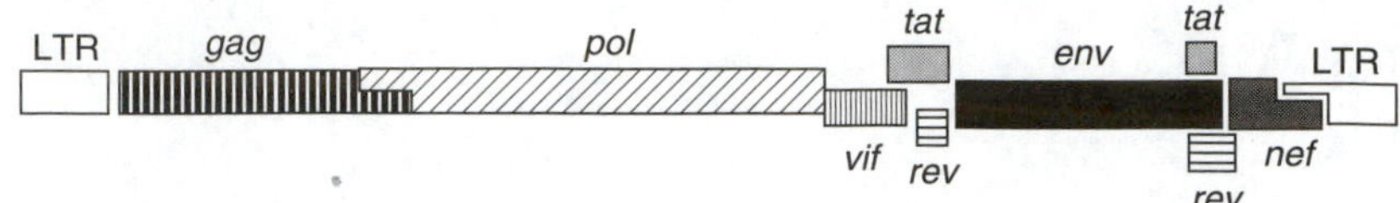

FIGURE 57-1. The HIV genome.

II. THE HUMAN IMMUNODEFICIENCY VIRUSES.

HIV-1 and -2 are retroviruses that belong to the Lentiviridae family. The viruses consist of two identical strands of +RNA associated with matrix proteins, a double protein capsid, and a lipid envelope with inserted glycoproteins.

A. The HIV genome.

The two strands of +RNA are linked near their 5′ ends. The HIV genome includes the following:

1. **Genes** (Figure 57-1)
   - **a.** The ***gag*** gene, which codes for a polyprotein that is cleaved postsynthetically into several immunogenic **structural proteins** (group-specific antigens)
   - **b.** The ***pol*** gene, which codes for the reverse transcriptase
     - **(1)** HIV reverse transcriptase is the most error-prone of all retrovirus reverse transcriptases. HIV isolates from serial passages of a single virus may differ by as much as 20% of their sequence.
     - **(2)** The *pol* gene product has several different enzymatic activities: it serves as a **polymerase,** a **ribonuclease,** and an **endonuclease.** The **integrase/ligase** activity of the endonuclease is critical for integrating the viral DNA into the host genome.
   - **c.** A gene located at the ***gag–pol*** **junction,** which is read in a different frame than the genes that code for the structural proteins, codes for a **protease** that cuts itself free from a larger polypeptide chain and proceeds to split the remaining polyprotein precursors into several other proteins and peptides
   - **d.** The ***env*** gene, which codes for the **envelope glycoproteins**
   - **e. Regulatory genes**
     - **(1)** The ***tat*** (transactivator of transcription) gene codes for a protein (p16) that binds to a region near the 5′ end of a nascent viral RNA strand known as TAR (transactivator response sequence) and promotes full transcription of that strand. The *tat* gene also seems to influence post-transcriptional events and to promote transcription of cellular genes.
     - **(2)** The ***rev*** (regulator of expression of viral proteins) gene codes for a second protein (p19) that promotes the expression of HIV-1 structural proteins.
     - **(3)** The ***vif*** (virion infectivity factor) gene codes for a protein (p23) that promotes viral expression. A virus that lacks *vif* is not infective.
     - **(4)** The ***nef*** (negative expression factor) gene codes for a protein that may decrease viral expression. However, in some cell lines, the *nef* gene seems to enhance replication.)
2. **Long terminal repeats (LTR)** flank the genes. The LTR regions contain TATA boxes and binding sites for nuclear factor kB (NFkB), a nuclear-binding protein. The *tat* gene product may enhance NFkB synthesis or modify NFkB to increase its affinity for the LTRs.

B. Structural proteins

1. Two **nomenclature systems** are used to describe the major structural components of HIV.
   - **a.** One system is based on chemical nature and molecular weight and uses "p" (for protein) or "gp" (for glycoprotein) with a number indicating the molecular weight in kilodaltons (e.g., p24, gp160).
   - **b.** The other system is based on the topography of the protein and uses the initials

MA (matrix), CA (capsid), SU (surface), or TM (transmembrane) followed by numbers indicating molecular weight (e.g., MA17).

2. The **major structural proteins** listed below are recognized by the immune system:
   a. **Glycoprotein gp160,** which consists of a transmembrane segment (gp41) noncovalently bound to the major external glycoprotein (gp120)
      (1) **gp120** is highly immunogenic and contains conserved and highly variable regions and a region that binds to the CD4 molecule of T cells.
      (2) **gp41** is believed to be analogous to the fusion-inducing proteins of paramyxovirus. Penetration of a cell by HIV may involve attachment of gp120 to CD4 and fusion mediated by gp 41. In addition, gp41 may mediate penetration in some cells lacking CD4.
   b. **Inner core capsid protein (p24** or **CA24)** forms the capsid.
   c. **Matrix protein (p17** or **MA17)** forms a layer between the viral core and the outer envelope.
   d. **Nucleic acid–binding proteins (p6, p7)**

C. Enzymes. HIV contains **reverse transcriptase** (a dimer of **p66** and **p51**) and an **endonuclease (p31).**

III. EPIDEMIOLOGY

A. Incidence

1. In 1993, over 600,000 cases of AIDS had been reported to the World Health Organization (WHO), which estimated that 2.5 million cases had actually occurred in that period. The estimates rose to 6.4 million infected individuals by 1995, and the projection for 2000 is that 110 million people will be infected and 25 million people will have AIDS. Between 80% and 90% of these cases will occur in third world countries, with large foci in South America, India, sub-Saharan Africa, and southeast Asia.

2. In the United States, at the end of 1994, 231,000 individuals were known to be HIV-positive, roughly half of them with clinical AIDS, and approximately 2% of them younger than 13 years of age. The Centers for Disease Control (CDC) estimates that the number of currently infected individuals in the United States exceeds 1 million.

B. Modes of transmission. The main modes of transmission of HIV in the United States are:

1. **Sexual contact**
   a. In the United States, the type of sexual contact carrying the greatest risk is **male-to-male,** followed by **male-to-female** and **female-to-male.** Heterosexual transmission is considerably more common in third-world countries but is on the rise in the United States.
   b. Factors associated with increased risk of venereal transmission include receptive anal intercourse, intercourse with a intravenous drug abuser, presence of genital ulcers, and multiple partners.

2. **Sharing of needles and syringes** among intravenous drug users

3. **Transplacental** or **perinatal** transmission from mother to child

4. **Blood** and **blood products.** Transmission is unlikely, because donated blood is tested for HIV and blood from potential donors who engage in high-risk activities or who are HIV-positive is declined.

5. **Organ transplantation.** Transmission is unlikely, because organ donors must be HIV-negative.

6. **Artificial insemination** and **maternal milk.** Evidence that HIV can be transmitted by maternal milk is inconclusive. In developed countries, HIV-infected women are advised to avoid breast-feeding. In regions of the world where infectious diseases and malnutrition are important causes of infant mortality, breast-feeding is still recommended.

C. AIDS exposure groups

1. Individuals with AIDS in the United States can be grouped according to risk factors or the probable mode of transmission. The ranking of exposure groups in most industrialized countries is similar.
   a. Homosexual or bisexual men (43%)
   b. Heterosexual intravenous drug users (26%)
   c. Homosexual or bisexual intravenous drug users (5%)
   d. Heterosexual individuals (10%)
   e. Children (1%)
   f. Recipients of blood, blood components, or organ transplants (2%)
   g. Hemophiliacs (1%)
   h. Other, or risk not reported or identified (6%)
2. In the United States, the fastest climbing rates of new HIV infection are in adolescents (especially gay males) and women.
3. Most children infected with HIV (90%) have a mother with or at risk for HIV infection (the risk of contracting HIV from an infected mother is approximately 30%). The remaining children acquire HIV through blood transfusion (10%) or through administration of coagulation factors.

IV. PATHOGENESIS

A. Infected cell populations

1. Once HIV enters the blood stream, it tends to infect **activated $CD4^+$ (helper) T cells,** using the CD4 molecule as a receptor. These cells express the CD4, $CD45RO^+$ phenotype of primed or memory T cells.
2. HIV also infects **monocytes, macrophages,** and **related cells** that express CD4-like molecules (expression of these molecules is much lower than CD4 expression in helper T cells). Monocytes and macrophages may also be infected by taking up virus–antibody complexes through Fc receptors. The infection of monocytes and macrophages is productive but not cytotoxic, and the infected cells become a source of persistent viral infection.
3. The **lymphoid tissues** (lymph nodes and peri-intestinal lymphoid tissue) are the main reservoirs for the virus in infected individuals. The virus replicates continuously, even in the early stages of asymptomatic disease.
4. In the central nervous system (CNS), the predominant infected cells are **microglial cells** of the monocyte-macrophage lineage. The significance of CNS infection in the pathogenesis of AIDS-associated dementia is unknown.
5. **Intestinal mucosal cells** are infected through an unknown receptor (perhaps membrane glycolipids). Intestinal infection may cause some forms of chronic AIDS-associated diarrhea.

B. Early viremic stage.

In the early stages of infection, the virus appears to replicate at a very low level for a variable period of time.

1. A transient decrease of total $CD4^+$ cells and an increase in circulating HIV-infected $CD4^+$ T cells may be detected. Soluble p24 may be detected in the circulation as early as 5–10 days after infection.

2. Circulating infectious virus is detectable for variable times, usually starting about the same time p24 appears, peaking 10–20 days after infection, and persisting until free anti-HIV antibody becomes detectable (**seroconversion**).

3. After seroconversion, integrated and soluble viral genomes are detectable by polymerase chain reaction (PCR) assay. Data collected from long-term survivors suggests that, in rare cases, the virus may be eliminated. Understanding why some individuals are long-term survivors while others develop AIDS rather swiftly is a major priority in AIDS research. At this point, it appears as if both host and microbial factors are involved:
   a. The genetic constitution of the individual may be critical. Differences in major histocompatibility complex (MHC) repertoire and transport-associated proteins are emerging as factors related to the evolution of HIV infection.
   b. The mode of exposure to HIV may play a significant role. Mucosal exposure to low virus loads seem to induce protective cell-mediated immunity (CMI) at the mucosal level, and the individuals may remain seronegative in spite of repeated exposures.
   c. At least in some cases, the long-term survivors seem to be infected by strains of reduced pathogenicity, which replicate less effectively and are associated with lower viral loads.
   d. Low virus loads (as determined by PCR assay) are associated with prolonged survival.

C. **Asymptomatic stage.** HIV-positive individuals remain asymptomatic for variable periods of time, often 10–15 years. During that period, the virus replicates but is kept in check by humoral and cellular immune responses.

1. **Humoral immune response to HIV.** Various types of antibodies are synthesized.
   a. **Neutralizing antibodies** directed against gp120 and gp41 inhibit the infectivity of free HIV in vitro.
      (1) The rate of progression to AIDS and the mortality rate are considerably higher in individuals lacking neutralizing antibodies.
      (2) However, neutralizing antibodies do not prevent infected individuals from eventually developing AIDS.
   b. **Antibody-dependent cell-mediated cytotoxicity (ADCC)–promoting antibodies** react with gp160 expressed on the membrane of infected cells.
   c. **Enhancing antibodies** react with gp41 antibodies and enhance HIV infectivity by an unknown mechanism. In some studies, the presence of HIV-enhancing antibodies appears to be correlated with progression toward AIDS.

2. **CMI** may either block infection or prevent the establishment of a productive infection. MHC-I–restricted $CD8^+$ T lymphocytes recognize a variety of epitopes in *gag, env, nef,* and *pol* proteins (the epitopes presumably correspond to short peptides captured during protein synthesis and expressed in association with MHC-I proteins).
   a. Cell-mediated cytotoxic reactions seem to be prominent in HIV-positive individuals who remain asymptomatic for prolonged periods.
   b. Evidence of specific anti-HIV cytotoxicity has been found in a group of 25 Nairobi prostitutes who have remained HIV-free (the rate of infection among Kenyan prostitutes in general is 90%).

D. **Immunosuppression**

1. **T cell activation and progressive depletion of $CD4^+$ T lymphocytes.** The evolution toward AIDS is associated with a progressive loss of immunologic protective mechanisms, particularly the progressive depletion of $CD4^+$ T lymphocytes. This decline is accompanied by increased HIV replication, suggesting that T-cell activation is essential for the replication of integrated HIV. *In vitro,* the replication of

integrated HIV is promoted by mitogenic or antigenic stimulation of infected T cells and by co-infection with viruses of the herpes family.

a. **T cell activation.** Several theories have been advanced about the cause of T cell activation that leads to enhanced replication of integrated HIV.
   (1) **Concurrent infection.** Infected macrophages and $CD4^+$ lymphocytes may be activated by concurrent infections (venereal or not).
   (2) **Superantigens.** Some viral components may act as superantigens, interacting directly with the $V\beta$ regions of specific T-cell receptors, thereby activating those cells.
   (3) **Activation of HIV-carrying dendritic cells.** Dendritic cells in the submucosa and lymphoid tissues may bind HIV without becoming infected. Activation of HIV-carrying dendritic cells could lead to clustering with noninfected T cells, which could receive activating signals and HIV from the dendritic cells.
   (4) **Cocaine use.** The addition of relatively low doses of cocaine to infected mononuclear cell cultures augments the replication of HIV, apparently by increasing the synthesis of transforming growth factor-β by the monocytes. This mechanism may contribute to the high incidence of AIDS in drug addicts.
   (5) **Tumor necrosis factor-α (TNF-α)** and **interleukin-6 (IL-6)** can promote HIV replication in monocytes, and TNF-α can promote HIV replication in infected T lymphocytes.
      (a) TNF-α induces the synthesis of a protein that binds to the NFkB-binding site on the LTR of the integrated viral genome. Binding promotes expression of the viral genome.
      (b) HIV-infected macrophages may release increased amounts of TNF-α and IL-6, thereby inducing HIV expression by both autocrine and paracrine mechanisms.

b. **Viremia.** Enhanced HIV replication leads to a second wave of viremia that is detectable as many as 14 months before the clinical evolution to AIDS. Coinciding with the second wave of viremia, antibody levels decline, particularly antibodies to p24. In terminal stages, both viremia and antibody levels may decrease again, perhaps reflecting total exhaustion of the $CD4^+$ cell population.

c. **T-cell depletion.** The causes of T-cell depletion are not well defined.
   (1) **Direct cytotoxicity** caused by virus replication is the simplest explanation. However, infection of T cells is not necessarily productive; the viral genome may integrate and remain unexpressed for long periods of time, while T cell numbers steadily decline.
   (2) **Apoptosis (programmed cell death).** Infected T cells express viral gp120 on the membrane, even when viral replication is minimal. Cell-surface gp120, soluble gp120, or virus-associated gp120 can interact with CD4 molecules on other infected or noninfected T cells. CD4–gp120 binding may stimulate apoptosis. Apoptosis can also be induced by antigenic stimulation of infected T cells.
   (3) **Syncytia formation.** The expression of gp120 on the surface of infected T cells promotes the fusion of the membranes of infected cells with the membranes of noninfected cells expressing CD4. The formation of syncytia allows direct cell–cell transmission of the virus and eventually leads to a reduction in the number of viable T cells. The emergence of strains with the syncytia-inducing sequences is usually a late event in the course of an HIV infection and is associated with a faster progression to AIDS (median of 23 months).
   (4) **Immune response.** The expression of viral glycoproteins in the membrane of infected T cells seems to trigger an immune response against those cells (mediated both by cytotoxic T cells and by ADCC mechanisms), which may contribute to $CD4^+$ T-cell depletion.

(5) **Co-infection.** *In vitro* co-infection of HIV-infected T cells with cytomegalovirus (CMV) or *Mycoplasma fermentans* has synergistic effects in the induction of viral replication and cell death.

(6) **Accumulation of unintegrated DNA** in the cytoplasm of infected cells is associated with vigorous HIV replication and cell death.

(7) **Infection of precursor cells.** Precursor cells in the thymus and bone marrow also are infected by HIV, which may account for the lack of regeneration of the declining $CD4^+$ lymphocyte pool.

2. Other factors contributing to the state of marked immunodepression associated with full-blown AIDS

a. When the $CD4^+$ lymphocyte count begins to fall, there is reduced activity of the TH_1 subset of T cells (there is no evidence that the activity of TH_2 cells increases). The imbalance of the TH_1 and TH_2 subsets (see Chapter 8 IV B) seems to precede the evolution toward AIDS. The patient becomes anergic, and the activities of cytotoxic T cells and natural killer (NK) cells decrease, owing to the lack of helper cells. B-cell responses also eventually decrease as the TH_2 subpopulation becomes numerically depleted.

b. Infected cells release soluble gp120, which binds to CD4 and prevents T cells from interacting with MHC-II antigens, thereby preventing the proper stimulation of helper T cells by antigen-presenting cells.

c. Immune complexes of viral antigens and the corresponding antibodies may also depress immune responses. For example, binding of complexes of gp120 and anti-gp120 to CD4 molecules on normal lymphocytes blocks activation via the T-cell receptor.

d. Infected monocytes can interact with noninfected $CD4^+$ macrophages and T lymphocytes, forming giant cells and contributing to the depletion of noninfected $CD4^+$ T lymphocytes. Chemotaxis, interleukin synthesis, and other accessory functions may be impaired in HIV-infected monocytes.

3. Humoral immunosuppression and stimulation of autoimmune responses

a. Impaired humoral responses to toxoids may result partly from the lack of helper T cells. In HIV infection, the B cell system seems to be in a state of permanent polyclonal activation, probably as a result of increased release of IL-6 by activated antigen-presenting cells and T cells.

b. Although many activated B cells produce antibodies to HIV antigens, polyclonal activation and loss of immunoregulatory mechanisms probably allow production of unrelated antibodies, including antinuclear autoantibodies and autoantibodies directed against platelets and lymphocytes. Anti-lymphocyte autoantibodies may be cross-reacting anti-viral antibodies. gp120 and the MHC molecule may have some structural similarities because both interact with CD4, and an immunodominant region of gp41 is homologous to the $\beta 1$ region of MHC-II.

E. **HIV escape from the immune response.** Despite the depletion of immunocompetent cells, most patients mount an anti-HIV humoral response that is still obvious when full-blown AIDS develops. Several factors may contribute to the escape of HIV from the host's immune response.

1. HIV can avoid the immune response by integrating its genome into host DNA with minimal expression of viral genes.

2. There are many subtypes of HIV, and HIV mutates at a much faster rate than most other viruses because HIV reverse transcriptase is error-prone and lacks proofreading activity. Mutations in epitopes of gp120 allow the virus to avoid recognition by preformed antibodies.

3. Humoral immune responses are less efficient than cell-mediated responses at eliminating virus-infected cells. Moreover, ADCC and lysis of infected cells after exposure to antibody and complement occur *in vitro* but may not be significant defense mechanisms *in vivo.* CMI is mostly responsible for keeping the infection under control, although its efficiency is limited.

V. CLINICAL STAGES OF HIV INFECTION.

Most patients with HIV infection develop AIDS. After a variable period without symptoms, 80%–100% of patients develop symptomatic HIV infection. Between 50% and 100% are predicted to develop clinical AIDS.

A. Five clinical stages of HIV infection are recognized.

1. **Acute illness associated with seroconversion**
   a. **Incubation time.** The typical incubation time is estimated to be 2–4 weeks. Viremia occurs during that time, and virus can be transmitted before antibodies are detected.
   b. **Clinical manifestations**
      (1) **Symptoms** are similar to those of infectious mononucleosis or the flu. The most common symptoms are **fever, sore throat, myalgia, headache, malaise,** and a **maculopapular rash.** Although 53%–93% of patients report these symptoms, the lack of specificity leads to frequent misdiagnoses. Most patients recover completely from the acute infection, although headaches and adenopathy may persist. It is not clear whether diagnosis and treatment at this stage can affect the long-term evolution of the disease.
         (a) During the latent period between exposure and production of detectable amounts of antibody, HIV infection can be diagnosed by detecting **virus** or **viral antigens.**
            (i) **Viral culture** and detection of viral RNA by **PCR** are the most reliable methods but are not available for routine diagnosis.
            (ii) **EIAs** for viral antigens, such as the p24 assay, have not proven to be very useful because of poor sensitivity.
      (2) **Serologic findings**
         (b) Seroconversion usually occurs 6 weeks after infection (antibodies to gp120 and gp41 are usually detected first, followed by antibodies to p24).
            (i) Because antibody tests are often negative during symptomatic primary infection, a seronegative patient who belongs to a high-risk group should be retested after 6 weeks.
            (ii) In rare cases, seroconversion can be delayed by 1 year or more.

2. **Asymptomatic HIV infection.** The patient remains seropositive with no symptoms or minimal symptoms (diffuse reactive lymphadenopathy and headache).
   a. **Clinical manifestations**
      (1) **Decreased $CD4^+$ lymphocyte count.** A progressive drop in the $CD4^+$ lymphocyte count is the most reliable indicator of clinically significant immunodeficiency.
         (1) Because $CD4^+$ lymphocyte counts are highly variable in an individual, repeated assays are needed.
         (2) The correlation between $CD4^+$ T-cell counts and the severity of clinical symptoms is less than perfect. Some individuals with extremely low counts remain asymptomatic, while others with much higher counts develop symptoms of AIDS.
      (2) **Detection of p24 antigen** in the blood is correlated with evolution toward AIDS, perhaps because it reflects viral replication unchecked by the immune system.
      (3) **Markers of leukocyte activation** become increasingly abundant as HIV infection progresses.
         (a) The markers include:

(i) Molecules released by activated T lymphocytes [β2-microglobulin, soluble interleukin-2 (IL-2) receptor, and soluble CD8]
(ii) Molecules released by activated monocytes (neopterin)
(iii) Expression of HLA-DR and CD38 (CD38 is expressed only by $CD8^+$ lymphocytes)

(b) Persistent increases in the levels of β_2 microglobulin and neopterin usually indicate a poor prognosis and evolution toward symptomatic infection. A combination of decreased $CD4^+$ cell numbers and increased β_2 microglobulin or neopterin levels or decreased $CD4^+$ cell numbers and detection of p24 antigen has better prognostic accuracy for evolution to AIDS than low $CD4^+$ lymphocyte counts alone.

b. An asymptomatic patient should be evaluated—and if necessary, treated—for other diseases seen in HIV-infected patients, such as syphilis, hepatitis B, and tuberculosis.

(1) Chemoprophylaxis of tuberculosis with isoniazid and immunoprophylaxis of influenza and pneumococcal pneumonia with the corresponding vaccines is indicated for patients at risk.

(2) *Toxoplasma* serology is also recommended, because it may identify patients at risk for developing severe toxoplasmosis at later stages of the disease. Eight percent to sixteen percent of HIV-infected individuals in urban areas have serologic evidence of infection with *T. gondii;* 80% develop toxoplasmosis when their $CD4^+$ counts drop consistently below 100/mm^3.

(3) In HIV-positive women, biannual pap smears are recommended, due to the increased frequency of infection with papillomaviruses, which is related to the development of cervical carcinoma.

3. Early symptomatic HIV infection

a. Fever, night sweats, fatigue, chronic diarrhea, disseminated lymphadenopathy, and **headache** in the absence of any specific opportunistic disease in a previously asymptomatic HIV-positive patient mark the transition toward symptomatic disease.

(1) Diarrhea is most likely caused by direct infection of the gastrointestinal mucosa by HIV.

(2) Disseminated lymphadenopathy, believed to represent a reactive response of all the nodal elements, is prominent in some patients and less obvious in others. Both T-and B-cell populations are expanded, and virus is not present in the reactive B lymphocytes.

b. Kaposi's sarcoma may appear relatively early.

(1) One etiologic theory is that release of IL-6, IL-1, TNF-α, and oncostatin M by activated macrophages is exaggerated, and that these factors act synergistically to promote the development of the vascular proliferative lesions typical of the tumor.

(2) Another theory is that the tumors are caused by a virus of the herpes family.

c. With time, **anergy** and other laboratory evidence of immunodeficiency may appear. Some **opportunistic infections** may develop, particularly **oral candidiasis, oral leukoplakia** (often asymptomatic), **upper** and **lower respiratory tract infections,** and **periodontal disease.**

4. Late symptomatic HIV infection. As $CD4^+$ cell counts progressively decline, the risk for developing **opportunistic infections** increases. The most common infections are listed in Table 57-1.

a. Opportunistic infections of greatest concern are ***Pneumocystis carinii* pneumonia,** whose frequency increases significantly when the $CD4^+$ lymphocyte count falls below 200/mm^3, and **toxoplasmosis,** which in AIDS patients often affects the brain.

b. As $CD4^+$ cell counts drop below 100/mm^3, infections with *Mycobacterium avium-intracellulare* or cytomegalovirus (CMV), esophageal candidiasis, cryptococcal pneumonitis and meningitis, recurrent herpes simplex infection, and

Table 57-1. Opportunistic Infections Characteristically Associated with AIDS

Pneumocystis carinii pneumonia (PCP)
Chronic cryptosporidiosis or isosporiasis causing intractable diarrhea
Toxoplasmosis
Extra-intestinal strongyloidosis
Candidiasis (oral candidiasis is considered a marker of progression toward AIDS; esophageal, bronchial, and pulmonary candidiasis are pathognomonic)
Cryptococcosis
Histoplasmosis
Infections caused by atypical *Mycobacteria,* such as *M.-avium intracellulare*
Pulmonary and extrapulmonary tuberculosis (often resistant to therapy)
Disseminated cytomegalovirus infection (may affect the retina and cause blindness)
Disseminated herpes simplex infection
Multidermatomal herpes zoster
Recurrent *Salmonella* bacteremia
Progressive multifocal leukoencephalopathy
Invasive nocardiosis

wasting increase in frequency. The release of TNF-α (cachectin) may participate in the wasting syndrome (known as "slim disease" in Africa) that characterizes advanced AIDS.

5. **Advanced HIV disease.** When $CD4^+$ lymphocyte counts fall below 50/mm^3, the immune system becomes severely dysfunctional, and the risk of death increases significantly. At this stage of the disease, all types of life-threatening opportunistic infections and complications are likely to occur.

B. AIDS. Full-blown AIDS is defined by the presence of one or several of the following features in an HIV-positive patient:

1. **Opportunistic infections** (see Table 57-1)
2. **Progressive wasting syndrome** (adults) or **failure to thrive** (infants)
3. **Unusually frequent** or **severe infections** not considered opportunistic, such as recurrent bacterial pneumonia or pulmonary tuberculosis. Recurrent bacterial infections are the most common infections in infants and children with AIDS.
4. Specific neoplastic diseases, such as **Kaposi's sarcoma, non-Hodgkin's lymphoma,** and **invasive cervical carcinoma**
5. Neuropsychiatric diseases such as **encephalopathy** (dementia) and **progressive multifocal leukoencephalopathy** (owing to reactivation of an infection with the JC virus) or significant developmental delays or deterioration in children
6. **Lymphocytic interstitial pneumonitis** in infants and children
7. A **$CD4^+$ cell count below 200/mm^3**

VI. DIAGNOSIS.

DIAGNOSIS. The combined accuracy of enzyme-linked immunosorbent assay (ELISA) and the Western blot test is greater than 99.5%.

A. ELISA is used to **screen** for HIV infection. ELISA uses either whole HIV antigens obtained from infected cell cultures or defined HIV antigens obtained using recombinant

DNA techniques. If the results of ELISA are positive, the assay is repeated to rule out errors or technical problems.

1. Serologic tests based on antibody detection are not fully reliable for early diagnosis of HIV infection. The median time from initial HIV infection to the development of antibody detectable using ELISA is 2.1 months; 95% of infected individuals develop antibody within 5.8 months of infection. Alternative approaches to the detection of early HIV infection include:
   - (a) Demonstration of viremia by culture and PCR
   - (b) Demonstration of antigenemia using a modified enzyme immunoassay (EIA) that detects p24 antigen after acid treatment of the serum to dissociate immune complexes
2. Serologic tests can be falsely negative late in disease, when antibody production ceases and viral replication is reduced because of depletion of host cells.
3. HIV infection is difficult to detect in neonates using antibody tests because maternal IgG antibodies may persist in the infant's serum for 1 year or longer. Alternative diagnostic approaches include:
   - a. **Viral culture and detection of genomic material by PCR.** Positive results are found in 35%–55% of infected neonates younger than 1 week of age and in 90%–100% of infants between the ages of 3 and 6 months.
   - b. **Assay for p24.** p24 is detected in 85%–95% of infected infants between the ages of 4 and 6 months, but in considerably fewer infected infants younger than 4 months.
   - c. **Measurement of plasma and urinary IgA antibody levels.** The IgA is fetal in origin because maternal IgA is not transferred across the placenta. In infected infants, the levels increase after 3 months. Positive results in uninfected neonates may result from transplacental transfer of some maternal IgA. Alternatively, the fetus may have reacted *in utero* to soluble HIV antigens that crossed the placenta.

B. Western blot (immunoblot) test. The Western blot test is used to **confirm** HIV infection. The test detects HIV-antigen—specific antibodies in the individual's serum. The Western blot is the only confirmatory test approved by the Food and Drug Administration (FDA) of the United States. A Western blot is considered positive if antibodies to p24, p31, and either gp41 or gp 120 are simultaneously detected.

VII. TREATMENT

A. Antiretroviral therapy. The drugs used to treat HIV-infected patients can be classified according to the stage of the HIV-replication cycle they affect.

1. **Drugs that inhibit reverse transcription**
   - a. **Zidovudine (ZDV), azidodideoxythymidine (AZT)**
     - (1) **Clinical use.** The usefulness of zidovudine in asymptomatic HIV-positive patients is controversial. Low doses of zidovudine reduce viremia and slow the progressive loss of $CD4^+$ cells, but these effects seem to wane after 2–3 years owing to the emergence of zidovudine-resistant HIV strains. There does not seem to be a significant increase in long-term survival, even though patients maintain higher $CD4^+$ cell counts for longer periods of time. As a rule, zidovudine is recommended in the following patients.
       - (a) **Those with $CD4^+$ cell counts below 500/mm^3**
       - (b) **Pregnant HIV-positive women and neonates born to HIV-positive women.** Zidovudine should be administered to pregnant HIV-positive women between weeks 14 and 34 of gestation (irrespective of $CD4^+$ cell counts), continued intrapartum, and administered to the neonate for 6 weeks. This treatment reduces the frequency of maternal–fetal transmission from 26% to 8%.
       - (c) **Individuals accidentally exposed to HIV** (e.g., by needle stick) can be

given a course of zidovudine, although there is no evidence supporting the benefits of prophylactic administration of zidovudine.

(2) **Side effects.** Zidovudine has serious side effects, such as anemia and neutropenia, that affect as many as 40% of the patients in later stages of the disease.

(a) When the side effects became troublesome, the usual alternatives are to reduce the zidovudine dosage and avoid the concomitant use of drugs that depress the bone marrow (e.g., trimethoprim–sulfamethoxazole) or to switch to a different antiretroviral drug.

(b) Zidovudine given in association with erythropoietin and granulocyte–monocyte colony stimulating factor (GM-CSF) to promote proliferation of erythrocyte and neutrophil precursors can extend the tolerance to zidovudine. However, GM-CSF is also toxic, causing anorexia and weight loss, anemia, fever, and thrombocytopenia.

(3) **Resistance to zidovudine** has been detected in patients treated for over 6 months. The resistance is associated with mutations in the gene for reverse transcriptase.

b. **Zalcitabine [dideoxycytidine (ddC)]** is particularly useful for cases of HIV that show resistance or fail to improve with zidovudine. However, zalcitabine has serious side effects, including painful sensorimotor peripheral axonal neuropathy and pancreatitis.

c. **Didanosine [dideoxyinosine (ddI)]** may increase survival time and may replace zidovudine in the treatment of presymptomatic HIV-positive patients.

d. **Stavudine** inhibits reverse transcriptase at levels similar to those of zidovudine but may be less toxic than zidovudine (although it is hepato- and neurotoxic).

e. **Nevirapine** is a nonnucleoside chain terminator that is bound to a hydrophobic pocket of the reverse transcriptase at a site different from the sites where other reverse transcriptase inhibitors bind. Thus, strains of HIV resistant to several of the other reverse transcriptase inhibitors are not cross-resistant to nevirapine.

2. **Drugs that interfere with HIV regulatory proteins**

a. Compounds that inactivate the *tat* and *rev* gene products are being tested.

b. Gene therapy with an adenovirus vector coding for an antisense mRNA that includes the TAR region (the target sequence in the viral genome for the *tat* protein) may inhibit viral replication.

3. **Protease inhibitors. Saquinavir, ritonavir,** and **indinavir** are synthetic, nonhydrolyzable peptides that behave as competitive inhibitors of the HIV protease. These compounds are being actively tested and their main therapeutic value may reside in their use in association with reverse transcriptase inhibitors.

4. **Drugs that inhibit viral assembly and budding.** Interferon-α (INF-α) seems to inhibit HIV budding and has been approved by the FDA for patients with Kaposi's sarcoma. The potential synergism of INF-α and inhibitors of reverse transcription is being investigated.

B. **Combination therapy.** Combinations of anti-HIV drugs, designed to circumvent the problems of drug resistance, appear to extend survival time. Two rationales are being followed:

1. The combination of two or more drugs targeting reverse transcriptase should reduce the likelihood of developing resistant strains, which would necessitate several simultaneous mutations in the reverse transcriptase gene. (Multiple mutations are more likely to produce a nonfunctional enzyme.)

2. The combination of two or more drugs targeting different points of the viral-replication cycle should reduce the likelihood of multiple resistance. An additional advantage is that the drugs' effects would be cumulative, permitting lower dosages of the individual antiretroviral agents, thereby decreasing the incidence and severity of side effects.

3. Early reports suggest that combination therapy with two reverse transcriptase inhibitors and a protease inhibitor often result in clinical improvement, marked reduction of viremia, and increases in CD4$^+$ T-cell counts.

Table 57-2. Antimicrobial Agents Used for Prevention of Infectious Complications of HIV/AIDS

Disease	Prevention
Pneumocystis carinii pneumonia	Trimethoprim–sulfamethoxazole (oral), dapsone (oral), or pentamidine (inhaled)
Tuberculosis infection (without active disease); (PPD > 5 mm induration)	Isoniazid daily for 1 year
Streptococcus pneumoniae pneumonia	Pneumovax every 5 years
Influenza A and B	Annual influenza vaccine
Recurrent oral candidiasis	Clotrimazole troche (dissolved in mouth)
Recurrent esophageal candidiasis	Fluconazole or ketoconazole (oral)
Recurrent herpes simplex or herpes zoster	Acyclovir
Cryptococcal meningitis	Amphotericin B for treatment of active disease; fluconazole for primary prevention or prevention of relapses
Cerebral toxoplasmosis	Pyrimethamine and sulfadiazine (or clindamycin); trimethoprim–sulfamethoxazole for primary prevention
Disseminated *Mycobacterium* complex	Rifabutin (clarithromycin also used)

PPD = purified protein derivative.

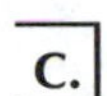
C. **Prophylactic therapy.** The successful treatment of symptomatic HIV infection requires antiretroviral therapy as well as prophylaxis for life-threatening opportunistic infections, as summarized in Table 57-2.

1. **Prevention of *P. carinii* pneumonia.** Prophylaxis for *P. carinii* pneumonia should be instituted in all patients with previous *P. carinii* pneumonia, $CD4^+$ cell counts consistently below $200/mm^3$ (in adults), or unexplained fever and thrush. Prophylaxis should be continued indefinitely.
   a. **Trimethoprim–sulfamethoxazole** is used to prevent *P. carinii* infection because of its low cost, convenient administration, and probable efficiency in the prevention of toxoplasmosis, nocardiosis, bacterial diarrhea, and bacterial respiratory tract infections. The main problem with trimethoprim–sulfamethoxazole is that it may cause bone marrow depression (a common side effect of zidovudine), so combinations of trimethoprim–sulfamethoxazole and zidovudine may not be tolerated.
   b. **Dapsone** and **pentamidine** are usually reserved for patients who do not respond to or do not tolerate trimethoprim–sulfamethoxazole.
2. **Prevention of CMV chorioretinitis. Foscarnet** and **ganciclovir,** which inhibit DNA polymerase, are effective for the prevention and treatment of CMV retinitis. An additional advantage of foscarnet is that it seems to inhibit both CMV and HIV replication.
3. **Prevention of mycobacterial infections.** Infections caused by *M. tuberculosis* and *M. avium-intracellulare* can be extremely difficult to treat because of the natural resistance of *M. avium-intracellulare* to tuberculostatic drugs and because of the emergence of multi-drug resistant strains of *M. tuberculosis.*
   a. **Isoniazid** is recommended for prophylaxis against *M. tuberculosis* in patients considered at risk.
   b. **Rifabutin** (a rifamycin, related to rifampin) is used for prophylaxis of infections by *M. avium-intracellulare* in patients with advanced AIDS or $CD4^+$ cell counts below $200/mm^3$.
4. **Prevention of bacterial and viral infections in children. Intravenous immunoglobulin (IVIg)** infusions given monthly reduce the incidence of bacterial and viral infection in HIV-infected children who are not receiving antiretroviral therapy. IVIg also slows the decline in $CD4^+$ lymphocyte counts.

VIII. IMMUNOPROPHYLAXIS.

Several approaches are being used to develop a vaccine for HIV. At present, there is no safe and effective HIV vaccine.

A. Types of HIV vaccines

1. **Attenuated vaccines** are made from genetically engineered strains lacking some crucial genes, so that the resulting virus causes a harmless infection. This approach has been tried successfully with simian immunodeficiency virus (SIV).
2. **Killed virus vaccines** do not induce protective anti-SIV immunity in animal trials. However, killed virus vaccines may prevent the emergence of clinical disease.
   - **a.** Monkeys vaccinated with killed SIV vaccines are less likely to develop disease but still become infected when challenged with live SIV.
   - **b.** In humans, it has been proposed that vaccination with low doses of killed HIV enhances TH_1 responses and favors the development of cell-mediated cytotoxicity. The benefits of therapeutic immunization in humans are not known. Evaluation is difficult because the end-point is a disease-free interval that is long and variable.
3. **Recombinant viral particles** made by inserting HIV glycoprotein genes in, for example, vaccinia-virus genomes induce neutralizing antibodies in animals. The overall effectiveness of recombinant vaccinia virus vaccines in humans has not been established.
4. **Component vaccines** have been prepared from isolated gp120, polymerized gp120, or gp120 peptides representing more conserved regions (such as the CD4-binding domain).

B. Unresolved Issues

1. **Efficiency.** Evaluation of HIV vaccine efficiency is complicated by the lack of adequate animal models (HIV can be transmitted to chimpanzees but does not cause clinical disease in these animals) and by the lack of adequate indices of protection in humans.
   - **a.** The efficiency of a vaccine is usually assessed by the quantity of protective antibodies. However, antibodies are not truly protective in the case of HIV. Therefore, an efficient vaccine should stimulate ADCC or CMI, which may be the only way to eliminate virus-infected cells.
     - **(1)** Certain conserved epitopes of gp120, gp41, and the *gag* protein may induce T-cell–mediated immunity.
     - **(2)** The assessment of cell-mediated cytotoxicity is much more laborious and expensive than the assessment of humoral immunity.
   - **b.** The lack of protection by antibodies results mostly from the variability of gp120. Different strains of HIV differ by as much as 20% in the structure of gp120, and antibodies elicited by one strain do not cross-react with other strains. However, some strains are more common than others (e.g., the MN strain accounts for approximately 30% of the HIV isolated in the United States), and it may be possible to prepare vaccines from mixtures of the most prevalent strains.
   - **c.** In an individual, HIV may undergo mutations. A single amino acid substitution in a critical epitope of gp120 may render the virus resistant to antibodies elicited earlier in the disease.
2. **Safety**
   - **a.** There is a remote possibility that genetically engineered, defective HIV strains could spontaneously revert to infectious, pathogenic strains.
   - **b.** An immune response directed against epitopes of gp120 could be cytotoxic to noninfected $CD4^+$ cells that bind soluble gp120.
   - **c.** The induction of antibodies may actually enhance the progression of disease by a variety of mechanisms (not yet proved):
     - **(1)** Antibodies may promote viral infection of macrophages by forming immune complexes that can be taken up through Fc receptors.

(2) Antibodies may help to "select" mutant viral strains.
(3) An ineffective humoral response may shield viral particles and infected cells from the more effective CMI mechanisms, resulting in the activation of dormant infections in asymptomatic HIV carriers.

d. Recombinant vaccines using vaccinia virus as a carrier may cause clinical disease in an asymptomatic but already immunocompromised patient.

3. Ethics and liability

a. Seronegative individuals who receive an HIV vaccine (which renders them seropositive for HIV by ELISA) must be protected against discrimination on the basis of seropositivity.

b. It would be difficult to evaluate the efficacy of a vaccine in volunteers, because these individuals may adopt behavioral changes that by themselves reduce the risk of HIV infection.

c. Possible adverse effects of a vaccine make liability of vaccine producers a major problem in industrialized countries.

Case 1: Revisited

The clinical presentation—a subacute febrile disease with cough, bloody sputum, weight loss, and consolidation of the right apex—strongly suggests that this patient has pulmonary tuberculosis. However, the facts that the patient has physical evidence of intravenous drug use, moved from an area with one of the highest incidences of HIV infection in the United States, and has disseminated lymphadenopathy and a very fast rate of deterioration makes the possibility that he is HIV-positive very likely. (It is actually recommended that all patients with active pulmonary tuberculosis living in areas of high HIV prevalence be tested). In addition, the patient's hepatosplenomegaly suggests that his infection may be disseminated. He may have been exposed to *Mycobacterium avium-intracellulare* as a result of his job on the poultry farm. This organism often causes disseminated infections in HIV-positive individuals.

Chest radiographs, blood and sputum cultures, and Gram and acid-fast stains of the sputum should be ordered to identify the extent and cause of the pulmonary disease. In addition, the HIV status of the patient needs to be determined, as well as his complete blood count with differential and the distribution of his lymphocyte subpopulations.

It is important to start therapy with antimicrobials as soon as possible. The choice of antimicrobials will depend on the precise etiology of the patient's lung infection. If *Mycobacterium tuberculosis* is identified, it should probably be considered potentially resistant to tuberculostatic drugs, given the fact that the patient moved from an area of high prevalence of those strains. In cases of confirmed resistance, therapy involves combinations of ethambutol, pyrazinamide, amikacin, and a fluoroquinolone. The treatment of *M. avium-intracellulare,* on the other hand, requires the use of different types of antimicrobials, such as clarithromycin. Finally, if the patient is proven to be HIV-positive and his blood count does not show neutropenia, treatment with zidovudine or with a combination of antiretroviral drugs should be initiated.

The prognosis largely depends on whether this patient has AIDS or not. However, proper treatment and institution of chemoprophylaxis, not only against *Mycobacteria,* but also against other opportunistic infections, is often associated with prolongation of life. The success of chemoprophylaxis, however, depends on many factors, and patient compliance is extremely important.

Summary Tables

Summary of the Major Bacteria

Genus	Identification	Gram Staining/ Morphology	Enzymes	Toxins	Capsule/ Surface Proteins	Epidemiology	Diagnosis	Diseases	Drug of Choice	Vaccine
Staphylococcus aureus	Mannitol-salt Coagulase positive Phage typing	+/•	Catalase, β-lactamase	Enterotoxins, TSST-1, Exfoliatin	Protein A	Person-to-person, carriers	Isolation, coagulase test	Skin infections, toxic shock syndrome, food poisoning, deep infections	Methicillin, oxacillin, vancomycin	No
Staphylococcus epidermidis	Coagulase negative	+/•	. . .	. . .	. . .	Opportunistic	Isolation, coagulase test	Bacteremia, endocarditis	. . .	No
Streptococcus pyogenes (group A)	Blood agar β hemolysis	+/•	Streptokinase, streptodornase, hyaluronidase, streptolysin O	Erythrogenic toxin, pyrogenic exotoxin A	Protein M	Person-to-person	Isolation, bacitracin sensitivity	Skin infections, pharyngitis, rheumatic fever, glomerulo-nephritis	Penicillin	No
Streptococcus agalactiae (group B)	Blood agar β hemolysis	+/•	Streptokinase, strepto-dornase, hyaluronidase, streptolysin O	. . .	. . .	Person-to-person, carriers	Isolation, bacitracin resistance	Neonatal meningitis	. . .	No
Streptococcus viridans	Blood agar α hemolysis	+/•	Streptokinase, strepto-dornase, hyaluronidase, streptolysin O	. . .	. . .	Person-to-person	Optochin resistance, bile insoluble	Endocarditis	. . .	No
Streptococcus pneumoniae	Blood agar α hemolysis	+/•	. . .	. . .	Poly-saccharide capsule	Person-to-person	Optochin sensitivity, bile soluble	Pneumonia, meningitis	Third-generation cephalo-sporin, penicillin	Yes
Neisseria meningitidis	Chocolate agar	−/•	IgA protease	Endotoxin	Poly-saccharide capsule	Inhalation	Oxidase reactivity, CSF agglutination	Meningitis, menin-goccemia	Penicillin	Yes
Neisseria gonorrhoeae	Thayer-Martin agar	−/•	β-lactamase (30%), IgA protease	. . .	Pili, no capsule	Sexual transmission	. . .	Gonorrhea, pelvic inflammatory disease	Ceftriaxone	No

Bacteroides fragilis	Anaerobic culture	−/■	β-lactamase	Endotoxin	Polysaccharide capsule	Opportunistic	. . .	Peritonitis, abscesses	Metro-nidazole, clindamycin	No
Vibrio cholerae	. . .	−/′	. . .	Cholera toxin	Adhesins	Fecal-oral, contaminated food and water	Usually clinical, oxidase reactivity	Profuse diarrhea	. . .	Yes
Vibrio para-haemolyticus	Halophilic	−/′	. . .	Enterotoxin	None	Contami-nated seafood	. . .	Watery diarrhea	. . .	No
Campylobacter fetus/jejuni	Thermophilic (*C. fetus*), micro-aerophilic	−/′	. . .	. . .	. . .	Fecal-oral, contaminated food	Isolation	. . .	. . .	No
Helicobacter pylori	. . .	−/′	Urease	. . .	. . .	Contami-nated food	Urease tests	Gastritis, gastric ulcer	Omeprazole, metronidazole, clarithromycin	No
Escherichia coli	MacConkey agar Lactose positive	−/■	. . .	ST, LT (ETEC); Verotoxin (EHEC)	Polysaccharide capsule	Fecal-oral, opportunistic, contaminated food	Indole positive	Watery diarrhea, dysentery	Ampicillin, trimethoprim–sulfa-methoxazole	No
Salmonella typhi	MacConkey agar Lactose negative	−/■	. . .	Endotoxin	Capsule (Vi)	Fecal-oral, contami-nated food	H_2S ±	Typhoid fever	Chloram-phenicol, ampicillin	Yes
Salmonella enteritidis	MacConkey agar Lactose negative	−/■	. . .	. . .	. . .	Contami-nated food (poultry)	H_2S positive	Salmonellosis, osteomyelitis	. . .	No
Shigella species	MacConkey agar Lactose negative	−/■	. . .	Hemolysin, Shiga toxin (*S. dysenteriae*)	. . .	Fecal-oral	H_2S negative nonmotile	Shigelosis, dysentery	Ampicillin, trimethoprim–sulfa-methoxazole	No
Klebsiella pneumoniae	MacConkey agar Lactose positive	−/■	. . .	Endotoxin	Polysaccharide capsule	Opportunistic	Mucoid colonies	Pneumonia, urinary tract infection	. . .	No
Proteus species	MacConkey agar Lactose negative	−/■	Urease	. . .	. . .	Opportunistic	Highly motile	Urinary tract infection, kidney stones	. . .	No

(continued)

(continued)

Genus	Identification	Gram Staining/ Morphology	Enzymes	Toxins	Capsule/ Surface Proteins	Epidemiology	Diagnosis	Diseases	Drug of Choice	Vaccine
Pseudomonas species	Lactose negative Oxidase positive	–/■	. . .	Toxin A, endotoxin	Slime (alginate) layer	Opportunistic	Pigments (pyocyanin, pyoverdin)	Burn infections, upper respiratory infections in cystic fibrosis patients	. . .	No
Brucella	Grow in 10% carbon dioxide	–/■	. . .	Endotoxin	. . .	Contaminated food (milk, cheese), contact	. . .	Brucellosis (undulating fever)	Tetracyclines	Yes (for herds)
Bacillus anthracis	Spore former	–/■	. . .	Anthrax toxin	D-glutamate	Contaminated animal products	. . .	Anthrax	Penicillin	Yes (for herds)
Bacillus cereus	Spore former	–/■	. . .	Enterotoxin	. . .	Contaminated food	. . .	Food poisoning	. . .	No
Clostridium botulinum	Spore former Anaerobic	–/■	. . .	Botulin (neurotoxin)	. . .	Contaminated food	. . .	Botulism (descending paralysis)	Antitoxin	No
Clostridium tetani	Spore former Anaerobic	–/■	. . .	Tetanospasmin	. . .	Soil-contaminated wounds	. . .	Tetanus (spastic paralysis)	Penicillin, antitoxin	Yes
Clostridium perfringens	Spore former Anaerobic	–/■	. . .	12 toxins: α toxin = lecithinase	. . .	. . .	. . .	Gas gangrene	. . .	No
Clostridium difficile	Spore former Anaerobic	–/■	. . .	Cyotoxic toxin	. . .	Endogenous opportunist	. . .	Antibacterial-induced enterocolitis	. . .	No
Haemophilus influenzae	Chocolate agar	–/■	IgA protease	. . .	Capsule (PRP)	Inhalation	Quellung reaction	Meningitis, epiglottitis, pneumonia	Ceftriaxone, ampicillin, chloramphen	Yes
Bordetella pertussis	. . .	–/■	. . .	Pertussis toxin	Capsule	Inhalation	. . .	Whooping cough, leukemoid reaction	. . .	Yes

Corynebacteria diphtheriae	. . .	+/■	. . .	Diphtheria toxin	. . .	Inhalation	. . .	Diphtheria	Antitoxin, penicillin	Yes
Legionella species	Charcoal-yeast extract agar + cysteine	N/A	β-lactamase	. . .	. . .	Opportun-istic, contaminated water	Direct immuno-fluorescence in tissues	Legionnaires' disease	Erythromycin	No
Mycoplasma pneumoniae	. . .	N/A	. . .	. . .	"Wall-less"	Person-to-person	Cold agglutinins	Atypical pneumonia	Erythromycin	No
Mycobacterium tuberculosis	Löwenstein-Jensen medium Aerobe	Acid-fast ■	. . .	. . .	Cord factor	Inhalation	Tuberculin test, isolation	Tuberculosis	Isoniazid ethambutol, rifampin (combinations)	Yes
Mycobacterium leprae	Cannot be cultured	Acid-fast ■	. . .	. . .	. . .	Person-to-person	Microscopy	Leprosy	Dapsone	No
Mycobacterium avium-intracellulare	Slow growth	Acid-fast ■	. . .	. . .	. . .	Opportunistic	Isolation	Tuberculosis-like infection	. . .	No
Treponema pallidum	Cannot be cultured	N/A ~	. . .	Endotoxin	. . .	Sexual transmission	Serologies	Syphilis	Penicillin	No
Borrelia burgdorferi	. . .	N/A ~	. . .	. . .	. . .	Tick	Serologies	Lyme disease	Tetracyclines	No
Chlamydia trachomatis	Cell cultures	N/A	. . .	Endotoxin	. . .	Sexual contact, person-to-person	Cytoplasmic inclusion, DNA probes	Trachoma, non-gonococcal urethritis, lympho-granuloma venereum	Tetracyclines, azithromycin	No
Chlamydia psitacci	Cell cultures	N/A	. . .	Endotoxin	. . .	Inhalation	Cytoplasmic inclusions, serologies	Atypical pneumonia	Tetracyclines	No
Rickettsia rickettsii	Cell cultures	N/A	. . .	Endotoxin	. . .	Tick	IFA, EIA, cDNA	Rocky Mountain spotted fever	Tetracyclines, chloram-phenicol	No
Rickettsia typhi	Cell cultures	N/A	. . .	Endotoxin	. . .	Flea	Weil-Felix reaction	Murine typhus	Tetracyclines	No
Coxiella burnetii	Cell cultures	N/A	. . .	Endotoxin	. . .	Inhalation	. . .	Q fever	Tetracyclines	No

• = coccus; ■ = rod; ′ = curved rod; ~ = spirochete; *cDNA* = complementary DNA; *CSF* = cerebrospinal fluid; *EIA* = enzyme immunoassay; *EHEC* = enterohemorrhagic *Escherichia coli; ETEC* = enterotoxigenic *Escherichia coli*; H_2S = hydrogen sulfide; IFA = immunofluorescent assay; *LT* = heat-labile toxin; *PRP* = phosphoribosyl ribitol phosphate; *ST* = heat-stable toxin; *TSST-1* = toxic shock syndrome toxin-1

Major Pathogenic Bacteria Organized by Type of Disease

Type of Disease	Bacteria
Skin infections	Staphylococci
	Streptococci
Upper respiratory tract infections	Group A *Streptococcus*
	Haemophilus influenzae
	Bordetella pertussis
	Corynebacterium diphtheriae
Otitis media	*Streptococcus pneumoniae*
	Moraxella (Branhamella) catarrhalis
	Haemophilus influenzae
	Group B *Streptococcus*
	Staphylococcus aureus
Lower respiratory tract infections	*Streptococcus pneumoniae*
	Haemophilus influenzae
	Mycoplasma pneumoniae
	Chlamydia psitacci
	Mycobacterium tuberculosis
	Klebsiella pneumonia
	Pseudomonas aeruginosa
	Staphylococcus aureus
	Anaerobic bacteria
Gastrointestinal infections	*Vibrio cholerae*
	Vibrio parahaemolyticus
	Escherichia coli
	Salmonella species*
	Shigella species
	Campylobacter species
	Helicobacter pylori
	Clostridium perfringens
	Clostridium difficile
	Bacillus cereus
Urinary tract infections	*Escherichia coli*
	Pseudomonas aeruginosa
	Enterobacter species
	Klebsiella species
	Proteus species
Venereal diseases	*Neisseria gonorrhoeae*
	Treponema pallidum
	Chlamydia trachomatis
	Haemophilus ducreyii
Meningitis	*Escherichia coli*
	Group B *Streptococcus*
	Listeria monocytogenes
	Haemophilus influenzae
	Neisseria meningitidis
	Streptococcus pneumoniae
Endocarditis	*Streptococcus viridans*
	Group D *Streptococcus* (enterococcus)
	Staphylococci
	Enterobacteriaceae and *Pseudomonas* species
Bone infections	*Staphylococcus aureus*
	Mycobacterium tuberculosis
	Salmonella typhi

* Except *Salmonella typhi* and *Salmonella typhimurium*, which cause enteric fever

Summary of the Major DNA Viruses

Family	Structure	Enzymes	Epidemiology	Disease	Treatment
Herpetoviridae	Double-stranded DNA, enveloped	None			
Herpes simplex virus type 1 (HHV-1)			Direct contact, latency, vertical	Gingivostomatitis, fever blisters, encephalitis, keratitis, congenital herpes	Acyclovir
Herpes simplex virus type 2 (HHV-2)			Sexual, vertical	Genital herpes Congenital/ neonatal herpes	Acyclovir
Varicella-zoster virus (HHV-3)			Respiratory, latency	Chickenpox, shingles, encephalitis	Acyclovir, varicella-zoster immunoglobulin
Epstein-Barr virus (HHV-4)			Respiratory, latency, oncogenic	Infectious mononucleosis, Burkitt's lymphoma, nasopharyngeal carcinoma	Supportive
Cytomegalovirus (HHV-5)			Respiratory, blood transfusion, latency, vertical	Hepatitis, kidney infections	Supportive, gancyclovir
Human herpesvirus type 6 (HHV-6)			Respiratory, latency	Exanthema subitum Lymphomas?	
Adenoviridae	Double-stranded DNA, naked	None	Respiratory, latency	Upper and lower respiratory infections, keratoconjunctivitis	Supportive
Papovaviridae	Double-stranded DNA, naked	None			
Papillomaviruses			Direct contact, latency, oncogenic	Warts, condyloma accuminata, cervical carcinoma	Removal, interferon-α (IFN-α)
Polyomavirus					
BK virus			?, Latency	Possible upper respiratory and kidney infections	
JC virus			?, Latency	Progressive multifocal leukoencephalopathy	Interferon-β (IFN-β)
Poxviridae	Double-stranded DNA, complex	RNA polymerase	Respiratory	Smallpox, molluscum contagiosum	
Hepadnaviridae	Incomplete double-stranded DNA, two capsids	DNA polymerase, reverse transcriptase	Blood, sexual, latency, oncogenic	Hepatitis, hepatoma	Supportive
Parvoviridae	Single-stranded DNA, naked	None	Respiratory?	Bone marrow aplasia, erythema infecciosum	Supportive

HHV = human herpesvirus.

Summary of the Major RNA Viruses

Family	Structure	Enzymes	Epidemiology	Disease	Treatment
Picornaviridae	Single-stranded +RNA, naked	None			
Rhinovirus			Respiratory	Common cold	Supportive
Enterovirus					
Picornavirus			Fecal-oral	Polio, meningitis	Supportive
Coxsackievirus			Fecal-oral	A: Herpangina, hand-foot-and-mouth disease B: Myocarditis, pericarditis, pleurodynia A&B: Meningitis	
Echovirus			Fecal-oral	Meningitis	Supportive
Hepatitis A virus			Fecal-oral	Acute hepatitis	Supportive
Togaviridae	Single-stranded +RNA, enveloped	None			
Alphavirus					
EEE, WEE, VEE			Mosquito	Encephalitis	Supportive
Flavivirus					
Yellow fever virus			Mosquito	Yellow fever	Supportive
Dengue virus			Mosquito	Arthralgia	
JBE, SLE virus			Mosquito	Encephalitis	
Hepatitis C virus			Blood, sexual	Non-A, non-B hepatitis, chronic active hepatitis	Interferon-α
Rubivirus					
Rubella virus			Respiratory, vertical	Rubella, postinfectious encephalitis, congenital rubella	Supportive
Coronaviridae	Single-stranded +RNA, enveloped	None	Respiratory	Upper respiratory tract infection, cold	Supportive
Caliciviridae	Single-stranded +RNA, naked	None			
Norwalk virus			Fecal-oral	Acute gastroenteritis, diarrhea (in adults)	Supportive
HEV	Single-stranded +RNA	?	Blood, fecal-oral	Hepatitis	
Orthomyxoviridae	Single-stranded −RNA, segmented, enveloped	RNA-RNA polymerase, endonuclease	Respiratory	Classic flu	Supportive, amantidine, rimantidine

(continued)

(continued)

Family	Structure	Enzymes	Epidemiology	Disease	Treatment
Paramyxoviridae	Single-stranded −RNA, enveloped	RNA-RNA polymerase			
Paramyxoviruses					
Parainfluenza virus	H&N, monotypic		Respiratory	Croup, bronchiolitis, upper respiratory infection	Supportive
Mumps virus	H&N, monotypic		Respiratory	Mumps, postinfectious encephalitis, meningitis	Supportive, mumps immuno-globulin
Morbilivirus					
Measles virus	H only, monotypic		Respiratory	Measles, pneumonia, postinfectious encephalitis, SSPE	Supportive, measles immuno-globulin
Pneumovirus					
Respiratory syncytial virus	No H or N		Respiratory	Upper and lower respiratory tract infection	Ribavirin
Rhabdoviridae	Single-stranded −RNA, enveloped	RNA-RNA polymerase	Direct contact (bite), inhalation (rare)	Rabies	Human rabies immune globin
Bunyaviridae	Single-stranded (−/+)RNA, enveloped	RNA-RNA polymerase			
California encephalitis virus			Mosquito	Encephalitis	Supportive
Hantavirus			Rodent excreta	Adult respiratory distress syndrome, hemorrhagic fever, kidney failure	Ribavirin?
Arenaviridae	Single-stranded (−/+)RNA, enveloped	RNA-RNA polymerase	Mosquito	Encephalitis	Supportive
Reoviridae	Double-stranded, segmented RNA, naked	RNA-RNA polymerase			
Reovirus			Fecal-oral	Diarrhea, upper respiratory tract infection	Supportive
Orbivirus			Tick	Colorado tick fever	Supportive
Rotavirus			Fecal-oral	Diarrhea (infants)	Supportive
Retroviridae HIV	Single-stranded +RNA	Reverse transcriptase, endonuclease	Sexual, needles, vertical	AIDS	Zidovudine
Unclassified Hepatitis D virus	Single-stranded −RNA, defective		Blood	Severe hepatitis	

EEE = Eastern equine encephalitis virus; JBV = Japanese B encephalitis virus; SLE = St. Louis encephalitis virus; VEE = Venezuelan equine encephalitis virus; WEE = Western equine encephalitis virus.

Summary of the Major Pathogenic Fungi

Organism	Disease	Morphology	Geographic Distribution	Treatment
Dermatophytes				
Trichophyton	Tinea (skin, head, nails)	Filamentous mycelia	Worldwide	Skin: Tolfnaftate, azoles Nails: Griseofulvin, itraconazole, allylamines
Microsporum species	Tinea (skin, head)	Filamentous mycelia	Worldwide	See *Trichophyton*
Epidermophyton floccosum	Tinea (skin, nails)	Filamentous mycelia	Worldwide	See *Trichophyton*
*Malassezia furfur**	Tinea versicolor	Masses of spores intermingled with mycelia ("spaghetti and meatballs")	Worldwide	Ketoconazole
Filamentous fungi				
Fonsecaea pedrosoi, F. compactum, Phialophora verrucosa	Chromomycosis	Sclerotic bodies in tissues	Warm climates (southern United States)	Azoles
Madurella mycetomatis, Phialophora jeanselmei, Pseudallescheria boydii	Mycetoma (lower extremities), Pseudalles cheriosis (lungs)	. . .	Warm climates	Ketoconazole
Rhizopus species, *Mucor* species, *Absidia* species	Zygomycosis (roof of mouth/ nose)	Nonseptate, ribbon-like hyphae	Worldwide	Amphotericin B
Aspergillus fumigatus, A. niger, A. flavus	Aspergillosis, aspergilloma (fungus ball)	Wide septate hyphae with dichotomic branching (45° angle)	Worldwide	Amphotericin B, surgery (for invasive lung disease)
Yeasts				
Candida albicans	Candidiasis	Gram-positive in tissues, yeast and pseudomycelial forms easily visualized	Worldwide	Skin, mucosa, gastrointestinal tract, vaginal infections: nystatin, azoles Systemic infections: Amphotericin B

Organism	Disease	Morphology	Geographic Distribution	Treatment
Cryptococcus neoformans	Cryptococcal meningitis, cryptococcosis	Capsulated yeast forms with narrow based-buds	Worldwide	Amphotericin B plus 5-Fluorocytosine, fluconazole for prophylaxis in immunocompromised individuals
Dimorphic fungi				
Blastomyces dermatidis	Blastomycosis	Thick walled yeast with single broad-based bud, septate hyphae	Eastern United States, Canada	Amphotericin B
Histoplasma capsulatum	Histoplasmosis	Exist as yeast in phagocytic cells, mycelia with tuberculate macroconidium in culture	Worldwide; high prevalence in the Ohio/ Mississippi River valley	Amphotericin B
Coccidioides immitis	Coccidioidomycosis	Spherules with endospores in tissues, arthrospores in the environment	Southwest desert regions in the United States, Central and South America	Amphotericin B, ketoconazole
Paracoccidioides brasiliensis	Paracoccidioidomycosis	Multiple, thin-walled yeasts with narrow based buds (captain's wheel)	Mexico, Central and South America, especially Brazil	Amphotericin B
Sporothrix schenckii	Sporotrichosis ("rose-grower's disease")	Cigar-shaped yeast forms in tissues	Worldwide	Cutaneous: Oral saturated potassium iodide Systemic: amphotericin B and itraconazole
Unclassified fungi				
Pneumocystis carinii	*Pneumocystis carinii* pneumonia (PCP)	Cysts with multiple sporozoites	Worldwide	Trimethoprim–sulfamethoxazole, pentamidine

* Not a dermatophyte, but causes skin infection.

Summary of the Major Human Pathogenic Parasites

Organism	Location	Transmission	Drug of Choice
Entamoeba histolytica	Large intestine	Fecal-oral, sexual	Metronidazole plus iodoquinol
Naegleria fowleri	Brain	Respiratory	None defined
Giardia intestinalis	Small intestine	Fecal-oral, many reservoir hosts	Quinacrine, metronidazole
Trichomonas vaginalis	Urogenital epithelium	Sexual	Metronidazole
Trypanosoma cruzi	Skeletal muscle, gastrointestinal tract	Kissing bug (*Triatoma*)	None defined
Leishmania species	Liver, spleen	Sandfly (*Phlebotomus*)	Pentavalent antimonials
Balantidum coli	Large intestine	Fecal-oral	Tetracycline
Plasmodium species	Red blood cells, liver	Female mosquito (*Anopheles*)	Chloroquine (plus primaquine if *P. vivax* or *P. ovale*); pyrimethamine plus sulfa, quinine (resistant strains)
Babesia	Red blood cells	Tick	None
Toxoplasma gondii	Brain, muscle	Ingestion	Pyrimethamine plus trisulfapyrimidines
Cryptosporidium	Small and large intestine	Fecal-oral	None
Ascaris lumbricoides (roundworm)	Small intestine	Ingestion	Pyrantel, pamoate, mebendazole
Necator americanus and *Ancyclostoma duodenale* (hookworm)	Small intestine	Cutaneous	Mebendazole, thiabendazole
Strongyloides stercoralis	Small intestine	Autoinfection	Thiabendazole
Trichuris trichiura (whipworm)	Large intestine, rectum	Ingestion	Mebendazole
Enterobius vermicularis (pinworm)	Cecum, ileum, sometimes appendix	Ingestion	Mebendazole
Trichinella spiralis	Muscle, intestine	Ingestion	Mebendazole
Wuchereria bancrofti	Blood, lymphatics	Mosquito	None defined
Onchocerca volvulus	Subcutaneous nodules	Black fly	None defined
Loa loa	Blood, eye	Horse fly	Diethylcarbamazine
Fasciola hepatica	Liver	Ingestion	None defined
Schistosoma	Superior and inferior mesenteric veins (*S. mansoni*), bladder (*S. hematobium*)	Cutaneous	Praziquantel
Taenia solium	Small intestine, brain	Ingestion	Niclosamide plus praziquantel
Taenia saginata	Small intestine	Ingestion	Niclosamide plus praziquantel
Echinoccus	Liver, lungs, kidneys, bones, brain	Ingestion	None defined

Pathogens Involved in Infections at Different Ages*

Infection	Newborn	Child	Adolescent	Adult < 60 Years	Adult > 60 Years
Osteomyelitis	*Staphylococcus aureus* Enterobacteriaceae Group A and B streptococci	**≤ 4 years:** *Haemophilus influenzae* *Streptococcus* species *Staphylococcus aureus* **> 4 years:** *Staphylococcus aureus* *Streptococcus* species *Haemophilus influenzae*	*Staphyloroccus aureus*	*Staphylococcus aureus*	*Staphylococcus aureus*
Meningitis	Group B and D streptococci Enterobacteriaceae *Listeria monocytogenes*	**1–3 months:** *Streptococcus pneumoniae* *Neisseria meningitidis* *Haemophilus influenzae* Neonatal pathogens **3 months–7 years:** *Streptococcus pneumoniae* *Neisseria meningitidis* *Haemophilus influenzae*	*Streptococcus pneumoniae* *Neisseria meningitids* *Listeria monocytogenes*	*Streptococcus pneumoniae* *Neisseria meningitids* *Listeria monocytogenes*	*Streptococcus pneumoniae*
Otitis media	Viral (?)† *Streptococcus pneumoniae* *Haemophilus influenzae* *Moraxella catarrhalis* Enterobacteriaceae Group B *Streptococci*	Viral (?) *Streptococcus pneumoniae* *Haemophilus influenzae* *Moraxella catarrhalis*	Viral (?) *Streptococcus pneumoniae* *Haemophilus influenzae* *Moraxella catarrhalis*	. . .	. . .
Septic arthritis	. . .	**< 3 months:** *Staphylococcus aureus* Enterobacteriaceae Group B streptococci **> 3 months:** *Staphylococcus aureus* *Haemophilus influenzae* *Streptococcus* species Enterobacteriaceae	*Staphylococcus aureus* *Haemophilus influenzae* *Streptococcus* species Enterobacteriaceae	*Staphylococcus aureus* Group A streptococci Enterobacteriaceae	. . .
Pneumonia	**< 5 days:** *Escherichia coli* Group A, B, and C, streptococci **> 5 days:** Group A and B streptococci *Escherichia coli* *Pseudomonas* species *Chlamydia trachomatis*	Viruses *Streptococcus pneumoniae* *Haemophilus influenzae* *Staphylococcus aureus*	Viruses *Mycoplasma* species *Chlamydia* *Streptococcus pneumoniae* *Haemophilus influenzae*	Viruses *Mycoplasma* species *Chlamydia* *Streptococcus pneumoniae* *Haemophilus influenzae* *Legionella* species	*Streptococcus pneumoniae* Group A streptococci *Legionella* species

* In decreasing order of frequency.
† Bacteria not recovered.
‡ The frequency of all *H. influenzae* infections is decreasing due to vaccination.

COMPREHENSIVE EXAM

QUESTIONS

DIRECTIONS: Each of the numbered items or incomplete statements in this section is followed by answers or by completions of the statement. Select the ONE lettered answer or completion that is BEST in each case.

1. A Spanish-speaking migrant worker is seen with complaints of chronic, intermittent bloody diarrhea of approximately 1 year's duration. Physical examination reveals hepatosplenomegaly. A peripheral blood examination shows eosinophilia. The patient's serum transaminase level is elevated. An upper gastrointestinal series reveals esophageal varicosities. Bacteriologic study of the feces shows normal flora. The treatment of this patient should include a drug that

(A) blocks γ-aminobutyric acid (GABA)
(B) blocks ribosomal function
(C) causes changes in intracellular calcium levels
(D) inhibits glutathione-S-transferase
(E) Is converted into products that alkylate DNA

2. A 22-year-old woman developed a urinary tract infection during her honeymoon. At the time she sought medical advice, she was febrile and complained of painful urination and flank pain. Her urine appeared "cloudy." Urine culture yields a lactose-fermenting, indole-positive, Gram-negative bacillus. The infectiveness of the organism responsible for this urinary tract infection is associated with specific

(A) exotoxins
(B) K antigens
(C) metabolic properties
(D) P fimbriae
(E) plasmids

3. A divorced mother of four tests positive for HIV-1 infection during investigation of a febrile illness with disseminated lymphadenopathy. A second enzyme immunoassay (EIA) is performed, and the results are the same. The woman denies intravenous drug use. She has dated several men since her divorce and cannot be positive about their sexual habits or use of intravenous drugs. What is the appropriate next step in the management of this patient?

(A) Treatment with zidovudine (azidothymidine, AZT) should be initiated
(B) All of the patient's close contacts should be tested for HIV antibodies
(C) The public health authorities should be notified
(D) A Western blot (immunoblot) test should be ordered
(E) The patient should be reassured and told that her disease is probably unrelated to AIDS

4. The survival of *Mycobacteria* after ingestion by macrophages is attributed to

(A) bacterial inhibition of complement activation via the alternative pathway
(B) bacterial inhibition of phagolysosome formation and interference with endosomal acidification
(C) the poor immunogenicity of the cell wall glycolipids
(D) the bacterium's rapid escape from the endosome into the cytoplasm of infected cells
(E) the bacterium's resistance to oxygen-active radicals released into the phagolysosome

5. In a chronic carrier of hepatitis B virus (HBV), which positive test is most indicative of high infectivity?

(A) Hepatitis B surface antigen (HBsAg)
(B) Hepatitis B core antigen (HBcAg)
(C) Hepatitis B e antigen (HBeAg)
(D) Anti-HBsAg
(E) Anti-HBeAg

6. A 27-year-old white man is brought to the hospital by emergency personnel. His complaints include chills, headache, backache, and nausea. His temperature is 104°F, and his arterial blood pressure is 100/60 mm Hg. There is evidence of vomit on his clothing. Upon questioning, the patient reveals that he recently participated in a Peace Corps project in Quito, Ecuador. Following admission to the hospital, gastric endoscopy reveals hemorrhagic areas of the stomach, small intestine, and colon. The patient's direct serum bilirubin level is 5 mg/dl. Assuming that this patient's symptoms are caused by a virus, what is the best tentative diagnosis?

(A) Dengue fever
(B) Malaria
(C) Typhoid fever
(D) Venezuelan equine encephalitis
(E) Yellow fever

7. Treatment of cells with a drug able to block DNA synthesis (e.g., actinomycin D) at the time of infection will prevent the replication of

(A) adenoviruses
(B) hepatitis A virus (HAV)
(C) rhabdoviruses
(D) polioviruses
(E) togaviruses

Questions 8–9

A 19-year-old white woman is temporarily employed at a day-care center, filling in time before going to college in the fall. For the past 5 days, she has suffered from increasingly debilitating diarrhea with cramps and borborygmus. Her stools are frequent, often explosive, fermentative, and foul smelling. The patient is an avid hiker and returned 2.5 weeks ago from a camping trip in Colorado. Physical examination reveals a distressed, but otherwise apparently fit, young woman. Her temperature is 99.1°F, her pulse is 78 beats per minute, her blood pressure is 115/65 mm Hg, and her respiratory rate is slightly increased. Ocular, oral, and chest examinations are normal. There is mild abdominal tenderness, but no enlargement of the liver or spleen. Wright's stain of the sediment of a fecal extract reveals the following organism:

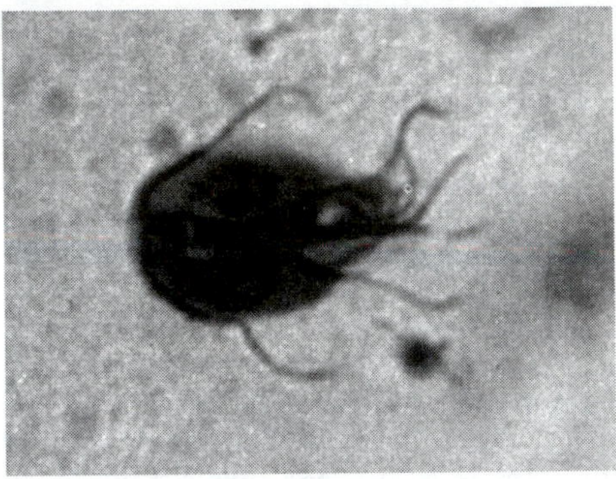

8. What is the main pathogenic mechanism responsible for this patient's diarrhea?

(A) Interference with the absorptive functions of duodenal villi
(B) Invasion of the mucosa and toxin production
(C) Invasion of the draining lymphatics, causing backflow into the intestine
(D) Secretion of proteases that destroy the intestinal villi
(E) Stimulation of electrolyte secretion by mucosal cells in the small intestine

9. Which one of the following therapeutic measures would be curative for this patient's diarrhea?

(A) Oral administration of metronidazole
(B) Oral administration of ampicillin
(C) Oral administration of nystatin
(D) A bland diet and plenty of electrolyte-replenishment sports beverages
(E) Intravenous fluid and electrolyte replacement

10. A retrovirus is found in a high proportion of laboratory animals of a given species. Most viremic animals are asymptomatic, but others develop a fatal wasting syndrome, and a few develop leukemia and other tumors after long periods of latency. The virus in question most likely lacks which one of the following genes?

(A) *gag*
(B) *pol*
(C) *env*
(D) *onc*

Questions 11–12

A sexually active 22-year-old college student presents to the local clinic with a localized vesicular eruption on the shaft of his penis. A scraping of the base of one of the vesicles is positive for Tzanck cells. The patient mentions that he had a similar eruption in the same area 2 months earlier.

11. The reappearance of this eruption may be explained by

(A) cell-mediated immunity (CMI) deficiency in the patient
(B) a prolonged period of viremia following the initial infection
(C) a second infection with a similar virus with a different serotype
(D) failure of the patient to comply with therapy prescribed at the initial episode
(E) reactivation of a latent infection

12. The mechanism of action of the agent used to treat this infection involves

(A) blocking of the active site of the cell's DNA-dependent RNA polymerases
(B) incorporation of a nucleoside analog into a nascent DNA chain
(C) induction of the synthesis and release of type I interferons
(D) inhibition of the release of viral nucleic acid into the host cell
(E) inhibition of viral messenger RNA (mRNA) capping

13. A 28-year-old woman seeks medical attention at the emergency room because she is having a very difficult menstrual period. In addition to bleeding profusely, she has had a fever that has been as high as 103°F and has felt extremely lethargic. She has had progressively severe diarrhea, which in the last day has been bloody. Physical examination shows a tachycardic, tachypneic female, with cold, damp skin and a blood pressure of 80/40 mm Hg. Faint, diffuse erythema is noted on her neck and the upper half of her thorax. The woman is admitted, bacteriologic tests are ordered, and both supportive therapy and administration of antibiotics are initiated. The organism most likely responsible for this woman's symptoms releases a toxin that

(A) dissolves lipid bilayer membranes
(B) causes epidermolysis
(C) causes hemolysis
(D) induces the massive release of proinflammatory cytokines
(E) causes persistent activation of adenylate cyclase in mucosal cells

Questions 14–15

The mother of a 3-year-old girl noted that her daughter was scratching her legs when she came in from playing in the backyard after a summer rain. Within a few days, the scratched area became oozy and covered with a honey-colored crust.

14. There are two major bacteria that could cause this type of skin infection in a child. Which one of the following characteristics is common to both?

(A) They turn red when counterstained with safranin
(B) They are difficult to grow in conventional bacteriologic culture media
(C) They frequently colonize the lower gastrointestinal tract as well as the skin
(D) Polysaccharide capsules are their main virulence factor
(E) They have peptidoglycan-rich cell walls

15. The choice of an oral antibiotic to treat this skin infection must take into consideration the

(A) synthesis of β-lactamases by one of the organisms potentially involved
(B) general patterns of antimicrobial susceptibilities for Gram-negative organisms
(C) innate resistance of the suspected organisms to hydrophilic compounds
(D) lack of effect of antibiotics that inhibit cell wall biosynthesis
(E) need to use an antimicrobial that accumulates in the stratum corneum

16. A 4-year-old boy receiving chemotherapy for acute lymphoblastic leukemia develops a persistent fever that is not affected by administration of broad-spectrum antibiotics. Physical examination shows extensive white plaques in the oral region and an erythematous rash in the perineal region. A complete blood count shows leukopenia (1000 leukocytes/μl, 70% lymphocytes with many blastic forms, 20% neutrophils, 8% monocytes, 2% basophils). What is the most likely cause of the fever in this patient?

(A) *Candida albicans*
(B) *Cryptococcus neoformans*
(C) Cytomegalovirus (CMV)
(D) Epstein-Barr virus
(E) *Pseudomonas aeruginosa*

17. A bacterium, grown in the presence of equal concentrations of glucose and lactose, uses glucose first. During this period of glucose utilization, the *lac* operon (Lac-O) is inactive as a result of

(A) the activation of a catabolite repressor gene
(B) the binding of glucose to the repressor, preventing proper removal from the operator
(C) the high levels of cyclic adenosine monophosphate (cAMP) generated during aerobic oxidation of glucose
(D) the failure of the catabolite activator protein (CAP) to bind to the Lac-O promoter
(E) lack of lactose uptake

18. Radiolabeled leucine, ribose, thymine, and uridine are added to the culture medium of a bacterial culture sensitive to rifampin, chloramphenicol, and nalidixic acid. Which one of the radiolabeled compounds will immediately fail to incorporate into the bacteria following the addition of nalidixic acid?

(A) Leucine
(B) Ribose
(C) Thymidine
(D) Uridine

19. Relapses of African trypanosomiasis are related to

(A) antigenic mimicry of host proteins by the trypanosome
(B) an inadequate host immune response
(C) inadequate therapy
(D) the periodic release of trypanosomes from red blood cells
(E) sequential antigenic variation of the trypanosome surface protein

20. Visceral larva migrans is usually acquired by contact with fecal materials from

(A) birds
(B) cattle
(C) dogs
(D) humans
(E) rodents

21. The role of bacterial capsules as virulence factors is usually related to their ability to interfere with

(A) antibody binding
(B) B lymphocyte activation
(C) antibacterial penetration of bacterial cells
(D) phagocytosis
(E) the release of interferon-γ (IFN-γ) and other macrophage-activating cytokines

22. The vaccine currently used for prevention of *Streptococcus pneumoniae* infections is made from

(A) a mixture of 23 recombinant *S. pneumoniae* strains
(B) killed *S. pneumoniae* of the 23 most prevalent *S. pneumoniae* serotypes
(C) capsular polysaccharides from 23 *S. pneumoniae* serotypes
(D) diphtheria toxoid conjugated with capsular polysaccharides from 23 *S. pneumoniae* serotypes
(E) M proteins from the cell wall of the 23 most prevalent *S. pneumoniae* serotypes

23. The chromosome of bacterium X is represented as follows:

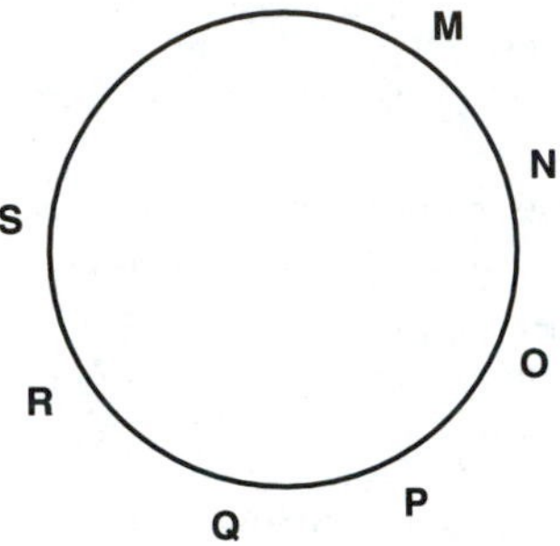

The letters represent genes on that bacterial chromosome that can be detected by plating on selective or differential media. There may be anywhere from 1 to 100 other genes between any of the marked genes. Bacterium X is mixed with bacterium Y, deficient in each of those genes designated by letters, in the presence of deoxyribonuclease (DNase). After a suitable period of time, a number of pure cultures of bacterium Y are obtained and analyzed for recombinants. The following recombinants are characterized:

Isolate 1 – M, N
Isolate 2 – P, Q
Isolate 3 – O, N
Isolate 4 – R, S

These results suggest that the genetic exchange between these bacteria involved

(A) conjugation
(B) generalized transduction
(C) high-frequency recombination
(D) specialized transduction
(E) transformation

24. A 32-year-old hepatitis B virus (HBV) carrier with a history of intravenous drug abuse is brought to the emergency room after collapsing in the street. He is deeply jaundiced, and has a fever of 101°F. He reports that he has had two other episodes of jaundice in the past 14 months for which he did not seek medical attention. He states that this is the worst he has ever felt, and admits to current intravenous drug use. The most likely diagnosis is superinfection with

(A) hepatitis A virus (HAV)
(B) hepatitis C virus (HCV)
(C) hepatitis D virus (HDV)
(D) hepatitis E virus (HEV)
(E) HIV

25. Penicillin is added to a culture of a Gram-positive rod. Twelve hours later, the number of bacteria has increased, and the organisms have assumed a round configuration. The most likely explanation for these observations is that the

(A) concentration of penicillin was insufficient
(B) culture was carried out in hypotonic medium
(C) organism carries a mutated transpeptidase
(D) organism is deficient in autolytic activity
(E) organism secretes penicillinase

26. A 56-year-old woman under treatment for inoperable breast cancer develops a painful, vesicular, hemorrhagic rash on her right buttock. Cytologic examination of scrapings from the base of one of the vesicles reveals cells with intranuclear inclusions. How is the virus responsible for these lesions best described?

(A) Enveloped, helical, DNA virus
(B) Enveloped, helical, RNA virus
(C) Enveloped, icosahedral, DNA virus
(D) Naked, helical, RNA virus
(E) Naked, icosahedral, DNA virus

27. Which one of the following is the infectious form of *Trichomonas vaginalis*?

(A) Quadrinucleated cyst
(B) Cyst with eight nuclei
(C) Egg
(D) Merozoite
(E) Trophozoite

28. The main advantage of passive immunization over active immunization is that passive immunization

(A) eliminates the risk of hypersensitivity reactions
(B) is effective against multiple organisms
(C) is more cost-effective as a public health measure
(D) provides immediate protection
(E) magnifies the specific immune response to the offending organism

29. A mutation in DNA gyrase is likely to result in resistance to which one of the following antibiotics?

(A) Amphotericin B
(B) Ciprofloxacin
(C) Penicillin
(D) Rifampin
(E) Streptomycin

30. Which one of the following properties is characteristic of a high-frequency recombinant (Hfr) bacterium?

(A) Frequent transfer of extrachromosomal resistance factors to recipient cells
(B) Incorporation of plasmid DNA into the bacterial chromosome
(C) Production of transducing particles
(D) Short doubling time
(E) Very frequent conjugation events

31. As a consequence of adding bacitracin to a growing cell, which peptidoglycan precursor(s) would accumulate in the cytoplasm?

(A) GlmNAc-MurNAc–pentapeptide-pentaglycine
(B) Lipid-P-P-MurNAc-pentapeptide
(C) Lipid-P-P-GlmNAc-MurNAc + pentapeptide
(D) UDP-MurNAc–pentapeptide + lipid P
(E) UDP-MurNAc–pentapeptide

32. Resistance of *Staphylococcus aureus* to methicillin is most often caused by

(A) alteration of the major target for the drug
(B) cell membrane impermeability
(C) decreased uptake of the antibiotic
(D) inactivation of autolysins
(E) synthesis of a potent β-lactamase

33. The molecular basis for the effect of cholera toxin on duodenal mucosal cells is

(A) activation of adenylate cyclase
(B) inactivation of a G_i protein
(C) increased activity of potassium pumps
(D) increased generation of cyclic adenosine monophosphate (cAMP)
(E) ribosylation of a guanosine triphosphate (GTP)-binding protein

34. What is the most common cause of aseptic meningitis of viral etiology?

(A) Enteroviruses
(B) Herpesviruses
(C) Arboviruses
(D) Retroviruses
(E) Orthomyxoviruses

35. The synthesis of erythrogenic toxin by specific strains of group A *Streptococcus* is determined by a

(A) bacterial chromosomal gene
(B) gene carried by a lysogenic phage
(C) specific virulence plasmid
(D) transposon

36. Which one of the following factors released by heating a suspension of sheep erythrocytes is required for the growth of *Haemophilus influenzae* in chocolate agar?

(A) Coagulase
(B) Nicotinamide adenine dinucleotide (NAD)
(C) Hemoglobin
(D) Hemolysin
(E) Protein A

37. Which one of the following properties is characteristic of cells transformed in culture by oncogenic viruses?

(A) Decreased agglutinability by lectins
(B) Decreased survival
(C) Increased rate of glucose transport across the cell membrane
(D) Increased expression of major histocompatibility complex (MHC) molecules
(E) Increased serum requirements

38. Which one of the following statements explains why nitroimidazoles are only effective against anaerobic organisms?

(A) Anaerobic fermentation lowers the pH to optimal values for imidazoles
(B) Catalase and superoxide dismutase inactivate the imidazoles
(C) Only anaerobes can generate active metabolites from imidazoles
(D) The DNA of aerobic bacteria is not sensitive to the imidazoles
(E) The imidazoles are quickly oxidized and inactivated by atmospheric oxygen

39. Which one of the following bacteria is most likely to be relatively resistant to antibiotics as a result of the relative impermeability of its cell wall?

(A) *Haemophilus influenzae*
(B) *Pseudomonas aeruginosa*
(C) *Staphylococcus aureus*
(D) *Streptococcus pneumoniae*
(E) *Streptococcus pyogenes*

40. A 32-year-old businessman presents with a penile lesion that is crateriform, moist, and peripherally indurated. Upon questioning, the patient reveals that the lesion has been present for approximately 10 days, and is not noticeably painful. Which one of the following tests should be performed to further narrow the diagnosis?

(A) Blood cultures
(B) Culture of the exudate
(C) Gram stain of the exudate
(D) Microhemagglutination *Treponema pallidum* (MHA-TP) test
(E) Venereal Disease Research Laboratory (VDRL) test

41. Which one of the following infection routes is most often involved in the neonatal transmission of hepatitis B virus (HBV)?

(A) Blood transfusion
(B) Fetal contact with infected blood during childbirth
(C) Ingestion of the virus via maternal breast milk
(D) Transmission of the virus from hospital personnel during childbirth
(E) Transplacental transmission of the virus

42. The finding of large, multinucleated, clumps of cells in the bronchial secretions of a 2-year-old girl with acute bronchopneumonia suggests that this infection is caused by

(A) *Bordetella pertussis*
(B) Epstein-Barr virus
(C) *Mycoplasma hominis*
(D) a rhinovirus
(E) respiratory syncytial virus

43. Which one of the following infections is most likely to be classified as opportunistic?

(A) Brucellosis in the child of a migrant worker
(B) *Escherichia coli* bacteremia in a leukemic patient receiving chemotherapy
(C) Group A streptococcal pharyngitis in a school-aged child
(D) Pulmonary anthrax in a wool sorter
(E) Pulmonary tuberculosis in a physician

44. A 45-year-old missionary is flown to Charleston, South Carolina from the Congo. He is in acute renal failure. Two months earlier, the patient had been diagnosed with malaria and treated with chloroquine. Recrudescence occurred after the first month of therapy. The recent deterioration in his kidney function followed a febrile crisis during which the patient noted that his urine was very dark. The most likely cause for this patient's acute renal failure is

(A) acute dehydration
(B) bilirubin toxicity
(C) deposition of immune complexes in the glomeruli
(D) massive intravascular hemolysis
(E) medicamentous renal toxicity

45. Which one of the following bacteria is most likely to be recovered from the cerebrospinal fluid (CSF) of a newborn with meningitis?

(A) *Escherichia coli*
(B) *Streptococcus agalactiae*
(C) *Haemophilus influenzae* type b
(D) *Listeria monocytogenes*
(E) *Streptococcus pneumoniae*

46. Which one of the following immunizations should be administered immediately after birth?

(A) Diphtheria–pertussis–tetanus (DPT) vaccine
(B) *Haemophilus influenzae* type b vaccine
(C) Hepatitis B vaccine
(D) HIV vaccine
(E) Oral polio vaccine

47. A 35-year-old migrant worker is admitted to the hospital with a high fever and malaise. When he started feeling weak 3 days ago, he checked his temperature and found it to be slightly elevated. Over the last 3 days, he has felt progressively worse and his temperature has reached 103°F. The resident on call in the emergency room observes a scanty maculopapular rash on the patient's trunk. The patient mentions that another worker in his group has been sick with similar symptoms. Which one of the following tests would be most likely to yield a diagnosis?

(A) Blood cultures
(B) Methylene blue staining of a fecal extract
(C) Serologic tests for *Brucella*
(D) Serologic tests for mumps virus, rubella virus, coxsackieviruses A and B, and echoviruses
(E) Stool cultures

48. Protection against influenza A virus in a nonimmune individual can be achieved through the administration of a drug that interferes with

(A) viral endonuclease activity
(B) binding of host messenger RNA (mRNA) caps by the viral P_1 protein
(C) synthesis of viral progeny RNA
(D) uncoating of nucleic acid
(E) viral adsorption and penetration

49. A 40-year-old mother of three children is readmitted to the hospital with general complaints of fever (102°F), malaise, anorexia, and flank pain. She had been released from the hospital 3 days previously following the removal of an ovarian cyst. The woman had been catheterized during her last admission, and review of her records reveals that she had a fever 24 hours after surgery. She was treated with ampicillin. A urine specimen was obtained through the catheter and was found to contain pus cells, casts, and numerous Gram-negative rods. A urine culture yielded colonies of an oxidase-positive bacteria; the colonies had a mucoid aspect and released a green, diffusible pigment. What is the etiologic agent of this condition likely to be?

(A) *Enterococcus*
(B) *Escherichia coli*
(C) *Klebsiella pneumoniae*
(D) *Proteus mirabilis*
(E) *Pseudomonas aeruginosa*

50. Which one of the following procedures is best for decontaminating a heat-sensitive reusable piece of equipment?

(A) Ethylene oxide gas sterilization
(B) Pasteurization
(C) Soaking in 3% hydrogen peroxide
(D) Soaking in alcohol
(E) Ultraviolet irradiation

51. Which *Streptococcus pyogenes* antigen is responsible for the induction of protective antibody?

(A) G protein
(B) Hyaluronidase
(C) M protein
(D) Polysaccharide capsular antigen
(E) Streptolysin

52. A veterinarian seeks medical attention, complaining of malaise and yellowing of the sclera. Physical examination confirms the existence of hepatomegaly and jaundice. Serologies for hepatitis A and B virus and blood cultures are negative. Renal function tests suggest moderate impairment of tubular function. The patient's serum creatinine kinase is elevated. The most likely diagnosis is

(A) hepatitis E
(B) leptospirosis
(C) Lyme disease
(D) malaria
(E) relapsing fever

53. A 10-year-old boy develops an ulcerated and indurated lesion on the base of his right thumb. He says that the lesion developed after he cut himself while cleaning his aquarium. Which one of the following best describes the organism that most likely caused this lesion?

(A) Acid-fast rod, grows best at temperatures below 37°C
(B) DNA virus with a nonenveloped icosahedral virion
(C) Gram-negative rod, strict aerobe, oxidase-positive, pyocyanin-producer
(D) Gram-negative, curvy rod, grows best in media with high salt concentration
(E) Pleomorphic, aerobic Gram-positive rod

54. A patient develops explosive, watery diarrhea 24 hours after eating seafood imported from South America. What bacterium is most likely involved?

(A) *Campylobacter fetus*
(B) *Salmonella typhimurium*
(C) *Shigella flexneri*
(D) *Vibrio cholerae*
(E) *Vibrio parahaemolyticus*

55. A new form of prophylaxis against the common cold is announced by the media. According to the press releases, it is based on a monoclonal antibody that successfully prevents the transmission of the common cold when administered by aerosol to healthy volunteers. Such antibody is likely to react with

(A) CD4
(B) CR2
(C) intercellular cell adhesion molecule-1 (ICAM-1)
(D) epithelial growth factor
(E) rhinovirus capsid proteins

56. A pregnant Vietnamese refugee presents for prenatal care. She mentions that she was sick 3 years previously, before emigrating to the United States, with jaundice that was accompanied by intestinal upset and followed by joint pains and generalized skin lesions that slowly subsided. She has felt well in the last 2 years. The possibility that this woman may still be harboring the infectious agent that caused her disease and that she could transmit it to her baby is considered. Which one of the following laboratory tests should be ordered next to investigate the cause of this woman's past infection?

(A) Hepatitis B surface antigen (HBsAg)
(B) IgG cytomegalovirus (CMV) antibody levels
(C) IgM antibody to hepatitis B core antigen (HBcAg)
(D) IgM antibody to HBsAg
(E) Quantitation of hepatitis A virus (HAV) IgM antibody

57. A mother brings her child to the pediatrician because the child has multiple vesicular eruptions on the mucous membranes of her mouth. The vesicles go away within 3 weeks. However, during the next 12 months, the child suffers several recurrent infections, characterized by blisters in the perioral region. Which type of drug is most likely to alleviate this child's symptoms?

(A) One that blocks nucleic acid release
(B) A reverse transcriptase inhibitor
(C) A viral protease inhibitor
(D) An activator of cellular ribonucleases
(E) An inhibitor of DNA synthesis

58. An alginate-producing, aerobic, oxidase-positive, Gram-negative bacillus is isolated from the sputum of a patient with cystic fibrosis. This organism is likely to be

(A) *Bacteroides fragilis*
(B) *Escherichia coli*
(C) *Klebsiella pneumonia*
(D) *Pseudomonas aeruginosa*
(E) *Streptococcus faecalis*

59. A laboratory technician has isolated an organism that grows in blood agar, forms round, smooth, pale yellow colonies surrounded by a narrow area of hemolysis, ferments mannitol, and is both catalase- and coagulase-positive. This organism is

(A) *Streptococcus pyogenes*
(B) *Streptococcus agalactiae*
(C) *Staphylococcus aureus*
(D) *Staphylococcus epidermidis*
(E) *Staphylococcus saprophyticus*

60. The most important pathogenic factor leading to the development of carditis in a patient with rheumatic fever is believed to be the

(A) induction of a specific autoimmune response to cardiac tissue
(B) persistent release of streptococcal antigens from silent infectious foci
(C) the release of a cardiotoxin
(D) the sharing of epitopes between streptococcal and cardiac tissue glycoproteins
(E) the tropism of group A streptococci for the cardiac valves

61. The bacterial agent most likely to be associated with meningitis in a 2-year-old child who has been properly immunized is

(A) *Escherichia coli*
(B) *Haemophilus influenzae* type b
(C) *Listeria monocytogenes*
(D) *Streptococcus agalactiae*
(E) *Streptococcus pneumoniae*

62. What is the cause of anemia associated with ancylostomiasis?

(A) Bone marrow depression caused by parasitic invasion
(B) Vitamin B_{12} deficiency caused by competitive absorption by the parasite
(C) Malabsorption of folic acid as a result of chronic diarrhea
(D) Massive hemoptysis during the initial phases of parasitic maturation
(E) Persistent iron loss

63. A graduate student tests positive on two enzyme immunoassays (EIAs) for HIV-1 antibody during investigation of a febrile illness with disseminated lymphadenopathy. The woman denies intravenous drug use, but has dated several men and cannot be positive about their sexual habits or use of intravenous drugs. The following diagram reproduces the results of Western blot tests for HIV antibodies performed with the sera of five individuals with positive results on EIAs for HIV antibody.

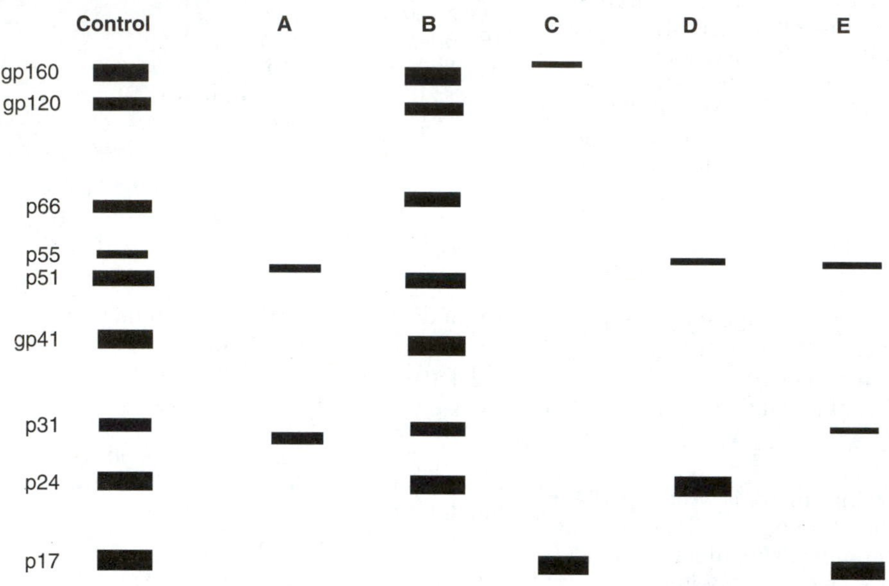

Which one of these patterns is most likely to correspond to this patient?

64. Bacteriologic examination of the cerebrospinal fluid (CSF) of a 6-year-old girl with suspected meningitis results in the isolation of a Gram-negative diplococcus that grows in chocolate agar and is oxidase positive. Which type of antibacterial should be selected for the treatment of this patient? One that will

(A) cause misreading of bacterial messenger RNA (mRNA)
(B) inactivate DNA-dependent RNA polymerase
(C) inhibit DNA gyrase
(D) inhibit peptidoglycan cross-linking
(E) prevent elongation of bacterial polypeptide chains

65. Which one of the following characteristics is common to most transforming genes found in DNA tumor viruses?

(A) The ability to induce the expression of genes controlling cell proliferation
(B) Activation as a result of chromosomal translocations
(C) Activation of second signal cascades
(D) Cytoskeletal disruption
(E) Inactivation of tumor suppressor gene products

66. A young man is admitted to the hospital with headaches, fever, and nuchal rigidity. A computed tomography (CT) scan of the head is normal and cerebrospinal fluid (CSF) examination shows mild leukocytosis with lymphocyte predominance. Agglutination tests and cultures for agents known to cause meningitis are negative. A tuberculin test is negative. What is the agent most likely to cause this type of clinical presentation?

(A) An enveloped +RNA virus
(B) An enveloped −RNA virus
(C) An enveloped DNA virus
(D) A naked +RNA virus
(E) A naked −RNA virus

67. Which end product is characteristic of fermentation by many streptococci?

(A) Acetic acid
(B) Butyric acid
(C) Lactic acid
(D) Propionic acid
(E) Pyruvic acid

68. Cultures of two neomycin-sensitive strains of *Escherichia coli* are mixed and cultured in the presence of neomycin. After 2 hours, the mixture is plated on neomycin-containing agar. A few neomycin-resistant colonies grow. The emergence of these resistant strains most likely resulted from

(A) conjugation
(B) penicillin-induced mutation
(C) spontaneous mutation
(D) transduction
(E) transformation

69. An auxotrophic strain of *Escherichia coli* with an inactive tryptophan operon mutates. What is the most easily detected manifestation of this mutation?

(A) Detection of the ability of some colonies to survive in tryptophan-depleted medium
(B) Detection of a change in the molecular weight of the repressor gene by Northern blot
(C) Detection of a normal repressor protein by Western blot
(D) Detection of intracellular tryptophan metabolites
(E) Detection of increased uptake of labeled tryptophan from the medium

DIRECTIONS: Each of the numbered items or incomplete statements in this section is negatively phrased, as indicated by a capitalized word such as NOT, LEAST, or EXCEPT. Select the ONE lettered answer or completion that is BEST in each case.

70. All of the following picornaviruses are resistant to the acidity of the stomach EXCEPT

(A) coxsackievirus A
(B) coxsackievirus B
(C) echoviruses
(D) polioviruses
(E) rhinoviruses

71. When susceptible cells are infected with type 12 adenovirus in the presence of vidarabine, all of the following viral components will be synthesized EXCEPT

(A) capsid proteins
(B) DNA polymerase
(C) DNA-binding protein
(D) E-1A protein
(E) major histocompatibility complex (MHC)-binding protein (gp19)

DIRECTIONS: Each set of matching questions in this section consists of a list of four to twenty-six lettered options (some of which may be in figures) followed by several numbered items. For each numbered item, select the ONE lettered option that is most closely associated with it. To avoid spending too much time on matching sets with large numbers of options, it is generally advisable to begin each set by reading the list of options. Then, for each item in the set, try to generate the correct answer and locate it in the option list, rather than evaluating each option individually. Each lettered option may be selected once, more than once, or not at all.

Items 72–74

(A) *Neisseria gonorrhoeae*
(B) *Treponema pallidum*
(C) *Salmonella typhi*
(D) *Rickettsia typhi*
(E) *Bordetella pertussis*

For each description, choose the appropriate organism.

72. Attaches to the ciliated epithelial cells of the trachea

73. Infects the endothelial cells of blood vessels

74. Causes persistent infection of the reticuloendothelial system

Items 75–76

(A) Herpes simplex virus (HSV)
(B) Papillomavirus
(C) Rhinovirus
(D) Rotavirus
(E) Rubella virus

For each method of dissemination, select the appropriate virus.

75. Hematogenous dissemination

76. Retrograde diffusion through nerve fibers

Items 77–79

(A) Large T antigen
(B) Small t antigen
(C) *tat* gene product
(D) *tax* gene product
(E) v-*src* gene product

For each effect, select the responsible antigen or gene product.

77. Upregulates the interleukin-2 (IL-2) receptor genes

78. Binds and inactivates retinoblastoma (Rb) gene product

79. Phosphorylates cytoskeleton proteins

Items 80–81

(A) DNA-dependent RNA polymerase
(B) RNA-dependent DNA polymerase
(C) RNA-dependent RNA polymerase
(D) RNase
(E) Thymidine kinase

For each virus, select the enzyme it is most likely to pack in its virion.

80. HIV

81. Respiratory syncytial virus

Items 82–83

(A) Bacitracin sensitivity
(B) Bile solubility
(C) Catalase positivity
(D) Coagulase positivity
(E) Factor X requirement
(F) Growth at 42°C
(G) Hydrogen sulfide (H_2S) production
(H) Indole production
(I) Lactose fermentation
(J) Urease activity

For each pair of organisms, select the reaction most likely to allow fast differentiation between them.

82. *Escherichia coli* and *Salmonella*

83. *Staphylococcus aureus* and group A streptococci

Items 84–85

(A) BK virus
(B) Epstein-Barr virus
(C) Hepatitis B virus (HBV)
(D) Hepatitis E virus (HEV)
(E) Herpes simplex virus (HSV)
(F) Human T lymphotropic virus-I (HTLV-I)
(G) Human herpesvirus type 6
(H) Human papillomavirus type 6
(I) JC virus

For each disease, select the virus with which it is most closely associated.

84. Progressive multifocal leukoencephalopathy

85. Genital warts

Items 86–88

(A) Aerosolized secretions
(B) Blood transfusion
(C) Contaminated food or water
(D) Contaminated saliva
(E) Mosquito bites
(F) Rodent excreta
(G) Soil contamination of an open wound
(H) Tick bites
(I) Transplacental transmission
(J) Venereal transmission

Match the general characteristics of each virus with its most likely mode of transmission.

86. Double-stranded RNA genome, can cause severe disease in infants

87. Negative RNA genome, causes acute respiratory distress syndrome

88. Enveloped virus with a +RNA genome, causes jaundice

Items 89–91

(A) Bats
(B) Birds
(C) Dogs
(D) Fleas
(E) Horses
(F) Monkeys
(G) Mosquitos
(H) Sandflies
(I) Ticks
(J) Tsetse flies

Match the infectious agent with its animal or arthropod vector.

89. St. Louis encephalitis virus

90. *Pasteurella multocida*

91. *Ehrlichia chaffeensis*

Items 92–93

(A) Acute gastroenteritis
(B) Flaccid paralysis
(C) Hemolytic–uremic syndrome
(D) Severe anaphylactic reactions
(E) Myocarditis
(F) Necrotizing fasciitis
(G) Protein synthesis inhibition
(H) Red blood cell lysis
(I) Spastic paralysis
(J) Watery diarrhea

Match each toxin with the appropriate pathologic effect.

92. Shiga-like toxin of *E. coli* serotype O157:H7

93. Group A streptococcus exotoxin B

Items 94-100

(A) *Bacteroides* species
(B) *Blastomyces dermatitidis*
(C) *Brucella melitensis*
(D) *Clostridium* species
(E) *Coccidioides immitis*
(F) *Entamoeba coli*
(G) *Entamoeba histolytica*
(H) Group A *Streptococcus*
(I) *Haemophilus ducreyi*
(J) *Haemophilus influenzae*
(K) HIV
(L) *Legionella pneumophila*
(M) *Mycobacterium kansasii*
(N) *Neisseria meningitidis*
(O) *Rhizopus oryzae*
(P) *Rickettsia prowazeckii*
(Q) *Rickettsia rickettsii*
(R) *Salmonella* species
(S) *Schistosoma haematobium*
(T) *Schistosoma mansonii*
(U) *Shigella dysenteriae*
(V) *Shigella* species
(W) *Sporothrix schenckii*
(X) *Staphylococcus aureus*
(Y) *Streptococcus pneumoniae*
(Z) *Treponema pallidum*

Match each clinical situation with the most likely causative agent.

94. A 47-year-old housewife scratched herself with a rose thorn 2 weeks ago while tending her garden. The scratch, which was located on the dorsal aspect of her left hand, took longer than 1 week to heal, and has left a bumpy scar. There is a red and bumpy track ascending from the scar to the forearm.

95. A 22-year-old man from Brazil who has been living in New York for the past year has developed chronic diarrhea, sometimes bloody, fever, hepatomegaly, and weight loss. Bacterial cultures of the stool have been repeatedly negative. A rectosigmoidoscopy reveals ulcerative lesions. Several antibiotic regimens have failed.

96. A 75-year-old man is admitted to the hospital complaining of shortness of breath, a productive cough, and a fever of 104°F, which had been preceded by a sudden and hard chill. A blood count reveals 20,000 white blood cells/μl, with a differential analysis of 75% neutrophils and 15% lymphocytes.

97. A 25-year-old boy scout leader is admitted to the hospital with fever, muscle aches, and headache. One week earlier, he had camped with his troop in the Smoky Mountains Park. Physical examination reveals a faint maculopapular rash covering his trunk and extremities, including the palms of the hands, and generalized muscle tenderness.

98. A 70-year-old man who smokes one pack of cigarettes per week makes an appointment with his physician because of the acute onset of a cough, fever (104°F), and diarrhea. The man has chronic bronchitis. Microscopic examination of a sputum sample shows polymorphonuclear lymphocytes and mononuclear cells, but no bacteria on Gram stain.

99. A 36-year-old woman becomes febrile after a Cesarean section. Her abdomen is tender and there is a foul-smelling vaginal discharge. The patient goes into septic shock. Administration of intravenous penicillin in high doses has no effect and the patient's condition continues to worsen.

100. An Ethiopian taxi driver in Washington, DC, complains of intermittent hematuria and progressive difficulties in passing urine. The following organism is visualized in the urinary sediment.

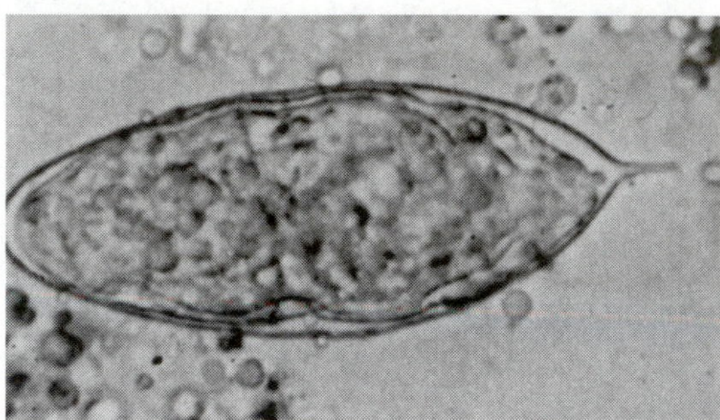

ANSWERS AND EXPLANATIONS

1. The answer is D [Chapter 44 III C 2 a (2) (a); Chapter 46 III B]. The Spanish-speaking migrant worker's presentation is typical of *Schistosoma mansonii* infection. This parasite, found in many regions of the world, including Mexico and Central America, reaches the liver through the systemic circulation and back-migrates to the intestinal wall. To complete the life cycle, eggs must migrate through the wall of intestinal blood vessels and through the intestinal musculature and mucosa to reach the lumen. This migration is responsible for the bloody diarrhea seen in this patient. In addition, eggs lodge In the liver, where they cause a granulomatous reaction, rich in eosinophils (hence the increased transaminases and eosinophilia), that eventually leads to cirrhosis, portal hypertension, and esophageal varicosities. The drug of choice to treat schistosomiasis is praziquantel, which inhibits the antioxidant enzyme glutathione-S-transferase (GST). GST has been shown to play an important role in the ability of trematodes and cestodes to survive within their hosts.

2. The answer is D [Chapter 16 II B 2 a (2); Chapter 51 II A 3 b, C 3]. The newlywed most likely has pyelonephritis, as evidenced by the dysuria, flank pain, and granular casts (the cause of her urine's "cloudy" appearance). *Escherichia coli,* a Gram-negative, lactose-fermenting, indole-positive rod, is the mostly likely organism responsible for her urinary tract infection. Unique fimbrial (P) antigens seem to be associated with the ability of certain *E. coli* strains to infect the upper portions of the urinary tract.

3. The answer is D [Chapter 29 II B 4 b]. The positive results of the patient's two enzyme immunoassays (EIAs) for HIV need to be confirmed using a Western blot (immunoblot) test before the patient is considered HIV-infected and treated as such. The Western blot tests for antibodies to HIV proteins and glycoproteins and is the most widely used confirmatory technique for a positive HIV antibody EIA.

4. The answer is B [Chapter 18 II B 2]. Sulfatides, special glycolipids located on the outer layers of *Mycobacterium tuberculosis,* inhibit phagolysosome formation and interfere with endosomal acidification, thereby ensuring the intracellular survival of this organism. As far as the other choices are concerned, *Listeria monocytogenes* rapidly escapes from the endosome into the cytoplasm of the infected cell, and *Salmonella typhi* is resistant to oxygen-active radicals released into the phagolysosome.

5. The answer is C [Chapter 55 I C 1 b (5)]. Chronic carriers of hepatitis B virus (HBV) have persistent antigenemia with undetectable antibody. Hepatitis B surface antigen (HBsAg), from the outer envelope, is found in all carriers, and is often the only viral protein synthesized by infected cells. The finding of hepatitis B e antigen (HBeAg), which corresponds to a capsid product, indicates that complete viral particles are being produced; therefore, the carrier is considered highly infective.

6. The answer is E [Chapter 34 II B 2, C 2]. The young Peace Corps volunteer probably contracted yellow fever during his trip to Ecuador. Yellow fever, a hemorrhagic syndrome, is characterized by a high fever, mucosal bleeding, hypotension, and elevated bilirubin levels, and is prevalent in Central and South America. Dengue fever, also caused by an arbovirus, is an arthralgia syndrome characterized by a "saddle back" fever and severe skeletomuscular pain. The patient does not have symptoms that would suggest encephalitis; therefore, Venezuelan equine encephalitis is unlikely. Malaria is caused by *Plasmodium,* a protozoan, and typhoid fever is caused by *Salmonella typhi,* a bacterium.

7. The answer is A [Chapter 23 II D 1; III B]. DNA viruses need to synthesize new DNA to be incorporated into their progeny. If DNA synthesis is inhibited, successful viral replication will not take place. In contrast, the replication cycle of most RNA viruses can proceed in spite of interference with DNA synthesis. Hepatitis A virus (HAV), rhabdoviruses, polioviruses, and togaviruses are RNA viruses replicate independently of DNA synthesis.

8–9. The answers are: 8- A [Chapter 45 III A 2 b (1), 3 a, b (2)], **9-A** [Chapter 45 III A 5]. The organism visualized in the feces is *Giardia lamblia (intestinalis),* a common parasite in the creeks of the mountains around Vail, Colorado. This parasite uses a ventral cusp to attach to the duodenal mucosa. When the number of parasites in the duodenum is sufficient to cover large areas of the intestinal mucosa, diarrhea develops because the parasites interfere with absorption by the duodenal villi.

Metronidazole is particularly effective against most flagellates, including *G. lamblia.* A bland diet and plenty of electrolyte-rich fluids could be beneficial, but not curative.

10. The answer is D [Chapter 27 III A 3, B 1]. The fact that the virus is widespread suggests horizontal transmission, and therefore, the virus must carry the genes essential for replication (*gag, pol, env*) on its genome. The fact that the development of malignancies is rare and occurs after a long latency period suggests that the virus does not carry an oncogene (otherwise, the incidence of tumors would be high) and that it causes malignancies by insertional mutagenesis.

11–12. The answers are 11-E [Chapter 30 II A 1 c, 2 b, C 2 a], **12-B** [Chapter 25 II B 3 a]. The college student's lesions are suggestive of genital herpes, both by their aspect (vesicular) and by their recurrence. This impression is confirmed by the finding of Tzanck cells (multinucleated giant cells) in the scraping from the base of the vesicle. Herpes simplex virus (HSV) causes latent infections of the nerve ganglia, and recurrences are associated with retrograde diffusion of the virus through the nerve fibers to the skin or mucosal surfaces innervated by those fibers.

Acyclovir is a nucleoside analog that is phosphorylated partly by a viral thymidine kinase. When taken up by the viral DNA polymerase, acyclovir blocks further elongation of the nascent DNA chain.

13. The answer is D [Chapter 12 I D 1, E 3 c]. The patient's clinical presentation is suggestive of toxic shock syndrome (TSS), which is caused by special strains of *Staphylococcus aureus* that release a potent exotoxin, toxic shock syndrome toxin-1 (TSST-1). This toxin behaves as a superantigen and cross-links major histocompatibility complex-II (MHC-II) molecules with T cell receptors on helper lymphocytes. Activation of the cross-linked cells leads to the massive release of proinflammatory cytokines, including interleukin-1 (IL-1), interleukin-8 (IL-8), and tumor necrosis factor-α (TNF-α). These cytokines induce fever, capillary leakage, circulatory collapse, and shock.

14–15. The answers are 14-E [Chapter 12], **15-A** [Chapter 12 I H 2]. The clinical scenario is suggestive of impetigo, which is usually caused by either *Staphylococcus aureus* or *Streptococcus pyogenes* (a group A streptococcus). Both bacteria have peptidoglycan-rich cell walls. They are Gram-positive; therefore, they do not take up safranin. They are easy to grow on conventional blood agar plates. They do not colonize the lower gastrointestinal tract. Their virulence factors include surface proteins and exotoxins, but not polysaccharide capsules.

S. aureus is often penicillin-resistant, a fact that must be taken into consideration when the decision has been made to initiate treatment before the organism involved has been identified and its susceptibility has been determined. Gram-positive bacteria are ideal targets for antibiotics that inhibit peptidoglycan cross-linking, thus disturbing cell wall biosynthesis.

16. The answer is A [Chapter 42 I A 1 b (1)]. This child's immune system is likely to be compromised as a result of the chemotherapy he is receiving to treat the leukemia. Low granulocyte counts and the administration of broad-spectrum antibiotics favor the development of opportunistic infections by agents not affected by antibiotics. In this patient, the white plaques in the mouth and erythematous rash in the perineal region strongly suggest that *Candida albicans* is overgrowing. It is likely that this organism has disseminated through the blood stream and is responsible for the patient's fever. *C. albicans* is not affected by any known antibacterial agent. Viral infections are also not affected by antibiotics, but usually are seen in patients with severe defects of cell-mediated immunity (CMI), rather than in patients with agranulocytosis.

17. The answer is D [Chapter 3 VII B; Figure 3-9]. Under the described conditions, the main factor preventing the expression of the *lac* operon (Lac-O) is the decrease in cyclic adenosine monophosphate (cAMP) level caused by the metabolism of glucose. As a result of the decreased cAMP level, the catabolite activator protein (CAP) does not bind to the promoter region, and in the absence of its enhancing activity, the operon is not expressed.

18. The answer is C [Chapter 4 II C 1 a, b (1)]. Nalidixic acid is an inhibitor of DNA gyrase and blocks DNA synthesis. Therefore, the incorporation of Thymidine into the bacterial DNA would be blocked by the addition of nalidixic acid to the bacterial culture.

19. The answer is E [Chapter 45 III E 1 c (1)]. The African trypanosomes have developed a genetic mechanism that allows them to change their outer antigens, thus evading the immune response. Each time the infecting trypanosomes change their outer antigenic coat, the patient suffers a relapse.

20. The answer is C [Chapter 46 I C 5]. Visceral larva migrans is caused by the larvae of *Toxocara canis,* a dog parasite. Human infection usually results from contact with fecal material from dogs.

21. The answer is D [Chapter 7 II]. Bacterial capsules, probably as a result of their poor immunogenicity and intrinsic negative charge, tend to interfere with phagocytosis. Some capsules have anticomplementary activity (e.g., they block the conversion of C3 or rapidly inactivate C3b), leading to decreased phagocytosis.

22. The answer is C [Chapter 12 II F 8]. The *Streptococcus pneumoniae* vaccine is a polyvalent vaccine made from the capsular polysaccharides of 23 serological groups. The capsular polysaccharide of *S. pneumoniae,* which has antiphagocytic properties, is the organism's main virulence factor. However, the immune system of normal adults responds to immunization with the polysaccharides, and the corresponding antibodies opsonize the bacteria and override the antiphagocytic effects of the capsule.

23. The answer is B [Chapter 3 V C 2 a]. Genetic exchange between bacterium X and bacterium Y most likely involved generalized transduction. Genetic exchange of chromosomal material between two bacteria has to involve high-frequency recombination, transduction, or transformation (conjugation only results in the transfer of plasmids). The fact that the genes from bacterium X seem to be transmitted to bacterium Y in pairs of close genes suggests that the transmission depends on the passage of randomly cut DNA segments of approximate size. This fact rules out specialized transduction, which usually results in the transfer of a gene or a few genes located in proximity to the site of insertion of the bacteriophage into the bacterial chromosome. High-frequency recombination usually results in the transfer of gene segments of unequal length, and those genes near the origin of replication tend to be always transferred, while distant genes are only rarely transferred. Generalized transduction or transformation could account for the transfer of genetic material as described in this experimental vignette. Transformation, however, would be affected by the presence of deoxyribonuclease (DNase) in the culture.

24. The answer is C [Chapter 38 V B 2]. Hepatitis D virus (HDV, delta agent) is an incomplete virus that infects hepatitis B virus (HBV)-infected individuals. It is usually transmitted through blood products (sharing of needles among intravenous drug users is a common mode of transmission) or sexual activities. Infection with HDV is associated with a symptomatic recrudescence.

25. The answer is D [Chapter 4 II A 1 a (2)]. The bactericidal effect of penicillin is based on two effects: inhibition of peptidoglycan cross-linking by transpeptidases and enhancement of peptidoglycan digestion by autolysins. If the organism is deficient in autolysins, the only effect of penicillin will be to prevent the proper cross-linking of nascent peptidoglycan. The bacterium will be able to replicate, but its cell wall will lack rigidity and, therefore, will assume a spherical configuration.

26. The answer is C [Chapter 30 III A 1 b, 2 b, C 1; Table 30-2] The clinical scenario is suggestive of shingles (herpes zoster) in an immunocompromised patient. The causative agent, varicella-zoster virus, is an enveloped DNA virus with an icosahedral nucleocapsid.

27. The answer is E [Chapter 45 III C 3 a]. The trophozoite is the infectious form of *Trichomonas vaginalis,* which is usually transmitted venereally. The trophozoite cannot survive for long in a dry environment. No cyst form has been described for *T. vaginalis.* The merozoite stage occurs during the life cycle of some sporozoa, but not flagellates.

28. The answer is D [Chapter 9 II D]. The administration of preformed antibodies (passive immunization) is associated with immediate, but short-lived, protection. Passive immunization is not as cost effective as active immunization, which can protect for many years. Furthermore, in some patients with antiimmunoglobulin antibodies, passive immunization can cause hypersensitivity reactions.

29. The answer is B [Chapter 4 II C 1 b; Table 5-3]. The fluoroquinolones (e.g., ciprofloxacin) are DNA gyrase inhibitors. A mutation that decreases ciprofloxacin's binding affinity for the bacterium but does not affect the enzyme functioning will result in resistance to this antibacterial agent.

30. The answer is B [Chapter 3 V A 2]. A high-frequency recombinant (Hfr) bacterium is one that has integrated a conjugative plasmid into its chromosome. As such, the Hfr bacterium becomes competent and engages in conjugation, but it mostly transfers bacterial chromosome pieces to the recipient bacteria, which do not possess the fertility (F) factor, or transfer factor (i.e., they remain unable undergo conjugation).

31. The answer is E [Chapter 2 II C 5 c; Figure 2-6]. Bacitracin inhibits the regeneration of lipid-P and, therefore, lipid P will be depleted and the formation of lipid-P-P-Mur-NAc–pentapeptide inhibited. The UDP-Mur-NAc–pentapeptide precursor accumulates in the cytoplasm.

32. The answer is A [Table 5-2]. Although in most cases, penicillin resistance is caused by the bacterial synthesis of β-lactamases, the resistance of *Staphylococcus aureus* to methicillin is caused by mutations in the methicillin-binding proteins of the bacterium. Alteration of this target results in decreased binding affinity for the antibiotic.

33. The answer is E [Chapter 16 III A 3 a; Figure 16-4]. Cholera toxin (choleragen) catalyzes the ribosylation of a guanosine triphosphate (GTP)-stimulatory protein, causing it to lose its guanosine triphosphatase (GTPase) activity. In other words, it becomes unable to deactivate itself by breaking down GTP. The persistent activation of the G_s protein results in activation of adenylate cyclase and exaggerated synthesis of cyclic adenosine monophosphate (cAMP), which in turn activates sodium-dependent chloride secretion and inhibits sodium and potassium absorption by the cell. The massive efflux of electrolytes into the intestinal lumen raises the tonicity of the intestinal contents and induces water hypersecretion, resulting in copious, watery diarrhea.

34. The answer is A [Chapter 49 IIIA 1 a]. The enteroviruses (including coxsackievirus A, echoviruses, and polioviruses) are by far the most common causes of viral meningitis. Arboviruses and herpes simplex virus (HSV) are more likely to cause encephalitis.

35. The answer is B [Table 7-2; Chapter 12 II B 1 d (1)]. Several major exotoxins of Gram-positive organisms (such as streptococcal erythrogenic toxins and diphtheria toxin) are produced by lysogenic strains, which carry prophages with the genes coding for the toxins.

36. The answer is B [Chapter 15 I A 1 a (1) (a)]. *Haemophilus influenzae* is a fastidious organism that requires two important growth factors: factor V (nicotinamide adenine dinucleotide, NAD) and factor X (protoporphyrin IX, hematin). Both of these factors are released by heating red blood cells, as takes place during the preparation of chocolate agar.

37. The answer is C [Chapter 27 I C 5]. The rate of glucose transport across the cell membrane increases in virus-transformed cells to support the transformed cells' growth requirements. Virus-transformed cells become immortalized and require fewer growth factors (such as those provided by serum). Agglutinability by lectins increases, because immortalized cells express more glycoproteins in their membranes, but express less of the normal cell membrane proteins, including major histocompatibility complex (MHC) molecules. (Some transforming viruses synthesize proteins that inhibit the transport of MHC molecules to the cell membrane; in other cases, the decreased expression results from the replacement of cellular membrane proteins by viral envelope proteins in the infected cell membrane.)

38. The answer is C [Chapter 4 II C 1 c]. Nitroimidazoles, such as metronidazole, become active after reduction, which converts them into DNA alkylating agents. Reduction is only observed in anaerobic organisms that use low redox potential compounds (i.e., ferredoxin) as electron acceptors.

39. The answer is B [Chapter 5 II A]. The cell wall of most Gram-negative organisms (such as *Pseudomonas aeruginosa*) is relatively impermeable to water-soluble antibiotics. *Haemophilus influenzae* is an exception to that rule; its resistance to penicillins is the result of plasmid-coded penicillinase synthesis.

40. The answer is E [Chapter 19 II C 2 a (1), E]. The businessman most likely has primary syphilis, caused by the spirochete *Treponema pallidum. T. pallidum* cannot be stained or cultured; therefore, diagnosis of primary syphilis usually relies on serologic tests or direct visualization of *Treponema* in chancre material using darkfield microscopy. The nonspecific tests, such as the Venereal Disease Research Laboratory (VDRL) test, tend to become positive sooner than the specific tests, such as the microhemagglutination *T. pallidum* (MHA-TP) test.

41. The answer is B [Chapter 38 III C 1 a]. The vertical transmission of hepatitis B virus (HBV) is believed to take place during birth (perinatal transmission), following contact of the newborn with maternally-infected blood. (Maternal blood can enter the fetal circulation directly when the placenta starts to detach.) For this reason, immunization immediately after birth may prevent the newborn from becoming infected.

42. The answer is E [Chapter 29 I A 3 c (1) (b); Chapter 36 IV]. Many bacteria and viruses can cause bronchopneumonia in young children, but only a few agents cause the formation of clusters of cells by membrane fusion. These syncytia appear microscopically as large, multinucleated clumps of cells. Syncytia formation is a common cytopathic effect of infection with paramyxoviruses, such as respiratory syncytial virus (RSV).

43. The answer is B [Chapter 11 III A 1; Figure 11-1]. *Escherichia coli,* part of the normal gastrointestinal flora, could behave as an opportunistic organism and cause bacteremia in an immunocompromised patient, such as a patient receiving cancer chemotherapy. An opportunistic agent, by definition, is present either as a commensal in the normal flora or in the environment, has limited virulence for immunocompetent individuals, and tends to infect those that are immunocompromised. The causative agents of the other infections listed (*Brucella, Streptococcus pyogenes, Bacillus anthracis,* and *Mycobacterium tuberculosis*) do not fulfill these criteria.

44. The answer is D [Chapter 45 V A 3 c (1)]. The missionary is most likely suffering from blackwater fever, a complication of malaria caused by *Plasmodium falciparum.* Massive intravascular hemolysis leads to hemoglobinuria, which causes darkening of the urine and acute renal failure.

45. The answer is B [Chapter 12 II C 1 b; Table 49-1]. Group B streptococci (e.g., *Streptococcus agalactiae*) are most common cause of neonatal meningitis, followed by *Escherichia coli. Listeria monocytogenes* and group D streptococcus, such as *Streptococcus pneumoniae,* are considerably less common causes. *Haemophilus influenzae* type B is a common cause of meningitis in children between the ages of 6 months and 2 years.

46. The answer is C [Table 9-1]. The vertical transmission of hepatitis B virus (HBV) takes place during birth and immediate vaccination appears to protect the newborn from becoming infected. The hepatitis B vaccine is the only vaccine recommended for administration to neonates. Infants should receive the diphtheria–pertussis–tetanus (DPT), oral polio, and *Haemophilus influenzae* type b vaccines at 2 months of age. A vaccine for HIV does not exist.

47. The answer is A [Chapter 16 II D 6 a]. The migrant worker most likely has typhoid fever. The clinical scenario (systemic febrile disease with a faint maculopapular rash on the trunk of an individual likely to live in primitive or semiprimitive conditions) is suggestive. Blood cultures are most likely to be positive at this stage of the disease. In the absence of symptoms suggestive of gastrointestinal involvement, tests on fecal material would not be useful. Brucellosis usually presents less acutely, with neurologic involvement, and runs a recurrent course. A viral etiology is possible, but the age of the patient and the severity of the symptoms argue against a viral etiology.

48. The answer is D [Chapter 25 II B 1 c]. Amantadine and rimantadine can be used to prevent influenza A infections in susceptible individuals. Both drugs inhibit the release of nucleic acids into the cell cytoplasm, thus preventing viral replication.

49. The answer is E [Chapter 17 I B 1 b, 2 a]. The patient appears to have contracted a nosocomial infection of the urinary tract in the hospital, caused by an oxidase-positive, ampicillin-resistant bacterium that grows in mucoid colonies. *Pseudomonas aeruginosa* most closely fits this description.

50. The answer is A [Chapter 6 II B 4]. Ethylene oxide gas sterilization is the best choice for decontaminating a heat-sensitive piece of equipment. Pasteurization employs mild heat. Diluted hydrogen peroxide (3%) is indicated for the disinfection of skin.

51. The answer is C [Chapter 12 II B 1 a (1)]. M protein is the major virulence factor of the group A streptococci. It is strongly immunogenic. However, there are more than 80 antigenic types of M protein, and immunity against one type may not be protective against another.

52. The answer is B [Chapter 19 IV]. The development of jaundice, hepatosplenomegaly, tubulopathy, and increased cardiac enzymes (e.g., creatinine kinase) is suggestive of leptospirosis. Dogs and cats can harbor *Leptospira,* making leptospirosis an occupational hazard for veterinarians.

53. The answer is A [Chapter 18 III F]. The granulomatous lesion and the association with the aquarium should immediately lead to the suspicion that *Mycobacterium marinum* is the causative agent. Like all *Mycobacteria, M. marinum* is an acid-fast rod. A defining characteristic of this organism is the fact that it grows at much lower temperatures than other *Mycobacteria* (30°C is the ideal temperature).

54. The answer is D [Chapter 16 III A 3, 4 a]. *Vibrio cholerae* is the most likely cause of this patient's enterocolitis. Peru is the epicenter of an ongoing cholera epidemic in South America. Cases of cholera resulting from the ingestion of imported, contaminated food (particularly shellfish) were reported at the onset of the epidemic. Cholera toxin, choleragen, induces copious, explosive, secretory diarrhea. *Escherichia coli* could also be considered in the list of possibilities.

55. The answer is C [Chapter 25 II B 1 b]. There are more than 100 antigenically distinct rhinoviruses; this great diversity impairs the development of protective antibodies directed against viral antigens. In contrast, blocking the viral receptor on mucosal cells [i.e., the intercellular cell adhesion molecule-1 (ICAM-1)] can protect against infection.

56. The answer is A [Chapter 38 III D 2 a (2) (b), (3), E; Chapter 55 III B]. The information provided by the Vietnamese refugee strongly suggests that she had hepatitis B; therefore, a major concern is that this woman is a chronic hepatitis B virus (HBV) carrier. The next step would be to measure hepatitis B surface antigen (HbsAg) levels. IgM antibodies are unlikely to persist 3 years after the infection, so measuring IgM antibody to hepatitis B core antigen (HBcAg) or HbsAg would be useless. Hepatitis A virus (HAV) is unlikely to cause chronic infection, and cytomegalovirus (CMV) does not fit the clinical picture.

57. The answer is E [Chapter 25 II B 3 a; Chapter 30 II A 2 a, D 1]. This child's symptoms are highly suggestive of infection with herpes simplex virus-1 (HSV-1). This virus can be treated with topical acyclovir, a target-activated nucleoside analogue that terminates DNA elongation.

58. The answer is D [Chapter 17 I B 4 b; Table 17-3]. *Pseudomonas aeruginosa* and other *Pseudomonas* species are frequently involved in pulmonary infections in patients with cystic fibrosis. The general characteristics of *Pseudomonas* include the production of an antiphagocytic alginate capsule, aerobic metabolism, oxidase positivity, and Gram-negative staining.

59. The answer is C [Table 12-2]. The organism is most likely *Staphylococcus aureus.* Of the three staphylococci mentioned (*Staphylococcus epidermidis, Staphylococcus saprophyticus,* and *S. aureus*), only *S. aureus* produces coagulase. Both *S. aureus* and *S. saprophyticus* are mannitol fermenters, but *S. aureus* colonies tend to be yellowish white, while *S. saprophyticus* colonies tend to be whitish gray. All three staphylococci are catalase positive and produce hemolysins.

60. The answer is D [Chapter 12 II B 3 a]. Rheumatic fever carditis may follow primary infection by group A streptococci and is a classic example of an autoimmune reaction. The autoimmune reaction is triggered as a consequence of molecular mimicry resulting from the sharing of antigenic structures between streptococcal and heart tissue glycoproteins.

61. The answer is E [Chapter 49 A 1 a]. *Streptococcus pneumoniae, Neisseria meningitidis,* and *Haemophilus influenzae* type b account for more than 80% of cases of bacterial meningitis in children. Prior to the introduction of highly effective conjugate vaccines, *H. influenzae* was the leading cause. However, at this time, *S. pneumoniae* outranks *H. influenzae,* closely followed by *N. meningitidis. Streptococcus agalactiae, Listeria monocytogenes,* and *Escherichia coli* are not common causes of infections in this age group.

62. The answer is E [Chapter 46 I B 4 c]. Hookworms (*Ancylostoma duodenale* and *Necator americanus*) have teeth that they use to attach to the mucosal surface, where they suck blood (approximately 150 ml/day/worm in the case of *A. duodenale,* and 40 ml/day/worm in the case of *N. americanus*). Over the long term, hookworm infestation causes persistent trauma and bleeding in the intestinal mucosa, leading to severe iron deficiency anemia.

63. The answer is B [Chapter 57 II B 2; VI B]. This patient is most likely HIV-positive; therefore, her Western blot results are most likely to resemble pattern B. True seropositive HIV-infected individuals show antibodies reactive with a wide variety of HIV antigens on the Western blot test, including envelope glycoproteins (gp160, gp120, gp41), enzymes (p66, p51), capsid proteins (p24), and matrix proteins (p17). All other patterns are considered indeterminate.

64. The answer is D [Chapter 4 II A 2 a (2) (a) (i); Chapter 14 I B 8 a (1)]. *Neisseria meningitidis* is a Gram-negative diplococcus that grows in chocolate agar and is oxidase positive. *N. meningitidis* is exquisitely sensitive to *β*-lactam antibiotics. The mechanism of action of these antibacterial agents involves inhibition of peptidoglycan cross-linking.

65. The answer is E [Chapter 27 II]. A common property of the proteins coded by several transforming genes defined in DNA tumor viruses is their ability to inactivate the products of tumor suppressor genes, such as p53 and the Rb gene product. In contrast, retroviral oncogene products tend to activate second signal cascades or to activate the expression of genes controlling cell proliferation.

66. The answer is D [Table 22-2; Chapter 49 III A 1 a; Table 49-2]. The clinical presentation is suggestive of viral meningitis, an impression that is reinforced by the negative results on tests used to detect bacteria and fungi involved in meningitis. The most common viral agents are enteroviruses, of the picornavirus group, which are naked +RNA viruses.

67. The answer is C [Chapter 2 II B 1 a (2) (a)]. Homolactic fermentation, in which pyruvate is converted into lactic acid, is characteristic of *Lactobacillus* species and many *Streptococcus* species.

68. The answer is C [Chapter 3 II A 1; Chapter 5 II B]. The emergence of strains resistant to neomycin most likely resulted from a spontaneous mutation. The transfer of genetic elements responsible for antibacterial resistance is impossible when the two original strains are sensitive to the antibacterial. Antibacterials do not cause mutations; rather, they represent a selective pressure for the development of spontaneous antibiotic-resistant mutants.

69. The answer is A [Chapter 3 VII C]. Although most choices are at least theoretically correct, the easiest way to determine whether a bacterium has become able to synthesize tryptophan is to test for its ability to grow in a tryptophan-depleted medium.

70. The answer is E [Chapter 33 I]. Rhinoviruses are acid-labile; these picornaviruses infect the upper respiratory tract. In contrast, echoviruses, polioviruses, and coxsackieviruses are enteroviruses. They resist stomach acidity and can be isolated from the feces.

71. The answer is A [Chapter 23 II D 1 a–b; Chapter 25 II B 2 a]. Vidarabine is a DNA chain terminator that inhibits the synthesis of progeny DNA. The late proteins of DNA viruses are synthesized from progeny DNA; therefore, in the presence of vidarabine, they will not be produced. Of all the listed adenoviral proteins, the capsid proteins are the only late proteins.

72–74. The answers are: 72-E [Chapter 15 II C 1], **73-D** [Chapter 21 III B 2], **74-C** [Figure 16-2; Table 21-1]. Adhesins, which mediate the attachment of *Bordetella pertussis* to ciliated epithelial cells of the trachea, are one of the major virulence factors of this organism, which causes whooping cough. Most of the other organisms on the list have adhesion factors, but they do not attach to the ciliated epithelial cells of the trachea.

Rickettsiae, such as *Rickettsia typhi,* are obligatory intracellular organisms that infect the vascular endothelium predominantly.

Many infectious organisms have the ability to survive phagocytosis and infect phagocytic cells of the reticuloendothelial system. *Salmonella typhi,* the etiologic agent of typhoid fever, is one of them.

75–76. The answers are 75-E [Chapter 34 III], **76-A** [Chapter 30 II A 1 c]. Many viruses, including rubella virus, spread to their target organs via a transient viremia.

Herpes simplex virus (HSV) latently infects neural sensory ganglia, and, when the infection is reactivated, reaches the target organ (i.e., the skin) by retrograde diffusion through the afferent nervous fibers.

77–79. The answers are: 77-D [Chapter 27 III E], **78-A** [Chapter 27 II A 3 a], **79-E** [Chapter 27 I C 3; III C 3 b]. The Tax protein of human T lymphotropic virus-I (HTLV-I) is believed to modify nucleoproteins [e.g., nuclear factor kB (NFkB)] involved in the control of the expression of interleukin and interleukin-receptor–coding genes. The overexpression of interleukin-2 (IL-2) and the corresponding receptor is believed to be the basis for the uncontrolled proliferation of T lymphocytes characteristic of the diseases caused by HTLV-1.

Large T antigen binds and inactivates the retinoblastoma (Rb) gene product. Normally, the Rb gene codes for a protein that binds and inactivates several transcription factors, preventing progression into the S phase of cell division. Therefore, inactivation of the Rb gene leads to uncontrolled cell proliferation.

The v-*src* gene product is a tyrosine kinase that phosphorylates cytoskeleton proteins, causing loss of contact inhibition of cell growth. Loss of contact inhibition is a major abnormality associated with malignant growth.

80–81. The answers are: 80-B [Chapter 23 IV A 3 a (1)], **81-C** [Chapter 23 IV B]. HIV, a retrovirus, needs to pack a reverse transcriptase (RNA-dependent DNA polymerase) in order to undergo the initial step of replication. Mammalian cells do not contain such an enzyme.

Respiratory syncytial virus is a -RNA virus. Therefore, in order to replicate, the virus must first transcribe a messenger +RNA strand. In order to do this, the virus needs to pack an RNA-dependent RNA polymerase. Like RNA-dependent DNA polymerase, RNA-dependent RNA polymerase is not available in mammalian cells.

82–83. The answers are 82-I [Tables 16-4 and 16-7], **83-C** [Tables 12-2 and 12-3]. One of the fastest and easiest ways to differentiate the coliforms (*Escherichia coli* and closely related enterobacteriaceae) from pathogenic enterobacteriaceae (such as *Salmonella* and *Shigella*) is by the organism's ability to ferment lactose. Coliforms are lactose fermenters, whereas *Salmonella* and *Shigella* are not. Other biochemical properties are used for final identification of these species, but lactose fermentation is a fast and easy initial screening test.

Staphylococcus aureus and group A streptococci are Gram-positive cocci that can be grown in similar media, under similar conditions. However, *S. aureus* is a catalase-positive aerobic organism, whereas Group A streptococci are catalase-negative facultative organisms.

84–85. The answers are 84-I [Chapter 31 III B 2 b], **85-H** [Table 31-1]. The JC virus is one of the two polyomaviruses that can infect humans (the other one is the BK virus). JC virus has been identified as the cause of progressive multifocal leukoencephalopathy.

Papillomaviruses can cause a variety of human diseases. Some genotypes are more frequently identified in association with some diseases than with others. Human papillomavirus type 6 is frequently associated with genital warts.

86–88. The answers are: 86-C [Chapter 37 VII A 1; Chapter 52 II A 1–2], **87-F** [Chapter 37 VI A, B 2 a], **88-B** [Chapter 38 IV A 1, B 1]. The only group of human viruses with a double-stranded DNA genome are the reoviruses, which includes the rotaviruses. Rotaviruses are a common cause of infantile diarrhea, and can lead to severe dehydration. Rotaviruses are transmitted via contaminated food or water.

The Sin nombre hantavirus, isolated in some states in the western United States, causes acute respiratory distress syndrome. Transmission involves exposure to materials contaminated with rodent excreta (the rodents in question act as reservoirs for the virus).

Among the many viruses that cause hepatitis, hepatitis C virus (HCV), a flavivirus, is the only one who has a positive-sense RNA genome and is enveloped. HCV is a major cause of posttransfusional hepatitis. In addition, HCV can be transmitted via dirty needles and venereally, but these are not the most common modes of transmission.

89–91. The answers are: 89-G [Chapter 34 II C 3 a], **90-C** [Chapter 17 II D], **91-I** [Table 21-5]. Most encephalitis viruses have animal reservoirs (e.g., birds, horses) and are transmitted by mosquitoes or ticks. Birds are the reservoir for St. Louis encephalitis virus, which is transmitted by mosquitoes to both humans and horses.

Pasteurella multocida is a zoonotic Gram-negative bacterium that infects dogs and cats, among other animals. It can be transmitted to humans via bite wounds from these animals.

Ehrlichia chaffeensis is a member of the Rickettsiaceae family and is transmitted by ticks. Ticks are also involved in the transmission of other rickettsioses, such as Rocky Mountain spotted fever and Lyme disease.

92–93. The answers are 92-C [Chapter 16 II B 3 a (1) (b)], **93-F** [Chapter 12 II B 1 d (3)]. *Escherichia coli* serotype O157:H7 produces a toxin that can be neutralized with antiserum against Shiga toxin, hence the name Shiga-like toxin. Both toxins can induce hemolytic-uremic syndrome, which has a high fatality rate, especially in young children.

Group A streptococci involved in necrotizing fasciitis release large amounts of exotoxin B, a cysteine protease that causes the extensive tissue damage seen in these patients.

94–100. The answers are 94-W [Chapter 42 II E], **95-G** [Chapter 45 II A], **96-Y** [Chapter 48 II A], **97-Q** [Chapter 21 II C 1], **98-L** [Chapter 20 I A], **99-A** [Chapter 53], **100-S** [Chapter 46 III B]. *Sporothrix schenckii* is found in soil and vegetation, including rose thorns. Skin abrasion introduces the fungus into the dermis. A pustule forms at the site of inoculation, spreading along the lymphatic vessels and usually ending at the regional lymph nodes. Sporotrichosis is also called rose grower's disease.

The association of chronic, sometimes bloody, diarrhea with hepatomegaly and ulcerative lesions in the distal colon in a patient from South America is extremely suggestive of intestinal amebiasis, caused by *Entamoeba histolytica*. *Entamoeba coli* is a commensal that does not cause clinical disease.

The clinical picture in the 75-year-old man (shortness of breath, productive cough, high temperature, hard chills) is suggestive of an acute bacterial infection of the lungs. At the age of this patient, pneumonia is most likely caused by *Streptococcus pneumoniae*. Another organism to be concerned with would be *Legionella pneumophila,* but the very acute presentation, the lack of predisposing factors, and the lack of other symptoms seen in legionellosis make this possibility less likely.

A fever accompanied by a maculopapular rash involving the palms of the hands in an individual who has been recently engaging in some type of outdoor activity should raise the hypothesis of Rocky Mountain spotted fever. The finding of a tick or a clear history of a tick bite are confirmatory, but the lack of these elements cannot be used to rule out the diagnosis.

The onset of pneumonia with diarrhea in a 70-year-old smoker with chronic bronchitis, peripheral blood neutrophilia, and a negative Gram stain of the sputum suggest infection caused by *Legionella pneumophila*. (The peripheral blood neutrophilia implies that the infection is caused by a bacterium.)

The woman recovering from a cesarean section most likely has a postsurgical anaerobic abscess (as suggested by the foul-smelling discharge). A Gram-negative organism is most likely the cause, because of the patient's rapid development of septic shock. The lack of response to penicillin suggests that *Bacteroides fragilis* may be involved, because approximately 85% of the isolates are β-lactamase producers.

The clinical picture of chronic hematuria in a patient of African origin should raise the suspicion of an infection with *Schistosoma haematobium*. The finding of oval eggs with a terminal spine in the urine confirms the diagnosis.

Index

Note: Page numbers in italic denote illustrations, those followed by *t* denote tables, those followed by Q denote questions, and those followed by E denote explanations.

A

Abortion, septic, 414
Abortive infection, 244, 293
Abscesses, 103
Acanthamoeba species, 373–374
Acellular vaccines, 140
Acetyltransferases, 56
Acid-fast rod organism, 540Q, 552E
Acid-fast staining, 18
Acquired immunodeficiency syndrome (AIDS), 510. (*See also* Human immunodeficiency virus (HIV))
  fungal infections in, 357
Actinomycetaceae
  Actinomycetaceae israelii, 190
  general properties, 189–190, 189*t*
  Nocardia asteroides, 190
  Nocardia brasiliensis, 190
  streptomycetes, 190–191
Actinomycetaceae israelii, 190
Active immunization, 83
Active tuberculosis, 169–170
Acyclovir, 236*t*
  administration of, 236
  clinical uses of, 236–237
  for herpes virus, 279, 496
  for HSV encephalitis, 439
  mechanism of action, 236, 535Q, 548E
  resistance to, 239
  for varicella-zoster virus, 280
Additive recombination, 28
Adenoviral pneumonia, 425
Adenoviruses
  assembly and release, 290
  clinical disease in, 289–290
  degree of tumorigenicity of adenovirus-transformed cells, 254
  diagnosis of, 290
  epidemiology of, 289
  general characteristics of, 289
  mechanism of transformation in, 254
  oncogenic potential of, 254
  pathogenesis of, 289
  prevention of, 290
  replication of, 534Q, 547E
  synthesis of, 217–218
  treatment of, 290
  type 2 as cause of urinary tract infections, 450
Adenylate cyclase-like toxin, 137
Adhesin-coding plasmids, 35
Adhesion colonization factors, 143, 161
Adhesions, 3, 65–66
Aerobic bacteria, 18–19
Aerobic respiration, 12, 13–14
Aerotolerant bacteria, 13
African trypanosomiasis, 379–380, 536Q, 549E
Agar
  blood, 133
  chocolate, 133
  Loeffler, 113
  Tindale, 113
Age, effect of, on outcome of viral infection, 243
Agglutination, 19
AIDS-associated dementia, 445
Air space pneumonia, 185–186
Alcoholic cirrhosis, 487
Alcohols, 61
  fermentation, 13
Alginate capsule, 161
Alkylating agents, 62
Allopurinol
  for *Trypanosoma cruzi,* 381
  for trypanosomiasis, 366
Allylamines
  in antifungal therapy, 342, 344
  for cutaneous mycoses, 344
Alphaviruses, 299
Alveolar pneumonia, 248
Amantadine
  for RNA viruses III, 307
  as synthetic antiviral agent, 234
Amebiasis, treatment of, 365–366
Amebic dysentery, 373
Amino acids, 12
  biosynthesis of, 14
Aminoglycosides, 49
  for pneumonia, 423
  for prostatitis, 453
Amoebae
  Acanthamoeba species, 373–374
  Entamoeba coli, 374
  Entamoeba gingivalis, 374
  Entamoeba hartmanni, 374
  Entamoeba histolytica, 371, 373
  Entamoeba nana, 374
  Lodamoeba butschlii, 374
  Naegleria fowleri, 374
Amorolfine in antifungal therapy, 342
Amoxicillin
  for disseminated infection, 132
  for *Haemophilus influenzae* infections, 135
  for *Shigella,* 148
  for urinary tract infection, 452
Amoxycillin
  for gram-negative bacteria, 46
  for gram-positive bacteria, 46
Amphotericin B
  for amebiasis, trichomoniasis, and giardiasis, 366
  in antifungal therapy, 340
  for blastomycosis, 351
  for candidiasis, 348
  for coccidioidomycosis, 354
  for cryptococcosis, 349
  for histoplasmosis, 352
  for meningitis, 438
  for paracoccidioidomycosis, 354
  for sporotrichosis, 355
  for streptomycetes, 191
Amphotericin for meningoencephalitis, 374
Ampicillin
  for gram-positive and gram-negative bacteria, 46
  for group B streptococci, 110
  for *Haemophilus influenzae,* 135
  for *Shigella,* 148
  for typhoid fever, 150–151
Anaerobic bacteria, 19
  distribution of, 465–466
  metabolic properties of, 465
  physical requirements of, 465
Anaerobic infections
  clinical manifestations, 469
  diagnosis of, 469–470, 469*t*
  epidemiology of, 466, 466*t*
  etiology, 468–469
  pathogenesis of, 466–468, 467*t*
  treatment of, 470
Anaerobic respiration, 14
Anamnestic response, 75–76
Anatomic location of normal flora, 98–100, *99*
Ancylostoma braziliense, 398
Ancylostoma caninum, 398
Ancylostoma duodenale, 391–392
Ancylostomiasis, 541Q, 553E
Anemia from sporozoans, 383
Angiomatosis, bacillary, 202
Anicteric infection, 325–326
Anionic agents, 61
Anisakis marina, 394–395
Ankylosing spondylitis, *Yersinia enterocolitica* in, 165
Anorectal gonorrhea, 130–131
Anterior nasal diphtheria, 115
Anthelmintic agents for parasitic infections, 368–369
Anthrax
  cutaneous, 123
  gastrointestinal, 123
  pulmonary, 123
Antibacterial agents
  versus antibiotics, 41, *42*
  bacterial resistance to, 53
    according to drug class, 57, 57*t*
    acquisition, 53–54, 54*t*
    antibiotic susceptibility testing, 58–60, *59*
    mechanisms, 54, 55–56*t*, 56–57

broad-spectrum, 41
classification of, 43, *45*
definitions, 41, *42*
for *Entamoeba histolytica,* 373
general criteria for effective antibiotic action, 41–42
general principles of effective antibacterial therapy, 42–43
in inhibiting nucleic acid synthesis, 48–49
in inhibiting nucleotide synthesis, 47–48
in inhibiting protein synthesis, 49–51, *50*
β-Lactam, 43, 46–47
narrow-spectrum, 41
for *Neisseria meningitidis,* 128
for opportunistic infection, 98
Antibiotic susceptibility testing, 58–60, *59*
Antibiotic therapy
for meningitis, 433
for *Vibrio cholerae,* 154
Antibiotic-associated diarrhea, 119
Antibiotics
versus antibacterial agents, 41
beta-lactam, 117
Antibodies
complement-fixing, 263
cross-reactive, 76
mucosal, 263
natural, 76
neutralizing, 263
Antibody-dependent cellular cytotoxicity (ADCC), 75
Antibody-mediated (humoral) immunity, 74–76
role of viral, in long-term, 264
types of antiviral, 263
Antibody-virus complexes, ingestion of, 264
Anticomplementary activity, 79
Antifungal therapy
agents in, 340–342
general principles in, 340, *341*
resistance to antimycotic agents, 342
Antigen load, 78
Antigenic determinants, 19
Antigenic drift, 305
Antigenic modulation, 266–267
Antigenic shift, 228, 305
Antigenic variation, 79–81, *80,* 266
Anti-infectious host defenses, 73
antibody-mediated (humoral) immunity, 74–76
cell-mediated immunity, 76–78, *77*
evasion of immune response, 78–81, 78*t*
nonspecific defense mechanisms, 73–74, 74*t*
Antimicrobial agents
chemical, 61–62
for meningitis, 436
physical, 62–63
Antimicrobial susceptibility testing, 95
Antimycotic agents, resistance to, 342
Antiparasitic agents, resistance to, 369
Antiphagocytic capsules, 79, 144
Antiphagocytic factor, 161
Antiprotozoal agents for parasitic infections, 365–368
Antiretroviral therapy for immunodeficiency virus infection, 511–512
Antiseptics, 61
α_1-Antitrypsin deficiency, 487
Antiviral agents
classes of, 233–234, *235, 236,* 236–238, *237*
resistance to, 239
Antiviral immune response
pathologic consequences of, 265–266
tissue damage as consequence of, 266
Apicomplexa, 363
Aplastic crisis, 291–292
Arboviruses, 299, 299*t,* 320
alphaviruses, 299
bunyaviruses, 299
clinical disease in, 299–301
control and prevention of, 302
diagnosis of, 301–302
epidemiology of, 301
flaviviruses, 299
and meningitis, 435
pathogenesis of, 299
reoviruses, 299
Arenaviruses
clinical disease in, 319
epidemiology of, 319
general properties, 319
Aromatic amino acids, 14
Arthralgia syndrome, 299
Arthritis
in Lyme disease, 182
Staphylococci infection in, 103, 109
Ascaris lumbricoides, 390–391
Ascending paralysis, 297
as complication of hypersensitivity reactions, 307
Aseptic meningitis, 294, 296, 297, 434, 434*t,* 538Q, 550E
fungal, 436–438
parasitic meningoencephalitis, 438
tuberculous, 435–436
viral, 435
Aspartate family, 14
Aspergillosis, 346
Athlete's foot, 343
Attenuated bacteria, 85
Attenuated virus vaccines, 84
for polio, 295
for varicella, 494
Attenuation, 39
Atypical measles, 492
Autoimmune hepatitis, 487
Autolysins, 7, *9*
Autolytic enzymes, 46
Autotrophic metabolism, 14
Autotrophs, 12
Auxotrophs, 12
Azithromycin
impact of, on protein synthesis, 51
for legionnaires' disease, 187
for treating *Chlamydiae trachomatis,* 198
for uncomplicated genital infection, 132
Azlocillin, 46
Azoles, 340–341
Aztreonam, 47

B

Babesia species, 385
Bacillary angiomatosis, 202
Bacillus
Bacillus anthracis
clinical disease in, 123
control and prevention of, 124
determinants of pathogenicity, 123
diagnosis of, 124
epidemiology of, 124
pathogenesis of, 123
treatment of, 124
Bacillus cereus
pathogenesis of and clinical disease in, 124
treatment of, 124
Bacillus subtilis, 124
Bacitracin, 47
sensitivity, 544Q, 554E
Bacteremia
Bacillus in, 123
clostridial, 414
diagnosis of, 410–411, 411*t*
Enterobacteriaceae in, 159, 160
gram-negative, 412–413
special types of, 413–414
gram-positive, 414–415
special types of, 415–416
Haemophilus in, 134–135
implications, 410
Listeria monocytogenes in, 117
Pseudomonas in, 162
sources of, 410
Staphylococci infection in, 103
Streptococci infection in, 108, 110
treatment of, 411–412
in urinary tract infections, 452
Bacteria, 5, 74, 518–521*t*
aerobic, 18–19
aerotolerant, 13
anaerobic, 19
attenuated, 85
DNA transfer between, 28, *29*
conjugation, 28, 30–31
transformation, 31–32
facultative, 19
gram-negative, 7–8, 9, *10,* 18, 54
gram-positive, 7, 9, 18, 54, 56
halophilic, 12
heterotrophic, 12
litotrophic, 12
mesophilic, 16
microaerophilic, 13
organotrophic, 12
psychrophilic, 16
thermophilic, 16
by type of disease, 522*t*
Bacteria mutation, origins, 22–23
Bacterial adherence to mucosal surfaces, 12
Bacterial classification
genetic relatedness, 19
metabolic activity, 18–19
morphologic features, 18
serologic reactivity, 19
staining properties, 18
Bacterial conjugation, 12
Bacterial dysentery, 147
Bacterial electron transport system, 7
Bacterial epiglottitis, acute, 134
Bacterial gene mapping, 32, 34
Bacterial genetic material
chromosomes, 21
plasmids, 21
transposable elements, 21–22, *22*
Bacterial growth
curves, 17
measurement of, 16
Bacterial infections, laboratory diagnosis of, 91
culture and isolation of microorganisms, 93–95
detection of pathogen-specific macromolecules, 92–93

microscopic examination of patient specimens, 91
serologic testing, 95–96
Bacterial lysis, 46
Bacterial meningitis, 92, 429–430
clinical manifestations, 431–432
diagnosis of, 432–433
epidemiology of, 430–431, 430*t*
etiology, 430
pathogenesis of, 431
prevention of, 433–434
prognosis, 434
treatment of, 433, 433*t*
Bacterial mutation
detection of, 23
types of, 23
Bacterial pathogenicity, genetic basis of
transmission of virulence genes among bacteria, 35
virulence factors, 34
Bacterial peritonitis, 487
Bacterial physiology
biosynthetic pathways, 14–16
energy metabolism, 13–14
growth, 16–18
nutritional requirements, 12–13
Bacterial pneumonia, 111
Bacterial prostatitis, 452–453
Bacterial resistance to antibacterial agents, 53
according to drug class, 57, 57*t*
acquisition, 53–54, 54*t*
antibiotic susceptibility testing, 58–60, *59*
mechanisms, 54, 55–56*t*, 56–57
Bacterial structure
cell envelope
cytoplasmic membrane, 7
wall, 7, *8*
cytoplasmic components, 11
external, 11
gram-negative, 7–8, *10*
gram-positive, 7
Bacterial translocation, 98
Bacterial virulence factors, 65–70
adhesions, 65–66
capsules, 65
exoenzymes, 66
invasiveness, 66
toxins, 67–68, 67*t*, 68*t*, *69*, 69*t*, 70
Bactericidal agents, 41, *42*
Bacteriophages, 32
types of infections, 32–33, *33*
Bacteriostatic agents, 41, *42*
Bacterium X, 536Q, 549E
Bacteroides fragilis, 466, 467, 469
Bacteroides species, 466, 545Q, 555E
Bacteroides thetaiotaomicron, 466
Bacteroides vulgatus, 466
Balantidium coli, 381–382
Bartonellaceae
clinical disease in, 201–202
epidemiology of, 202, 202*t*
laboratory diagnosis of, 202
treatment of, 202
B-cell lymphoma, human herpesvirus-6 virus as cause of, 283
Benzimidazoles for nematode infections, 368
Beta-lactam antibiotics, 117
Beta-lactamase, 129
Bile solubility testing, 112
Binary fission, 5
Biosynthesis
macromolecule, 14–15
nucleotide, 14
Biphasic growth, 18
Bithionol
for cestode and trematode infections, 369
for *Fasciola* infections, 405
for *Paragonimus westermani,* 406
BK virus, 246, 252, 286
Blackwater fever, 539Q, 551E
Bladder cancer, 403
Blastomyces dermatitidis, 349
Blastomycosis
clinical disease in, 350
diagnosis of, 350–351
epidemiology of, 349
treatment of, 351
Blocking factors, 81
Blood agar, 94, 133
Blood cultures, 539Q, 551E
Blood dyscrasias, 50
Bloody diarrhea, 457, 463, 533Q, 547E
Bordetella pertussis, 543Q, 553–554E
clinical disease in, 137
determinants of pathogenicity, 136–137, *138*
epidemiology of, 139
general properties, 136, 136*t*
immunity, 139–140
immunoprophylaxis, 140
laboratory diagnosis of, 139
pathogenesis of, 137
therapy, 139
in whooping cough, 136
Borrelia
Borrelia burgdorferi
clinical disease in, 181–182
determinants of pathogenicity, 181
epidemiology of, 182
laboratory diagnosis of, 182–183
pathogenesis of, 181
treatment of, 183
Borrelia recurrentis
clinical disease in, 180–181
distribution, 181
epidemiology of, 181
laboratory diagnosis of, 181
pathogenesis of, 180
Botulinum toxin, 67
Botulism, 120
infant, 121
wound, 121
Breakbone fever, 300
Breath test, 156
Broad-spectrum antibacterial agents, 41
Broad-spectrum nucleoside analogues, 238
Bronchiolitis, 289–290, 309
Bronchitis, 111, 420
chronic, 135, 297
Bronchopneumonia, 420
Brucella
clinical disease in, 163, *163*
control and prevention of, 164
determinants of pathogenicity, 162–163
epidemiology of, 164
general properties, 162, 163*t*
laboratory diagnosis of, 164
pathogenesis of, 163
treatment of, 164
Budding, 5
Bulbar poliomyelitis, 294
Bulbospinal poliomyelitis, 294
Bulbous impetigo, 103
Bullous lesions, 490
Bunyaviruses, 299
clinical disease in, 319–320
general properties, 319
Burkitt's lymphoma, 254
chromosomal translocation in, 255
Epstein-Barr virus as cause of, 281
Burns, severe, 357

C

C substance, 106, 107
Calcium dipicolinate, 17
Caliciviruses
clinical disease in, 318
diagnosis of, 318
epidemiology of, 317
general properties, 317
pathogenesis of, 317
prevention of, 318
treatment of, 318
Calmette, 83
Campylobacter, 166
classification of, 155
clinical disease in, 155–156
epidemiology of, 155
general properties, 155, 155*t*
laboratory diagnosis of, 156
treatment of, 156
Campylobacteriaceae, 141
Candida albicans, 475, 535Q, 548E
Candida as cause of urinary tract infections, 450
Candidemia, 347, 348
Candidiasis, 474
clinical disease in, 347
diagnosis of, 347–348, 476
epidemiology of, 347
treatment of, 348, 477
Capillaria hepatica, 394
Capillaria philippinensis, 394
Capnophilic bacteria, 12
Capsid proteins, 205, 214, 217, 543Q, 553E
Capsomeres, 207
Capsular polysaccharide, 133–134
Capsules, 3, 65, 126
alginate, 161
antiphagocytic, 79
hyaluronic, 107
polysaccharide, 110–111
Captain's wheel, 354
Carbapenems, 47
Carbenicillin, 46
Carbohydrates, 12
utilization of, 19
Carbon in bacterial physiology, 12
Carboxypeptidases, 46
Carbuncles, 103
Carcinoma
cervical, 285
hepatocellular, 326, 486
nasopharyngeal, 254, 255, 281
Cardiohepatic toxin, 107
Cardiolipin, laboratory diagnosis of, 178
Carditis, 541Q, 552–553E
Carrión's disease, 201
Catabolite repression, 38
Catalase, 13
Catalase positivity, 544Q, 554E
Cationic agents, 61
Cat-scratch disease, 201–202
CD8 suppressor cells, activation of, 78
Ceepryn chloride, 61
Cefaclor, 46
Cefazolin, 46
Cefixime, 132

Cefotaxime, 46, 132
Cefoxitin, 46
Ceftriaxone, 46, 128, 132
Cefuroxime, 46
Cell cultures, 271
 detecting viral growth in, 271–272
 tests, 67
Cell membrane, 7
Cell transformation, role in, 258
Cell tropism, 243
Cell wall, 7, *8*
 modification of permeability, 56–57
 removal of, 9
 teichoic acid, 101
Cell-mediated immunity (CMI), 76–78, *77*
 immunocompetent cells, 264
 inhibition of, 185
 viral interaction with immunocompetent cells, 264–265
Cells lacking MHC-I antigens, infection of, 266
Cell-to-cell spread, 116
Cellulitis, 108, 118, 134
Central nervous system (CNS) infections, 353
Cephalexin, 46
Cephalic tetanus, 121
Cephalosporins
 chemistry of, 46
 classification of, 46–47
 for pneumonia, 421, 423
 for prostatitis, 453
 for *Staphylococci* infections, 105
 for *Streptococci* infections, 109
 third-generation, 112, 135
 for urinary tract infection, 452
Cephalothin, 46
Cerebral toxoplasmosis, 438
Cerebrospinal fluid (CSF)
 examination of, 127
 findings in diagnosing meningitis, 432, 432*t*
Cervical carcinoma, papillomaviruses as cause of, 285
Cervicitis, 130
 mucopurulent, 196–197
Cestodes (tapeworms), 363
 Diphyllobothrium latum, 399
 Dipylidium caninum, 401
 Echinococcus granulosus, 401–402
 Echinococcus multilocularis, 401–402
 Hymenolepis diminuta, 399–400
 Hymenolepis nana, 399–400
 Taenia saginata, 400–401
 Taenia solium, 400–401
 treatment of infection, 369
Chagas' disease, 380
Chancre, 175
Chancroid, 136
Chemical antimicrobial agents, 61–62
Chemical mutagenesis, 23
Chemoprophylaxis, 128, 136
Chickenpox (varicella), 84
 clinical manifestations, 494
 complications, 494
 immunity, 494
 prevention of, 494
 treatment of, 494
 varicella-zoster virus as cause of, 279–280
 Chlamydia trachomatis, 474
 Chlamydiae, 193–194, 194*t*
  Chlamydiae pneumoniae, 195
  Chlamydiae psittaci, 194–195
  Chlamydiae trachomatis, 195
   clinical disease in, 195–197
   control and prevention of, 198
   epidemiology of, 197
   laboratory diagnosis of, 197
   serotypes, 195
   treatment of, 197–198
Chloramphenicol
 Francisella tularensis in, 166
 impact on protein synthesis, 11, 50
 for *Neisseria* infections, 128
Chloramphenicol acetyltransferase, 56
Chloroquine
 for malaria, 367
 for *Plasmodium* species, 384
Chocolate agar, 94, 125, 133
Cholera toxin, 67, 538Q, 550E
Chorea, 109
Chromatographic analysis in identification of mycobacteria, 168
Chromomycoses, 344–345
Chromosomes and bacterial genetics, 21
Chronic fatigue syndrome
 Epstein-Barr virus as cause of, 281
 human herpesvirus-6 virus as cause of, 283
Ciliates, *Balantidium coli,* 381–382
Ciliophora, 363
Ciprofloxacin, 537Q, 550E
 for *Bartonella,* 202
 impact of, on nucleic acid synthesis, 48
 for *Neisseria* infections, 128, 132
 for *Salmonella,* 150
Circulatory collapse, 410
Cirrhosis, 326, 482
 association between hepatocellular carcinoma and, 486
 complications of, 487
Citrobacter, 160
Clarithromycin
 impact of, on protein synthesis, 51
 for legionnaire's disease, 187
 for uncomplicated genital infection, 112
Clavulanic acid, 46
Clindamycin
 for *Babesia* species, 385
 for *Bacillus* infection, 124
 for *Cryptosporidium parvum,* 387
 for *Plasmodium* species, 384
 for *Pneumocystis carinii* infections, 368
 and protein synthesis, 51
 for *Staphylococcal* infections, 105
 for *Toxoplasma gondii,* 386
Clofazimine in treating leprosy, 174
Clonorchis species, 404–405
Clostridial bacteremia, 414
Clostridium
 Clostridium botulinum
  determinants of pathogenicity, 120
  diagnosis of, 121
  epidemiology of, 121
  pathogenesis of and clinical disease in, 120–121
  treatment of, 121
 Clostridium difficile
  determinants of pathogenicity, 119
  diagnosis of, 120
  epidemiology of, 119–120
  pathogenesis of and clinical disease in, 119
  treatment of, 120
 Clostridium perfringens
  determinants of pathogenicity, 118
  diagnosis of, 119
  pathogenesis of and clinical disease in, 118–119
  treatment of, 119
 Clostridium tetani
  clinical disease in, 121–122
  control and prevention of, 122
  determinants of pathogenicity, 121
  epidemiology of, 122
  pathogenesis of, 121
  treatment of, 122, 123*t*
Clostridium botulinum, 468
Clostridium difficile, 468
Clostridium difficile diarrhea, 119
Clostridium perfringens type C toxoid, 85
Clostridium species, 468
Clostridium tetani, 468
Clotrimazole
 for *Acanthamoeba* infections, 374
 for candidiasis, 348
 for cutaneous mycoses, 344
CMV chorioretinitis, prevention of, 513
Coagulase, 19
Coagulase test, 105
Coccidioidal meningitis, 437
Coccidioidomycosis
 clinical disease in, 353
 diagnosis of, 353–354
 epidemiology of, 352
 intraocular, 353
 life cycle of, 352–353
 pulmonary, 353
Colitis, pseudomembranous (necrotizing), 119
Colonization factor antigens (CFAs), 66, 143–144
Colorado tick fever virus, 320
Commensal organisms, 3
Common cold, 289, 296, 297, 309
Community perspective, viral diseases from, 242
Complement fixation tests, 96, 273
 in diagnosing blastomycosis, 350, 352, 353
 in diagnosing coccidioidomycosis, 353
 in diagnosing histoplasmosis, 352
 in diagnosing *Rickettsia rickettsii,* 201
Complement-fixing antibodies, 263
Complement-mediated lysis, 74
Component vaccines, 84–85
Conditioned lethal mutants, 225–226
Condylomata acuminata (genital warts), 474, 476
Confluent lesions, 490
Congenital cytomegalovirus (CMV) infection, 265
Congenital infections, 241
Congenital rubella, 302
Congenital syphilis, 479
Congenital transmission
 for cytomegalovirus, 282
 perinatal, 278–279
Conjugate vaccines, 128
Conjugation, 28, 30–31
Conjugative plasmids, 21
Conjunctivitis, 290, 311
 neonatal, 478
Contagious pustular dermatitis (orf), 291
Corneal blindness as complication from herpes simplex virus, 278
Coronaviruses
 clinical disease in, 317
 diagnosis of, 317

epidemiology of, 317
general properties, 317
pathogenesis of, 317
prevention of, 317
therapy, 317
Corticosteroids
for meningitis, 436
for *Taenia* infections, 401
for *Toxocara canis,* 398
for *Trichinella* species, 394
Corynebacterium as cause of urinary tract infections, 450
Corynebacterium diphtheriae
clinical presentation, 115
control and prevention of, 116
determinants of pathogenicity, 113–114
diagnosis of, 115
epidemiology of, 115
general characteristics of, 113
pathogenesis of, 114–115
treatment of, 115–116
Coryza, 311
Coulter counter, 16
Cowpox, 291
Coxiella burnetii, 199–200
Coxsackieviruses, 243
classification of, 296
clinical disease in, 296
general characteristics of, 296
prevention of, 296
treatment of, 296
Craniofacial alterations in congenital syphilis, 177
Creutzfeldt-Jakob disease, 445–446, 446*t*
Crosslinking, 16
Cross-reactive antibodies, 76
Cross-reactive immune reaction, 490
Cryptococcal meningitis, 348, 436–437
Cryptococcosis
clinical disease in, 348
determinants of pathogenicity, 348
diagnosis of, 348–349
epidemiology of, 348
treatment of, 349
Cryptococcus neoformans, 348
Cryptosporidium parvum, 387
Crystal violet, 18
Cutaneous anthrax, 123
Cutaneous infections, 348
Cutaneous leishmaniasis, 378
Cutaneous mycoses
dermatophytoses, 343–344
tinea versicolor, 344
Cutaneous route, 241
Cycloserine, 47
Cysticercosis, 400
Cystitis, 451
hemorrhagic, 290
Cytokine therapy for *Leishmania* species, 378
Cytomegalovirus (CMV)
clinical disease in, 281–282
diagnosis of, 282
and meningitis, 435
pathogenesis of, 281
transmission of, 282
treatment of, 282
Cytoplasmic components, 11
Cytoplasmic membrane, 7
antigens, 107
Cytotoxic T lymphocytes, 264
Cytotoxins, 67

D

D-alanyl carboxypeptidase, 16
Dane particle, 324
Dapsone
for human immunodeficiency virus, 513
for leprosy, 174
Darkfield examination, 91
Deep organ, 103
Defective interfering (DI) particles, 229–231, 246
Defective oncoviruses, 257
Defective virus particles, 226
Degenerative brain diseases, 441–442
caused by unconventional agents, 445–447
progressive multifocal leukoencephalopathy, 443–444, 443*t*
retroviral, of central nervous system, 444–445
AIDS-associated dementia, 445
progressive spastic paraparesis, 444–445
subacute sclerosing panencephalitis, 442–443
unconventional agents in, 445–447
Degenerative retroviral diseases of central nervous system
AIDS-associated dementia, 445
progressive spastic paraparesis, 444–445
Deletion mutants, 226
Dematiaceous fungi, 345
Denaturing agents, 61–62
Dengue fever, 299–300, 301
Dental caries, 110
Dermatophytoses, 343–344
Desferrioxamine for *Plasmodium* species, 384
Deuteromycetes, 335
Dexamethasone for meningitis, 433
Diabetes, 357
Diarrhea, 145, 290, 456, 534Q, 548E
antibiotic-associated, 119
bloody, 457, 463, 533Q, 547E
infantile, 296
parasitic, 461, 462*t*
profuse secretory, 456
traveler's, 145
viral, 460–461, 461*t*
Didanosine (dideoxyinosine) (ddI), 238
for human immunodeficiency virus, 512
Dientamoeba fragilis, 376
Diethylcarbamazine citrate (DEC)
for *Ancylostoma* infections, 398
for *Loa loa,* 397
for nematode infections, 369
for *Toxocara canis,* 398
for *Wuchereria bancrofti,* 396
Dimorphic fungi infections, 335
blastomycosis
clinical disease in, 350
diagnosis of, 350–351
epidemiology of, 349
treatment of, 351
coccidioidomycosis
clinical disease in, 353
diagnosis of, 353–354
epidemiology of, 352
life cycle, 352–353
histoplasmosis
clinical disease in, 351
diagnosis of, 351–352
epidemiology of, 351
immunity, 351
pathogenesis of, 351
paracoccidioidomycosis
clinical disease in, 354
diagnosis of, 354
epidemiology of, 354
pathogenesis of, 354
treatment of, 354
sporotrichosis, 354
clinical disease in, 355
diagnosis of, 355
epidemiology of, 355
pathogenesis of, 355
treatment of, 355
Diphtheria
anterior nasal, 115
pharyngeal, 115
tonsillar, 115
Diphtheria antitoxin, 116
Diphtheria toxin, 67
Diphtheria toxoids, 85
Diphtheria-pertussis-tetanus (DPT) vaccine, 116
Diphyllobothriasis, 399
Diphyllobothrium latum, 399
Diploid cultures, 271
Dipylidium caninum, 401
Direct cell-to-cell propagation, 79, 266
Direct contact with vesicular discharge in transmission of herpes simplex virus, 278
Direct immunofluorescence
in diagnosing bacterial infections, 91
in diagnosing *Bordetella pertussis,* 139
in diagnosing *Chlamydiae trachomatis,* 197
in diagnosing *Haemophilus influenzae,* 133
in diagnosing *Rickettsiaceae,* 201
in diagnosing viral infections, 272–273, 274
Discrete lesions, 490
Disinfectants, 61
high-level, 61
low-level, 61
Disseminated disease, 351
Disseminated endothelial damage, 184
Disseminated infection, 131
Disseminated intravascular coagulation (DIC), 299, 410
development of, 413
Disseminated (miliary) tuberculosis, 170
DNA, 11
DNA hybridization, 274–275
DNA polymerase, agents that inhibit, 234
DNA polymerase I, 25
DNA synthesis, 541Q, 552E
DNA transfer between bacteria, 28, *29*
conjugation, 28, 30–31
transformation, 31–32
DNA tumor viruses, 251, 542Q, 553E
adenoviruses
degree of tumorigenicity of adenovirus-transformed cells, 254
mechanism of transformation in, 254
oncogenic potential of, 254
hepatitis B
mechanism of transformation in, 256
oncogenic potential of, 255–256

herpesviruses
mechanism of transformation in Epstein-Barr virus-related malignancies, 255
oncologic potential, 254
papillomaviruses
mechanism of transformation in, 254
oncogenic potential of, 253–254
polyoma, and simian virus 40 (SV40)
conditions that may contribute to transformation, 252–253
mechanism of transformation in, 253
oncogenic potential of, 252
DNA tumor viruses and retroviruses, 251
characteristics of transformed cells, 251–252
identifying viral oncogenic behavior, 252
DNA vaccines, 86
DNA viruses, 208, 212–214, *213,* 225, 523*t,* 537Q, 549E
recombination between, 226–227, *227*
replication cycle of major human
adenoviruses, 217–218
hepatitis B virus (HBV), 219
herpesvirus, *213,* 218
papovaviruses, 216–217, *217*
poxviruses, 218–219
DNA viruses I
cytomegalovirus (CMV), 281–283
Epstein-Barr virus, 280–281
herpes simplex virus (HSV), 277–279
varicella-zoster virus, 279–280
DNA viruses II
adenoviruses, 289–290
papillomaviruses, 285–286, 286*t*
parvoviruses, 291–292
polyomaviruses, 286–287
poxviruses, 290–291
DNA-dependent RNA polymerase, 542Q, 553E
Doxycycline
for *Bartonella,* 202
for *Chlamydia trachomatis,* 132
for *Chlamydiae trachomatis,* 198
for *Pneumocystis carinii* infections, 368
for *Rickettsiae rickettsii,* 201
Drug class, bacterial resistance according to, 57, 57*t*
Drug-resistant mutants, 226
Duponol LS, 61
Dynamic theory, 277
Dysentery, 456

E

Ear infections, *Pseudomonas* in, 162
Early proteins, 212
EBNA-2, 255
EBNA-5, 255
Ebola virus, 318, 318*t*
Ecchymosis, 490
Echinococcosis (hydatid disease), 401–402
Echinococcus granulosus, 401–402
Echinococcus multilocularis, 401–402
Echoviruses, 243
clinical disease in, 297
treatment of, 297
Eczema herpeticum as complication from herpes simplex virus, 278
Eflornithine
for *Trypanosoma* species, 380
for trypanosomiasis, 366
Ehrlichia chaffeensis, 200, 545Q, 555E
Ehrlichiosis, 200
Electron acceptors in bacterial physiology, 12
Electron donors in bacterial physiology, 12
Electron transport, 57
Elek's test, 115
Elephantiasis, 395
Empiric therapy, 135
Enanthem, 490
Encephalitis, 429
acute, 491
as complication of measles, 491
as complication from herpes simplex virus, 278
as complication in mumps, 310
distribution of, 301
and echoviruses, 297
and herpes, 236
incidence of, 301
mortality rates from, 301
and poliovirus infection, 294
postinfectious, 302, 312
primary viral, 249
secondary viral, 249
transmission of, 301
viral, 439
Encephalitis syndrome, 301
Encephalopathy, 487
Endarteritis, 175
Endocarditis, 117, 347
acute, 103
Endonucleases, 208
Endotoxins, 3, 68, 70
and *Bordetella pertussis,* 137
and Enterobacteriaceae, 143
and *Neisseria gonorrhoeae,* 129
Entamoeba coli, 374
Entamoeba gingivalis, 374
Entamoeba hartmanni, 374
Entamoeba histolytica, 371, 373, 545Q, 555E
Entamoeba nana, 374
Enteritis necroticans, 118
Enterobacter, 159
Enterobacteriaceae, 141, 141*t*
as cause of urinary tract infections, 450
Citrobacter, 160
Enterobacter, 159
Escherichia coli, 160
control and prevention of, 146–147
determinants of pathogenicity, 144–145
diagnosis of, 145–146
epidemiology of, 145
general properties, 144, 144*t*
pathogenesis of and clinical disease in, 145
treatment of, 146
general properties
classification of, 141
determinants of pathogenicity, 142–144
features, 141, 142*t*
genetic exchange, 141–142
virulence factors, 143–144
Klebsiella, 159, 160*t*
Morganella, 160
Proteus, 160, 160*t*
Providencia, 160
Salmonella
classification of, 148
clinical disease in, 149
control and prevention of, 151
determinants of pathogenicity, 149
epidemiology of, 149–150
general properties, 148, 148*t*
laboratory diagnosis of, 150
pathogenesis of, 149
treatment of, 150–151
Serratia, 159
Shigella
clinical disease in, 147
control and prevention of, 148
determinants of pathogenicity, 147, 147*t*
epidemiology of, 147–148
general properties, 147
laboratory diagnosis of, 148
pathogenesis of, 147
treatment of, 148
Enterobius vermicularis, 389–390
Enterocolitis (salmonellosis), 149, 456
Enterohemorrhagic (verotoxin-producing), 144
Enteropathogenic *Escherichia coli,* 145
Enterotoxin-coding plasmids, 35
Enterotoxins, 67, 102, 118, 144
Enterovirus type 70, 297
Enterovirus type 72, 297
Enteroviruses, 243, 293, 538Q, 550E
Entner-Doudoroff pathway, 13
Envelope glycoproteins, 256
Envelope proteins, 214
Enveloped viruses, 214, 216
Enzyme immunoassay (EIA)
in detecting pathogen-specific macromolecules, 92
in diagnosing *Bordetella pertussis,* 139
in diagnosing *Chlamydiae trachomatis,* 197
in diagnosing hepatitis C, 330
Enzyme-deficient mutants, 226
Enzyme-linked immunosorbent assay (ELISA) to screen for human immunodeficiency virus infection, 510–511
Enzymes, 208
production of, 19
Enzymoimmunoassays, 273
Eosinophilia, tropical pulmonary, 395
Epidemic diarrhea, *Klebsiella* in, 159
Epidemic keratoconjunctivitis, 290
Epidemic typhus, 199
Epidemics, periodicity of, 242
Epidermodysplasia verruciformis, papillomaviruses as cause of, 285–286
Epidermophyton floccosum, 343
Epididymitis, 196
Epididymoorchitis as complication in mumps, 310
Epiglottitis, acute bacterial, 134
Epithelial cell necrosis, 490
Epstein-Barr nuclear antigen-1 (EBNA-1), 255
Epstein-Barr virus, 254
chronic
clinical disease in, 280–281
diagnosis of, 281
pathogenesis of, 280
transmission of, 281
treatment of, 281
clinical disease in, 280–281
diagnosis of, 281
pathogenesis of, 280
transmission of, 281
treatment of, 281

Epstein-Barr virus-related malignancies, mechanism of transformation in in, 255
Ergosterol, 336
Erysipelas, 108
Erythema infectiosum (fifth disease), 292
 clinical manifestations, 493
 complications, 493
 incubation period, 492–493
Erythema migrans in Lyme disease, 181–182
Erythema multiforme (erythema multiforme minor), 497
Erythema nodosum, 109
Erythematous, 493
Erythematous maculopapular exanthem, 492
Erythrogenic toxins, 107
Erythromycin
 for *Borrelia,* 181
 for *Chlamydiae trachomatis,* 197
 for *Giardia lamblia,* 376
 impact of, on protein synthesis, 51
 for legionnaires' disease, 187
 for pneumonia, 423
 for staphylococcal toxin diseases, 105, 109
 for streptococci infections, 109
Escherichia coli, 160, 543Q, 544Q, 553E, 554E
 in bacteremic infections, 412
 in urinary tract infections, 450
Escherichia coli bacteremia, 539Q, 551E
Esophageal candidiasis, 348
Ethanol, 61
Ethylene oxide, 62
Ethylene oxide gas sterilization, 540Q, 552E
Eukaryotes, 4*t,* 5
Exanthem, 490
 nonspecific febrile illness with, 493
Exfoliatins, 102
Exoantigen test, 350
Exoenzymes, 3, 66
Exonuclease, 25
Exotoxin A, 107
Exotoxin B, 107, 108
Exotoxins, 3, 68*t*
 and *Clostridium perfringens,* 118
 and Enterobacteriaceae, 143
 functional classification of, 67
 genetics in, 67
 and group A streptococci, 107
 identification of, 67–68
 pyrogenic, 101–102
 structure of, 67
Extended-spectrum penicillins, 46

F

Factor V, 133
Factor X, 133
Facultative anaerobes, 12
Facultative bacteria, 19
Failure to thrive, 510
Famciclovir, 237
 for herpes simplex virus, 279
Fansidar (sulfadoxine-pyrimethamine)
 for malaria, 367
 for *Plasmodium* species, 384
Fasciola gigantica, 405
Fasciola hepatica, 405
Fasciolopsis buskii, 406
Fc receptors, 211
Fecal-oral route, 241
Fermentation, 12
Fermentative metabolism, 13
Ferriprotoporphyrin for malaria, 367
Fifth disease. (*See* Erythema infectiosum (fifth disease))
Filamentous fungi, 335
Filoviruses
 clinical disease in, 318
 epidemiology of, 318
 general properties, 318
 pathogenesis of, 318
Filtration, 63
Fimbrial antigens, 143
5-Fluorocytosine (5-FC)
 in antifungal therapy, 342
 for cryptococcosis, 349
 for meningitis, 438
Flaccid paralysis, 545Q, 555E
Flagella, 11
Flagellates
 Dientamoeba fragilis, 376
 Giardia lamblia, 374–376
 Leishmania species, 377–379
 Trichomonas species, 376–377
 Trypanosoma species, 379–381
Flatworms (flukes). (*See* Trematodes (flatworms, flukes))
Flaviviruses, 299
Flocculation tests, 96
Fluconazole
 for candidiasis, 348
 for meningitis, 438
Flukes. (*See* Trematodes (flatworms, flukes))
Flu-like syndrome, 300
Fluorescent treponemal antibody absorption test (FTA-ABS), 96
 in diagnosing syphilis, 178
Fluoroquinolones, 48
 for *Mycoplasmataceae hominis,* 189
 for prostatitis, 453
 for uncomplicated genital infections, 132
 for *Urealyticum,* 189
 for urinary tract infection, 452
Folinic acid for *Toxoplasma gondii,* 386
Follicular keratitis, 195–197
Folliculitis, 103
Food, contamination of, 104
Food poisoning, 459–460
 for *Bacillus* infections, 124
 clinical manifestations of, 460
 Clostridium botulinum in, 120, 121
 Clostridium perfringens in, 118–119
 diagnosis of, 460
 staphylococcal, 104
 treatment of, 460
 Vibrio parahaemolyticus in, 154
Food-borne transmission, 145
Foscarnet
 clinical uses of, 238
 for cytomegalovirus, 282
 for human immunodeficiency virus, 513
 mechanisms of action of, 238
Frameshift mutations, 23, *24*
Francisella tularensis, 166
Fructose-6-phosphate dehydrogenase, 13
Fulminant hepatic failure, 482
Fungal disease. (*See also* Antifungal therapy)
 diagnosis of, 339–340
Fungal meningitis, 436–438
Fungi, 5, 526–527*t*
 dematiaceous, 345
Furazolidone for *Giardia lamblia,* 376
Furuncles, 103
Fusion proteins, 246
Fusobacterium necrophorum, 465–466
Fusobacterium nucleatum, 465–466, 468

G

Gallbladder, surgical removal of, 151
Gambian sleeping sickness, 379–380
Ganciclovir
 administration of, 237
 clinical uses of, 237
 for cytomegalovirus, 282
 for human immunodeficiency virus, 513
 for pneumonia, 425
 resistance to, 239
Gangrene, 127
Gardnerella vaginalis, 475
Gardnerella vaginalis vaginitis, 476
Gas gangrene (myonecrosis), 118, 119
Gastroenteritis, 455, 463
 Campylobacter in, 155
 clinical presentation, 456
 definitions, 456
 diagnosis of, 457–458, 458*t*
 epidemiology of, 456
 pathogenesis of bacterial diarrhea, 457
 prevalence, 456
 treatment of, 459
 Yersinia enterocolitica in, 165
Gastrointestinal anthrax, 123
Gastrointestinal tract, normal flora in, 100
Generalized tetanus, 121
Genetic basis of bacterial pathogenicity
 transmission of virulence genes among bacteria, 35
 virulence factors, 34
Genetic factors, effect of, on outcome of viral infection, 243
Genetic homology, 141
Genetic variation, role of, in evolution of viruses, 231
Genital herpes, 474
 herpes simplex virus as cause of, 278
Genital warts, 544Q, 554E
 papillomaviruses as cause of, 285
Genomic integration, 266
Germ theory of disease, 4
Gerstmann-Sträussler disease, 445
Giant cell pneumonia, 311
Giant multinucleated cells, 246
Giardia lamblia, 374–376, 534Q, 548E
Giardiasis, treatment of, 365–366
Gigantobilharzia, 404
Ginghausu for *Plasmodium* species, 384
Glomerulonephritis, acute poststreptococcal, 109
Glutamate family, 14
Glutaraldehyde, 62
Glutathione-S-transferase, 533Q, 547E
Glycolytic (Embden-Meyerhof) pathway, 13
Glycoprotein oligosaccharides, increased content of, 252
Gonococcal pelvic inflammatory disease, 132

Gonorrhea, 473, 475, 476, 477
anorectal, 130–131
pharyngeal, 131
gp120, immunodominant domain of, 231
Gram negative rods I. *(See Haemophilus)*
Gram staining, 18
Gram-negative bacteria, 7–8, 9, *10,* 18, 54
Gram-negative cocci. *(See Moraxella; Neisseria)*
Gram-negative rods II. (*See* Opportunistic bacteria; Zoonotic bacteria)
Gram-positive bacteria, 7, 9, 18, 54, 56
Gram-positive cocci. *(See Staphylococci; Streptococci)*
Gram-positive rods. *(See Bacillus; Clostridium; Corynebacterium diphtheriae; Listeria monocytogenes)*
Granulomatous cervical lymphadenitis, 172
Granulomatous ulcers, 371
Gray baby syndrome, 50
Griseofulvin
in antifungal therapy, 341
for cutaneous mycoses, 344
Group A streptococci, 538Q, 544Q, 550E, 554E
Group antigens, 256
Group D streptococci as cause of urinary tract infections, 450
Growth cycles, 17
Growth factor activity, 258
Guarnieri bodies, 248, 291
Guérin, 83
Guillain-Barré syndrome, 155
as complication of hypersensitivity reactions, 307

H

H antigens, 142–143
Haemophilus aegyptius, 136
Haemophilus ducreyi, 136
Haemophilus influenzae, 133, 134*t,* 422, 538, 550E
classification of, 133
clinical disease in, 134–135, 134*t*
determinants of pathogenicity, 133–134
epidemiology of, 135
general properties, 133
immunity, 135
laboratory diagnosis of, 135
pathogenesis of, 134
prophylaxis, 135–136
treatment of, 135
Haemophilus parainfluenzae, 136
Haemophilus influenzae meningitis, 50
Halofantrine for *Plasmodium* species, 384
Halophilic bacteria, 12
Hand-foot-and-mouth disease, 296
Hand-foot-and-mouth syndrome
clinical manifestations, 495
incubation period, 495
treatment of, 495
Hantaan virus, 319
Hantaviruses, 242
Heat-labile toxins, 67, 144
Heat-stable toxin (ST), 67, 144
Heavy metals, 62
Helical nucleocapsids, 207
Helicobacter
classification of, 155
clinical disease in, 155–156
epidemiology of, 155
general properties, 155, 155*t*
laboratory diagnosis of, 156
treatment of, 156
Helicobacter pylori, 100
clinical disease in, 156
determinants of pathogenicity, 156
diagnosis of, 156–157
general properties, 156, 156*t*
treatment of, 157
Helix distortion mutations, 23
Helminths, 363
Helper T cells, depletion of, 265
Helper T lymphocytes, 264
Hemadsorption, 271–272
Hemadsorption inhibition, 272
Hemagglutination, 272
Hemagglutination inhibition, 273
Hematogenous dissemination, 410
α-Hemolysin, 102
Hemolysins, 19, 102, 161
α-Hemolytic streptococci, 106
β-Hemolytic streptococci, 106
γ-Hemolytic streptococci, 106
Hemolytic-uremic syndrome, 145, 147, 457, 545Q, 555E
Hemorrhagic colitis, 145
Hemorrhagic cystitis, 290
Hemorrhagic diathesis, 302
Hemorrhagic fever, 319
Hemorrhagic syndrome, 300
Hepatic amebiasis, 373
Hepatis, peliosis, 202
Hepatitis. (*See also* Viral hepatitis)
acute, 482
chronic, 482
as complication in mumps, 310
Hepatitis A virus (HAV), 297, 324*t,* 482*t,* 483
clinical disease in, 323
diagnosis of, 483
epidemiology of, 323
immunity, 324
laboratory diagnosis of, 323–324
prevention of, 324
treatment of, 324
vaccination for, 484
Hepatitis B surface antigen (HBsAg), 85, 541Q, 552E
Hepatitis B vaccine, 85, 539Q, 551E
Hepatitis B virus (HBV), 219, 324, 324*t,* 482*t,* 483, 534Q, 547E
carriers of, 265
classification of, 325
clinical disease in, 325–326
diagnosis of, 326–327, 327*t, 328,* 483
epidemiology of, 325
etiology for, 486
general properties, 324–325
infection, 265
oncogenic potential of, 255–256
pathogenesis of, 325, 486
prevention of, 327, 329
serologic tests, 487
vaccination for, 484
Hepatitis C virus (HCV), 324*t,* 329, 482*t,* 483
clinical presentation, 329
diagnosis of, 483
epidemiology of, 329
etiology for, 486
general properties, 329
laboratory diagnosis of and screening, 330
pathogenesis of, 486
prevention of, 330
serologic tests, 487
treatment of, 330
vaccination for, 484
Hepatitis D virus (HDV), 324*t,* 330, 482*t,* 483, 537Q, 549E
clinical disease in, 331
diagnosis of, 483
epidemiology of, 330
etiology for, 486
general properties, 330
laboratory diagnosis of, 331
pathogenesis of, 331, 486
prevention of, 331
Hepatitis E virus (HEV), 482*t,* 483
classification of, 331
clinical disease in, 331
diagnosis of, 332, 483
epidemiology of, 331
general properties, 331
pathogenesis of, 331
treatment of, 332
Hepatocellular carcinoma, 326
association between cirrhosis and, 486
Hepatomegaly, 184
Hepatosplenomegaly, 302
in congenital syphilis, 177
Hepatotoxic drug, 487
Herd immunity, 242
Herpangina, 296
clinical manifestations, 495
complications, 495
differential diagnosis of, 495
incubation period, 495
treatment of, 495
Herpes, neonatal, 479
Herpes encephalitis, 236, 279
Herpes simplex virus (HSV), 544Q, 554E
clinical disease in, 277–278
diagnosis of, 279
and meningitis, 435
pathogenesis of, 277
transmission of, 278–279
treatment of, 279, 477
and vaginal discharge, 475
Herpes virus infections, 87
Herpes zoster. (*See* Shingles (herpes zoster))
Herpesviruses, *213,* 218, 278*t*
cytomegalovirus (CMV), 281–283
Epstein-Barr virus, 280–281
herpes simplex virus (HSV), 277–279
mechanism of transformation in Epstein-Barr virus-related malignancies, 255
oncologic potential, 254
varicella-zoster virus, 279–280
Herpetic gingivostomatitis
clinical manifestations, 495–496
complications, 496
herpes simplex virus as cause of, 277–278
treatment of, 496
Heterobilharzia, 404
Heteroploid cultures, 271
Heterotrophic bacteria, 12
Heterotrophs, 12
Hexachlorophene, 61
Hfr conjugation, 28

High-frequency recombinant (Hfr) bacterium, 537Q, 550E
High-frequency recombinant (Hfr) cells, 28, *30*
High-frequency recombinant (Hfr) conjugation, 31
Histidine, 14
Histoplasmosis
clinical disease in, 351
diagnosis of, 351–352
epidemiology of, 351
immunity, 351
pathogenesis of, 351
HIV vaccines, 84
HIV-1 infection, 501, 533Q, 547E
HIV-2 infection, 501
Homogeny, 31
Homolactic fermentation, 13
Homology, genetic, 141
Honeymoon cystitis, 145
Hookworms. *(See Ascaris lumbricoides)*
Host defenses, 3
Host-dependent mutants, 225
Host-range mutants, 226
Hot mutants, 226
HSV encephalitis, 439
HTLV-1, 259–260
HTLV-2, 259–260
Human diploid cell vaccine (HDCV), 316
Human herpesvirus-6 (HHV-6, HBLV)
clinical disease in, 283
epidemiology of, 283
Human immunodeficiency virus (HIV), 86, 87, 544Q, 554E
clinical stages of, 508–510
diagnosis of, 510–511
enzymes, 503
epidemiology of, 503–504
genome, 502, *502*
immunoprophylaxis, 514–515
pathogenesis of
asymptomatic stage, 505
early viremic stage, 504–505
escape from immune response, 507–508
immunosuppression, 505–507
infected cell populations, 504
structural proteins, 502–503
treatment of, 511–513
Human papillomavirus type 6, 544Q, 554E
Human rabies immune globulin (HRIG), 316
Humoral immunity, 135
Hutchinson's triad in congenital syphilis, 177
Hyaluronic capsule, 107
Hydrogen peroxide, 62
Hydronephrosis, 403
Hydrops fetalis, 292
Hymenolepis diminuta, 399–400
Hymenolepis nana, 399–400
Hyperbilirubinemia in congenital syphilis, 177
Hypotension, 127

I

Icosahedral nucleocapsids, 207
Icteric infection, 326
Icteric leptospirosis (Weil's syndrome), 184
Idoxuridine (IDU), 236
IgA, 75
IgA proteases, 126, 129
IgG antibodies, 75
IgM antibodies, 75
Ileal loop test, 67
Imidazoles, 340–341
Imipenem, 47
Immortalization, 251
Immune effector mechanisms, inhibition of, 267
Immune reaction, 490
cross-reactive, 490
Immune response
determination of, 78
evasion of, 78–81, 78*t*, 266
impaired, 111
interference with, 81
Immune system and viruses, 263–266
Immunity
humoral, 135
natural, 3
Immunization
active, 83
mass, 242
passive, 83
schedules, 86*t*, 87
Immunoassay, enzyme, 139
Immunocompetent cells, infection of, 265
Immunocompromised status, 98
Immunodiffusion assays, 96
Immunodiffusion precipitin test, in diagnosing blastomycosis, 350
Immunodiffusion test
in diagnosing coccidioidomycosis, 353
in diagnosing histoplasmosis, 352
in diagnosing paracoccidioidomycosis, 354
Immunodominant domain of gp120, 231
Immuno-electron microscopy, 273
Immunofluorescence, direct, 133, 139
Immunoprophylaxis, 65, 128, 135–136
history of, 83
Immunotherapeutic agents, vaccines as, 86–87
Impaired immune response, 111
Impetigo, 108
Inapparent infections, 242, 246
Inclusion bodies, 213, 248
Inclusion conjunctivitis, 197
India ink test, 349
Indinavir, 238
for human immunodeficiency virus, 512
Indirect fluorescence (EIA) in diagnosing *Rickettsia rickettsii,* 201
Indirect immunofluorescence tests, 96
Inducible operons, 37
Infant botulism, 120–121
Infantile diarrhea, 296
Infection
abortive, 244, 293
neonatal, 110
persistent, 244, 246, 246*t*, 289
temperate, 33
Infections
acute, 263
anaerobic
clinical manifestations, 469
diagnosis of, 469–470, 469*t*
epidemiology of, 466, 466*t*
etiology, 468–469
pathogenesis of, 466–468, 467*t*
treatment of, 470
chronic, 263
latent, 242, 246, 246*t*
nosocomial, 104, 119–120
parasitic
diagnosis of, 363–365
helminths, 363
protozoa, 363
treatment of
anthelmintic agents, 368–369
antiprotozoal agents, 365–368
general principles, 365
Infectious mononucleosis, Epstein-Barr virus as cause of, 280–281
Influenza A pneumonia, 424–425
Influenza A virus, 539Q, 551E
Influenza vaccine, 84
Inoculation, 241
Inorganic ions in bacterial physiology, 12
Insect viruses, 85
Insertion sequences (IS elements), 21–22, *22*
Intercellular cell adhesion molecule-1 (ICAM-1), 540Q, 552E
Interferon-α (IFN-α), 73, 233, 234, 327
for hepatitis B, 487
for hepatitis C, 487
Interferon-β (IFN-β), 73, 233
Interferon-γ (IFN-γ), 73, 233, 234
Interferons
production of, 73
regulation of expression, 233
type I, 233
type II, 233–234
types of, 233
Interleukin-1 (IL-1), 73
Interleukin-2 (IL-2) receptor genes, 544Q, 554E
Interleukin-6 (IL-6), 73
Internalin, 116
Interstitial pneumonia, 248
Intestinal fluke. *(See Fasciolopsis buskii)*
Intestinal nematodes
Ancylostoma duodenale, 391–392
Anisakis marina, 394–395
Ascaris lumbricoides, 390–391
Capillaria hepatica, 394
Capillaria philippinensis, 394
Enterobius vermicularis, 389–390
Necator americanus, 391–392
Strongyloides stercoralis, 392
Trichinella species, 392–394
Trichuris trichiura, 390
Intestinal tract, anaerobic bacteria in, 466
Intracellular bacteria. (*See* Bartonellaceae; Chlamydiae; Rickettsiaceae)
Intracellular digestion, avoidance of, 79
Intracellular parasites, 205
Intraocular coccidioidomycosis, 353
Intravenous immunoglobulin (IVIg), 513
Invasion plasmid antigens (Ipa), 66
Invasiveness-coding plasmids, 35
Iodoquinol for amebiasis, trichomoniasis, and giardiasis, 365–366
Isoniazid, for mycobacterial infections, 169, 513
Isopropyl alcohol, 61
Isospora species, 387
Itraconazole
for meningitis, 438
for sporotrichosis, 355

Ivermectin
for *Brugia malayi,* 395–396
for nematode infections, 368–369
for *Onchocerca volvulus,* 396
for *Strongyloides stercoralis,* 392

J

Jarisch-Herxheimer reaction, 180
Jaundice, 482, 545Q, 554E
JC virus, 246, 252, 286–287, 544Q, 554E
Jenner, 83
Jock itch, 343
JV virus, 443–444

K

K antigens, 142
Kaposi's sarcoma, 254
Kaposi's varicelliform eruption as complication from herpes simplex virus, 278
Keratitis as complication from herpes simplex virus, 278
Keratoconjunctivitis, epidemic, 290
Ketoconazole
for blastomycosis, 351
for candidiasis, 348
for histoplasmosis, 352
for tinea versicolor, 344
Kidney stones, *Proteus* in, 160
Killed vaccine, for polio, 295
Killed vaccines, 84
Kirby-Bauer technique, 58–59
Kitasato, 83
Klebsiella, 159, 160*t*
Klebsiella pneumoniae, 422, 469
as cause of urinary tract infections, 450
Koch, Robert, 4
Koch postulates, 4
Koplik spots, 311, 491
Kuru, 445
Kynuon stain, 18

L

Laboratory diagnosis of
bacterial infections, 91
culture and isolation of microorganisms, 93–95
detection of pathogen-specific macromolecules, 92–93
microscopic examination of patient specimens, 91
serologic testing, 95–96
Klebsiella in, 159
serologic testing, 95–96
Lac operon (Lac-O), 37–38, 536Q, 548–549E
β-Lactam antibacterial agents, 43, 46–47
β-Lactamase inhibitors, 46
β-Lactamase tests, 59–60
β-Lactamases, 46, 54, 535Q, 548E
Lactate compound, 12
Lactation, transmission during, 241
Lactic acid, 542Q, 553E
Lactobacillic as cause of urinary tract infections, 450
Lady Montagu, 83
Lamivudine (2′-deoxy-3′-thiacytidine) (3TC), 238, 327
Lancefield system, 106
Large granular lymphocytes (K cells), 75
Large T antigen, 544Q, 554E
Large-cell pneumonia as complication from varicella-zoster virus, 280
Laryngeal warts, papillomaviruses as cause of, 285
Laryngotracheobronchitis (croup), 309
Lassa fever virus, 319
Late proteins, 213
Late syphilis, 478
Latent infections, 242, 246, 246*t*
Latex agglutination tests, 349, 352, 353
Legionella pneumophila, 185, 422, 545Q, 555E
Legionellaceae, 185
Legionellaceae pneumophila, 185, 186*t*
clinical disease in, 185–186
determinants of pathogenicity, 185
epidemiology of, 186
general properties, 185
laboratory diagnosis of, 186
prevention of, 187
treatment of, 186–187
other species, 187
Legionnaires' disease, 185–186
Leishmania species, 377–379
Leishmaniasis
cutaneous, 378
mucocutaneous, 378
treatment of, 366–367
visceral, 378
Lentivirus, 256
Lepromatous leprosy, *Mycobacterium leprae* in, 173
Leprosy, 87
lepromatous, 173
tuberculoid, 173
Leptospira, 183, 183*t*
clinical disease in, 183–184
epidemiology of, 184
general properties, 183
laboratory diagnosis of, 184
treatment of, 184
Leptospirosis, 183–184, 540Q, 552E
Leukemia, acute T cell, 259
Leukocidin, 102
LGV, 196
Ligases, 25, 208
Lincomycin, 51
Lincosamides, 51
Lipoligosaccharide, membrane, 133
Lipopolysaccharide (LPS), 8, *10,* 56, 68, 70, 126
Lipopolysaccharide (LPS) side chains, 66
Listeria monocytogenes
clinical disease in, 117
determinants of pathogenicity, 116–117
diagnosis of, 117
epidemiology of, 117
general characteristics of, 116, 116*t*
immunity, 117–118
pathogenesis of, 117
treatment of, 117
Listeriolysin, 116
Listeriosis, neonatal, 117
Litotrophic bacteria, 12
LMP-1, 255
LMP-2, 255
Lobar pneumonia, 420
Local tetanus, 121
Lodamoeba butschlii, 374
Loeffler agar, 113
Loeffler's syndrome, 390, 391–392
Lomefloxacin, 48
Long terminal repeats (LTRs), 257
Lower respiratory tract infections, 289–290
Lumbar puncture in diagnosing meningitis, 432
Lung fluke. *(See Paragonimus westermani)*
Lung infections, causes of, 420
Lyme disease, 181
epidemiology of, 182
laboratory diagnoses of, 182–183
treatment of, 183
Lymph node enlargement, 492
Lymphadenopathy in congenital syphilis, 177
Lymphoblastic leukemia, acute, 535Q, 548E
Lymphocytes, 264
Lysogeny, 35
Lysozyme, 7
Lytic infection, 289
Lytic life cycle, 33
Lytic viruses, 246

M

M protein, 66, 79, 106, 107, 540Q, 552E
MacConkey agar, 94
Macrolides
impact of, on protein synthesis, 51
for *Mycoplasmataceae hominis,* 189
for *Urealyticum,* 189
Macromolecule biosynthesis, 14–15
Macrophage membranes, virus receptors on, 264
Macrophages, 73, 533Q, 547E
activation of, 234
Macula, 490
Maculopapular rash, 492
acute viral disease with
atypical measles, 492
erythema infectiosum (fifth disease), 492–493
measles (rubeola), 491
roseola (exanthem subitum), 492
rubella (German measles), 492
Major histocompatibility complex-I (MHC-I) molecules, 244
Malaria, 81, 86
treatment of, 367
Malassezia furfur, 344
Malignant transformation, two-hit theory of, 260–261
Mannose receptors, 73
Mantoux test, 171
Marburg virus, 318, 318*t*
Mass immunization, 242
Mastoiditis, 108
Matrix proteins, 213
Measles (rubeola), 84, 309
as cause of subacute sclerosing panencephalitis (SSPE), 442–443
clinical disease in, 311–312
clinical manifestations, 491
complications, 491
diagnosis of, 312
epidemiology of, 312
prevention of, 312, 491
treatment of, 491
Measles (rubeola) pneumonia, 311, 425

Mebendazole
for *Ascaris lumbricoides,* 391
for *Capillaria philippinensis,* 394
for *Enterobius vermicularis,* 390
for *Necator americanus,* 392
for nematode infections, 368
for *Strongyloides stercoralis,* 392
for *Trichinella* species, 394
for *Trichuris trichiura,* 390
Medical helminthology, 389–406
Medical microbiology
historical significance, 4
interaction with host, 3
microorganisms, 3
Medical protozoology
amoebae
Acanthamoeba species, 373–374
Entamoeba coli, 374
Entamoeba gingivalis, 374
Entamoeba hartmanni, 374
Entamoeba histolytica, 371, *373*
Entamoeba nana, 374
Lodamoeba butschlii, 374
Naegleria fowleri, 374
ciliates, *Balantidium coli,* 381–382
flagellates
Dientamoeba fragilis, 376
Giardia lamblia, 374–376
Leishmania species, 377–379
Trichomonas species, 376–377
Trypanosoma species, 379–381
Pneumocystis carinii
clinical disease in, 388
epidemiology of, 387–388
laboratory diagnosis of, 388
treatment of and prevention of, 388
sporozoans
Babesia species, 385
Cryptosporidium parvum, 387
Isospora species, 387
Plasmodium species, 382–384
Toxoplasma gondii, 385–387
Medicine and retroviruses, 260
Mefloquine for *Plasmodium* species, 384
Melarsoprol
for *Trypanosoma* species, 380
for trypanosomiasis, 366
Membrane fusion, 211
Membrane lipoligosaccharide, 133
Membrane transport properties, changes in, 252
Membrane transport proteins, 56
Membrane-attack complex (MAC), 74
Membranous glomerulonephritis, 326
Meningitis
aseptic, 294, 296, 297, 429, 434, 434*t,* 435–438, 538Q, 550E
fungal, 436–438
parasitic meningoencephalitis, 438
tuberculous, 435–436
viral, 435
and *Bacillus anthracis,* 123
bacterial, 92, 429–430
clinical manifestations, 431–432
diagnosis of, 432–433
epidemiology of, 430–431, 430*t*
etiology, 430
pathogenesis of, 431
prevention of, 433–434
prognosis, 434
treatment of, 433, 433*t*
as complication from herpes simplex virus, 278
as complication from varicella-zoster virus, 280
as complication in mumps, 310
cryptococcal, 348
Group B streptococci in, 110
Haemophilus influenzae in, 134
Listeria monocytogenes in, 117
Neisseria meningitidis in, 126, 134
neonatal, 145
Streptococcus pneumoniae in, 111
viral, 249
Meningococcemia, 414
acute, 127
Meningoencephalitis, 290, 296, 429
primary amoebic, 373
treatment of, 374
Mepacrine for *Giardia lamblia,* 376
Mercurochrome, 62
Merthiolate, 62
Mesophilic bacteria, 16
Mesosomes, 7
Metabolism
autotrophic, 14
fermentative, 13
respiratory, 13–14
Metaphyseal radiolucencies, 302
Methanol, 61
Metrifonate for *Schistosoma* species, 404
Metronidazole, 48–49, 534Q, 548E
for amebiasis, trichomoniasis, and giardiasis, 365–366
for *Entamoeba histolytica,* 373
for *Giardia lamblia,* 376
for *Trichomonas* species, 377
MHC molecules, interference with expression of, 79
MHC-viral peptide complex expression, inhibition of, 266
Miconazole for cutaneous mycoses, 344
Microaerophilic bacteria, 13
Microbial flora, 3
Microbial virulence, 3
Microorganisms, 3
classes of pathogenic, 4–6
culture and isolation of, 93–95
Microsporum, 343
Migratory arthritis, 302
Minimal inhibitory concentration (MIC), 58
methods of determination, 58–59, *59*
Missense mutations, 23, *24*
Mixed acid fermentation, 13
Mixed component (acellular) vaccines, 85
Molluscum contagiosum, 476
Monkeypox, 291
Monobactams, 47
Monocytes, activation of, 234
Monotrichus flagellum, 11
Moraxella, 132
Morbilliform (measles-like) rash, 297, 311, 490
Morganella, 160
Morpholines in antifungal therapy, 342
Morphologic examination, 272
Mosquitoes, diseases transmitted by, 242
Motility, genetic control of, 11
Mucocutaneous leishmaniasis, 378
Mucopurulent cervicitis, 196–197
treatment of, 197–198
Mucosal antibodies, 263
Mucosal surfaces, bacterial adherence to, 12
Multiple organ failure, 127, 410
Multisystemic disease of newborn, 296
Mumps virus, 84, 309
clinical disease in, 310
diagnosis of, 310
epidemiology of, 310
and meningitis, 435
prevention of, 311
treatment of, 311
Mutagenesis
chemical, 23
radiation, 23
Mutation repair mechanisms
dark repair, 24–25, *26*
DNA glycosylase-mediated repair, 25–26
light repair, 23, *25*
post-replication recombination repair, 26–27
SOS, 27
Mutation suppression
DNA transfer between bacteria, 28, *29*
conjugation, 28, 30–31
transformation, 31–32
extragenic, 27–28
genetic basis of bacterial pathogenicity
transmission of virulence genes among bacteria, 35
virulence factors, 34
intragenic, 27
transduction, 32–33, *33*
Mutational resistance, 53
Mutations, 243
frameshift, 23, *24*
helix distortion, 23
inactivating regulatory gene, 39
missense, 23, *24*
nonsense, 23
reversion, 23
same sense (silent), 23, *24*
single-base (point), 23, *24*
spontaneous, 22–23
Mycelia, 335
Mycetismus, 336
Mycetoma, 190, 345
Mycobacteria, 533Q, 547E
culture and isolation, 167–168
general properties, 167
identification, 168
pathogenesis of, 167
prevention of infections, 513
Mycobacteria other than tuberculosis (MOTT)
clinical disease in, 171
diagnosis of, 172
epidemiology of, 171, 172*t*
Mycobacterium avium-intracellulare complex, 172
Mycobacterium fortuitum complex, 172
Mycobacterium kansasii, 172
Mycobacterium marinum, 172
Mycobacterium scrofulaceum, 172
Mycobacterium leprae
control and prophylaxis, 174
diagnosis of, 173–174
epidemiology of, 173
pathogenesis of and clinical disease in, 173
treatment of, 174
Mycobacterium tuberculosis, 100
control and prevention of, 171
determinants of pathogenicity, 169
epidemiology of, 170
general properties, 168, 168*t*
laboratory diagnosis of, 170
pathogenesis of and clinical disease in, 169–170
treatment of, 170–171, 170*t*

Mycology
characteristics of and classification of fungi, 335
epidemiology of, 337
morphology, 335, 336*t*
pathogenesis of, 336–337
structure, 335–336
Mycoplasma, 474
Mycoplasma pneumoniae, 420
pneumonia caused by, 423
Mycoplasmataceae, 187, 187*t*
historical information, 187
Mycoplasmataceae pneumoniae
clinical disease in, 187–188
diagnosis of, 188–189
epidemiology of, 188
immunity, 188
pathogenesis of, 187
Mycoplasmataceae hominis
clinical disease in, 189
diagnosis of, 189
epidemiology of, 189
treatment of, 189
Mycoses
cutaneous, 343–344
filamentous fungi as causes of, 345–346
subcutaneous, 344–345
Mycotoxicosis, 336
Myocarditis
as complication of respiratory syncytial virus, 313
Corynebacterium diphtheriae in, 296
Coxsackie B virus in, 296

N

N-acetylglucosamine, 7
N-acetylmuramic acid, 7
Naegleria fowleri, 374
Naftifine
in antifungal therapy, 342
for dermatophytoses, 344
Naked viruses, 214, 216
Nalidixic acid, 48
Narrow-spectrum antibacterial gents, 41
Nasopharyngeal carcinoma, 254, 255
Epstein-Barr virus as cause of, 281
Natural antibodies, 76
Natural antiviral compounds, 233–234
Natural immunity, 3
Natural killer (NK) cells, 74, 264
activation of, 234
Necator americanus, 391–392
Necrosis, 127
Necrotizing fasciitis, 108, 545Q, 555E
Negri bodies, 248
Neisseria
classification of, 125
culture and isolation, 125
epidemiology of, 125
general characteristics of, 125, 126*t*
Neisseria gonorrhoeae, 129, *129*
classification of, 129
clinical disease in, 130–131
determinants of pathogenicity, 129
diagnosis of, 131–132
epidemiology of, 131
immunity, 130
pathogenesis of, 130
treatment of, 132
Neisseria meningitidis
classification of, 125–126
clinical disease in, 126–127
control and prevention of, 128
determinants of pathogenicity, 126
diagnosis of, 127–128
epidemiology of, 127
immunity, 126
pathogenesis of, 126
treatment of, 128
Neisseria gonorrhoeae, 475
Nematodes (roundworms), 363
filarial
Brugia malayi, 395–396
Dirofilaria species, 397
Loa loa, 397
Onchocerca volvulus, 396–397
Toxocara canis, 397–398
Wuchereria bancrofti, 395–396
intestinal
Ancylostoma duodenale, 391–392
Anisakis marina, 394–395
Ascaris lumbricoides, 390–391
Capillaria hepatica, 394
Capillaria philippinensis, 394
Enterobius vermicularis, 389–390
Necator americanus, 391–392
Strongyloides stercoralis, 392
Trichinella species, 392–394
Trichuris trichiura, 390
treatment of infections, 368–369
Neonatal conjunctivitis, 478
Neonatal herpes, 479
Neonatal infection, 110
Neonatal listeriosis, 117
Neonatal meningitis, 145
Neonatal ophthalmia (ophthalmia neonatorum), 131
Neonatal pneumonia, 478
Neonatal transmission of hepatitis B virus (HBV), 538Q, 551E
Neuropathy, peripheral, 114
Neurotoxins, 67
Neutralization, 272
Neutralizing antibodies, 263
Neutrophils, 130
Nevirapine (dipyridodiazepinone), 238
for human immunodeficiency virus, 512
resistance to, 239
Niclosamide
for cestode and trematode infections, 369
for *Diphyllobothrium latum,* 399
for *Dipylidium caninum,* 401
for *Taenia* infections, 401
Nifurtimox
for *Trypanosoma cruzi,* 381
for trypanosomiasis, 366
Niridazole for *Schistosoma* species, 404
Nitroimidazoles, 48–49, 538Q, 550E
Nocardiosis
pulmonary, 190
subcutaneous, 190
Nodule, 490
Nodulectomy for *Onchocerca volvulus,* 396
Nonbacterial prostatitis, 453
Non-Burkitt B cell lymphoma, 255
Nonconjugative plasmids, 21
Nondefective oncoviruses, 257
Nongonococcal urethritis, 196, 196*t,* 474, 477
laboratory diagnosis of, 476
Mycoplasmataceae hominis in, 189
treatment of, 197–198, 477
Urealyticum in, 189
urethral discharge in, 475
Nonionic agents, 61
Nonobstructive pyelonephritis, acute, 451
Nonphotochromogens, 168
Nonsense mutations, 23
Norfloxacin, 150
Normal flora, 97
anatomic location of, 98–100, *99*
as pathogens, 97–98
role of, 97
Nosocomial infections, 104, 119–120
Novobiocin, 48
Nucleic acid
antibacterial agents that inhibit synthesis, 48–49
detection of sequences, 92–93
hybridization in identification of mycobacteria, 168
probe tests, 92, 350
progeny, 213
replication, 32
of viruses, 207
Nucleic acid core, 205
Nucleocapsids, 205
Nucleoid, 11
Nucleotidases, 56
Nucleotide biosynthesis, 14
Nucleotide excision repair system, 24–25, *26,* 27
Nucleotide synthesis, antibacterial agents that inhibit, 47–48
Nutrition, effect of, on outcome of viral infection, 243
Nystatin in antifungal therapy, 340

O

O antigens, 143
Obligate aerobes, 12
Obligate anaerobes, 12
Ocular disease, 195–197
Ocular histoplasmosis, 351
Ofloxacin, 48
Oltipraz for *Schistosoma* species, 404
Onc, 534Q, 548E
Oncogenes, identification of, 258–259, 259*t*
Oncogenic viruses, 538Q, 550E
Oncoviruses, 256
defective, 257
nondefective, 257
Onychomycosis, 343
Oophoritis as complication in mumps, 310
Operons, 35, *36–37,* 38–39
inducible, 37
lac, 37–38
repressible, 37
tryptophan, 39
Opisthotonos, 121
Opportunistic bacteria
Enterobacteriaceae
Citrobacter, 160
Enterobacter, 159
Escherichia coli, 160
Klebsiella, 159, 160*t*
Morganella, 160
Proteus, 160, 160*t*
Providencia, 160
Serratia, 159
Pseudomonas, 160
clinical disease in, 162
determinants of pathogenicity, 161
diagnosis of, 162
epidemiology of, 162
general properties, 161, 161*t*
pathogenesis of, 162
prevention of, 162
treatment of, 162

Opportunistic infection, 97–98
Opportunistic mycoses
clinical disease in, 358–359
diagnosis of, 359
etiology, 357
predisposing conditions, 357, 358, 358*t*
treatment of, 359
Opportunistic organisms, 3
Opsonins, 73, 75
Opsonization, 75
Optochin sensitivity testing, 112
Oral cavity
anaerobic bacteria in, 465–466
normal flora in, 99–100
Oral vaccine for polio, 295
Orbiviruses, 320
Organic nutrients in bacterial physiology, 12
Organotrophic bacteria, 12
Ornithosis, 194
Oropharyngeal infections, 348
Oroya fever, 201
Orthomyxoviruses, 222–223, *223*
classification of, 305
complications, 307
diagnosis of, 306–307
epidemiology of, 305–306
pathogenesis of and clinical disease in, 306
prevention of, 307–308
structure, 305
treatment of, 307
Osteomyelitis, 103, 149
Otitis media
as complication of respiratory syncytial virus, 313
Group A streptococci in, 108
Haemophilus influenzae in, 134
Moraxella in, 132
rhinoviruses in, 297
Streptococcus pneumoniae in, 111
Oxamniquine for *Schistosoma* species, 404
Oxidase, 19
Oxidase test, 19
Oxidizing agents, 62
Oxygen in bacterial physiology, 12

P

P fimbriae, 533Q, 547E
Pancreatitis as complication in mumps, 310
Papillomaviruses
clinical disease in, 285
epidemiology of, 285
mechanism of transformation in, 254
oncogenic potential of, 253–254
treatment of, 286
Papovaviruses, 216–217, *217,* 285
papillomaviruses, 285–286, 286*t*
polyomaviruses, 286–287
Papula, 490
Paracoccidioidomycosis
clinical disease in, 354
diagnosis of, 354
epidemiology of, 354
pathogenesis of, 354
treatment of, 354
Paragonimus westermani, 405–406
Parainfluenza viruses, 309
Paralysis, ascending, 297, 307
Paralytic poliomyelitis, 294
Paramyxoviruses, 309
classification of, 309
general characteristics of, 309
measles (rubeola)
clinical disease in, 311–312
diagnosis of, 312
epidemiology of, 312
prevention of, 312
mumps
clinical disease in, 310
diagnosis of, 310
epidemiology of, 310
prevention of, 311
treatment of, 311
parainfluenza, 309
respiratory syncytial
clinical disease in, 313
diagnosis of, 313
epidemiology of, 313
pathogenesis of, 313
prevention of, 313
treatment of, 313
Paraparesis, spastic tropical, 259
Parasites, 6, 75, 528*t*
intracellular, 205
Parasitic diarrhea, 461, 462*t*
Parasitic infections
diagnosis of, 363–365
helminths, 363
protozoa, 363
treatment of
anthelmintic agents, 368–369
antiprotozoal agents, 365–368
general principles, 365
Parasitic meningitis, 438
Parasitic sexually transmitted diseases, 477
Paromomycin for *Entamoeba histolytica,* 373
Parotitis, 310
Parrot fever, 194
Particle agglutination, 92
Parvoviruses, 205, *206*
clinical disease in, 291–292
epidemiology of, 291
structure, 291
Passive immunization, 83, 537Q, 550E
Pasteur, 83
Pasteurella multocida, 166, 545Q, 555E
Pasteurization, 62
Pathogens, 3
involved in infections at different ages, 529*t*
normal flora as, 97–98
Pathogen-specific macromolecules, detection of, 92–93
Pathologic consequences of antiviral immune response, 265–266
Peliosis hepatis, 202
Pelvic inflammatory disease (PID), 130, 197, 478
Mycoplasmataceae hominis in, 189
Urealyticum in, 189
Penicillin, 537Q, 549E
for *Bacillus subtilis,* 124
bacterial resistance in, 46
for *Borrelia,* 181
chemistry of, 43, *45*
for *Corynebacterium diphtheriae,* 116
extended-spectrum, 46
for leptospirosis, 184
mechanism of action, 43, 46
for *Pasteurella multocida,* 166
penicillinase-resistant, 105
prophylactic, 109
semisynthetic β-lactamase-resistant, 46
spectrum of activity, 46
for *Streptococcus pneumoniae,* 112
toxicity of, 46
for treating syphilis, 179–180
Penicillin G, 128
for *Actinomyces israelii,* 190
for pneumonia, 421
Penicillinase susceptible, 46
Penicillinase-resistant penicillin, 105
Penicillin-binding proteins (PBPs), 43, 46
Pentamidine
for human immunodeficiency virus, 513
for *Pneumocystis carinii* infections, 368, 388
for pneumonia, 426
Pentavalent antimonials for *Leishmania* species, 378
Pentose phosphate shunt, 13
Peptidoglycan, *7, 8,* 101, 129
Peptidoglycan biosynthesis, *15,* 15–16
Peptidoglycan crosslinking, *7, 9*
Peptidoglycan structure, *7*
Peptidoglycan-rich cell walls, 535Q, 548E
Pericarditis, 296
Perihepatitis (Fitz-Hugh–Curtis syndrome), 131
Perinatal transmission, 241
for cytomegalovirus, 282
of herpes simplex virus, 278
Peripheral neuropathy, 114
Peritonitis, bacterial, 487
Peritrichous flagella, 11
Permissive cells, 205
Persistent infection, 244, 246, 246*t,* 289
Pertussis toxin, 137
Petechiae, 490
Petechial or purpuric lesions, acute viral disease with, 496, 497*t*
Petroff-Hauser chamber, 16
Phage typing, 104
Phagocytosis, 536Q, 549E
cell types in, 73–74
mechanisms by which capsules prevent, 65
Pharyngeal diphtheria, 115
Pharyngeal gonorrhea, 131
Pharyngitis, 108, 127
Phenolic compounds, 61
Phenotypic masking, 229
Phenotypic mixing, 228–229, *230*
Phosphofructokinase, 13
Phospholipases, 116
Phosphorylases, 56
Phosphorylates, cytoskeleton proteins, 544Q, 554E
Photochromogens, 168
Photolyase, 23, *25*
Photophobia, 311
Photosynthesis, 14
Physical antimicrobial agents, 62–63
Picornaviruses, 219–220
enteroviruses, 293
coxsackieviruses, 296, 296*t*
echoviruses, 296–297
polioviruses, 293–295
rhinoviruses, 293
Pili, 12, 66, 130
Pinworm. *(See Enterobius vermicularis)*
Piperacillin, 46
PLa protease, 79
Plaque-size mutants, 226
Plasma membrane, 7
Plasmids, 11
adhesin-coding, 35

and bacterial genetics, 21
conjugative, 21
enterotoxin-coding, 35
integration, 28
invasiveness-coding, 35
nonconjugative, 21
resistance, 35
resistance (R), 54
transmission of, 35
virulence, 35
Plasmodium species, 382–384
Pleurodynia, 296
Pleuro-pneumonia-like organism (PPLO), 187
Pneumocystis carinii, 363
clinical disease in, 388
epidemiology of, 387–388
laboratory diagnosis of, 388
prevention of, 388
treatment of, 367, 388
Pneumocystis carinii pneumonia, 425–426, 513
Pneumonia, 419
adenoviral, 289–290, 425
alveolar, 248
bacterial, 111, 420–423
Enterobacteriaceae in, 160
giant cell, 311
Group B streptococci in, 108, 110
Haemophilus influenzae in, 135
influenza A virus, 424–425
interstitial, 248
Klebsiella in, 159
measles, 311
measles (rubeola), 425
Neisseria meningitidis in, 127
neonatal, 197, 478
parainfluenza viruses in, 309
protozoal, 425–426
respiratory syncytial virus, 425
Staphylococci in, 103
viral, 423–425
Pneumonitis, 302, 420
Pneumovirus, 309
Point of mutations, 225–226
Polar flagella, 11
Polio vaccine, 84
Poliomyelitis
bulbar, 294
bulbospinal, 294
paralytic, 294
spinal, 294
Polioviruses, 243
clinical disease in, 293–295
epidemiology of, 293
laboratory diagnosis of, 295
pathogenesis of, 293
prevention of, 295, 295*t*
Polyarteritis nodosa, 326
Polyhexamethylene biguanide, 374
Polymerase chain reaction (PCR), 275
clinical applications, 93
in identification of mycobacteria, 168
limitations, 93
technique, 93
Polymorphonuclear leukocytes, 73
Polyomaviruses
BK virus, 286
JC virus, 286–287
Polypeptide capsule, 11
Polysaccharide capsule, 110–111, 133–134
Polysaccharide core, 143–144
Polysaccharides, 84
complex, 11
Polysegmented genome, 207
Polyvalent vaccine, 112
Pontiac fever, 185, 186
Porins, 56
Postinfectious encephalitis, 302, 312
as complication from varicella-zoster virus, 280
Postpolio syndrome, 294–295
Poststreptococcal glomerulonephritis, acute, 109
Poxviruses, 218–219
diseases caused by orthopoxviruses, 290–291
diseases caused by parapoxviruses, 291
diseases caused by unclassified poxviruses, 291
structure, 290
Praziquantel
for cestode and trematode infections, 369
for *Clonorchis* species, 405
for *Diphyllobothrium latum,* 399
for *Dipylidium caninum,* 401
for *Echinococcus* infections, 402
for *Fasciolopsis buskii,* 406
for *Hymenolepis diminuta,* 400
for *Paragonimus westermani,* 406
for *Schistosoma* species, 404
for *Taenia* infections, 401
Pregnant women, rubella in, 303
Premalignant and malignant lesions, treatment of, 286
Prevotella bivia, 466
Prevotella disiens, 466
Prevotella melaninogenica, 466, 467, 468, 470
Prevotella oralis, 466
Primaquine
for malaria, 367
for *Plasmodium* species, 384
Primary amoebic meningoencephalitis, 373
Primary cultures, 271
Primary hepatoma, 255–256
Primary response, 75
Primary viral encephalitis, 249
Productive infection, 244
Profuse secretory diarrhea, 456
Progeny nucleic acid, 213
Progressive multifocal leukoencephalopathy (PML), 287, 443*t,* 544Q, 554E
clinical manifestations, 444
diagnosis of, 444
etiology, 443
pathogenesis of, 443–444
predisposing factors, 443
prevention of, 444
treatment of and prognosis, 444
Progressive muscle wasting, 487
Progressive spastic paraparesis, 444–445
Progressive wasting syndrome, 510
Proguanil for malaria, 367
Proinflammatory cytokines, 535Q, 548E
Prokaryotes, 4*t,* 5, 6
Propamidine isethionate
for *Acanthamoeba* species, 374
for amebiasis, trichomoniasis, and giardiasis, 366
Prophylactic penicillin, 109
Prophylactic therapy for human immunodeficiency virus, 513
Propionic fermentation, 13
Prostatitis
clinical manifestations, 453
complications, 453
diagnosis of, 453
etiology, 452–453
treatment of, 453
Protease inhibitors, 238
Proteases, 161, 208
Protein A, 102
Protein F, 107
Protein G, 107
Protein kinases, 258
autoactivation of, 258
Protein-denaturing compounds, 61–62
Proteins
antibacterial agents that inhibit synthesis, 49–51, *50*
capsid, 217
early, 212
fusion, 246
late, 213
matrix, 213
regulatory, 212, 217–218
transactivating, 258
viral, 208
viral surface, 231
Proteolytic (toxic) enzymes, 19
Proteus, 160, 160*t*
as cause of urinary tract infections, 450
Protoplasts, 9
Protozoa, 363
Protozoal pneumonia, 425–426
Providencia, 160
Pruritus ani, 389
Pseudocowpox (milkers' nodule), 291
Pseudomembranous (necrotizing) colitis, 119
Pseudomonas, 160
as cause of urinary tract infections, 450
clinical disease in, 162
determinants of pathogenicity, 161
diagnosis of, 162
epidemiology of, 162
general properties, 161, 161*t*
pathogenesis of, 162
prevention of, 162
treatment of, 162
Pseudomonas aeruginosa, 538Q, 540Q, 541Q, 551E, 552E
in bacteremic infections, 412
Pseudomonas toxin A, 67
Pseudotype formation, 229
Psittacosis, 194
Psychrophilic bacteria, 16
Puerperal fever, 108
Mycoplasmataceae hominis in, 189
Urealyticum in, 189
Pulmonary anthrax, 123
Pulmonary coccidioidomycosis, 353
Pulmonary disease, 351
Pulmonary syndrome hantavirus ("Sin Nombre" strain), 319–320
Purine nucleotides, 14
Purines, 12
Purpura, 490
Pyelonephritis
as complication of bacterial prostatitis, 453
end-stage chronic, 452
Pyocyanin, 161
Pyoderma (impetigo), 103, 108
Pyogenic cocci, pneumonia caused by, 422
Pyoverdin, 161
Pyrantel
for *Ascaris lumbricoides,* 391
for nematode infections, 369

Pyrantel pamoate
for *Enterobius vermicularis,* 390
for *Necator americanus,* 392
Pyrimethamine
for *Toxoplasma gondii,* 386
for toxoplasmosis, 367
Pyrimidine nucleotides, 14
Pyrimidines, 12
Pyrogenic exotoxins, 101–102
Pyruvate compound, 12
Pyruvate family, 14

Q

Q fever, 199–200
Qinghaosu (artemisinin) for malaria, 367
Quadrivalent vaccine, 128
Quellung reaction, 112, 133
Quinacrine hydrochloride
for amebiasis, trichomoniasis, and giardiasis, 365–366
for *Giardia lamblia,* 376
Quinine
for *Babesia* species, 385
for *Plasmodium* species, 384
Quinolones
in inhibiting nucleic acid synthesis, 48, 150, 151
for pneumonia, 423
for typhoid fever, 150, 151

R

R protein, 106
Rabies virus, 242
and meningitis, 435
Radiation, 63
Radiation mutagenesis, 23
Radioimmunoassays, 273
Rapid plasma reagin (RPR), 96
in diagnosing syphilis, 178
Rash, morbilliform, 311
Reactive arthritis, *Yersinia enterocolitica* in, 165
Receptor-mediated endocytosis (viropexis), 211
Recombinant immunoblot assay (RIBA) in diagnoses of hepatitis C, 330
Recombinant intercellular cell adhesion molecule-1 (ICAM-1), 234
Recombinant vaccines, 85
Recombinant vaccinia viruses, 85
Recombinase A *(recA),* 27
Red blood cell lysis, 545Q, 555E
Regulatory gene, mutations inactivating, 39
Regulatory proteins, 212, 217–218
Reiter's syndrome, 196
Reoviruses, 299
classification of, 320
orbiviruses, 320
rotaviruses, 320–321
structure, 320
Replicative recombination, 21
Repressible operons, 37
Resistance genes, acquisition of, 53–54, 54*t*
Resistance plasmids, 35
Resistance (R) plasmids, 54
Respiration, aerobic, 13–14
Respiratory disease, 135
Respiratory distress syndrome, 544Q, 554E
Respiratory metabolism, 13–14
Respiratory route, 241
for cytomegalovirus, 282
Respiratory syncytial virus, 309, 539Q, 551E
clinical disease in, 313
diagnosis of, 313
epidemiology of, 313
pathogenesis of, 313
prevention of, 313
treatment of, 313
Respiratory syncytial virus pneumonia, 425
Reticulocytopenia, 493
Reticuloendothelial system, 211, 264
Retinoblastoma (Rb) gene product, 544Q, 554E
Retroviruses, 220–222, *221*
HTLV-1, 259–260
HTLV-II, 259–260
mechanisms of transformation, 259
and medicine, 260
oncogenes, 258–259
oncogenic potential of, 257–258
structure and classification of, *256,* 256–257
Reverse transcriptase, agents that inhibit, 237–238
Reverse transcription, 220
Reversion mutations, 23
Reye's syndrome
as complication from varicella-zoster virus, 280
as complication of hypersensitivity reactions, 307
Rhabdoviruses, 222
clinical disease in, 316
control of, 316
general properties of, 315
pathogenesis of, 315–316
prevention of, 316
treatment of, 316
Rheumatic fever, 109, 541Q, 552–553E
Rhinorrhea in congenital syphilis, 177
Rhinoviruses, 243, 293, 543Q, 553E
diagnosis of, 298
epidemiology of, 297
immunity, 298
pathogenesis of and clinical disease in, 297
treatment of, 298
Rhizopoda (amoebae), 363
Rhodesian sleeping sickness, 379–380
Ribavirin, 238, 313
for pneumonia, 425
Ribosomes, 11
Rickettsia prowazekii, 199
Rickettsia rickettsiae, 199
Rickettsia rickettsii, 545Q, 555E
Rickettsia typhi, 543Q, 553–554E
Rickettsiaceae, 194*t,* 198
clinical disease in, 199–200
epidemiology of, 200, 200*t*
general properties, 198, 198*t*
laboratory diagnosis of, 200–201
pathogenesis of, 198–199
treatment of, 201
Rifabutin for mycobacterial infections, 513
Rifampin, 128, 136
for *Bartonella,* 202
for meningitis, 433
for mycobacteria, 169
for treating leprosy, 174
Rimantadine, 234
for RNA viruses II, 307
as synthetic antiviral agent, 234
Ringworm, 343
Risus sardonicus, 121
Ritonavir, 238
for human immunodeficiency virus, 512
RNA genome, 544Q, 554E
RNA viruses, 208, 225, 524–525*t*
arboviruses, 299–302, 300*t*
recombination between, 227–228
replication cycle of major human, 219, *220*
+RNA viruses, 219–222
−RNA viruses, *222,* 222–223
+RNA virus, 542Q, 553E
rubella virus, 299, 302–303
+RNA viruses, 208, *214,* 214–215, 219–222
−RNA viruses, 208, *215,* 215–216, *222,* 222–223
RNA viruses I, enteroviruses, 293
coxsackieviruses, 296, 296*t*
echoviruses, 296–297
polioviruses, 293–295, 295*t*
rhinoviruses, 297–298
RNA viruses II
classification of, 305
complications, 307
diagnosis of, 306–307
epidemiology of, 305–306
pathogenesis of and clinical disease in, 306
prevention of, 307–308
structure, 305
treatment of, 307
RNA viruses IV
classification of, 309
general characteristics of, 309
measles (rubeola)
clinical disease in, 311–312
diagnosis of, 312
epidemiology of, 312
prevention of, 312
mumps
clinical disease in, 310
diagnosis of, 310
epidemiology of, 310
prevention of, 311
treatment of, 311
parainfluenza, 309
respiratory syncytial
clinical disease in, 313
diagnosis of, 313
epidemiology of, 313
pathogenesis of, 313
prevention of, 313
treatment of, 313
RNA viruses V
arenaviruses
clinical disease in, 319
epidemiology of, 319
general properties, 319
bunyaviruses
clinical disease in, 319–320
general properties, 319
caliciviruses
clinical disease in, 318
diagnosis of, 318
epidemiology of, 317
general properties, 317
pathogenesis of, 317
prevention of, 318
treatment of, 318
coronaviruses
clinical disease in, 317
diagnosis of, 317
epidemiology of, 317

general properties, 317
pathogenesis of, 317
prevention of, 317
therapy, 317
filoviruses
clinical disease in, 318
epidemiology of, 318
general properties, 318
pathogenesis of, 318
reoviruses
classification of, 320
orbiviruses, 320
rotaviruses, 320–321
structure, 320
rhabdoviruses
clinical disease in, 316
control, 316
general properties, 315
pathogenesis of, 315–316
prevention of, 316
treatment of, 316
RNA-dependent DNA polymerase, 544Q, 554E
RNA-dependent RNA polymerase, 222, 544Q, 554E
Rocky Mountain spotted fever, 50, 199
Romaña's sign, 380
Roseola infantum (exanthema subitum)
clinical manifestations, 492
human herpesvirus-6 virus as cause of, 283
incubation period, 492
treatment of, 492
Rotaviruses, 320–321
Round worms, 363
Roux, 83
Rubella (German measles, three-day measles), 84, 302
clinical disease in, 302
clinical manifestations, 492
complications, 492
diagnosis of, 303
epidemiology of, 302–303
and meningitis, 435
prevention of, 303, 492
treatment of, 303, 492

S

Sabin, 83
Sabin's oral polio vaccine, 84
Safranin, 18
St. Louis encephalitis virus, 545Q, 555E
Salmonella, 544Q, 554E
Salmonella typhi, 543Q, 553–554E
Salmonella typhimurium, 79
Salmonellosis, 149, 150
Salpingitis, 478
Same sense (silent) mutations, 23, *24*
Saprophytes, 5
Saquinavir, 238
for human immunodeficiency virus, 512
Sarcomastigophora, 363
Satellitism, 133
Scalded skin syndrome, 103–104
Scarlet fever, 108
staphylococcal, 104
Schistosoma haematobium, 545Q, 555E
Schistosoma species (blood flukes), 402–404
Schistosomatium, 404
Schistosomes, 81
Scotochromogens, 168
Secondary viral encephalitis, 249
Selective permeability, 7
Semisynthetic β-lactamase-resistant penicillins, 46
Sepsis
implications, 410
sources, 410
Septic abortion, 414
Septic shock
in acute meningococcemia, 127
and bacteremia, 410, 452
pathogenesis of, *69,* 69*t,* 70
treatment of, 412
Septicemia
Klebsiella in, 159
Proteus in, 160
Staphylococci in, 103
Serine family, 14
Serologic techniques, 272, 273–274
Serologic tests, 67–68, 95–96, 112
Serotyping, 19
Serratia, 159
as cause of urinary tract infections, 450
Serum sickness-type syndrome, 326
Sex pilus, 28
Sexual transmission of herpes simplex virus, 278
Sexually transmitted diseases (STDs), 473, 474*t*
approach to patient
clinical manifestations, 475–476
history, 474–475
physical examination, 475
complications, 478–479
epidemiology of
gonorrhea, 473
nongonococcal urethritis, 474
laboratory diagnosis of, 476–477
prevention of, 477–478
treatment of
candidiasis, 477
gonorrhea, 477
herpes simplex, 477
parasitic, 477
syphilis, 477
Shiga-like toxin, 145
Shingles (herpes zoster)
clinical manifestations, 494–495
complications, 495
prevention of, 495
treatment of, 495
Silver nitrate, 62
Single-base (point) mutations, 23, *24*
Sinusitis, 108, 111, 132, 297
Skin, normal flora in, 98–99
Skin purpura, 127
Skin warts
papillomaviruses as cause of, 285
treatment of, 286
Sleeping sickness, 80
Smallpox, 290–291
Sodium hypochlorite (bleach), 62
Soft tissue infections, 119
Solid-phase immunoassays, 273
SOS repair, 27
Spastic paralysis, 121
Spastic tropical paraparesis, 259
Specialized transduction, 34
Spectinomycin, 132
Spheroplasts, 9
Spinal poliomyelitis, 294
Spiramycin
for *Cryptosporidium parvum,* 387
for *Toxoplasma gondii,* 386
Spirochetes, 175. *(See also Borrelia; Leptospira, Treponema)*
Splanchnic ischemia, 98
Spontaneous mutations, 22–23, 543Q, 553E
Sporothrix schenckii, 545Q, 555E
Sporotrichosis, 354
clinical disease in, 355
diagnosis of, 355
epidemiology of, 355
pathogenesis of, 355
treatment of, 355
Sporozoans, 363
Babesia species, 385
Cryptosporidium parvum, 387
Isospora species, 387
Plasmodium species, 382–384
Toxoplasma gondii, 385–387
Sporulation, 17
Spumaviruses, 256
Staphylococcal bacteremia, 415
Staphylococcal food poisoning, 104
Staphylococcal scarlet fever, 104
Staphylococcal toxic shock syndrome (TSS), 415
Staphylococcal toxin diseases, 103–104
Staphylococci
classification of, 101, 102*t*
clinical disease in, 103–104
control and prevention of, 105
determinants of pathogenicity, 101–103
epidemiology of, 104
general properties, 101, 101*t, 102*
laboratory diagnosis of, 104–105
structure, 101
treatment of, 105
Staphylococcus aureus, 415, 537Q, 541Q, 544Q, 550E, 552E, 554E
as cause of urinary tract infections, 450
penicillins for, 46
in primary lung abscess, 468–469
in staphylococcal infections, 101
Staphylococcus aureus peptidoglycan, *9*
Staphylococcus epidermidis, 101, 415
Staphylococcus saprophyticus, 101
as cause of urinary tract infections, 450
Static theory, 277
Stavudine, 238
for human immunodeficiency virus, 512
Steric hindrance, 263
Sterilization, 61
Stevens-Johnson syndrome (erythema multiforme major), 497–498
Sties, 103
Streptococcal pharyngitis, 92
Streptococcal toxic shock syndrome, 108
Streptococci
classification of, 106
determinants of pathogenicity, 106, 106*t*
general properties, 105, *105,* 105*t*
group A, 107–109, 109*t*
group B, 109–110
group D, 110
laboratory diagnosis of, 106–107, 107*t*
Streptococcus pneumoniae, 110–112, 110*t, 111*
viridans, 110
Streptococcus agalactiae, 539Q, 551E
Streptococcus pneumoniae infections, 468, 536Q, 541Q, 545Q, 549E, 553E, 555E
pneumonia caused by, 420–422

Streptococcus pyogenes, 469
Streptolysin O, 107
Streptolysin S, 108
Streptomycetes, 190–191
Streptomycin, 11
Francisella tularensis in, 166
String test, 375
Strongyloides stercoralis, 392
Subacute bacterial endocarditis, 110
Subacute sclerosing panencephalitis (SSPE), 312
clinical manifestations, 442
as complication of measles, 491
diagnosis of, 442
epidemiology of, 442
etiology, 442
pathogenesis of, 442
prevention of, 443
treatment of and prognosis, 442
Subcutaneous mycoses
chromomycoses, 344–345
mycetoma, 345
Sulbactam, 46
Sulfadiazine, 48
for *Toxoplasma gondii,* 386
Sulfamethoxazole, 48
Sulfamethoxazole-trimethoprim, 48
Sulfamethoxydiazine, 48
Sulfatides for mycobacteria, 169
Sulfisoxazole, 48
Superantigens, 101
Superoxide dismutase, 13
Suramin
for *Trypanosoma* species, 380
for trypanosomiasis, 366
Sylvatic yellow fever, 301
Syncytia, 246, 271
Synthetic antiviral agents, 234, *235, 236,* 236–238, *237*
Synthetic oligopeptide vaccines, 85–86
Syphilis, 175, *176,* 177, 474, 477
adult, 178–179, 179–180
primary, 175
secondary, 175, 177
tertiary, 177
treatment of, 179–180, 179*t*
congenital, 177, 479
laboratory diagnoses of, 179
treatment of, 180
late, 478
primary and secondary, 178–179
laboratory diagnoses of, 178–179
tertiary, 179
laboratory diagnoses of, 179

T

T cell leukemia, acute, 259
T protein, 106
Taenia saginata, 400–401
Taenia solium, 400–401
Taeniasis, 400
Tapeworms. (*See* Cestodes (tapeworms))
Target-activated nucleoside analogues, 236
Tax gene product, 544Q, 554E
Temperate (lysogenic) infection, 33
Temperature-sensitive mutants, 225
Terbinafine
in antifungal therapy, 342
for cutaneous mycoses, 344
Tetanospasmin, 121
Tetanus
cephalic, 121
generalized, 121
local, 121
Tetanus toxin, 67
Tetanus toxoids, 85
Tetracyclines, 11
for *Borrelia,* 181
chemistry of, 49, *50*
for *Chlamydiae pneumoniae,* 195
for *Chlamydiae psittaci,* 195
for *Francisella tularensis,* 166
for leptospirosis, 184
for *Mycoplasmataceae hominis,* 189
for *Pneumocystis carinii* infections, 368
for pneumonia, 423
toxicity, 49–50
for *Urealyticum,* 189
Thalidomide in treating leprosy, 174
Thayer-Martin agar, 94
Thayer-Martin medium, 125
Thermophilic bacteria, 16
Thiabendazole
for *Ancylostoma* infections, 398
for *Capillaria philippinensis,* 394
for nematode infections, 368
for *Strongyloides stercoralis,* 392
for *Toxocara canis,* 398
Third-generation cephalosporins, 112, 135
Thrombocytopenia, 299
Thrombocytopenic purpura ("blueberry muffin" baby), 302
Thymidine, 536Q, 549E
Ticarcillin, 46
Tindale agar, 113
Tinea barbae, 343
Tinea capitis, 343
Tinea corporis, 343
Tinea cruris, 343
Tinea pedis, 343
Tinea unguium, 343
Tinea versicolor, 344
Tinidazole for *Giardia lamblia,* 376
Tissue damage as consequence of antiviral response, 266
Togaviruses, 220
Tolnaftate
for candidiasis, 348
for fungal infections, 344
Tonsillar diphtheria, 115
Total antibody assays, 273
Toxic shock syndrome, 104
staphylococcal, 415
Toxic shock syndrome toxin-1 (TSST-1), 102
Toxin neutralization, 75
Toxins, 67–68, 67*t,* 68*t, 69,* 69*t,* 70, 161
adenylate cyclase-like, 137
diphtheria, 67
heat-labile, 144
heat-stable, 144
pertussis, 137
Toxoid-polysaccharide conjugates, 85
Toxoids, 84–85
Toxoplasma gondii, 385–387
Toxoplasmosis
cerebral, 438
treatment of, 367
Tracheal cytotoxin, 137
Trachoma, 195–197
treatment of, 197–198
Transactivating proteins, 258
Transcription, 221–222
Transduction, 32–33, *33*
specialized, 34
types of, 33–34
Transformation, 31–32, 251
Transformed cells, characteristics of, 251–252
Transforming infection, 289
Translocation, bacterial, 98
Transmission during lactation, 241
Transpeptidase, 16
Transplacental transmission, 241
Transposable genetic elements and bacterial genetics, 21
Transposons, 22
Traveler's diarrhea, 145
Trematodes (flatworms, flukes), 363
Clonorchis species, 404–405
Fasciola gigantica, 405
Fasciola hepatica, 405
Fasciolopsis buskii, 406
Gigantobilharzia, 404
Heterobilharzia, 404
Paragonimus westermani, 405–406
Schistosoma species (blood flukes), 402–404
Schistosomatium, 404
treatment of infection, 369
Trichobilharzia, 404
Treponema
clinical disease in, 175
determinants of pathogenicity, 175
epidemiology of, 177
general properties, 175, 176*t*
immunity, 177–178
laboratory diagnosis of, 178
pathogenesis of, 175
treatment of, 179–180
Treponema pallidum immobilization (TPI) test in diagnosing syphilis, 178
Triazoles, 340–341
Trichinella species, 392–394
Trichobilharzia, 404
Trichomonas species, 376–377
Trichomonas vaginalis, 474, 475, 537Q, 549E
Trichomoniasis, 376–377, 474, 476
treatment of, 365–366
Trichophyton, 343
Trichuris trichiura (whipworm), 390
Trimethoprim-sulfamethoxazole
for human immunodeficiency virus, 513
in inhibiting nucleotide synthesis, 48
for *Isospora* species, 387
for *Nocardia* infections, 190
for *Plasmodium* species, 384
for *Pneumocystis carinii* infections, 367
for pneumonia, 426
for *Shigella,* 148
for streptomycetes, 191
for *Toxoplasma gondii,* 386
for toxoplasmosis, 367
for typhoid fever, 150
for urinary tract infection, 452
Trismus (lockjaw), 121
Triton K-12, 61
Triton W-30, 61
Trophozoites, 371
Tropical pulmonary eosinophilia, 395
Trypanosoma brucei gambiense, 379–380
Trypanosoma brucei rhodesiense, 379–380
Trypanosoma cruzi, 380–381
Trypanosoma species, 379–381
Trypanosomiasis, treatment of, 366
Tryptophan operon, 39
Tuberculoid leprosy, *Mycobacterium leprae* in, 173

Tuberculosis, 87
active, 169–170
disseminated (miliary), 170
Tuberculous meningitis, 435–436
Tularemia, *Francisella tularensis* in, 166
Tumor necrosis factor-α (TNF-α), 73
Tumor viruses, 251
Tumor-associated retroviruses, 251
Tumor-associated surface antigens, expression of, 252
Two-hit theory of malignant transformation, 260–261
Type I interferons, 233
Type II interferons, 233–234
Typhoid fever
chloramphenicol for, 149–150
transmission of, 149–150
Typhoid vaccine, 84
Typhus, epidemic, 199
Tzanck cells, 246, 280, 535Q, 548E

U

UDP-MurNAc-pentapeptide, 15, 537Q, 550E
UDP-MurNAc-tripeptide, 15
Ulcerative keratitis, 373
Ulcerative lesions, 475
Ulcers, 490
granulomatous, 371
Ultrasonic energy, 63
Upper respiratory tract, normal flora in, 100
Urban yellow fever, 301
Ureaplasma, 474
Ureaplasma urealyticum
clinical disease in, 189
diagnosis of, 189
epidemiology of, 189
treatment of, 189
Urease activity, tests of, 156
Urethral discharge, 475
Urethritis, 130, 450
nongonococcal, 196, 196*t*
Urinary tract infections, 533Q, 547E
clinical manifestations, 450–451
complications in, 452
diagnosis of, 451
epidemiology of, 449–450
Escherichia coli in, 145
etiology, 450
Klebsiella in, 159
Proteus in, 160
treatment of, 451
Urine, microscopic examination of uncentrifuged, 451
Urine cultures, 451
Urine samples, 451
Urogenital tract, normal flora in, 100
Urticaria, 490
Urticarial lesions, acute viral disease with, 496, 496*t*

V

Vaccines, 128
acellular, 140
attenuated virus, 84
component, 84–85
conjugate, 128
definition of, 83
diphtheria-pertussis-tetanus (DPT), 116
DNA, 86
as immunotherapeutic agents, 86–87
killed (inactivated), 84
polyvalent, 112
quadrivalent, 128
recombinant, 85
for RNA viruses II, 308
for rubella virus, 303
synthetic oligopeptide, 85–86
Vagina, anaerobic bacteria in, 466
Vaginal candidiasis, 348
Vaginitis, 475
Vancomycin
and bacterial cell wall synthesis, 47
for methicillin-resistant staphylococci, 105, 112
for pneumonia, 421
Varicella. (*See* chickenpox (varicella))
Varicella-zoster immune globulin (VZIG), 494
Varicella-zoster virus
clinical disease in, 279–280
diagnosis of, 280
immunoprophylaxis, 280
pathogenesis of, 279
transmission of, 280
treatment of, 280
Variola major, 290–291
Variola minor, 291
Variolation, 83
Vasculitis, 184
Veillonella species, 466
Venereal Disease Research Laboratory (VDRL), 96, 538Q, 551E
Venereal Disease Research Laboratory (VDRL) test in diagnosing syphilis, 178
Venereal route, 241
Venereal transmission for cytomegalovirus, 282
Venereal warts, treatment of, 286
Vero cells, 67
Verocytotoxin, 145
Verotoxin, 145
Verruciformis, epidermodysplasia, 285–286
Vesicles, 490
Vesicular eruption, 535Q, 548E
Vesicular rash, 490
of chickenpox, 279–280
Vesicular rash, acute viral disease with, 493, 493*t*
chickenpox (varicella), 494
hand-foot-and-mouth syndrome, 495
herpangina, 495
herpetic gingivostomatitis, 495–496
shingles (herpes zoster), 494–495
Vibrio cholerae, 142*t,* 151, 151*t,* 540Q, 552E
classification of, 151
determinants of pathogenicity, 152, *152*
epidemiology of, 154
laboratory diagnosis of, 154
pathogenesis of, 152, *153,* 154
prevention of, 154
treatment of, 154
Vibrionaceae, 141
Vibrio cholerae, 142*t,* 151, 151*t*
classification of, 151
determinants of pathogenicity, 152, *152*
epidemiology of, 154
laboratory diagnosis of, 154
pathogenesis of, 152, *153,* 154
prevention of, 154
treatment of, 154
Vibrio parahaemolyticus
determinants of pathogenicity, 154
epidemiology of, 155
general properties, 154
treatment of, 155
Vibrio vulnificus
epidemiology of and clinical disease in, 155
general properties, 155
Vidarabine (adenine arabinoside), 234
Viral diarrhea, 460–461, 461*t*
Viral diseases
acute
associated with erythema multiforme and Stevens-Johnson syndrome, 497–498, 497*t*
with maculopapular rash
atypical measles, 492
erythema infectiosum (fifth disease), 492–493
measles (rubeola), 491
roseola (exanthem subitum), 492
rubella (German measles), 492
with vesicular rash, 493, 493*t*
chickenpox (varicella), 494
hand-foot-and-mouth syndrome, 495
herpangina, 495
herpetic gingivostomatitis, 495–496
shingles (herpes zoster), 494–495
from community perspectives
periodicity of epidemics, 242
public health concerns, 242
role of resistance, 242
horizontal transmission
cutaneous route, 241
fecal-oral route, 241
inoculation, 241
respiratory route, 241
venereal route, 241
pathogenesis of, determinants of, 243
seasonal fluctuation, 242–243
vertical transmission, 241
during lactation, 241
perinatal, 241
transplacental transmission of, 241
zoonotic, 242
Viral encephalitis, 439
Viral envelope, 205
Viral exanthematic diseases, 489–490
acute, with maculopapular rash, 491–493, 491*t*
acute, with petechial or purpuric lesions, 496, 497*t*
acute, with urticarial lesions, 496, 496*t*
acute, with vesicular rash, 493–496
mechanisms of mucocutaneous reactions to viruses, 490
Viral genetics
genomes
DNA viruses, 225
RNA viruses, 225
interactions between
complementation, 228–229, *229, 230*
defective interfering particle, 229–231
effects of infection of cell on behavior of other viruses, 230–231
reassortment, 228, *228*
recombination, 226–228, *227*
mutation
general characteristics of, 225
types of, 225–226
Viral genomes, 205, 207

interactions between, 226–228, *227*
possession of, 251
Viral hemagglutinin, 231
Viral hepatitis, 481–482
acute, 484–485
chronic, 486–487
diagnostic tests, 483
epidemiology of, 482–483, 482*t*
prevention of, 483–484
Viral hepatitis, acute, 484–485
Viral-induced immunosuppression, 111
Viral infections
diagnosis of
culture, 271–272
isolation, 272–273
diagnosis of serology, 273–274
DNA hybridization, 274–275
effects of, on behavior of other viruses, 230–231
host factors that influence outcome of, 243
pathology
causes of cell death in viral-infected cells, 248
cytopathic effects, 247–248, 247*t*
histopathic effects, 248–249
sequence of events in, 244, *245*
types of, 244, 246, 246*t*
Viral meningitis, 249, 435, 439
Viral mutation
general characteristics of, 225
types of, 225–226
Viral nucleic acid, uncoating of, 211–212
Viral pneumonia, 423–425
Viral polymerases, 208
Viral replication
cycle of major human DNA viruses
adenoviruses, 217–218
hepatitis B virus (HBV), 219
herpesvirus, *213*, 218
papovaviruses, 216–217, *217*
poxviruses, 218–219
relationship between virus and host cell, 211
replication cycle of major human RNA viruses, 219, *220*
+RNA viruses, 219–222
−RNA viruses, *222*, 222–223
stages of
adsorption, 211, 212*t*
penetration, 211
synthesis, 212–216, *213, 214, 215*
uncoating of nucleic acid, 211–212
Viral structure, 205
capsid
composition, 207
functions, 207
nucleocapsid symmetry, 207
resistance, 207
envelope
composition, 207
denaturation, 207
nucleic acid core, 207
proteins, 208, 208*t*
Viral surface proteins, 231
Viral thymidine kinase, 236
Viral-coded glycoproteins, 207
Viral-coded polymerases, 213
Viremia, 244, 299
initial, 293
second, 293
Viridans, 106
Virions, 205
Viroceptors, 267
Virulence factors, 3
bacterial, 65–70
Virulence plasmids, 35
Virulent (lytic) infection, 32–33, *33*
Virus neutralization, 75
Virus-antibody complex deposition, 265
Virus-antibody complex facilitation of infection, 265
Viruses, 74
DNA, 208
general characteristics of
host specificity, 205
replication, 205
size, 205
and immune system, 263–266
insect, 85
main families of human, 209, 209*t*
nomenclature, 208–209
recombinant vaccinia, 85
of reduced virulence, 246
reproduction, 4–5
RNA, 208
+RNA, 208, *214*, 214–215
−RNA, 208, *215*, 215–216
role of genetic variation in evolution of, 231
taxonomic classification of, 209
Visceral larva migrans, 536Q, 549E
Visceral leishmaniasis, 378
Vitamins, 12
Von Behring, 83
V-src gene product, 544Q, 554E

W

Warts
genital, 285
laryngeal, 285
skin, 285, 286
venereal, 286
Wassermann test in diagnosing syphilis, 178
Waterhouse-Friderichsen syndrome, 127, 414
Weil-Felix test in diagnosing *Rickettsia rickettsii*, 201
Western blot (immunoblot) test, 274, 533Q, 547E
to confirm human immunodeficiency virus infection, 511
Western blot (immunoblot) tests, 542Q, 553E
Wheals, 490
Whooping cough, 136, 139
vaccine for, 84
Wilson's disease, 487
Wound botulism, 121
Wound infections, *Proteus* in, 160

X

Xeroderma pigmentosum, 25

Y

Yeast infections, 348
candidiasis
clinical disease in, 347
diagnosis of, 347–348
epidemiology of, 347
treatment of, 348
cryptococcosis
clinical disease in, 348
determinants of pathogenicity, 348
diagnosis of, 348–349
epidemiology of, 348
treatment of, 349
Yeasts, 335
Yellow fever, 301, 534Q, 547E
vaccine for, 84
Yersin, 83
Yersinia enterocolitica
Campylobacter, 166
clinical disease in, 165
determinants of pathogenicity, 165
epidemiology of, 165–166
Francisella tularensis, 166
Pasteurella multocida, 166
Yersinia pestis
clinical disease in, 165
determinants of pathogenicity, 164–165
epidemiology of, 165
general properties, 164, 164*t*
historical significance, 164
treatment of, 165

Z

Zalcitabine (dideoxycytidine, ddC), 238
for human immunodeficiency virus, 512
Zephiran, 61
Zidovudine (azidothymidine, AZT), 237, *237*
resistance to, 239
Zidovudine dideoxythymidine (AZT), 511–512
Ziehl-Neelsen stain, 18, 168
Zoomastigophorea (flagellates), 363
Zoonosis, 124
Zoonotic bacteria, 162
Brucella
clinical disease in, 163, *163*
control and prevention of, 164
determinants of pathogenicity, 162–163
epidemiology of, 164
general properties, 162, 163*t*
laboratory diagnosis of, 164
pathogenesis of, 163
treatment of, 164
Yersinia enterocolitica
Campylobacter, 166
clinical disease in, 165
determinants of pathogenicity, 165
epidemiology of, 165–166
Francisella tularensis, 166
Pasteurella multocida, 166
Yersinia pestis
clinical disease in, 165
determinants of pathogenicity, 164–165
epidemiology of, 165
general properties, 164, 164*t*
historical significance, 164
treatment of, 165
Zoonotic organisms, 3
Zoonotic transmission, 242
Zygomycetes, 335
Zygomycosis, 345–346